Pediatric Autoimmunity and Transplantation

AF729048

Farzaneh Rahmani • Nima Rezaei
Editors

Pediatric Autoimmunity and Transplantation

A Case-Based Collection with MCQs, Volume 3

Springer

Editors
Farzaneh Rahmani
Student's Scientific Research Center (SSRC)
Tehran University of
Medical Sciences (TUMS)
Tehran
Iran

NeuroImaging Network (NIN)
Universal Scientific Education and
Research Network (USERN)
Tehran
Iran

Nima Rezaei
Department of Immunology, School of
Medicine
Research Center for Immunodeficiencies
(RCID)
Children's Medical Center
Tehran University of Medical Sciences
(TUMS)
Tehran
Iran

Network of Immunity in Infection
Malignancy and Autoimmunity (NIIMA)
Universal Scientific Education and Research
Network (USERN)
Tehran
Iran

ISBN 978-3-030-26282-2 ISBN 978-3-030-26280-8 (eBook)
https://doi.org/10.1007/978-3-030-26280-8

© Springer Nature Switzerland AG 2020
This work is subject to copyright. All rights are reserved by the Publisher, whether the whole or part of the material is concerned, specifically the rights of translation, reprinting, reuse of illustrations, recitation, broadcasting, reproduction on microfilms or in any other physical way, and transmission or information storage and retrieval, electronic adaptation, computer software, or by similar or dissimilar methodology now known or hereafter developed.
The use of general descriptive names, registered names, trademarks, service marks, etc. in this publication does not imply, even in the absence of a specific statement, that such names are exempt from the relevant protective laws and regulations and therefore free for general use.
The publisher, the authors, and the editors are safe to assume that the advice and information in this book are believed to be true and accurate at the date of publication. Neither the publisher nor the authors or the editors give a warranty, expressed or implied, with respect to the material contained herein or for any errors or omissions that may have been made. The publisher remains neutral with regard to jurisdictional claims in published maps and institutional affiliations.

This Springer imprint is published by the registered company Springer Nature Switzerland AG
The registered company address is: Gewerbestrasse 11, 6330 Cham, Switzerland

Preface

Immunology has found its way well into the practice of pediatrics. Years after publication of the first pediatric textbooks, footprints of immunology can be found in diagnosis and practice of almost all pediatric disorders. Delivering a magnificent contribution is the advent of novel diagnostic methods in molecular genetics in pediatric practice. Genetic diagnosis is now an indispensable part of the routine practice of primary immunodeficiency disorders, inborn metabolic errors, and monogenic malformations, making way into diagnostic criteria of some as well. It won't go far wrong to state that the science of pediatrics has entered into an era of interdisciplinary practice with genetics and immunology. The rapid flow of discovery of biological drugs during the last decade, availability of next-genome and whole-exome sequencing methods, and the outstanding boost in the rate of success of hematopoietic and solid organ transplantation are all affirmative to this notion. Thanks to molecular genetic methods, an increasing number of the newly introduced "autoinflammatory disorders" are being characterized, donors and recipients are being cross-matched using intricate phenotypic cross matching, and immunotherapy for allergy benefits from state-of-the-art characterization of culprit epitopes in peptide scales. This book tries to strike a balance between cutting-edge science of immunology and clinical practice of pediatrics, through a series of meticulously chosen case discussions, presented by pediatric practitioners and immunology experts.

Pediatric Immunology Series is a three-volume book series and a collection of well-presented case discussions in pediatric medicine. Volume I, *Pediatric Allergy*, is focused on diagnosis and practice of allergy, asthma, atopy, and relevant disorders. Volume II, *Pediatric Immunology*, thoroughly addresses cases on primary immunodeficiency disorders; and finally, Volume III, *Pediatric Autoimmunity and Transplantation*, is a constellation of cases in autoimmune and rheumatologic disorders of childhood, secondary immunodeficiency conditions, and real cases with hematopoietic and solid organ transplantation.

Volume III of this series is the final frame and a diverse constellation of case discussions, from autoimmunity and pediatric rheumatologic disorders to immunohematology and transplantation, to autoimmune skin disorders, and finally to secondary conditions causing immunodeficiency. Chapters 1–19 and 82–83 showcase case discussions with childhood-onset rheumatologic disorders, adult rheumatic disorders with pediatric onset, and disorders of potential autoimmune origin such as idiopathic thrombocytopenia. Cutaneous immune-related conditions and cutaneous manifestations of systemic disorders are a must know for every pediatric practitioner and are hence addressed in Chaps. 57–81. Secondary conditions that mimic presentations of primary immunodeficiency disorders comprise heterogeneous entities that are the main focus of the few cases presented in Chaps. 20–34. Finally, the fine art of recipient, i.e., donor matching in hematopoietic stem cell and solid organ transplantation, is skillfully discussed in Chaps. 35–56 of this volume.

The Pediatric Immunology Series is the result of a multinational collaboration of more than 350 scientists from more than 100 well-known universities/institutes worldwide. I would like to hereby acknowledge the expertise of all contributors for their generous devotion of time and effort in preparing each of the chapters. I would also like to extend my gratitude to the Springer publication for providing me the opportunity to publish the book.

We are hopeful that this book provides an exemplary touch to the fast-growing intersection of pediatrics and immunology, and a useful guide for pediatric practitioners worldwide.

Tehran, Iran — Farzaneh Rahmani
Tehran, Iran — Nima Rezaei

Abbreviations

3TC	Lamivudine
4CmenB	4-Component meningococcal serogroup B vaccine
AA	Alopecia areata
ABC	Abacavir
ACE	Angiotensin-converting enzyme
ACLE	Acute cutaneous lupus erythematosus
ACPA	Anti-citrullinated protein antibody
ACR	American College of Rheumatology
AD	Autosomal dominant
ADCC	Antibody-dependent cellular cytotoxicity
AECA	Anti-endothelial cells
AGEP	Acute generalized exanthematous pustulosis
aGVHD	Acute GVHD
AIDS	Acquired immunodeficiency syndrome
AIHA	Autoimmune hemolytic anemia
ALDY	Annular lichenoid dermatitis of youth
ALL	Acute lymphoblastic leukemia
ALPS	Autoimmune lymphoproliferative syndrome
AML	Acute myeloid leukemia
AMR	Antibody-mediated rejection
ANA	Antinuclear antibody
ANC	Absolute neutrophil count
ANCA	Anti-neutrophil cytoplasmic antibodies
Anti-CCP	Anti-cyclic citrullinated peptide
Anti-dsDNA	Anti-double-stranded DNA
Anti-EMA	Anti-endomysial antibodies
Anti-ENA	Anti-extractable nuclear antigens
Anti-eTG	Anti-epidermal transglutaminase
Anti-MDA5	Anti-melanoma differentiation-associated gene 5 antibodies
Anti-TG	Anti-thyroglobulin

Anti-TPO	Antithyroid peroxidase
Anti-tTG	Tissue transglutaminase antibody
APC	Antigen-presenting cells
APECED	Autoimmune polyendocrinopathy-candidiasis-ectodermal dystrophy
APGAR	Appearance, pulse, grimace, activity, and respiration
APS-1	Autoimmune polyendocrine syndrome type 1
AR	Autosomal recessive
ARF	Acute rheumatic fever
ART	Anti-retroviral therapy
A-T	Ataxia-telangiectasia
AT1R	Anti-angiotensin II type 1 receptor
ATG	Anti-thymocyte globulin
ATN	Acute tubular necrosis
ATR	Ataxia-telangiectasia and Rad3 related
AZT	Zidovudine
BB-UVB	Broadband ultraviolet B
BCG	Bacillus Calmette-Guérin
BD	Behçet's disease
BMT	Bone marrow transplantation
BMZ	Basement membrane zone
BNP	Brain natriuretic peptide
BP	Blood pressure
BPAg2	Bullous pemphigoid antigen
bpm	Beats per minute
BSA	Body surface area
BSLE	Bullous SLE
CAJDM	Clinically amyopathic juvenile dermatomyositis
c-ANCA	Cytosolic anti-neutrophil cytoplasmic antibodies
CARRA	Childhood Arthritis and Rheumatology Research Alliance
CAT	Cutaneous assessment tool
CBC	Complete blood count
CBDC	Chronic bullous disease of childhood
CBT	Cord blood transplantation
CCLE	Chronic cutaneous lupus erythematosus
CD	Cluster of differentiation
CDC	Complement-dependent cytotoxicity
CGD	Chronic granulomatous disease
CHAQ	Childhood Health Assessment Questionnaire
CHB	Congenital heart block
CHS	Chediak-Higashi syndrome
CID	Combined immunodeficiency
CLAD	Childhood linear IgA disease
CM	Cutaneous mastocytosis
CMAS	Childhood Myositis Assessment Scale

CMC	Chronic mucocutaneous candidiasis
CMG2	Capillary morphogenesis gene 2
CML	Chronic myeloid leukemia
CMP	Cartilage matrix protein
cMPO	Myeloperoxidase deficiency
CMV	Cytomegalovirus
CNIs	Calcineurin inhibitors
CRP	C-reactive protein
CsA	Cyclosporine A
CSF	Cerebrospinal fluid
CT	Computed tomography
CTL	Cytotoxic T-lymphocytes
CVID	Common variable immune deficiency
CWD	Common and well-documented alleles
CXCR4	CXC chemokine receptor 4
CXR	Chest X-ray
DAT	Direct antiglobulin test
DCM	Diffuse cutaneous mastocytosis
DFA	Direct fluorescent antibody
DGP	Gliadin-derived peptides
DH	Dermatitis herpetiformis
DIF	Direct immunofluorescence
DIHS	Drug-induced hypersensitivity syndrome
DIRA	Deficiency of interleukin-1 receptor antagonist
DLE	Discoid lupus erythematosus
DLI	Donor lymphocyte infusion
DMARDs	Disease-modifying antirheumatic drugs
DNA	Deoxyribonucleic acid
DOCK8	Dedicator of cytokinesis 8
DRESS	Drug reaction with eosinophilia and systemic symptoms
DSA	Donor-specific antibodies
dsDNA	Double-stranded DNA antibodies
Dsg	Desmoglein
DT	Diphtheria and tetanus toxoids full strength
dT	Diphtheria-tetanus toxoids with reduced content of diphtheria
DtaP	Diphtheria-tetanus acellular pertussis vaccine
DTaP3	Diphtheria-tetanus-3-component acellular pertussis vaccine
DTaP5-IPV-Hib	Diphtheria-tetanus-3-component acellular pertussis-inactivated polio haemophilus influenzae type b
DTaP-IPV-HBV+Hib	Hexavalent diphtheria-tetanus-acellular pertussis-inactivated polio-hepatitis B vaccine
E	Ethambutol
EB	Epidermolysis bullosa

EBV	Epstein-Barr virus
ECDS	En coup de sabre
ECP	Extracorporeal photopheresis
EFE	Endocardial fibroelastosis
ELE	Erysipelas-like erythema
ELISA	Enzyme-linked immunosorbent assay
EM	Erythema multiforme
EmA	Anti-endomysium
EMG	Electromyography
EMM	Erythema multiforme major
ERK	Extracellular signal-regulated kinases
ES	Evans syndrome
ESID	European Society for Immunodeficiencies
ESR	Erythrocyte sedimentation rate
ESRD	End-stage renal disease
ETaR	Anti-endothelin-1 type A receptor
EULAR	European League Against Rheumatism
FACS	Fluorescence-activated cell sorting
Fas	First apoptosis signal
FCXM	Flow cytometric crossmatch
FDA	Food and Drug Administration
FFP	Fresh frozen plasma
FHLH/FHL	Familial hemophagocytic lymphohistiocytosis
FIA	Flow injection analysis
FiO2	Fraction of inspired oxygen
FISH	Fluorescence in-situ hybridization
FLAMSA	Fludarabine, cytarabine, amsacrine
Flt3L	FMS-like tyrosine kinase 3 ligand
FOXP3	Forkhead box protein 3
FS-MPGN	Focal segmental membranoproliferative glomerulonephritis
FTT	Failure to thrive
FUMHD	Febrile ulceronecrotic Mucha-Habermann disease
G6PD	Glucose-6-phosphatase deficiency
GATA2	GATA-binding factor 2
G-CSF	Granulocyte colony-stimulating factor
GI	Gastrointestinal
GM-CSF	Granulocyte-macrophage colony-stimulating factor
GPCR	G protein-coupled receptor
GU	Genitourinary
GVHD	Graft versus host disease
GvL	Graft-versus-leukemia
H	Isoniazid
HAART	Highly active anti-retroviral therapy
HAV	Hepatitis A vaccine

Hb	Hemoglobin
HBV	Hepatitis B virus
HCT	Hematopoietic cell transplantation
HCV	Hepatitis C virus
HFS	Hyaline fibromatosis syndrome
Hib	Haemophilus influenza type b vaccine
HiDAC	High-dose cytarabine
HIGM	Hyper-IgM syndrome
HIV	Human immunodeficiency virus
HLA	Human leukocyte antigens
HLA-B27	Human leukocyte antigen-B27
HLH	Hemophagocytic lymphohistiocytosis
HNIG	Human normal immunoglobulin
HPA	Hereditary papulotranslucent acrokeratoderma
HPLC	High-performance liquid chromatography
HPS	Hermansky-Pudlak syndrome
HPS2	Hermansky-Pudlak type 2
HPV	Human papilloma virus
HRCT	High-resolution computed tomography
HSC	Hematopoietic stem cells
HSCT	Hematopoietic stem cell transplantation
HSE	Herpes simplex encephalitis
HSP	Henoch-Schönlein purpura
HSV	Herpes simplex virus
HUS	Hemolytic uremic syndrome
HUV	Hypocomplementemic urticarial vasculitis
HUVS	Hypocomplementemic urticarial vasculitis syndrome
IA	Idiopathic anaphylaxis
IBD	Inflammatory bowel disease
ICU	Intensive care unit
IFN	Interferon
IFN-γ	Interferon-γ
IgA	Immunoglobulin A
IgE	Immunoglobulin E
IgG	Immunoglobulin G
IgM	Immunoglobulin M
IHC	Immunohistochemistry
IIF	Indirect immunofluorescence
IIV	Inactivated influenza vaccine
IL	Interleukin
IL-12	Interleukin-12
ILAR	International League Against Rheumatism
ILD	Interstitial lung disease
IM	Intramuscular
IMA	Inherited maternal antigens/haplotype

IMGT	International ImMunoGeneTics information
Inf	Influenza vaccine
INH	Isoniazid
IPA	Inherited paternal antigens/haplotype
IPSS	International Prognostic Scoring System
IPV	Inactivated polio vaccine
ITK	IL-2 inducible tyrosine/T-cell kinase
ITP	Idiopathic thrombocytopenic purpura
IV	Intravenous
IVIG	Intravenous immunoglobulin
JDM	Juvenile dermatomyositis
JIA	Juvenile idiopathic arthritis
JPsA	Juvenile psoriatic arthritis
kD	Kilodalton
KD	Kawasaki disease
kg	Kilogram
KS	Kaposi sarcoma
LABD	Linear IgA bullous disease
LAD	Leukocyte adhesion deficiency
LAIV	Live attenuated influenza vaccine
LDH	Lactate dehydrogenase
LE	Lupus erythematosus
LEKTI	Kazal-type-related inhibitor
LFT	Liver function test
LOF	Loss-of-function
LP	Lumbar puncture
LPV	Lopinavir
LQTS	Long QT syndrome
LRD	Living-related donor
LSc	Localized scleroderma
LSS	Lymphocyte steroid sensitivity
LTs	Leukotrienes
LTT	Lymphocyte transformation test
LYST	Lysosomal trafficking regulator protein
MAC	Membrane attack complex
MAPK	Mitogen-activated protein kinases
MAS	Macrophage activation syndrome
MBEH	Monobenzyl ether of hydroquinone
MCV	Mean corpuscular volume
MDR-AML	Myelodysplasia-related-AML
MDS	Myelodysplastic syndrome
MDS/AML	Myelodysplastic syndrome/acute myeloid leukemia
Men	Meningococcal vaccine
MenCV4	4-Valent (A,C,W-135,Y) conjugate meningococcal vaccine

MF	Mycosis fungoides
MFI	Mean fluorescence intensity
MIS	Mastocytosis in the skin
MIV	Marginal inflammatory vitiligo
MMF	Mycophenolate mofetil
mmHg	Millimeter of mercury
MMR	Measles-mumps-rubella
MODS	Multi-organ dysfunction syndrome
MOTT	Mycobacteria other than tuberculosis
MPO	Myeloperoxidase
MRI	Magnetic resonance imaging
MRSA	Methicillin-resistant *Staphylococcus aureus*
MSA	Myositis-specific autoantibodies
Msc/MSCs	Mesenchymal stem cells
MSH6	mutS homolog 6
MSMD	Mendelian susceptibility to mycobacterial disease
mTOR	Mechanistic target of rapamycin
MUD	Matched unrelated donors
WHIM syndrome	Warts, hypogammaglobulinemia, infections, and myelokathexis
NASH	Nonalcoholic steatohepatitis
NAT	Nucleic acid testing
NBT	Nitroblue tetrazolium
NB-UVB	Narrowband ultraviolet B
NEC	Necrotizing enterocolitis
NEMO	NF-kB essential modulator
NIH	National Institutes of Health
NIMA	Non-inherited maternal HLA antigen/haplotype
NIPA	Non-inherited paternal HLA antigen/haplotype
NK cell	Natural killer cell
NKT cells	Natural killer T cells
NLE	Neonatal lupus erythematosus
NLRs	NOD-like receptor
NMDP	National Marrow Donor Program
NOTA	National Organ Transplantation Act
NPV	Nevirapine
NRTI	Nucleoside reverse transcriptase inhibitors
NSAIDs	Nonsteroidal anti-inflammatory drugs
NTM	Non-tuberculous mycobacteria
NT-proBNP	N-terminal proBNP
NUV	Normocomplementemic urticarial vasculitis
OCA	Oculocutaneous albinism
OLT	Orthotopic liver transplantation
OPO	Originating organ procurement organization
OPV	Oral polio vaccine

OS	Omenn's syndrome
PAF	Platelet-activating factor
PAN	Polyarteritis nodosa
p-ANCA	Perinuclear anti-neutrophil cytoplasmic antibodies
PAP	Pulmonary alveolar proteinosis
PAPA	Pyogenic sterile arthritis, pyoderma gangrenosum, and acne
PBSCT	Peripheral blood stem cell transplantation
PCP	*Pneumocystis jirovecii* pneumonia
PCR	Polymerase chain reaction
PCV	Pneumococcal conjugate vaccine
PF	Pemphigus foliaceus
PG	Pyoderma gangrenosum
PKCδ	Protein kinase C-delta
PL	Pityriasis lichenoides
PLC	Pityriasis lichenoides chronica
PLE	Protein-losing enteropathy
PLEVA	Pityriasis lichenoides et varioliformis acuta
PMA	Phorbol 12-myristate 13-acetate
PO	Per os/oral
PPSV	Pneumococcal polysaccharide vaccine
PRCSG	Pediatric Rheumatology Collaborative Study Group
PRI	Potential repigmentation index
PRINTO	Paediatric Rheumatology International Trials Organisation
PRP	Pityriasis rubra pilaris
PRS	Parry-Romberg syndrome
PUVA	Psoralen and ultraviolet A
PV	Pemphigus vulgaris
R	Rifampicin
RA	Rheumatoid arthritis
RAST	Radioallergosorbent test
RBC	Red blood cell
RF	Rheumatoid factor
RIC	Reduced-intensity conditioning
ROS	Reactive oxygen species
RV	Rotavirus vaccine
SAA	Serum amyloid A
SAB	Single-antigen antibody
SAM	Severe acute malnutrition
SBEG	Suction blister epidermal grafts
SBS	Short bowel syndrome
SCID	Severe combined immunodeficiency
Scl-70	Anti-toposiomerase I
SCLE	Subacute cutaneous lupus erythematosus
sIL-2R or sCD25	Soluble interleukin-2 receptor

sIL-2Rα	Soluble IL-2 receptor alpha
SIRS	Systemic inflammatory response syndrome
SJIA	Systemic juvenile idiopathic arthritis
SJS	Stevens-Johnson syndrome
SLE	Systemic lupus erythematosus
SLICC	Systemic Lupus International Collaborating Clinics
SM	Systemic mastocytosis
SMA II	Spinal muscular atrophy type 2
SoJIA	Systemic-onset juvenile idiopathic arthritis
SPD	Subcorneal pustular dermatosis
SPINK5	Serine protease inhibitor, Kazal type 5
SPT	Skin prick test
SSc	Systemic sclerosis
SSLR	Serum sickness-like reaction
SSSS	Staphylococcal scalded skin syndrome
STEC	Shiga toxin-producing strains of *Escherichia coli*
STR	Short tandem repeat
T	Tetanus toxoid
TACO	Transfusion associated volume overload
TA-TMA	Transplant-associated thrombotic microangiopathy
TBI	Total body irradiation
TCE	T-cell epitopes
TCR	T-cell receptor
TCRαβ	Alpha/beta T-cell receptor
TCRγδ	Gamma/delta T-cell receptor
Tdpa	Tetanus-diphtheria-acellular pertussis with reduced content of diphtheria an pertussis antigens
TEN	Toxic epidermal necrolysis
TG	Triglyceride
Th1	T helper 1
Th17	T helper 17
Th2	T helper 2
TIA	Transient ischemic attack
TIV	Trivalent influenza vaccine
TKI	Tyrosine kinase inhibitor
TMA	Thrombotic microangiopathy
TORCH	Toxoplasmosis, other (syphilis, varicella-zoster, parvovirus B19), rubella, cytomegalovirus, and herpes
TPMT	Thiopurine *S*-methyltransferase
TPN	Total parenteral nutrition
TPO	Thyroid peroxidase
TRALI	Transfusion-associated lung injury
TREC	T-cell receptor excision circles
UA	Urinary analysis
UC	Ulcerative colitis

UCB	Umbilical cord blood
UNOS	United Network for Organ Sharing
UP	Urticaria pigmentosa
URI	Upper respiratory tract infection
UV	Ultraviolet
UVA-1	Ultraviolet-A1
V(D)J	Variable, diversity, joining
Var	Varicella vaccine
VASI	Vitiligo Area Severity Index
VETF	Vitiligo European Task Force
VIDA	Vitiligo Disease Activity Score
VOD	Veno-occlusive disease
VZIG	Varicella-zoster immune globulin
VZV	Varicella zoster virus
WAS	Wiskott-Aldrich syndrome
WBC	White blood cell
WES	Whole-exome sequencing
XLP	X-linked lymphoproliferative disease
XLP1	X-linked proliferative disorder type I
Z	Pyrazinamide

Contents

1 **Introduction to Autoimmunity, Secondary Immunodeficiency, and Transplantation** 1
Terry Harville, Soumya Pandey, Piyush Kumar, Marco Antonio Yamazaki-Nakashimada, Larry Ngek Tangie, Farzaneh Rahmani, and Nima Rezaei

2 **Fever and Cervical Lymphadenopathy** 17
Berenise Gamez-Gonzalez and Marco Antonio Yamazaki-Nakashimada

3 **Prolonged Refractory High Fever** 25
Ross Petty and Farhad Salehzadeh

4 **Pain in Both Knees** 31
Ross Petty and Farhad Salehzadeh

5 **Challenging Pain in Knee and Ankle** 35
Peter Jandus

6 **Fever and Urticarial Rash** 43
Mojgan Kianiamin

7 **Knee Swelling and Rash** 47
Ross Petty and Farhad Salehzadeh

8 **Malaise, Weight Loss and Intermittent Fever** 53
Ross Petty, Farhad Salehzadeh, and Marco Antonio Yamazaki-Nakashimada

9 **Anemia, Microhematuria and Proteinuria** 57
Živanović S. Snežana, Ivana Djuric-Filipovic, and Zorica Živković

10 **Fever, Anasarca and Arthralgia** 61
Erika Sifuentes-Rodriguez, Francisco Rivas-Larrauri, and Marco Antonio Yamazaki-Nakashimada

11 **Bradycardia in a Neonate** ... 65
Ross Petty and Farhad Salehzadeh

12 **Annular Rash in a Neonate** ... 71
Yan Ling Kong and Emily Yiping Gan

13 **Itchy Facial Rash** ... 77
Yan Ling Kong and Emily Yiping Gan

14 **Muscle Weakness and Fever** ... 85
Piyush Kumar and Anupam Das

15 **Pruritic Erythematous Rashes on Face and Eyelids** ... 91
Selcen Kundak and Malik Ergin

16 **Edema of Hands and Hypopigmented Lesions on Her Neck and Cheeks** ... 97
Ana Luisa Rodríguez-Lozano and Marco Yamazaki-Nakashimada

17 **Asymptomatic Atrophic Plaque on the Face** ... 103
Yan Ling Kong and Emily Yiping Gan

18 **Morbiliform Rash and Fever** ... 109
Luciana Paula Samorano, João Avancini, and Marcella Soares Pincelli

19 **Recurrent Interstitial Keratitis and Audiovestibular Dysfunction** ... 115
Kristina A. Dzhuma, Oleg B. Iaremenko, and Maksym I. Situkho

20 **Breathlessness and Weight Loss** ... 121
Sowmya Shashidhara, H. Koushik, and Sangita Trivedi

21 **Neck Swelling and Fever** ... 127
Sowmya Shashidhara, H. Koushik, and Sangita Trivedi

22 **Puffy Face and Abdominal Distension** ... 133
Sowmya Shashidhara, H. Koushik, and Sangita Trivedi

23 **Hematuria and Abdominal Mass** ... 139
Sowmya Shashidhara, H. Koushik, and Sangita Trivedi

24 **Pitting Edema and Desquamation** ... 143
Sowmya Shashidhara, H. Koushik, and Sangita Trivedi

25 **Fever and Cutaneous Nodules** ... 149
Sowmya Shashidhara, H. Koushik, and Sangita Trivedi

26 **Neck Stiffness and Fever** ... 153
Tangie Ngek Larry and Derrick Tembi Efie

27 **Rash and Generalized Body Pains** ... 157
Tangie Ngek Larry and Derrick Tembi Efie

28 Positive HIV and Violet Macular Rash . . . 161
Tangie Ngek Larry and Derrick Tembi Efie

29 Weight Loss and Tuberculin Skin Test Anergy . . . 165
Léila Dangou, Medeton Grâce Hounkpe, Josephiel Fortunato, and Crescent Darius Cossou-Gbeto

30 Edema on Lower Limbs . . . 169
Medeton Grâce Hounkpe, Léila Dangou, Josephiel Fortunato, and Crescent Darius Cossou-Gbeto

31 Asthenia and Fatigue . . . 173
Dominique M. A. Bullens and Isabelle Meyts

32 Infections, Whitish Skin Papules and Subcutaneous Nodules . . . 179
Delara Babaei

33 Recurrent Pneumonia and History of Transplantation . . . 185
Sonia de Arriba-Méndez, Eva Macías, and Ignacio Dávila

34 Painful Skin Nodules, Prolonged Fever and Cervical Lymphadenopathy . . . 189
Michelle N. G. Ying, Emily Yiping Gan, and Jean Aan Mark Koh

35 Malaise, Laryngitis and Fever . . . 197
Claus-Philipp Maier and Dominik Schneidawind

36 Acute Myeloid Leukemia Requiring Hematopoietic Stem Cell Transplantation . . . 203
Soumya Pandey and Terry Harville

37 Discrepant Cytomegalovirus Serology Between Donor and Recipient in Hematopoietic Stem Cell Transplantation . . . 207
Soumya Pandey and Terry Harville

38 Suspected Immunodeficiency . . . 211
Soumya Pandey and Terry Harville

39 Linkage Disequilibrium Between HLA Alleles in Hematopoietic Stem Cell Transplantation . . . 217
Soumya Pandey and Terry Harville

40 T-Lymphoblastic Lymphoma . . . 223
Soumya Pandey and Terry Harville

41 No Lymphocytes in an Infant . . . 229
Beatriz Morillo-Gutierrez and Mary Slatter

42 DOCK8 Deficiency and No Matched Donor . . . 237
Beatriz Morillo-Gutierrez and Mary Slatter

43 Diarrhea Post-HSCT . . . 241
Beatriz Morillo-Gutierrez and Mary Slatter

44 Follow-Up of a Severe Combined Immunodeficiency, Who Received Bone-Marrow Transplantation Four Decades Ago 247
Romina Dieli-Crimi and Teresa Español

45 Nonalcoholic Steatohepatitis Referred for Liver Transplantation ... 251
Laura Cooling

46 Acute Respiratory Distress During Stem Cell Infusion 255
Laura Cooling

47 Acute Dyspnea After Platelet Transfusion 259
Laura Cooling

48 Requiring Immunization After Rescue Autologous HSCT 265
Darko Richter

49 Fever and Abdominal Pain 273
Esraa M. Eloseily and Randy Q. Cron

50 Prolonged Fever, Rash and Mucosal Bleeding 281
Beata Derfalvi

51 Recurrent Infections, Diarrhea and Hypereosinophilia 289
Haskologlu Sule, Islamoglu Candan, and Ikinciogullari Aydan

52 Liver Transplantation Who Developed Pancytopenia Post-transplantation 295
Soumya Pandey and Terry Harville

53 Kidney Transplant Candidate Showing Presence of Pre-formed Donor-Specific Antibodies Against a Prospective Living Donor 305
Soumya Pandey and Terry Harville

54 Heart Transplant Candidate Who Required Extra-Corporal Membrane Oxygenation (ECMO) 311
Soumya Pandey and Terry Harville

55 Acute Antibody-Mediated Rejection of Transplantation with Negative Prospective Crossmatch Results 319
Soumya Pandey and Terry Harville

56 Kidney Transplantation in a Patient with End Stage Renal Disease (ESRD) Secondary to Focal Segmental Glomerulosclerosis 325
Soumya Pandey and Terry Harville

57 Itchy Violaceous Plaques 329
Yan Ling Kong and Emily Yiping Gan

58 Photosensitivity and Bullous Lesions 337
Ashi and Piyush Kumar

59 **Recurrent Bullous Lesions** . . . 345
Santoshdev P. Rathod and Piyush Kumar

60 **Refractory Blisters and Erosions** . . . 349
Ziying Vanessa Lim and Emily Yiping Gan

61 **Annular Blisters and Erosions** . . . 357
Soner Uzun and Aslı Bilgic-Temel

62 **Vesicular Pruriginous Lesions** . . . 363
Dario Didona and Biagio Didona

63 **Widespread Vesiculobullous Rash** . . . 369
Soner Uzun and Aslı Bilgic-Temel

64 **Itchy Skin Rashes** . . . 375
Marzieh Tavakol

65 **Blisters on Back and Upper Extremities** . . . 381
Gulsen Akoglu

66 **Itchy Blisters** . . . 387
Yan Ling Kong and Emily Yiping Gan

67 **Sudden Onset Grouped Blisters** . . . 393
Soner Uzun and Aslı Bilgic-Temel

68 **Pruritic Blisters** . . . 399
Anupam Das and Piyush Kumar

69 **Widespread Depigmented and Hypopigmented Patches** . . . 403
Piyush Kumar and Sunil K. Kothiwala

70 **Whitish Patches** . . . 409
Gulsen Akoglu

71 **Hyperpigmented Patches** . . . 415
Yan Ling Kong and Emily Yiping Gan

72 **Outbreaks of Erythematous and Necrotic Papules with Hemorrhagic Crusts** . . . 421
Selcen Kundak and Malik Ergin

73 **Persistent, Annular Urticarial Plaque** . . . 427
Selcen Kundak and Malik Ergin

74 **Yellow, Reddish Brown Skin Lesions** . . . 433
Alireza Shafiei

75 **Erythroderma** . . . 435
Wojciech Baran and Jacek Szepietowski

76 **Erythematous Scaly Plaques** . . . 439
Sunil K. Kothiwala and Piyush Kumar

77 Multiple Circinate, Sterile, Flaccid, Relapsing Pustules 445
Selcen Kundak and Malik Ergin

78 Purpuric Macules and Oral Erosions 451
Dipak Kr. Agarwalla and Piyush Kumar

79 Diffuse Skin Rash and Mucosal Lesions 459
Marzieh Tavakol

80 Painful Facial Ulceration 465
Dario Didona and Biagio Didona

81 Patchy Hair Loss 469
Anupam Das and Piyush Kumar

82 Concerning Weight Loss Over Three Weeks 475
Farzaneh Rahmani and Nima Rezaei

83 Toddler with Bruising on Knees 479
Farzaneh Rahmani and Nima Rezaei

Index 483

Contributors

Dipak Kr. Agarwalla Department of Dermatology, Gauhati Medical College and Hospital, Guwahati, Assam, India

Gulsen Akoglu, MD, MSc Gulhane Training and Research Hospital, Dermatology and Venereology Clinic, University of Health Sciences, Ankara, Turkey

Ashi Gauhati Medical College, Guwahati, Assam, India

João Avancini, MD Department of Dermatology, Hospital das Clínicas of the University of São Paulo Medical School, São Paulo, Brazil

Ikinciogullari Aydan, MD Department of Pediatric Allergy and Immunology, Ankara University School of Medicine, Ankara, Turkey

Delara Babaei, MD Department of Allergy and Clinical Immunology, Mofid Children's Hospital, Shahid Beheshti University of Medical Sciences, Tehran, Iran

Wojciech Baran, MD, PhD Department of Dermatology, Venereology and Allergology, Wroclaw Medical University, Wrocław, Poland

Aslı Bilgic-Temel, MD Seydisehir State Hospital, Dermatology Clinic, Konya, Turkey

Dominique M.A. Bullens, MD, PhD Allergy and Clinical Immunology Research Group, KU Leuven, Leuven, Belgium

Islamoglu Candan, MD Department of Pediatric Allergy and Immunology, Ankara University School of Medicine, Ankara, Turkey

Laura Cooling, MD, MS Department of Pathology, University of Michigan, Ann Arbor, MI, USA

Crescent Darius Cossou-Gbeto, MD Internal Medicine, Hematology and Oncology Department, Aix-en-Provence Hospital Center, Aix-en-Provence, France

Randy Q. Cron, MD, PhD Division of Rheumatology, Department of Pediatrics, University of Alabama at Birmingham, Birmingham, AL, USA

Léila Dangou, MD Pediatric Department, Bethesda Hospital in Cotonou, Cotonou, Benin

Anupam Das Department of Dermatology, KPC Medical College, Kolkata, West Bengal, India

Ignacio Dávila, MD, PhD Faculty of Medicine, Department of Biologic and Diagnostics Sciences, University of Salamanca, Salamanca, Spain

Allergy Service, University Hospital of Salamanca, Salamanca, Spain

Sonia de Arriba-Méndez, MD, PhD Pediatric Service, University Hospital of Salamanca, Salamanca, Spain

Faculty of Medicine, Department of Biologic and Diagnostics Sciences, University of Salamanca, Salamanca, Spain

Beata Derfalvi, MD, PhD Department of Pediatrics, Dalhousie University/IWK Health Centre, Halifax, NS, Canada

Biagio Didona, MD First Division of Dermatology, Istituto Dermopatico dell'Immacolata-IRCCS, Rome, Italy

Dario Didona, MD Department of Dermatology and Allergology, Philipps University, Marburg, Germany

Romina Dieli-Crimi, MD, PhD Clinical Immunologist, Immunology Unit, Hospital Universitario Vall d'Hebron, Barcelona, Spain

Ivana Djuric-Filipovic, MD, PhD Children's Hospital for Lung Diseases and Tuberculosis, Medical Center "Dr Dragiša Mišović", Belgrade, Serbia

Kristina A. Dzhuma, MD Bogomolets National Medical University, National Specialized Children's Hospital, Kyiv, Ukraine

Derrick Tembi Efie, MD Tokombere District Hospital, Tokombere, Cameroon

Health and Human Development Research Network, Douala, Cameroon

Esraa M. Eloseily, MD, MRCPCH Division of Rheumatology, Department of Pediatrics, University of Alabama at Birmingham, Birmingham, AL, USA

Division of Rheumatology, Department of Pediatrics, Assiut University Children's Hospital, Assiut, Egypt

Malik Ergin, MD Department of Pathology, Dr. Behçet Uz Children's Hospital, İzmir, Turkey

Teresa Español, MD, PhD Clinical Immunologist, Immunology Unit, Hospital Universitario Vall d'Hebron, Barcelona, Spain

Josephiel Fortunato, MD Pediatric Department, Goho Hospital Center of Abomey, Abomey, Benin

Berenise Gamez-Gonzalez, MD Hospital Infantil de Especialidades de Chihuahua, Chihuahua, Mexico

Emily Yiping Gan, MBBS, MRCP, MD Dermatology Service, KK Women's and Children's Hospital, Singapore, Singapore

National Skin Centre, Singapore, Singapore

Terry Harville, MD, PhD Departments of Pathology and Laboratory Services, Pediatrics, and Internal Medicine, University of Arkansas for Medical Sciences, Little Rock, AR, USA

Medeton Grâce Hounkpe, MD ENT Department, University Hospital Hubert Koutoucou Maga of Cotonou, Cotonou, Benin

Oleg B. Iaremenko, MD, PhD Department of Internal Medicine, Bogomolets National Medical University, Kyiv, Ukraine

Peter Jandus, MD Division of Immunology and Allergology, Department of Medicine, University Hospital and Medical Faculty, Geneva, Switzerland

Mojgan Kianiamin, MD Chamran Medical Hospital, Tehran, Iran

Clinic of immunology and Allergy, Chamran General Hospital, Army Medical University, Tehran, Iran

Jean Aan Mark Koh, MB, BS Dermatology Service, KK Women's and Children's Hospital, Singapore, Singapore

Yan Ling Kong, MBBS National Skin Centre, Singapore, Singapore

Sunil K. Kothiwala, MD SkinEva Clinic, Jaipur, Rajasthan, India

H. Koushik, MBBS, MD Department of Pediatrics, Kasturba Medical College, Manipal University, Manipal, Karnataka, India

Piyush Kumar, MD Department of Dermatology, Katihar Medical College, Katihar, Bihar, India

Selcen Kundak, MD Department of Dermatology, Dr. Behçet Uz Children's Hospital, İzmir, Turkey

Tangie Ngek Larry, MD Faculty of Medicine and Biomedical Sciences, University of Yaounde 1, Yaounde, Cameroon

Ziying Vanessa Lim, MBBS, MRCP (UK), M.Med (Int Med) National Skin Centre, Singapore, Singapore

Eva Macías, MD, PhD Faculty of Medicine, Department of Biologic and Diagnostics Sciences, University of Salamanca, Salamanca, Spain

Allergy Service, University Hospital of Salamanca, Salamanca, Spain

Claus-Philipp Maier, MD Department of Internal Medicine II, University Hospital Tuebingen, Tuebingen, Germany

Isabelle Meyts, MD, PhD Inborn Errors of Immunity, KU Leuven, Leuven, Belgium

Beatriz Morillo-Gutierrez, MD Translational Paediatrics and Infectious Diseases Unit, Santiago de Compostela University Hospital, Santiago de Compostela, Spain

Soumya Pandey, MD Department of Pathology and Laboratory Services, University of Arkansas for Medical Sciences, Little Rock, AR, USA

Ross Petty, MD, PhD Pediatric Rheumatology, University of British Columbia, Vancouver, BC, Canada

Marcella Soares Pincelli, MD Department of Dermatology, Hospital das Clínicas of the University of São Paulo Medical School, São Paulo, Brazil

Farzaneh Rahmani, MD, MPH Students Scientific Research Center (SSRC), Tehran University of Medical Sciences, Tehran, Iran

NeuroImaging Network (NIN), Universal Scientific Education and Research Network (USERN), Tehran, Iran

Santoshdev P. Rathod Department of Dermatology, Smt. NHL Municipal Medical College, Ahmedabad, Gujarat, India

Nima Rezaei, MD, PhD Department of Immunology, School of Medicine, Research Center for Immunodeficiencies (RCID), Children's Medical Center, Tehran University of Medical Sciences (TUMS), Tehran, Iran

Network of Immunity in Infection, Malignancy and Autoimmunity (NIIMA), Universal Scientific Education and Research Network (USERN), Tehran, Iran

Darko Richter, MD, PhD Pediatric Allergy and Clinical Immunology, University Hospital Center Zagreb, Zagreb, Croatia

Outpatient and Emergency Service, Department of Pediatrics, University Hospital Center Zagreb, Zagreb, Croatia

Francisco Rivas-Larrauri, MD Clinical Immunology Department, Instituto Nacional de Pediatría, Mexico City, Mexico

Ana Luisa Rodríguez-Lozano, MD, MSc Clinical Immunology Department, Instituto Nacional de Pediatria, Mexico City, Mexico

Farhad Salehzadeh, MD Pediatric Rheumatology, Bouali Children's Hospital, ARUMS, Ardabil, Iran

Luciana Paula Samorano, MD Department of Dermatology, Hospital das Clínicas of the University of São Paulo Medical School, São Paulo, Brazil

Dominik Schneidawind, MD Department of Internal Medicine II, University Hospital Tuebingen, Tuebingen, Germany

Alireza Shafiei Bahrami Children's Hospital, Tehran, Iran

Sowmya Shashidhara, MBBS, MD Department of Pediatrics, Kasturba Medical College, Manipal University, Manipal, Karnataka, India

Network of Immunity in Infection, Malignancy and Autoimmunity (NIIMA), Universal Scientific Education and Research Network (USERN), Manipal, Karnataka, India

Erika Sifuentes-Rodriguez, MD Clinical Immunology Department, Instituto Nacional de Pediatría, Mexico City, Mexico

Maksym I. Situkho, MD, PhD O. Kolomijchenko Otolaryngology Institute, Kyiv, Ukraine

Mary Slatter, MD Department of Paediatric Immunology, Great North Children's Hospital, Royal Victoria Infirmary, Newcastle upon Tyne, UK

Institute of Cellular Medicine, Newcastle University, Newcastle upon Tyne, UK

Živanović S. Snežana, MD, PhD Pediatric Internal Diseases Clinic, Clinical Center of Nis, Faculty of Medicine, University of Nis, Nis, Serbia

Haskologlu Sule, MD Department of Pediatric Allergy and Immunology, Ankara University School of Medicine, Ankara, Turkey

Jacek Szepietowski, MD, PhD Department of Dermatology, Venereology and Allergology, Wroclaw Medical University, Wrocław, Poland

Larry Ngek Tangie, MD Faculty of Medicine and Biomedical Sciences, University of Yaounde, Yaounde, Cameroon

Marzieh Tavakol, MD Non-communicable Diseases Research Center, Alborz University of Medical Sciences, Karaj, Iran

Department of Allergy and Clinical Immunology, Shahid Bahonar Hospital, Alborz University of Medical Sciences, Karaj, Iran

Sangita Trivedi, MBBS, MD Department of Pediatrics, Government Medical College, Veer Narmad South Gujarat University, Surat, Gujarat, India

Soner Uzun, MD Department of Dermatology and Venereology, School of Medicine, Akdeniz University, Antalya, Turkey

Marco Antonio Yamazaki-Nakashimada, MD Clinical Immunology Department, Instituto Nacional de Pediatría, Mexico City, Mexico

Michelle N.G. Ying, MB, BS Dermatology Service, KK Women's and Children's Hospital, Singapore, Singapore

Zorica Živković, MD, PhD Children's Hospital for Lung Diseases and Tuberculosis, Medical Center "Dr Dragiša Mišović", Belgrade, Serbia

Faculty of Pharmacy, University Business Academy in Novi Sad, Novi Sad, Serbia

Chapter 1
Introduction to Autoimmunity, Secondary Immunodeficiency, and Transplantation

Terry Harville, Soumya Pandey, Piyush Kumar, Marco Antonio Yamazaki-Nakashimada, Larry Ngek Tangie, Farzaneh Rahmani, and Nima Rezaei

This book is a constellation of case discussions on pediatric autoimmune disorders, rheumatological diseases, secondary immunodeficiency disorders, and case discussions on hematopoietic stem cell and solid organ transplantations. The following is an overview and head start of the content related to each topic.

T. Harville (✉)
Departments of Pathology and Laboratory Services, Pediatrics, and Internal Medicine, University of Arkansas for Medical Sciences, Little Rock, AR, USA
e-mail: harvilleterryo@uams.edu

S. Pandey
Department of Pathology and Laboratory Services, University of Arkansas for Medical Sciences, Little Rock, AR, USA

P. Kumar
Department of Dermatology, Katihar Medical College, Katihar, Bihar, India

M. A. Yamazaki-Nakashimada
Clinical Immunology Department, Instituto Nacional de Pediatría, Mexico City, Mexico

L. N. Tangie
Faculty of Medicine and Biomedical Sciences, University of Yaounde, Yaounde, Cameroon

F. Rahmani
Student's Scientific Research Center (SSRC), Tehran University of Medical Sciences, Tehran, Iran

NeuroImaging Network (NIN), Universal Scientific Education and Research Network (USERN), Tehran, Iran

N. Rezaei
Department of Immunology, School of Medicine, Research Center for Immunodeficiencies (RCID), Children's Medical Center, Tehran University of Medical Sciences (TUMS), Tehran, Iran

Network of Immunity in Infection, Malignancy and Autoimmunity (NIIMA), Universal Scientific Education and Research Network (USERN), Tehran, Iran

© Springer Nature Switzerland AG 2020
F. Rahmani, N. Rezaei (eds.), *Pediatric Autoimmunity and Transplantation*,
https://doi.org/10.1007/978-3-030-26280-8_1

Human immune system is trained to recognize self from non-self-tissue. Adaptive or pathologic changes in self-antigens, acquired functions in the immune system or lack of proper initial training to the immune system, can all result in **autoimmunity**. Clinical manifestations depend on the organ(s) affected, which in turn depends on nature and type of autoimmunity reaction, autoantibodies and autoreactive T cells.

Pediatric **rheumatologic disorders** are good examples of autoimmune disease in childhood that bear substantial health burden considering the high prevalence of systemic manifestations and the more severe course in this age group. The hallmark pathology of rheumatological disorders is "inflammatory response against self-antigens", the same as other autoimmune disorders. Unfortunately, chronicity might leave a full picture of the disease only to be revealed during adulthood and presents early diagnosis in pediatric patients.

Practice of adult rheumatologic disorders in the pediatric population puts forward a number of special health issues related to this age group. As an example, the higher prevalence of certain complications such as uveitis in children with juvenile idiopathic arthritis, mandates close follow-up with ophthalmologic consult, and growth problems associated with treatment side-effects might restrict the use of corticosteroids and biologic agents in children with rheumatologic disorders.

Juvenile idiopathic arthritis (JIA) is a chronic inflammatory disease and a prototype of rheumatic disorders in pediatric patients [1]. Systemic-onset juvenile idiopathic arthritis is now classified as an autoinflammatory disorder and discussed in volume II of this series. Henoch-Schönlein purpura (HSP) and Kawasaki disease (KD) are two prototypic childhood vasculitides. Frequency of Kawasaki disease has been increasing worldwide over the years, raising serious concern knowing that up to 50% of untreated infants and toddlers face the threat of developing coronary artery aneurysms, a serious condition with lifelong morbidity and mortality. It is worth mentioning that 20% percent of patients with systemic lupus erythematosus (SLE) first manifest during childhood, often by cutaneous symptoms, making it crucial to make an early diagnosis. JIA, HSP, KD and SLE along with a number of other pediatric rheumatologic disorders are given special attention in the first chapters of this volume (Chapters 1–19, 82 and 83). Examples of autoimmune conditions that affect the skin as a single organ system such as vitiligo, alopecia areata, and pemphigus, or cutaneous manifestations of the more common multi-systemic autoimmune conditions such as SLE or dermatomyositis [2], are discussed the final chapters of the book (Chapters 57–81).

Right before getting through chapters describing patients with hematopoietic cell transplantation, we have gathered a series of case discussion of patients with **secondary immunodeficiency disorders** (Chapters 20–34). Immune defects observed in secondary immunodeficiency are usually heterogeneous in their clinical presentation, and their prognosis depends on the severity of the primary condition [3]. Secondary immunodeficiency conditions could be classified into three broad classes based on the etiologic factor:

1. Immunosuppression combined with non-immune disorders: malnutrition, cancer and infection are three major factors that cause secondary immunodeficiency in children. There are strong evidence that malnutrition can adversely impact

immune system. Childhood malignancies such as Hodgkin's disease often destroy cell mediated and humoral immunities, thereby reducing the capacity of the immune system to fight infections. All infective agents, from *Mycobacterium tuberculosis* to HIV virus can give rise to secondary immunodeficiency.
2. Iatrogenic factors: immunosuppressive agents are the most common cause of iatrogenic immunodeficiency. Two most common indication are treatment of autoimmune disorders or prevent transplant rejection.
3. Physiological factors: physiological factors such as immaturity of the immune system in preterm infants, could predispose to secondary immunodeficiency.

Worldwide, protein-calorie malnutrition is the leading cause of secondary immunodeficiencies, considering more than 200 million children being wasted or stunted in WHO reports in 2016 [4, 5]. Unfortunately, limited access to food sources in the main etiology of malnutrition, followed by chronic diseases that induce cachexia, chronic infections and neoplastic conditions.

HIV infection is a global challenge, and among leading causes of secondary immunodeficiency in children and adolescents. HIV infection follows the inevitable course eventually leading to acquired immunodeficiency syndrome (AIDS) state that is characterized by combined immunodeficiency, lymphopenia, increased susceptibility to infections with opportunistic pathogens. Something about 1,990,000 children under 15 years old need anti-retroviral therapy worldwide, less than 30% of which are currently under coverage [6].

Immune defects, aberrations in laboratory tests, and clinical presentation of secondary immunodeficiencies are heterogeneous in nature. Fortunately the immune impairment generally improves with the resolution of the primary condition. A series of case presentations regarding conditions associated with secondary immunodeficiency are presented and discussed in Chapters 20–34.

Hematopoietic Cell Transplantation (HCT) (originally known as Bone Marrow Transplantation or BMT, and also been known as **Hematopoietic Stem Cell Transplantation or HSCT**) began as a successful endeavor in 1968, by Dr. Robert A Good in an infant with severe combined immunodeficiency (SCID). Several things had to come to pass to allow for this. A better understanding of human leukocyte antigens (HLA), and in particular the ability to "type" patients and donors were the foremost essentials for appropriate donor selection [7]. Dr. Paul Terasaki developed a cellular-based typing system, in part based on the work of Dr. Bernard Amos, who had led the way for a better understanding of HLA in the 1950s and early 1960s [8–21]. In the following paragraphs of this writing readers are provided with a head start introduction on HLA and the complex donor selection process for HCT. The aim is to provide prerequisite knowledge for the reader to get ready for the real-life examples of donor-patients selection for HCT presented in Chapters 35–51 of this volume.

The HLA gene locus found on chromosome 6p21, can be divided into Class I (A, B, and C Loci) and Class II (DR, DQ, and DP Loci) (Figs. 1.1, 1.2, 1.3, 1.4, 1.5, and 1.6). Class I HLA are responsible for presenting "endogenous" antigens to $CD8^{+}$ T lymphocytes and are found to be expressed on essentially all nucleated cells in

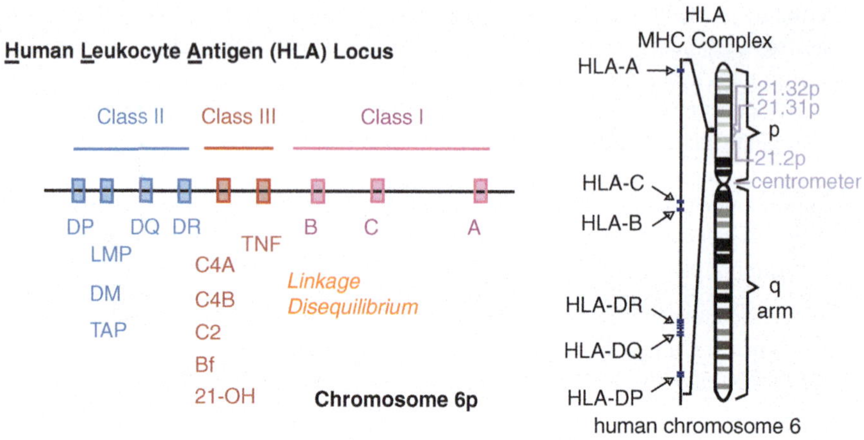

Fig. 1.1 HLA Gene Locus on Chromosome 6p21. Linkage disequilibrium is the concept that "the genes remain inherited together" more than expected form normal chromosome crossover events during meiosis and gametogenesis

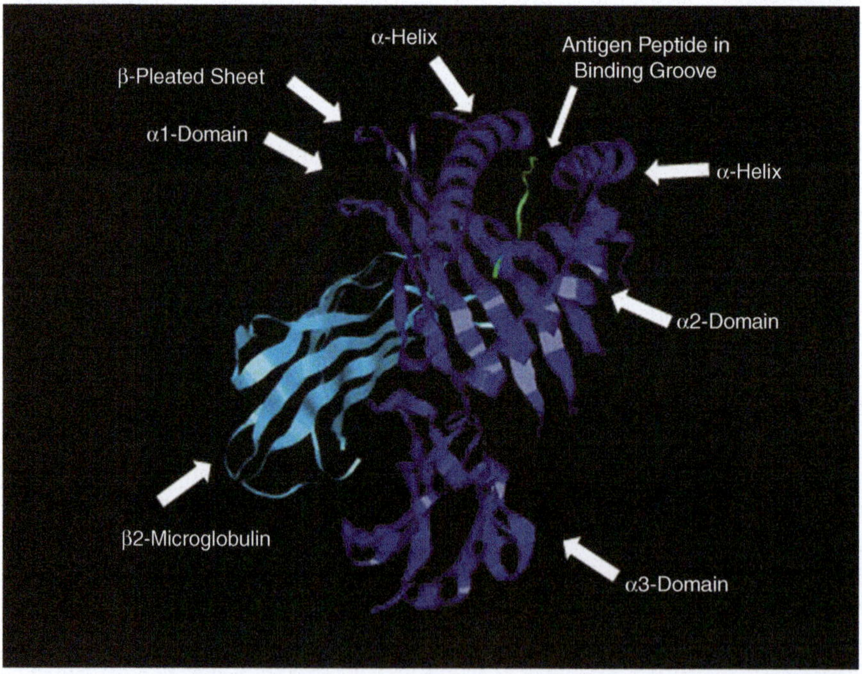

Fig. 1.2 The ultrastructure of HLA Class I molecule (Image constructed from data from the RCSB Protein Data Bank (http://www.rcsb.org/pdb/protein) using RasWin. Components are labelled and discussed in the text. Most of the diversity resides in amino acid substitutions in the α-helices, with some in the β-pleated sheet. HLA class I is comprised of the polymorphic α-chain and the non-covalently attached non-polymorphic β2-microglobulin. The antigen-binding groove resides between the α-helices on top of the β-pleated sheet between the α1- and α2-domains)

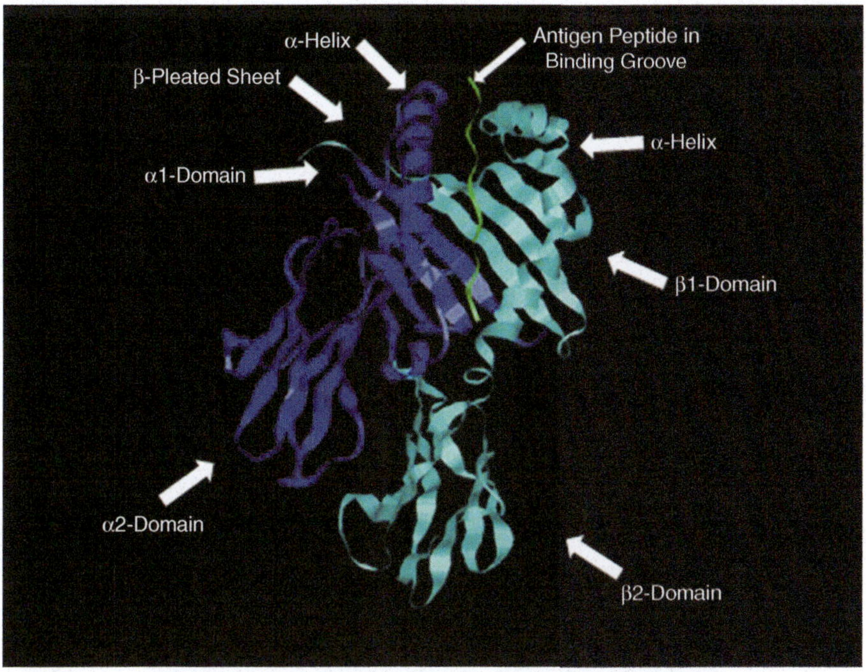

Fig. 1.3 The ultrastructure of HLA Class II molecule (Image constructed from data from the RCSB Protein Data Bank (http://www.rcsb.org/pdb/protein) using RasWin. Components are labelled and discussed in the Text. Most of the diversity resides in amino acid substitutions in the α-helices and some in the β-pleated sheet. HLA class II is comprised of the polymorphic β-chain and the non-covalently attached relative non-polymorphic α-chain, for DR, and two polymorphic α- and β-chains each for DQ and DP. The antigen-binding groove resides between the α-helices on top of the β-pleated sheet between the α1- and β2-domains)

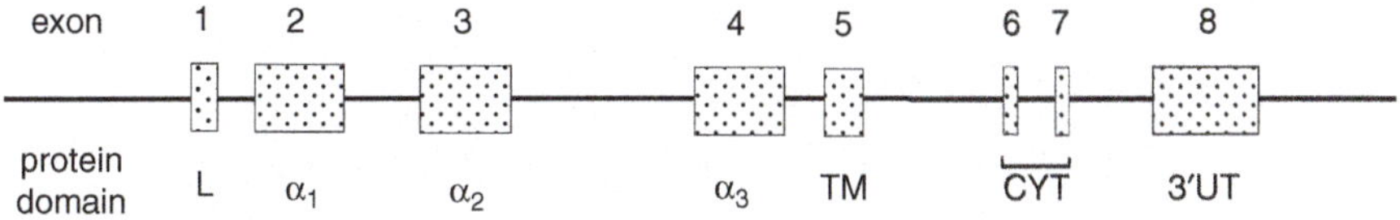

Fig. 1.4 HLA Class I Gene Structure Organization (Exons and introns are shown for class I HLA. The corresponding protein domains are depicted, indicating the exon location. The polymorphisms in exons 2 and 3 (α1 and α2 domains, respectively) generate the main diversity of HLA class I)

humans. To "complete" the molecule for cell-surface expression, β2-microglobulin is non-covalently complexed with HLA class I. Human RBCs do not express HLA, except for some "remnant" occasional expression. These are known as Bennett-Goodspeed (Bg) antigens (Bg^a, HLA-B7; Bg^b, HLA-B17; which includes B57 and B58 subtypes, and Bg^c, HLA-A28; which includes A68 and A69 subtypes). Importantly, platelets express class I HLA proteins. Class II are typically responsi-

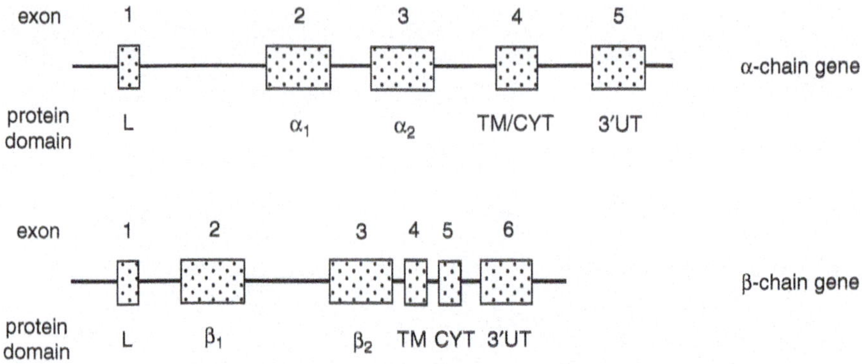

Fig. 1.5 HLA Class II Gene Structure Organization (Exons and introns are shown for class II HLA, A and B gene components, α and β subunit proteins, respectively. The corresponding protein domains are depicted, indicating the exon location. The polymorphisms in exons 2 of the α and β protein subunits (α1 and β1 domains, respectively) generate the main diversity of HLA class II, for DQ and DP, and the β1 domain for DR, since the α1 domain of DR is not very polymorphic)

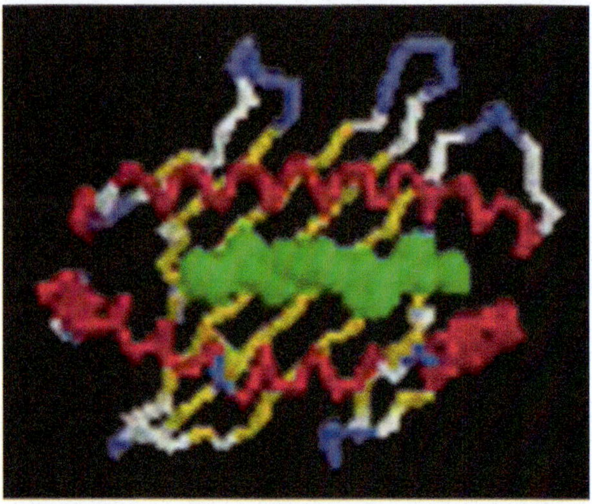

Fig. 1.6 Antigen-Binding Region of HLA: "Looking down" on the top of an HLA molecule, the view "seen" by the T cell receptor. The polymorphic regions include the α-helices and the β-turns of the β-pleated sheet. These are the areas "exposed", for which antibodies can be generated and can elicit T lymphocyte reactivity. These are the areas, which define the "name" of the specific HLA component present. These are the regions, which "must" be matched in order to have successful HCT

ble for presenting "exogenous" antigens to CD4⁺ T lymphocytes, and are found on the cell surface of "professional" antigen presenting cells (APC). Major APCs include dendritic cells, macrophage/monocytes and B lymphocytes. Also included are Kupffer cells in the liver, microglial cells in the brain, and renal peritubular and glomerular capillary cells in the normal human kidney.

An additional consideration is that mesenchymal stem cells (Msc SC) express lower than normal levels of class I HLA and do not express detectable levels of class II HLA. Human hematopoietic stems cells (HSC) are thought to have variable amounts of HLA expression. Lower levels are thought to be present on undifferentiated HSC, with increasing levels as the cells become more differentiated. A progenitor cell may have as much as 80% of HLA expression as that of a fully-differentiated cells.

The diversity of HLA antigens is generated by polymorphisms primarily in the α-helices and β-pleated sheet of the α1 and α2 domains (exons 2 and 3) for class I HLA and the α1 and β1 domains (exons 2 of the A and B gene products) for class II HLA (Figs. 1.2, 1.3, 1.4, 1.5, and 1.6).

Originally, patients and donors were typed at serologic level determination of the HLA type, while now, molecular-level typing is being increasingly performed. The original typing was typically for a 6 of 6 HLA-A, HLA-B, and HLA-DR match which meant matching of both sets of alleles from the patient and the donor. This has expanded to 8 of 8 (HLA-A, -B, -C, and -DR), 10 of 10 (HLA-A, -B, -C, −DR, and -DQ), and finally 12 of 12 (HLA-A, -B, -C, −DR, −DQ, and -DP). As described below, some may consider 10 of 10 matching, with HLA-A, -B, -C, -DRB1, and -DPB1, since HLA-DQB1 mismatches are not believed to influence HCT outcomes, whereas HLA-DPB1 mismatching may influence the outcomes. The greater the extent of overall matching is thought the overall better are outcomes. Note that HLA-DRB3, -DRB4, and -DRB5 are not considered in the matching process.

Mendelian genetics predicts that 25% of sibling donors would be HLA-matched. Yet, in most programs, only 10–15% of patients have an HLA-identical sibling. To deal with issue, the National Marrow Donor Program (NMDP) was established to act as an entity to enroll potential non-related HLA-matched donors (matched-unrelated donors; MUD). More than seven million potential donors are in the registry. Additionally, there are registries in Europe and elsewhere in the world. Umbilical Cord Blood Registries (UCB) came into existence in the early 1990s, as an alternative source of HSC for MUD transplants.

The registries maintain information about the potential donors, including age, ethnicity, ABO status, CMV status, availability to donate, as well as, the HLA typing results. The donor typing results in the registry may be as little as HLA-A, -B, and -DR at the serologic designation, or may be a complete molecular type. When potential donors are selected from the registries, specimens are sent for typing and verification that the potential donor has the correct HLA type to be considered for the patient.

HLA Nomenclature

The original HLA typing by serologic techniques was developed by Amos and Terasaki in the 1950s and 1960s. However, as molecular biologic techniques were developed in the 1970s and 1980s, it became obvious that the serologic determination was inadequate to fully define an individual HLA type. Newer, molecular based typing approaches began in the 1990s, but only came into widespread use after 2005.

Tables 1.1, 1.2, and 1.3 indicate the current numbers of alleles determined by gene sequencing for each of the HLA components. Since most amino acids have multiple triplet codons, "wobble", differences in the third base will produce different DNA sequences, but not changes in the protein structure. These genes will generate different names though, since the naming is based on the DNA sequence, although producing the same proteins. Therefore, a new nomenclature was developed to deal with these issues.

The original nomenclature was based on serologic determinations and names, for example, HLA-A2. The original "molecular" naming merely converted the values to a "four-digit" number, for example, HLA-A0201. Soon though, greater than 100 A2s were found, so that a new system was required.

The current nomenclature takes the same concept but uses digits in "fields" separated by colons (:), so that as many digits as needed could reside in a field between the colons. For example, A∗0101 would become A∗01:01 (Fig. 1.7), but A∗01:714 is also allowed (http://hla.alleles.org/).

Currently, for transplantation purposes, only the Field 1 and Field 2 components are used in donor-patient selection (e.g. A∗01:01). This is also known as "four-digit" in the old concept and "two-field" in the new concept.

The current nomenclature could produce a type such as HLA-A∗01:01:01:01. As noted in Fig. 1.7, the first two digits or first field are derived from the original serow-

Table 1.1 Class I allele frequencies

	A	B	C
Number of alleles	3997	4859	3605
Number of null alleles	186	147	131
Number of proteins	2792	3518	2497

http://www.ebi.ac.uk/ipd/imgt/hla/stats.html and http://www.allelefrequencies.net/

Table 1.2 Class II DR allele frequencies

	DRA	DRB1	DRB3	DRB4	DRB5
Number of alleles	7	2122	145	66	54
Number of null alleles	0	52	4	7	3
Number of proteins	2	1532	119	52	48

http://www.ebi.ac.uk/ipd/imgt/hla/stats.html and http://www.allelefrequencies.net/

Table 1.3 Class II DQ and DP allele frequencies

	DQA1	DQB1	DPA1	DPB1
Number of alleles	92	1152	56	942
Number of null alleles	3	31	0	22
Number of proteins	35	779	26	655

http://www.ebi.ac.uk/ipd/imgt/hla/stats.html and http://www.allelefrequencies.net/

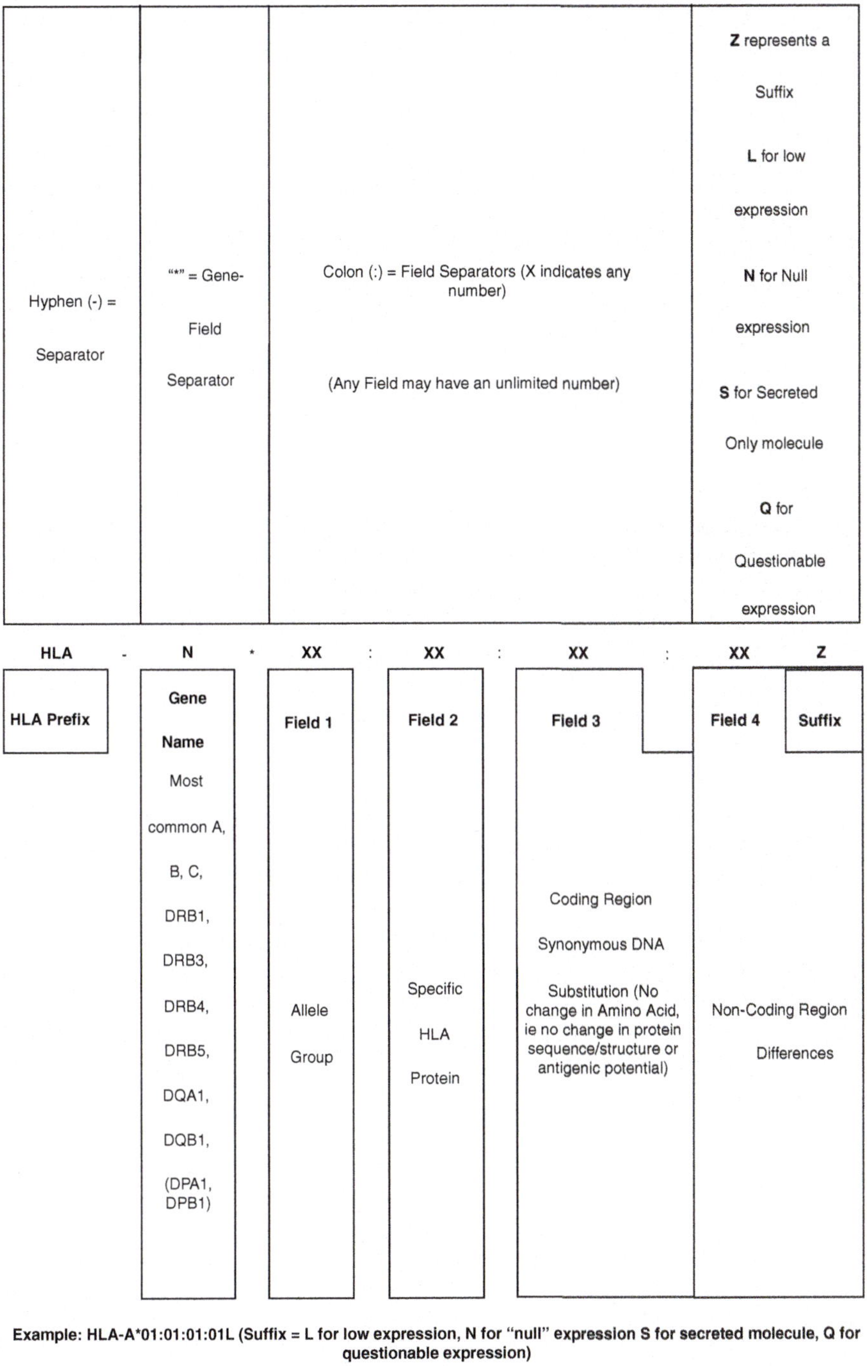

Fig. 1.7 Modern nomenclature system for HLA

logic typing (e.g. A1 to provide A*01). The second field (second group of digits) corresponds to the specific polymorphisms, generated from exons 2 and 3, for class I from exon 2 for class II. These are identified as variants or polymorphisms from the original prototypical HLA type. The third field is used to indicate DNA differences in the triplet codons, which do not alter the protein sequence. The fourth field is used to indicate differences in DNA sequences essentially outside of exons 2 and 3 for class I, and exon 2 for class II. As noted, for matching purposes, only the first two fields are used. In the past, this was frequently stated as a "four-digit" match, but is now considered a "two-field" match.

Specific Donor Selection Issues

Overall HCT outcomes are related to the extent of HLA matching. There is ~10% decrease in survival for each additional HLA locus mismatch when considering an 8 of 8 match. Interestingly, HLA-DQ mismatching has not been shown to have a detrimental effect and is not considered as a criteria to exclude potential donors.

Other HLA locus mismatching may have deleterious effects, from resistance-to-engraftment at one end, to acute graft versus host disease (GVHD) at the other. HLA-B locus mismatching results in greater risk for GVHD, HLA-DR mismatching results in greater risks for resistance-to-engraftment and HLA-A and C locus mismatches individually result in risk for GVHD and resistance to engraftment. Overall, most consider that HLA-DR must be matched to begin the process of a successful outcome.

HLA-C is recognized by the KIR ligands on NK cells. If an HLA-C mismatched donor appears to be otherwise the best donor to select, the favorable outcomes of HLA-C-KIR mismatches shall be considered in donor selection process as it confers better tumorocidal characteristics.

HLA-DP is complex to consider and discuss and was last discovered compared to the rest of HLA family. HLA-DP was originally not thought to elicit antibody responses, which further led to the concept that antibody reactivity was not important in eliciting rejection in cases with HLA-DP mismatch. More recently, it has been shown that HLA-DP does elicit antibodies as well as T lymphocyte reactivity, both influencing outcomes.

The issue of T cell epitopes (TCE) matching should also be considered along with HLA-DPB1 matching. The T lymphocyte reactivity can be defined in terms of specific epitope reactivity, called TCE. Each donor HLA-DPB1 can be defined as matched, if it is the identical HLA-DPB1 as the patient. Further, if there is HLA-DPB1 mismatch between the patient and the donor, a permissive or non-permissive mismatch based on the TCE type(s) present can be assigned. Permissive mismatches share TCE, whereas non-permissive do not. Bottom-line to this discussion is that matched HLA-DPB1 and permissive mismatches appear to provide similar long-term outcomes, and therefore, permissive mismatches may be acceptable for donor selection. It is not easy to know whether the mismatched HLA-

DPB1 is permissive or non-permissive. Thus, a "web-based" algorithm process is available: https://www.ebi.ac.uk/ipd/imgt/hla/dpb.html.

Therefore, the hierarchy for consideration of a potential donor will be an 8 of 8 match at the minimal. The best scenario is considered to be a 12 of 12, HLA-A, -B, -C, -DRB1, -DQB1, and -DPB1, match, followed by 10 of 10, HLA-A, -B, -C, -DRB1, and -DPB1, match. The next best may be 9 of 10, HLA-A, -B, -C, and -DRB1 with one HLA-DPB1 TCE permissive mismatch, and then 8 of 10 with two HLA-DPB1 TCE permissive mismatches. Once again note, the NMDP data indicate that HLA-DQ mismatches do not greatly influence HCT outcomes, and HLA-DRB3, -DRB4, and -DRB5 are not considered in the matching process.

Additional Issues Regarding Donor Selection

Anti-HLA antibodies in the recipient may have a deleterious role on the outcome of HCT, resulting in resistance-to-engraftment. Having a high number of anti-HLA antibodies, by itself, is not an issue with HCT, as long as the antibodies are not directed to any of the donor HLA components. Yet, high levels of anti-HLA antibodies could result in difficulty finding compatible platelet donors subsequent to transplantation. Elevated levels of anti-HLA antibodies, not directed toward the donor, do not result in poorer outcomes. In contrast, donor-specific antibodies (DSA) result in engraftment failure or resistance to engraftment in the setting of mismatched donor HCT.

Individuals inherit one haplotype of HLA from each parent. These are commonly referred to as inherited maternal antigens/haplotype (IMA) and inherited paternal antigens/haplotype (IPA), respectively. During pregnancy, the fetus is exposed to the non-inherited maternal HLA haplotype (NIMA, non-inherited maternal antigens), while being un-exposed to non-inherited paternal HLA haplotype (NIPA, non-inherited paternal antigens). The fetal exposure to NIMA results in generation of tolerance to those HLA components, while the mother is becoming partially tolerized to the IPA in the fetus. In contrast, the lack of exposure to NIPA does not allow for tolerization. Thus if a related HLA-mismatched donor is all that is available, demonstrating that the mismatched HLA component is a NIMA could result in successful transplantation. This is particularly true with UCB transplants, where a greater extent of HLA mismatching may be present in the potential donors. To determine the NIMA and NIPA for a patient, both parents must have HLA typing performed.

The Process of Donor Selection

In general, only sibling donors would be expected to have a matched HLA type with the patient. In some families though, other relatives could possibly be matched though, when members of the same family have married in prior generations.

Typically, the family members being typed are initially typed for class I (as a cost saving option). If an HLA Class I match is found with the patient, the match is confirmed by HLA class II typing.

MUD require additional typing and scrutiny. First, the patient is required to be typed twice, on different specimens to confirm the results. The MUD donor's HLA type is also confirmed to be equivalent to that in the registry at the transplantation center prior to the transplantation.

Summary of the Donor Selection Considerations

The algorithm for donor selection has specific items to consider. Perhaps foremost is the extent of the match. Donor gender and age and CMV status are somewhat important. Donor blood type is not so important, but may receive consideration in ultimate selection. Finally, if the donor is listed as inactive or unavailable, then consideration should not be given, and a separate donor should be sought.

When the NMDP search results are examined, the group of potential available donors with the highest expectation for matching, are placed on the consideration list. Amongst these, typically the youngest are considered as highest. If the patient is CMV positive, then a CMV positive donor is recommended/required. If the patient is CMV negative, a CMV negative donor is required. Male versus female donor is also important, with use for specific situations. When the underlying indication for HCT is highly treatable and curable, e.g. a non-complicated male patient with acute lymphoblastic leukemia (ALL), a sex-matched donor may be the best choice to reduce some of the risk for GVHD. Yet, in high-risk acute myeloid leukemia (AML), especially in resistant cases, using a female donor for a male patient could result in a greater extent of "graft-versus-leukemia" (GvL) effect and afford a better outcome.

The first successful **solid organ transplantation** was a kidney transplant performed in 1954 between twins, where immunosuppressive therapy was not needed. Subsequent attempts between non-twins were not so successful. The barriers to successful transplantation were ABO-incompatibility and HLA-incompatibility. ABO typing was well established at that time, but not so for HLA. Histocompatibility concepts began with studies on mice in the late nineteenth century, and greatly expanding in the 1940s and 1950s with Peter Medawar leading the way. Studies expanded on the human major histocompatibility complex, with the first International Workshop on HLA organized by Bernard Amos in 1964. At that time, Paul Terasaki had developed the complement-dependent cytotoxicity (CDC or microcytoxicity) assay, which allowed HLA typing to be accomplished, and could be used for detection of anti-HLA antibodies. During 1965, Paul Terasaki worked with Thomas Starzl to use the CDC assays to identify suitable donors for patients requiring renal transplantation. Additionally, corticosteroids and azathioprine had been identified along with reasonably good anti-rejection medications yielding to the first successful solid organ transplantation. In 1968, Christiaan Barnard performed the first cardiac transplant with some success. Cyclosporine A was introduced in 1970s, improving the overall success of the anti-rejection medication regimen, and decreasing the extent of HLA matching required for successful transplantation. In 1977, the first computer-based matching system was developed and named United Network for Organ Sharing (UNOS). In 1984, the National Organ Transplantation Act (NOTA) was initiated. Strict use of HLA matching as criteria for donor selection led to bias in the transplantation of non-minority patients. As calcineurin inhibitors reduced the need for HLA matching, more equitable allocation of available deceased-donor organs could be accomplished, which was one of the goals of UNOS and NOTA. Over the ensuing decades, much knowledge on HLA and the immunity of tolerance and rejection accumulated. This has allowed for continuous improvement in testing procedures and success rate in transplantation. A major component was the recognition of the role for anti-HLA antibodies, and improvement in antibody detection systems. Currently most centers use some form of single-antigen antibody (SAB) technique, most commonly using the Luminex® platform.

Serologic level typing (e.g. HLA-A2) has been conventionally used for the donor allocation purposes. More recently, as anti-HLA antibodies can be detected at the allele level (e.g. Anti-HLA-A∗02:01, as compared with anti-HLA-A∗02:06, which do not share the same exposed epitopes and thereby must bind to different epitopes), there has become more interest in defining patients and donors HLA typing at the molecular level. The traditional serologic typing of HLA-A, -B, and -DR is being replaced by allele-level recognition, considering the role of anti-HLA antibodies to HLA-C, HLA-DQB1, HLA-DQA1, HLA-DPB1, and possibly HLA-DPA1. These concepts continue to be implemented in assay and interpretation by the UNOS, all resulting in better transplantation outcomes. Read Chapters 52–56 for examples on how molecular technology is changing the practice of organ transplantation.

References

1. Petty RE, Southwood TR, Manners P, Baum J, Glass DN, Goldenberg J, He X, Maldonado-Cocco J, Orozco-Alcala J, Prieur AM, Suarez-Almazor ME, Woo P. International League of Associations for Rheumatology classification of juvenile idiopathic arthritis: second revision, Edmonton, 2001. J Rheumatol. 2004;31(2):390–2.
2. Wang L, Wang FS, Gershwin ME. Human autoimmune diseases: a comprehensive update. J Intern Med. 2015;278(4):369–95.
3. Nicholson AA, Sapru I, Densmore M, Frewen PA, Neufeld RW, Theberge J, McKinnon MC, Lanius RA. Unique insula subregion resting-state functional connectivity with amygdala complexes in posttraumatic stress disorder and its dissociative subtype. Psychiatry Res. 2016;250:61–72.
4. Woroniecka M, Ballow M. Office evaluation of children with recurrent infection. Pediatr Clin N Am. 2000;47(6):1211–24.
5. Ashtari M. Anatomy and functional role of the inferior longitudinal fasciculus: a search that has just begun. Dev Med Child Neurol. 2011;54(1):6–7.

6. Von Der Heide RJ, Skipper LM, Klobusicky E, Olson IR. Dissecting the uncinate fasciculus: disorders, controversies and a hypothesis. Brain J Neurol. 2013;136(6):1692–707.
7. Confer D. HLA Matching guidelines 2012 HLA matching guidelines for selecting unrelated donors and CBUs for HCT. In: National Marrow Donor Program. 2012. https://bethematchclinical.org/Resources-and-Education/Education-Courses-and-Events/Allogeneic-HCT-Education/HLA-Matching-Guidelines/
8. Harville TO. HLA typing for cellular product characterization and identity testing. Cellular therapy: principles, methods, and regulations. Bethesda: AABB; 2016.
9. Petersdorf EW, Hansen JA, Martin PJ, Woolfrey A, Malkki M, Gooley T, Storer B, Mickelson E, Smith A, Anasetti C. Major-histocompatibility-complex class I alleles and antigens in hematopoietic-cell transplantation. N Engl J Med. 2001;345(25):1794–800.
10. Rosenbaum EPS, Harville TO, Drobena GA, Cottler-Fox M. Flow cytometric panel-reactive antibody results and the ability to find transfusion-compatible platelets after antibody-desensitization for allogeneic bone marrow transplant. Ann Clin Lab Sci. 2016;46(6):662–5.
11. Pandey S, Rosenbaum E, Cottler-Fox M, Harville TO. Percent cPRA (calculated Panel Reactive Antibody) value predicts percent of positive platelet crossmatches. Ann Clin Lab Sci. 2017;47(3):315–8.
12. Buckley RH, Schiff RI, Schiff SE, Markert ML, Williams LW, Harville TO, Roberts JL, Puck JM. Human severe combined immunodeficiency: genetic, phenotypic, and functional diversity in one hundred eight infants. J Pediatr. 1997;130(3):378–87.
13. Pandey S, Rhodes-Clark B, Borja-Cacho D, Jethava Y, Harville T. P159 high-resolution HLA-typing can confirm diagnosis of graft versus host disease after orthotopic liver-transplantation. Hum Immunol. 2016;77:153.
14. Lee SJ, Klein J, Haagenson M, Baxter-Lowe LA, Confer DL, Eapen M, Fernandez-Vina M, Flomenberg N, Horowitz M, Hurley CK, Noreen H, Oudshoorn M, Petersdorf E, Setterholm M, Spellman S, Weisdorf D, Williams TM, Anasetti C. High-resolution donor-recipient HLA matching contributes to the success of unrelated donor marrow transplantation. Blood. 2007;110(13):4576–83.
15. Spellman S, Setterholm M, Maiers M, Noreen H, Oudshoorn M, Fernandez-Vina M, Petersdorf E, Bray R, Hartzman RJ, Ng J, Hurley CK. Advances in the selection of HLA-compatible donors: refinements in HLA typing and matching over the first 20 years of the National Marrow Donor Program Registry. Biol Blood Marrow Transplant. 2008;14(9 Suppl):37–44.
16. Bray RA, Hurley CK, Kamani NR, Woolfrey A, Muller C, Spellman S, Setterholm M, Confer DL. National marrow donor program HLA matching guidelines for unrelated adult donor hematopoietic cell transplants. Biol Blood Marrow Transplant. 2008;14(9 Suppl):45–53.
17. Crocchiolo R, Ciceri F, Fleischhauer K, Oneto R, Bruno B, Pollichieni S, Sacchi N, Sormani MP, Fanin R, Bandini G, Bonifazi F, Bosi A, Rambaldi A, Alessandrino PE, Falda M, Bacigalupo A. HLA matching affects clinical outcome of adult patients undergoing haematopoietic SCT from unrelated donors: a study from the Gruppo Italiano Trapianto di Midollo Osseo and Italian Bone Marrow Donor Registry. Bone Marrow Transplant. 2009;44(9):571–7.
18. Woolfrey A, Klein JP, Haagenson M, Spellman S, Petersdorf E, Oudshoorn M, Gajewski J, Hale GA, Horan J, Battiwalla M, Marino SR, Setterholm M, Ringden O, Hurley C, Flomenberg N, Anasetti C, Fernandez-Vina M, Lee SJ. HLA-C antigen mismatch is associated with worse outcome in unrelated donor peripheral blood stem cell transplantation. Biol Blood Marrow Transplant. 2011;17(6):885–92.
19. Petersdorf EW, Gooley T, Malkki M, Horowitz M. Clinical significance of donor-recipient HLA matching on survival after myeloablative hematopoietic cell transplantation from unrelated donors. Tissue Antigens. 2007;69(Suppl 1):25–30.

20. Pidala J, Lee SJ, Ahn KW, Spellman S, Wang HL, Aljurf M, Askar M, Dehn J, Fernandez Vina M, Gratwohl A, Gupta V, Hanna R, Horowitz MM, Hurley CK, Inamoto Y, Kassim AA, Nishihori T, Mueller C, Oudshoorn M, Petersdorf EW, Prasad V, Robinson J, Saber W, Schultz KR, Shaw B, Storek J, Wood WA, Woolfrey AE, Anasetti C. Nonpermissive HLA-DPB1 mismatch increases mortality after myeloablative unrelated allogeneic hematopoietic cell transplantation. Blood. 2014;124(16):2596–606.
21. Eapen M, Klein JP, Ruggeri A, Spellman S, Lee SJ, Anasetti C, Arcese W, Barker JN, Baxter-Lowe LA, Brown M, Fernandez-Vina MA, Freeman J, He W, Iori AP, Horowitz MM, Locatelli F, Marino S, Maiers M, Michel G, Sanz GF, Gluckman E, Rocha V. Impact of allele-level HLA matching on outcomes after myeloablative single unit umbilical cord blood transplantation for hematologic malignancy. Blood. 2014;123(1):133–40.

Chapter 2
Fever and Cervical Lymphadenopathy

Berenise Gamez-Gonzalez and Marco Antonio Yamazaki-Nakashimada

A previously healthy 17-month-old girl was admitted to the hospital with a 4-day history of fever, irritability and a left cervical lymphadenopathy. One day later she presented maculopapular rash on the trunk and extremities, severe nausea and vomiting episodes. She received antibiotics without any improvement. On physical examination she was febrile with a temperature of 38.3 °C, tachycardic and tachypneic. Weight, height, and head circumference were all within normal range. She also had generalized irritability, bilateral conjunctival injection with reddened and cracked lips, mild erythema of the pharynx, strawberry tongue, and cervical adenopathy (>1.5 cm diameter). BCG scar erythema was also noted (Fig. 2.1).

Laboratory tests showed: Hb 11 g/dL, WBC count 11,240/μL (neutrophils 7.76/μL and lymphocytes 1570/μL), platelet count 281,000/μL, CRP: 1 mg/dL, creatinine: 0.6 mg/dL, ESR: 14 mm/h, AST: 418 IU/L, ALT: 501 IU/L, total bilirubin: 3.1 mg/dL, with 1.77 mg/dL direct bilirubin and albumin: 3.7 g/L.

Diagnosis of Kawasaki disease (KD) was made on the basis of the clinical manifestations and laboratory results. Treatment with intravenous immunoglobulin (IVIG) (2 g/kg) and aspirin was immediately started (80 mg per kg day). Echocardiography on the day of admission was normal. After first course of IVIG administration the patient remained febrile, with no resolution of the mucocutaneous manifestations and deterioration of general condition. A second course of IVIG was given along with methylprednisolone pulse (30 mg/kg/day) while the aspirin dose was reduced to 5 mg/kg/day. After the second dose of IVIG and steroid treatment, her fever subsided and cutaneous lesions progressively faded with normalization of inflammatory parameters. On the tenth day since initiation of the symptoms, thrombocytosis, along with desquamation of the fingers was observed. She was discharged on day 11 with a stable condition and with low dose aspirin continued.

B. Gamez-Gonzalez
Hospital Infantil de Especialidades de Chihuahua, Chihuahua, Mexico

M. A. Yamazaki-Nakashimada (✉)
Clinical Immunology Department, Instituto Nacional de Pediatría, Mexico City, Mexico

© Springer Nature Switzerland AG 2020
F. Rahmani, N. Rezaei (eds.), *Pediatric Autoimmunity and Transplantation*,
https://doi.org/10.1007/978-3-030-26280-8_2

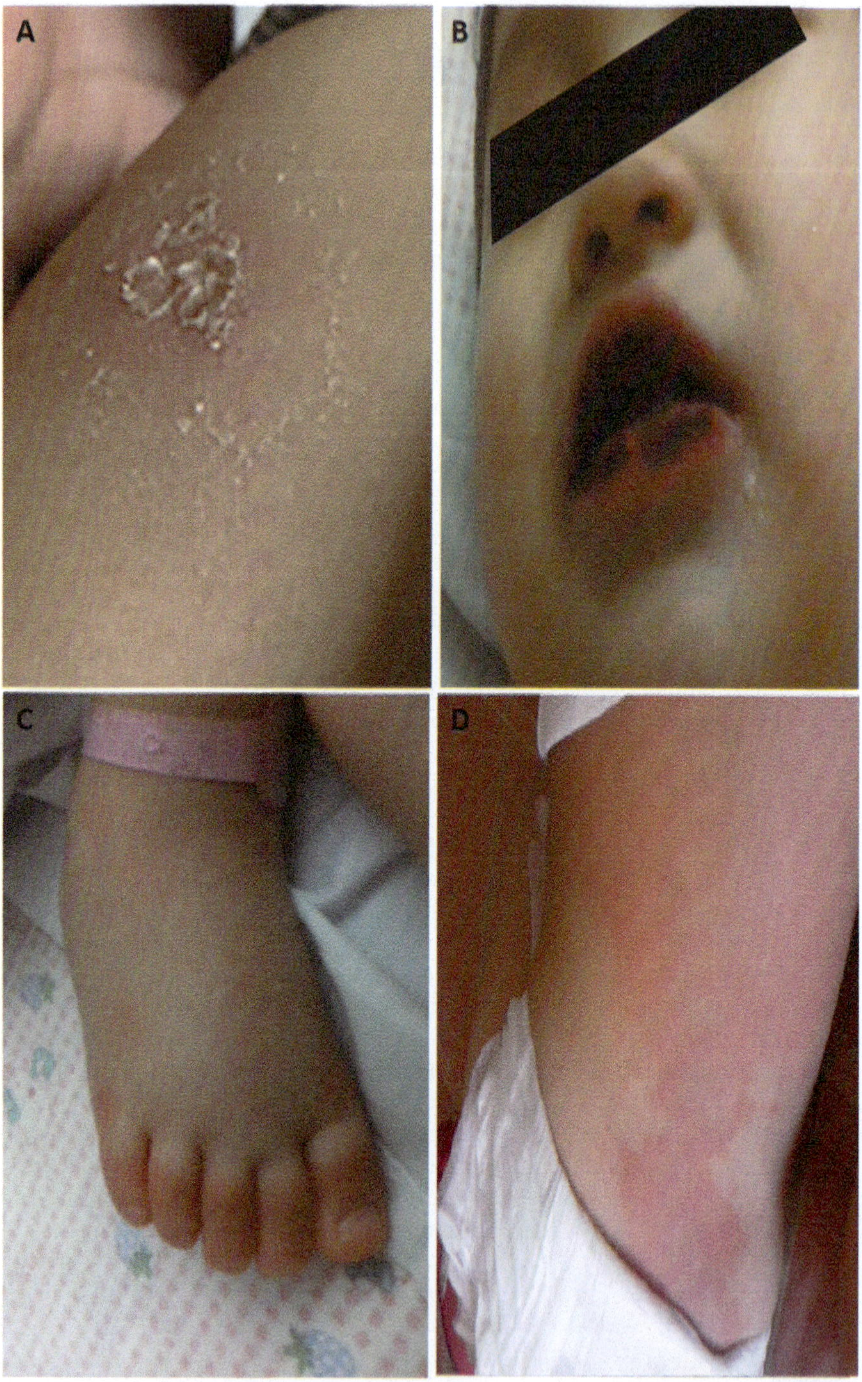

Fig. 2.1 Skin peeling, cracked lips, redness in extremities, and generalized rash in a girl with fever and a cervical lymphadenopathy

Q1. At her first admission and according to the clinical criteria of KD, the patient presentation is compatible with which of the following forms of Kawasaki disease?

A. Incomplete Kawasaki disease
B. Typical Kawasaki disease
C. Severe Kawasaki disease
D. Kawasaki disease shock syndrome
E. Refractory Kawasaki disease

Answer: *The correct answer is* ***B.***

Based on clinical findings the patient had a classic presentation KD (typical or complete KD). The diagnosis of KD can be made with 4 days of fever when at least 4 of the principal clinical features are present. A careful history could help reveal that the principal clinical features were present during the illness but have resolved by the time of evaluation [1]. Some clinical features may have abated in patients who present 1–2 weeks after the initiation of fever and a careful interrogation of prior signs and symptoms of the disease can help establish the diagnosis [1, 2]. Patients who lack all the clinical features of classic KD have to be evaluated for incomplete KD. If coronary abnormalities are detected, the diagnosis of KD is confirmed.

Cervical lymphadenopathy is a less common feature in KD, but can be the only initial clinical finding. Persistence of fever can give a clue to rule out bacterial lymphadenitis, a common misdiagnosis of cervical lymphadenopathy in KD. Beside the typical clinical criteria for KD, other clinical findings might be helpful. A reaction at the site of BCG vaccination is an early and specific clinical sign and although not included in the classical criteria provides strong support for the diagnosis [3]. An erythematous desquamating perineal eruption is also a valuable early clinical finding facilitating the diagnosis of the disease.

Q2. What is the best diagnosis in a patient with KD who has persistent fever despite initial intravenous immunoglobulin administration?

A. Recurrent KD
B. Non-IVIG responder patient with KD
C. Scarlet fever
D. Atypical or severe KD

Answer: *The correct answer is* ***B.***

When a patient with KD develops persistent fever within 36 hours after the last dose of IVIG infusion, IVIG resistance has to be considered, i.e. refractory IVIG or non-response to IVIG (2). These patients are at higher risk of developing coronary artery lesions [4]. The immunologic basis of IVIG resistance is unknown. Polymorphisms in the Fc gamma receptor may play a role in initial response or resistance to IVIG [5].

KD patients are classified as recrudescent if they begin having symptoms and fever within 2 weeks of the disease, and recurrent if there is a new episode of the disease after at least 2 months since the onset of the first symptoms [6]. Atypical KD is a term that should be reserved for patients who have an unusual complication, such as renal impairment that is generally not seen in KD. Incomplete and atypical KD are sometimes used interchangeably.

Q3. According to the Japanese Predictive System for IVIG resistance, which of the following series of conditions confer a high risk of IVIG resistance in this patient?

A. Fever ≤ 4 days; AST ≥ 100 UI/L; ALT ≥ 80 UI/L; total bilirubin ≥ 0.9 mgdL
B. C-reaction protein ≥ 1 mg/dL; albumin ≥ 3 g/L. Na ≤ 135 mmol/L.
C. Fever days ≤ 4; neutrophils ≥ 60%; age > 6 months
D. Fever ≤ 4 days; AST ≥ 200 UI/L; ALT ≥ 80 UI/L; platelets ≥ 300,000/μL
E. Fever ≤ 4 days; neutrophils ≥ 60%; AST ≥ 100 UI/L; ALT ≥ 80 UI/L; Na ≤ 135 mmol/L.

***Answer:** The correct answer is **A**.*

Scoring systems have been constructed to identify patients who are likely to be resistant to IVIG and who may benefit from a more aggressive initial treatment (Table 2.1). Kobayashi, Egami and Sano are the three principal Score System used in Japanese population [7–9]. Although current risk prediction models for Japanese population are not as accurate to be used in other countries [10], all three scoring systems could identify our patient as potentially IVIG unresponsiveness. Predictive models are therefore warranted to be evaluated for non-Japanese population.

Q4. Which of the below answers is the therapy of choice in patients with refractory disease despite IVIG treatment?

A. Methylprednisolone pulse (30 mg/kg/day) in 3 days
B. Infliximab and other TNF-α inhibitors
C. Prednisone 1–2 mg/kg/day for 2 weeks
D. A second dose of IVIG infusion
E. All of the above

***Answer:** The correct answer is **E**.*

Table 2.1 Risk scores for predicting IVIG resistance in patients with Kawasaki disease

Kobayashi (7 variables)	Egami (5 variables)	Sano (3 variables)
Low risk 0–3 points; high risk ≥4)	Low risk 0–2 points; high risk ≥3)	Low risk 0–1 points; high risk 2)
2 points: • AST ≥ 100 UI/L • Sodium ≤ 133 mmol/L, fever days ≤ 4% neutrophils: ≥80% 1 point: • CRP ≥ 10 mg/dL • Age ≤ 1 year • Platelets ≤ 30 × 10^4/mm^3	2 points: • AST ≥ 200 UI/L 1 point: • Fever days ≤ 4 • CRP ≥ 8 mg/dL • Age ≤ 6 months • Platelets ≤ 30 × 10^4/mm^3	1 point: • ALT ≥ 80 UI/L • Total bilirrubin ≥ 0.9 mg/dL • CRP ≥ 7 mg/dL

The optimal treatment of patients with refractory KD has not been determined. Most experts recommend administration of a second dose of IVIG as recommended by the American Heart Association consensus guidelines [3, 11]. Although there are no controlled studies demonstrating its effectiveness, a second dose is a common practice and appears effective in many patients. Corticosteroids have also been used to treat patients who have failed to respond to initial therapy [1]. Treatment with IVIG plus steroids has significantly lowered rates of persistent of fever and elevated laboratory inflammatory parameters, but no difference in the incidence of coronary artery lesions has been seen in patients receiving steroids compared with second dose IVIG. Both pulsed and long-term steroid treatment could be considered as a regimen option along with second infusion of IVIG or for treatment of patients with KD who have had recurrent or recrudescent fever after additional IVIG [1]. Unless high-risk patients are reliably identified, steroids cannot be recommended routinely as a component of initial therapy.

TNF-α inhibitors have potent anti-inflammatory effects and are used in the treatment of various forms of vasculitis. Infliximab can be considered as an alternative to a second dose of IVIG. Patients with refractory KD receiving infliximab have been shown to have shorter hospitalization and fever duration, but similar coronary artery outcomes compared to IVIG-treated patients [4, 12]. Further prospective trials are needed to define the exact role of TNF-α blockers in IVIG resistant KD. Given the role of activated T cells in the pathogenesis of vasculitis in patients with KD, T cell inhibitors like cyclosporine are considered as treatment options for refractory KD [13, 14].

Q5. Which of the following conditions is suspected when a patients with KD has persistence of systemic inflammation along with hepatosplenomegaly, high grade fever, and pancytopenia?

A. Severe Kawasaki disease with toxic shock
B. Kawasaki disease shock syndrome
C. Atypical Kawasaki disease
D. Immunoglobulin resistance Kawasaki disease
E. Macrophage activation syndrome

Answer: *The correct answer is* ***E****.*

Macrophage activation syndrome (MAS) is a potentially fatal complication of rheumatic diseases. It occurs usually in the context of systemic juvenile idiopathic arthritis (SJIA), but it may occur also, in systemic lupus erythematosus (SLE) and KD [15]. Incidence of MAS in children with KD has been estimated to be 1.1% [16]. MAS can result in progressive multi-organ failure and fatal outcomes if unrecognized. Early recognition of MAS is often challenging given the lack of a single pathognomonic clinical or laboratory feature. The clinical findings and laboratory tests of MAS and KD overlap, and unfortunately, histopathological features of hemophagocytosis may not be present during the initial stages [17]. MAS can be detected in any stage of KD, i.e. acute, subacute or convalescence, or develop even before the diagnosis of KD is made. Most frequently, KD-associated MAS develops simultaneously with the clinical initiation of KD. Persistence of fever with splenomegaly, hyperferritinemia, thrombocytopenia and elevated AST should prompt consideration of MAS complicating KD [18].

Q6. Which one of the following provides a better support to the diagnosis of KD, when incomplete Kawasaki disease is suspected?

A. Serum CRP ≥ 3 mg/dL and Serum ESR ≥ 40 mm/h
B. High N-terminal moiety of B-type natriuretic peptide serum level
C. High serum procalcitonin levels
D. Presence of severe hemolytic anemia
E. Platelet count less than 450,000/μL after the 7th day of fever

Answer: *The correct answer is* ***A***.

KD should be considered in the differential diagnosis of prolonged unexplained fever associated with any of the principal clinical features. These patients have to be evaluated with a suspicion of incomplete KD with echocardiogram and laboratory parameters. Normal echocardiogram does not rule out the diagnosis of KD.

A markedly elevated CRP and ESR is common in a majority of patients, and could prove useful to support the diagnosis [2, 3, 19, 20]. Although no laboratory test is diagnostic for KD, many are characteristic for the disease including: leukocytosis with neutrophil predominance and normocytic normochromic anaemia. Hyponatraemia can be present and has been associated with worse coronary artery outcomes. Mildly elevated serum liver enzymes and hyperbilirubinemia could also be present [21]. Hypoalbuminemia is common and associated with severe disease. Thrombocytosis is a characteristic feature in the subacute phase 2–4 weeks after onset of fever. Thrombocytopenia can be a sign of severe KD with disseminated intravascular coagulation and is a risk factor for the development of coronary artery lesions as well [22].

Brain-derived natriuretic peptide (BNP) and its N-terminal moiety (NT-proBNP) are elevated at the onset of symptoms in some patients, but do not have sufficient discriminative ability to differentiate KD [23, 24]. Prospective large cohort studies are needed to help determine best cut-off values and further clarify the role of NT-proBNP in the diagnosis of KD.

Practical Points

- KD should be considered in the differential diagnosis of any prolonged unexplained fever in childhood
- Cervical lymphadenopathy is a less common principal clinical features in KD, but can be the only initial clinical finding
- When a patient with KD develops new fever within 36 hours after the last dose of IVIG infusion, IVIG resistance has to be considered
- Macrophage activation syndrome is a potential complication of KD
- Treatment of refractory KD includes repeated IVIG infusions with infliximab and/or corticosteroids

References

1. Newburger JW, Takahashi M, Gerber MA, Gewitz MH, Tani LY, Burns JC, Shulman ST, Bolger AF, Ferrieri P, Baltimore RS, Wilson WR, Baddour LM, Levison ME, Pallasch TJ, Falace DA, Taubert KA. Diagnosis, treatment, and long-term management of Kawasaki disease: a statement for health professionals from the Committee on Rheumatic Fever, Endocarditis, and Kawasaki Disease, Council on Cardiovascular Disease in the Young, American Heart Association. Pediatrics. 2004;114(6):1708–33.
2. McCrindle BW, Rowley AH, Newburger JW, Burns JC, Bolger AF, Gewitz M, Baker AL, Jackson MA, Takahashi M, Shah PB, Kobayashi T, Wu MH, Saji TT, Pahl E. American Heart Association Rheumatic Fever, Endocarditis, and Kawasaki Disease Committee of the Council on Cardiovascular Disease in the Young; Council on Cardiovascular and Stroke Nursing; Council on Cardiovascular Surgery and Anesthesia; and Council on Epidemiology and Prevention. Diagnosis, treatment, and long term management of Kawasaki disease: a scientific statement for health professionals from the American Heart Association. Circulation. 2017;135(17):e927–99.
3. Gamez-Gonzalez LB, Hamada H, Llamas-Guillen BA, Ruiz-Fernandez M, Yamazaki-Nakashimada M. BCG and Kawasaki disease in Mexico and Japan. Hum Vaccin Immunother. 2017;13(5):1091–3.
4. Tremoulet AH, Best BM, Song S, Wang S, Corinaldesi E, Eichenfield JR, Martin DD, Newburger JW, Burns JC. Resistance to intravenous immunoglobulin in children with Kawasaki disease. J Pediatr. 2008;153(1):117–21.
5. Shrestha S, Wiener HW, Olson AK, Edberg JC, Bowles NE, Patel H, Portman MA. Functional FCGR2B gene variants influence intravenous immunoglobulin response in patients with Kawasaki disease. J Allergy Clin Immunol. 2011;128(3):677–80.
6. Hirata S, Nakamura Y, Yanagawa H. Incidence rate of recurrent Kawasaki disease and related risk factors: from the results of nationwide surveys of Kawasaki disease in Japan. Acta Paediatr (Oslo, Norway : 1992). 2001;90(1):40–4.
7. Sano T, Kurotobi S, Matsuzaki K, Yamamoto T, Maki I, Miki K, Kogaki S, Hara J. Prediction of non-responsiveness to standard high-dose gamma-globulin therapy in patients with acute Kawasaki disease before starting initial treatment. Eur J Pediatr. 2007;166(2):131–7.
8. Egami K, Muta H, Ishii M, Suda K, Sugahara Y, Iemura M, Matsuishi T. Prediction of resistance to intravenous immunoglobulin treatment in patients with Kawasaki disease. J Pediatr. 2006;149(2):237–40.
9. Kobayashi T, Inoue Y, Takeuchi K, Okada Y, Tamura K, Tomomasa T, Kobayashi T, Morikawa A. Prediction of intravenous immunoglobulin unresponsiveness in patients with Kawasaki disease. Circulation. 2006;113(22):2606–12.
10. Sleeper LA, Minich LL, McCrindle BM, Li JS, Mason W, Colan SD, Atz AM, Printz BF, Baker A, Vetter VL, Newburger JW. Evaluation of Kawasaki disease risk-scoring systems for intravenous immunoglobulin resistance. J Pediatr. 2011;158(5):831–835.e833.
11. Burns JC, Capparelli EV, Brown JA, Newburger JW, Glode MP. Intravenous gamma-globulin treatment and retreatment in Kawasaki disease. US/Canadian Kawasaki Syndrome Study Group. Pediatr Infect Dis J. 1998;17(12):1144–8.
12. Burns JC, Best BM, Mejias A, Mahony L, Fixler DE, Jafri HS, Melish ME, Jackson MA, Asmar BI, Lang DJ, Connor JD, Capparelli EV, Keen ML, Mamun K, Keenan GF, Ramilo O. Infliximab treatment of intravenous immunoglobulin-resistant Kawasaki disease. J Pediatr. 2008;153(6):833–8.
13. Tremoulet A, Pancoast P, Franco A, Bujold M, Shimizu C, Onouchi Y, Tamamoto A, Erdem G, Dodd D, Burns J. Calcineurin inhibitor treatment of intravenous immunoglobulin-resistant Kawasaki disease. J Pediatr. 2012;161(3):506–12.
14. Hamada H, Suzuki H, Abe J, Suzuki Y, Suenaga T, Takeuchi T, Yoshikawa N, Shibuta S, Miyawaki M, Oishi K, Yamaga H, Aoyagi N, Iwahashi S, Miyashita R, Honda T, Onouchi Y, Terai M, Hata A. Inflammatory cytokine profiles during Cyclosporin treatment for immunoglobulin-resistant Kawasaki disease. Cytokine. 2012;60(3):681–5.

15. Bracaglia C, Prencipe G, De Benedetti F. Macrophage Activation Syndrome: different mechanisms leading to a one clinical syndrome. Pediatr Rheumatol Online J. 2012;15(1):5.
16. Wang W, Gong F, Zhu W, Fu S, Zhang Q. Macrophage activation syndrome in Kawasaki disease: more common than we thought? Semin Arthritis Rheum. 2015;44(4):405–10.
17. Bode S, Lehmberg K, Maul-Pavicic A, Vraetz T, Janka G, Stadt U, Ehl S. Recent advances in the diagnosis and treatment of hemophagocytic lymphohistiocytosis. Arthitis Res Ther. 2012;14(3):213.
18. García-Pavón S, Yamazaki-Nakashimada M, Báez M, Borjas-Aguilar K, Murata C. Kawasaki disease complicated with macrophage activation syndrome: a systematic review. J Pediatr Hematol Oncol. 2017;36(9):445–51.
19. Burns J, Glode M. Kawasaki syndrome. Lancet (London, England). 2004;364(9433):533–44.
20. Rowley A. Incomplete (atypical) Kawasaki disease. Pediatr Infect Dis J. 2002;21(6):563–5.
21. Tremoulet A, Jain S, Chandrasekar D, Sun X, Sato Y, Burns J. Evolution of laboratory values in patients with Kawasaki disease. Pediatr Infect Dis J. 2011;30(12):1022–6.
22. Nofech-Mozes Y, Garty B. Thrombocytopenia in Kawasaki disease: a risk factor for the development of coronary artery aneurysms. Pediatr Hematol Oncol. 2003;20(8):597–601.
23. Dahdah N, Siles A, Fournier A, Cousineau J, Delvin E, Saint-Cyr C, Spiegelblatt L, Bonny Y, Vartian M, Montigny M. Natriuretic peptide as an adjunctive diagnostic test in the acute phase of Kawasaki disease. Pediatr Cardiol. 2009;30(6):810–7.
24. Lin K, Chang S, Yu C, Lin S, Liu S, Chao H, Lee M, Wu J, Lee C. Usefulness of natriuretic peptide for the diagnosis of Kawasaki disease: a systematic review and meta-analysis. BMJ Open. 2015;5(4):e006703.

Chapter 3
Prolonged Refractory High Fever

Ross Petty and Farhad Salehzadeh

An 11-month-old, previously healthy, white male infant was admitted to the hospital because of refractory high fever for 1 week. He had developed non-purulent bilateral conjunctivitis, erythematous truncal rash and fissured lips since and was extremely irritable on admission. He was given an antipyretic and a 5 day course of oral cephalexin with no response. His family members were all healthy.

In physical examination, weight, height, and head circumference were at the 50th percentile. His heart rate was 125/min, respiratory rate: 22/min, and blood pressure 70/40 mmHg and he was febrile *T*: 39.5 °C from axillary measurement. The infant was very irritable, and appeared unwell. He had a widespread polymorphous rash on his trunk and perineum with red and vertically cracked lips and conjunctival injection. Aside from a tachycardia, the cardiovascular examination was normal. There was one large non-tender lymph node in the submandibular region, but no other lymphadenopathy or organomegaly.

Initial laboratory investigations revealed, WBC: 15,500/μL with 65% PMN and 37% lymphocyte, Hb was 9.6 g/dL and platelets were 570,000/μL. ESR was 45 mm/h, CRP: 30 mg/dL and albumin was 3 g/dL.

In urinalysis, 15 WBC were seen in each HPF and urine culture was negative. Due to his extreme irritability a lumbar puncture was performed showing: WBC: 25/μL with PMN: 5% and 95% lymphocytes, glucose: 65 g/dL and protein: 2.4 g/dL, in CSF analysis.

Q1. What is the most likely diagnosis in this patient?

A. Systemic onset juvenile idiopathic arthritis
B. Severe viral or bacterial infection

R. Petty
Pediatric Rheumatology, University of British Columbia, Vancouver, BC, Canada

F. Salehzadeh (✉)
Pediatric Rheumatology, Bouali Children's Hospital, ARUMS, Ardabil, Iran

© Springer Nature Switzerland AG 2020
F. Rahmani, N. Rezaei (eds.), *Pediatric Autoimmunity and Transplantation*,
https://doi.org/10.1007/978-3-030-26280-8_3

C. Kawasaki disease
D. Stevens-Johnson syndrome

Answer: *The correct answer is* ***C.***

Kawasaki disease (KD), is one of the most common vasculitides of childhood, and is self-limited, but may cause significant long-term morbidity because of dilatation or aneurysms of the coronary and other major arteries. It is characterized by persistent high fever, rash, and conjunctivitis, occasionally associated with uveitis, swollen cracked lips, oral mucositis, transient arthritis, edematous extremity changes, and cervical lymphadenopathy, which is usually unilateral. Vasculitis of the coronary arteries may be detected by echocardiography in up to one-quarter of the patients. The average age at onset is 3 years, and three-quarters of affected children are below the age of 5 years (Table 3.1).

Laboratory tests typically reveal normal or elevated WBC count with neutrophil predominance and elevated acute phase reactants during the acute phase. Low serum sodium and albumin levels, elevated serum liver enzymes, and sterile pyuria can also be present. In the second week after fever onset, thrombocytosis is a characteristic finding.

It is important to note that children who only partially fulfill the diagnostic criteria (incomplete KD) have an equal or higher risk of developing coronary artery aneurysms compared to those who fulfill the criteria. Younger patients are less likely to meet the classic criteria and are at greatest risk of developing coronary artery abnormalities.

McCrindle et al. [2], have proposed an approach to evaluation of a child with incomplete Kawasaki disease. In a child with high fever and 2 or 3 criteria for the diagnosis of Kawasaki disease, or the infant with 7 days or more of unexplained fever, demonstration of CRP <3 mg/dL or ESR < 40 mm/h suggests a low probability of KD, and the child should be carefully monitored clinically and with repeat CRP or ESR measurements if the fever persists. However, if the child has elevated acute phase reactants (CRP ≥ 3 mg/dL or ESR ≥ 40 mm/h), the demonstration of 3 or more of the following laboratory abnormalities indicates the need for treatment as KD: anemia (adjusted for age), platelet count ≥ 450,000/μL after the seventh day of fever, albumin ≤3 g/dL, elevated ALT, WBC ≤ 15,000/μL, urine WBC ≥ 10 /hpf,

Table 3.1 Criteria for the diagnosis of Kawasaki disease [1]

Fever for >5 days (4 days if treatment with intravenous immunoglobulin eradicates fever) plus at least 4 of the following signs not explained by another disease process[a]:
• Bilateral conjunctival injection (80–90%)
• Changes in oropharyngeal mucous membranes including one or more of injected and/or fissured lips, strawberry tongue, injected oropharynx (80–90%)
• Changes in peripheral extremities including erythema/edema of dorsum of hands and/or feet (acute phase); periungual desquamation (later phase) (80%)
• Polymorphous rash, primarily truncal; non-vesicular (>90%)
• Cervical lymphadenopathy with at least one node >1.5 cm (50%)

[a]If coronary artery abnormalities are present, fewer than 4 criteria are required

or an abnormal echocardiogram. Echocardiographic abnormalities of the coronary artery diameter are expressed as Z scores, the number of standard deviations above the normal mean. Echocardiography is considered abnormal if any of three conditions are met: (a) Z-score of diameter of left anterior descending coronary artery or right coronary artery is equal or above ≥2.5, (b) a coronary artery aneurysm is observed, or (c) if ≥3 other suggestive features exist, including; decreased left ventricular function, mitral regurgitation, pericardial effusion, or Z scores in left anterior descending coronary artery or right coronary artery is between 2 and 2.5.

Characteristics that suggest a high probability of another diagnosis include exudative conjunctivitis, exudative pharyngitis, ulcerative intraoral lesions, bullous or vesicular rash, generalized adenopathy, or splenomegaly.

Exanthematous viral and bacterial infections, systemic juvenile rheumatoid arthritis (SJIA), Stevens-Johnson syndrome, and toxic shock syndrome, are among the most important differential diagnoses of KD. Viral illnesses such as measles, especially when atypical or occurring after vaccination, EBV, and adenovirus infections share many of the signs of mucocutaneous involvement, but they typically lack evidence of systemic inflammation or extremity changes of KD. Toxin-mediated illnesses, especially scarlet fever, staphylococcal scalded skin syndrome, and toxic shock syndrome lack the ocular and articular involvements typical of KD. Drug reactions, such SJIA as those in Stevens-Johnson syndrome or serum sickness, may mimic KD but have subtle differences in the ocular and mucosal manifestations.

The pattern of fever, persistent instead of intermittent, localized rather than generalized lymphadenopathy, absence of organomegaly, and the presence of ocular and oral mucosal makes SJIA unlikely. KD may be confused with polyarteritis nodosa, but renal abnormalities, hematuria, hypertension, characteristic of PAN are unlikely in patients with KD, although children with KD may have sterile pyuria. Desquamation of the tips of digits and perineum after the acute phase is highly characteristic of KD (Table 3.2).

Q2. Which of the following evaluations has the highest priority in this patient?

A. Electrocardiogram
B. Urine culture
C. PCR study of CSF
D. Echocardiography

Answer: *The correct answer is* ***D.***

Echocardiography is indicated in every child with suspected KD to exclude involvement of the coronary arteries. Increased echogenicity of the artery walls, dilatation or aneurysms of the arteries are common findings in echocardiography. An ECG may be useful in documenting the ischemic effects of coronary artery disease, but in most instances is normal in children with KD.

Imaging study such as sonography and brain scan will not be helpful in this patient. CSF findings may indicate an aseptic meningitis in KD. Bone marrow aspiration is a useful tool to rule out malignancy, especially leukemia. This patient does not have clinical or laboratory features suggestive of a malignancy. Although it is

Table 3.2 Differential diagnoses of Kawasaki disease [3][a]

Infections
Viruses
Adenovirus
Measles
Parvovirus
Cytomegalovirus
Herpes simplex
Rickettsia
Rocky Mountain spotted fever
Spirochetes
Leptospirosis
Bacteria
Streptococcus, including post-streptococcal rheumatic fever
Staphylococcus
Immune reactions
Stevens-Johnson syndrome
Toxic shock syndrome
Serum sickness
Rheumatic diseases
Systemic onset juvenile idiopathic arthritis
Polyarteritis Nodosa

[a]Adapted from Son, MB, and Sundel RP.: Kawasaki disease. In Petty R, Laxer R, Lindsley C, Wedderburn L: Textbook of Pediatric Rheumatology 7th Ed. Elsevier 2016

highly unlikely, it is reasonable to rule out infection by CSF culture. Urine culture would also be appropriate since there is low grade sterile pyuria.

Q3. What is the treatment of choice in this patient?

A. Broad spectrum antibiotics
B. Intravenous immunoglobulin and aspirin
C. Corticosteroids
D. Cytotoxic agents

Answer: *The correct* answer *is* ***B.***

Treatment with aspirin and intravenous immunoglobulin (IVIG) (Table 3.3) should be initiated promptly in hospital in a child with KD or in children in whom the diagnosis is strongly suspected, even if criteria for diagnosis are not fulfilled. Investigations for other causes can be undertaken simultaneously, but should not delay treatment. The risk of delaying treatment of KD significantly outweighs the risk of side-effects of treatment with IVIG and aspirin. Antibiotics are not indicated, except in the child with a concurrent bacterial infection [3]. The role of corticosteroids in management of KD is still somewhat controversial but may have a place in resistant or recurrent KD. Cytotoxic agents are not indicated. The role of biologic agents such as anti-TNF monoclonal antibodies is not established.

Table 3.3 Evaluation and management of a child with Kawasaki disease [4][a]

Evaluation
General physical examination
Evaluation of cardiac status: Echo, (if normal, repeat at 6–8 weeks), ECG
Ophthalmologic examination (exclude uveitis)
Hematologic and inflammatory parameters
WBCC and differential, hemoglobin, platelet count, ESR or CRP (monitor at 2 week intervals until stable, then 1 month intervals until normal
AST, ALT, bilirubin, creatinine, electrolytes, urinalysis
Treatment
Aspirin
If child is febrile, give 80–100 mg/kg/day in 4 doses
If child is afebrile, give 3–5 mg/kg/day in one dose
IVIG 2 g/kg administered over 8–12 h
Keep in hospital until afebrile for 24 h:
If fever persists or returns, repeat IVIG 2 g/kg
If inadequate clinical response, consider oral prednisone 2 mg/kg/day, or I.V. Methylprednisolone 30 mg/kg/dose on 1–3 consecutive days. Role of infliximab is uncertain

[a]Adapted from Son M.B., Sundel RP. Kawasaki disease. In Petty R, Laxer R, Lindsley C, Wedderburn L. Textbook of Pediatric Rheumatology 7th Edition. Elsevier 2016

Recommendations regarding restrictions on physical activity and long-term follow-up have been outlined by the Council on Cardiovascular Disease in the Young of the American Heart Association [1].

Maintain low dose aspirin until ESR and platelet count are normal if there are no coronary abnormalities, for 2 years if coronary artery abnormalities have resolved, "forever" if coronary artery disease persists.

Practical Points

- Vasculitis of the coronary arteries is a life-threatening complication of Kawasaki disease (KD) and is detected in echocardiography of up to one-quarter of the patients
- Younger patients are less likely to meet the classic criteria and are at greatest risk of developing coronary artery abnormalities
- In a child with high fever and 2 or 3 criteria for the diagnosis of Kawasaki disease, or the infant with 7 days or more of unexplained fever, demonstration of CRP <3 mg/dL or ESR < 40 mm/h suggests a low probability of KD
- Treatment with aspirin and intravenous immunoglobulin should be initiated promptly in hospital in a child with KD or in children in whom the diagnosis is strongly suspected, even if criteria for diagnosis are not fulfilled

References

1. Newburger JW, Takahashi M, Gerber MA, Gewitz MH, Tani LY, Burns JC, Shulman ST, Bolger AF, Ferrieri P, Baltimore RS, Wilson WR, Baddour LM, Levison ME, Pallasch TJ, Falace DA, Taubert KA. Diagnosis, treatment, and long-term management of Kawasaki disease: a statement for health professionals from the Committee on Rheumatic Fever, Endocarditis, and Kawasaki Disease, Council on Cardiovascular Disease in the Young, American Heart Association. Pediatrics. 2004;114(6):1708–33.
2. McCrindle BW, Rowley AH, Newburger JW, Burns JC, Bolger AF, Gewitz M, Baker AL, Jackson MA, Takahashi M, Shah PB, Kobayashi T, Wu MH, Saji TT, Pahl E. Diagnosis, treatment, and long-term management of Kawasaki disease: a scientific statement for health professionals from the American Heart Association. Circulation. 2017;135(17):e927–e99.
3. Son MB, Sundel RP. Kawasaki disease textbook of pediatric rheumatology. 7th ed. Philadelphia: Elsevier; 2011.
4. Benseler SM, McCrindle BW, Silverman ED, Tyrrell PN, Wong J, Yeung RS. Infections and Kawasaki disease: implications for coronary artery outcome. Pediatrics. 2005;116(6):e760–6.

Chapter 4
Pain in Both Knees

Ross Petty and Farhad Salehzadeh

A 4-year-old girl is referred to the pediatric rheumatology clinic because of a 7-month history of swelling and pain in both knees, left ankle, and right wrist. She has morning stiffness lasting more than 15 min in the affected joints. She suffers from an occasional low grade fever. She does not have a rash, history of recent travel, or a positive family history of autoimmune disease. Her parents are not related.

Physical examination showed a well-appearing girl. Her symptomatic joints were swollen, and painful at the end of restricted range of motion. They were slightly warm but not erythematous. She walked with a limp and guarded her right wrist. The remainder of her examination was normal.

Laboratory investigations revealed a hemoglobin of 11.5 g/dL, and an ESR of 40 mm/h. Anti-nuclear antibody (ANA) was detected at a titer of 1:160. Rheumatoid factor (RF) was present at low titer on one occasion, but was negative on repeat testing. HLAB27 was negative.

Q1. Which type of JIA (Juvenile idiopathic arthritis) is the most likely diagnosis in this patient?

A. Polyarthritis rheumatoid factor negative JIA
B. Oligoarthritis JIA
C. Psoriatic arthritis
D. Undifferentiated JIA

Answer: *The* **correct** *answer is* ***B.***

Children under the age of 16 years who have persistent arthritis for at least 6 weeks, satisfy the ILAR classification criteria for JIA, providing other diagnoses

R. Petty
Pediatric Rheumatology, University of British Columbia, Vancouver, BC, Canada

F. Salehzadeh (✉)
Pediatric Rheumatology, Bouali Children's Hospital, ARUMS, Ardabil, Iran

© Springer Nature Switzerland AG 2020
F. Rahmani, N. Rezaei (eds.), *Pediatric Autoimmunity and Transplantation*,
https://doi.org/10.1007/978-3-030-26280-8_4

Table 4.1 ILAR classification of juvenile idiopathic arthritis [1]

Systemic
Oligoarthritis
Persistent
Extended
Polyarthritis
Polyarthritis rheumatoid factor negative
Polyarthritis rheumatoid factor positive
Psoriatic arthritis
Enthesitis related arthritis
Undifferentiated arthritis
Fits no category
Fits more than one category

have been excluded. The classification recognizes seven categories of JIA (Table 4.1), defined by type of disease in the first 6 months unless features characteristic of systemic JIA, i.e. typical quotidian fever, typical rash, generalized lymphadenopathy, hepatosplenomegaly, pericarditis or pleural effusions, are present. This classification depends on the number of inflamed joints, i.e. each joint is counted separately, except for the joints of the cervical spine, the carpus, and tarsus, any of which is counted as one joint, and the presence of extra-articular features: psoriasis, enthesitis or the systemic features of systemic JIA.

An affected joint is defined as one with limitation of range of motion with evidence of past or current inflammation, warmth, swelling, pain on motion or tenderness.

Joint swelling or effusion is sufficient to define active arthritis. The criteria are based on physical examination.

This patient has arthritis in 4 joints, 7 months after onset of symptoms, and fulfills criteria for oligoarticular JIA with 4 or fewer affected joints, which is most common in young girls. The presence of rheumatoid factor on one occasion does not alter this classification. However, if there were two positive tests for RF or anti-cyclic citrullinated peptide (anti-CCP) at least 3 months apart, the diagnosis would be undifferentiated JIA, and progression to RF positive polyarthritis would be a possibility. If a patient with oligoarticular onset JIA develops arthritis in more than 4 joints after the first 6 months of disease, the classification under the ILAR criteria would be "extended oligoarthritis", rather than polyarthritis.

In polyarthritis there are more than four inflamed joints during the first 6 months of disease, often including small joints of the hands [2]. Presence of RF on two occasions at least 3 months apart distinguishes RF positive polyarthritis from RF negative polyarthritis.

In systemic-onset JIA (SoJIA or Still's disease) high daily spiking, quotidian fever lasting 1 week or longer, in association with arthritis, characteristic rash, lymphadenopathy, pericarditis, and organomegaly are characteristic findings. SoJIA is considered to be an autoinflammatory disorder by some investigators [3] and is presented in Volume 2 of this book. SoJIA has no sexual predilection. Enthesitis-related arthritis (ERA) is defined by arthritis and enthesitis, particularly in large joints of the lower extremities, and can eventually affect the spine and sacroiliac joint. An enthesis is defined as the site of attachment of ligament, tendon or fascia to bone. ERA It is more common in adolescent boys and is characterized by the absence of RF, and has a strong association with the human leukocyte antigen-B27 (HLA-B27).

Juvenile psoriatic arthritis is defined as arthritis associated with either psoriasis or with two of the following: dactylitis, nail pitting or onycholysis, or psoriasis in a first-degree relative. Under ILAR criteria the classification of juvenile psoriatic arthritis cannot be made if the patient has a positive test for RF or HLA-B27. The absence of HLA-B27 makes ERA less likely, and a negative family history of psoriasis, make juvenile psoriatic arthritis unlikely.

Q2. What is the significance of a positive ANA test in children with oligoarticular JIA?

A. It is necessary for the diagnosis of JIA
B. It is important to predict the prognosis of JIA
C. It helps choose the best treatment option for JIA
D. It help predict certain complications of JIA

Answer: *The correct answer is* ***D.***

In children with oligoarticular JIA, the presence of ANA detected by a fluorescence assay is strongly associated with susceptibility to chronic asymptomatic anterior uveitis. In such children, ophthalmologic evaluation with slit lamp biomicroscopy is indicated every 3–4 months [4]. A high ANA titer in association with arthritis could suggest the possibility of systemic lupus erythematosus (SLE). ANA is not associated with ERA or systemic juvenile rheumatoid arthritis (SJIA).

Q3. What is the significance of a positive test for rheumatoid factor in this patient?

A. It is similar to anti-citrullinated peptide antigen in adult rheumatoid arthritis
B. It is associated with severity of joint injury
C. It is associated with extra-articular complications of JIA
D. It influences therapy decision in JIA and intraarticular injection

Answer: *The correct answer is* ***B.***

The correlation between RF and anti-citrullinated protein antibody (ACPA), i.e. anti-cyclic citrullinated peptide (anti-CCP), in JIA varies from one study to another [5, 6]. As RF can be present transiently following viral infections, the presence of two positive tests at least 3 months apart is required by the ILAR classification for the definition of RF positive polyarthritis. RF is strongly associated with severe erosive arthritis, and to a lesser degree, with rheumatoid nodules. The ILAR criteria does not consider ACPA and as a result, the rare RF negative ACPA positive patients with polyarthritis would be classified as having RF negative polyarthritis. However, studies showing a correlation between ACPA positivity with erosive arthritis in children with JIA [7], suggest that a strongly positive ACPA test should alert the physician to the possibility of progressive erosive arthritis. ACPA may occasionally be positive in other types of JIA including ERA, SJIA, oligo-extended, and poly-RF-negative JIA.

Practical Points

- Children under the age of 16 years who have persistent arthritis for at least 6 weeks, satisfy criteria for juvenile idiopathic arthritis (JIA)
- Involvement of 4 or more than 4 joints in the first 6 months after the appearance of symptoms indicates polyarthritic JIA and with fewer than 4 joints the diagnosis would be oligoarticular JIA
- Children with oligoarticular JIA, and positive ANA detected by a fluorescence assay are particularly susceptible to chronic asymptomatic anterior uveitis
- Positive rheumatoid factor in children with polyartheritic JIA is associated with severe erosive arthritis and with progression to adult rheumatoid arthritis

References

1. Petty RE, Southwood TR, Manners P, Baum J, Glass DN, Goldenberg J, He X, Maldonado-Cocco J, Orozco-Alcala J, Prieur AM, Suarez-Almazor ME, Woo P. International League of Associations for Rheumatology classification of juvenile idiopathic arthritis: second revision, Edmonton, 2001. J Rheumatol. 2004;31(2):390–2.
2. Naidu SH, Ostrov BE, Pellegrini VD. Small hand joint involvement in juvenile rheumatoid arthritis. J Pediatr. 2000;136(1):134–5.
3. De Benedetti F, Schneider R. Systemic juvenile idiopathic arthritis. Textbook of pediatric rheumatology. 7th ed. Philadelphia: Elsevier; 2011.
4. Heiligenhaus A, Niewerth M, Ganser G, Heinz C, Minden K. Prevalence and complications of uveitis in juvenile idiopathic arthritis in a population-based nation-wide study in Germany: suggested modification of the current screening guidelines. Rheumatology (Oxford). 2007;46(6):1015–9.
5. Peckham H, Cambridge G, Bourke L, Sen D, Radziszewska A, Leandro M, Ioannou Y. Antibodies to cyclic citrullinated peptides in patients with juvenile idiopathic arthritis and patients with rheumatoid arthritis: shared expression of the inherently autoreactive 9G4 idiotype. Arthritis Rheumatol (Hoboken, NJ). 2017;69(7):1387–95.
6. Tebo AE, Jaskowski T, Davis KW, Whiting A, Clifford B, Zeft A, McNally B, Hill HR, Bohnsack J, Prahalad S. Profiling anti-cyclic citrullinated peptide antibodies in patients with juvenile idiopathic arthritis. Pediatr Rheumatol Online J. 2012;10:29.
7. Pang SY, Liu HY, Huang YJ, Liu YF, Dai YM, Zeng P, Zeng HS. Diagnostic performance of anti-citrullinated protein/peptide antibodies in juvenile idiopathic arthritis. Genet Nol Res. 2016;15(2). https://doi.org/10.4238/gmr.15028641.

Chapter 5
Challenging Pain in Knee and Ankle

Peter Jandus

A 12-year-old Caucasian boy presented to our clinic with progressive recurrent pain of his right knee and ankle, and a diffuse muscle pain in the hips. The pain had worsened in his foot in the last 6 weeks. He had no fever, skin lesions or a history of infections. Initially, his pain was treated with paracetamol which appeared to be ineffective after a while. The knee was swollen and painful with a reduced range of motion. The pain restricted his mobility and prevented him from playing football.

Q1. Which one of the following is the most appropriate next step in the evaluation and management of this patient's condition?

A. Acquisition of a detailed medical history with growth and weight curves
B. Assessment of the family history would be not contributive
C. Immunology work-up would be not helpful at this stage
D. Physical examination
E. Knee joint aspiration and assessment

Answer: *The correct answers are* ***A*** *and* ***D.***

A. A detailed medical history about the boy's growth and weight curves would give information if his development was appropriate until now.
B. A family history is important as it might give us an idea about hereditary. There is no consanguinity in the family. His 10-year-old sister has no problems and his father had uveitis.
C. In children with a history of chronic/recurrent arthritis an immunologic work-up is mandatory.
D. The physical examination is the key to the patients' diagnosis.
E. A puncture at this time without any signs of sepsis or other red flags would be excessive at the moment.

P. Jandus (✉)
Division of Immunology and Allergology, Department of Medicine,
University Hospital and Medical Faculty, Geneva, Switzerland
e-mail: peter.jandus@hcuge.ch

© Springer Nature Switzerland AG 2020

F. Rahmani, N. Rezaei (eds.), *Pediatric Autoimmunity and Transplantation*,
https://doi.org/10.1007/978-3-030-26280-8_5

The boy's growth and weight curves were always in the same percentile; 75% and developmental milestones were reported as within normal range. Physical examination disclosed normal heart sounds, no dyspnea, no lymphadenopathy, or organomegaly and normal skin and oral mucosa. He had a swollen, tender and warm right knee and ankle with a reduced range of motion along with bilateral tenderness in plantar fascia and a painful left Achilles tendon. Repeated laboratory work-up at two occasions 3 months apart showed negative rheumatoid factor (RF), anti-cyclic citrullinated peptide (anti-CCP), and anti-nuclear antibody (ANA). He also had elevated CRP: 13 mg/L (reference < 10), and normal leukocyte count with differentials. He was also found to be positive for HLA-B27.

Q2. What is the most likely cause of this patient's presentations?

A. Overuse arthritis
B. Behçet disease
C. Juvenile idiopathic arthritis
D. Familial Mediterranean fever
E. Osgood-Schlatter disease

Answer: *The correct answer is* ***C.***

A. Overuse, especially during sport activities which involve running or jumping may lead to joint pain and tendonitis. The boy has pain even during rest and after stopping sport activities after weeks, making this an unlikely diagnosis.
B. Enthesopathy and arthritis can be found in Behçet disease. The boy's father had uveitis, but no other characteristic features of Behçet as painful mouth or genital sores, erythema nodosum or cutaneous pustules. The boy himself had none of the above symptoms.
C. The boy might present a subtype of the juvenile idiopathic arthritis. The disease is typically seen among males, after the age of six. The main characteristics of the patients include negative RF and ANA. HLA-B27 positivity is reported in 65–80% of patients. Patients report enthesopathy and asymmetric arthritis of the lower extremities.
D. The boy's presentation with enthesopathy and large joint pains could be compatible with familial Mediterranean fever. However other typical features as periodic fever, abdominal attacks, scrotal pain or pleuritic chest pain were absent.
E. Osgood–Schlatter disease is an inflammation of the patellar ligament at the tibial tuberosity. Children present a painful edema below the knee that exacerbates with activity and alleviates with rest. An episode of pain typically lasts a few months. One or both knees may be affected and flares may reoccur. Osgood-Schlatter cannot explain the boy's enthesopathy.

The ILAR proposed classification criteria for juvenile idiopathic arthritis (JIA) with last update in 2001. This classification criteria is not ideal but still widely used [1]. According to ILAR classification criteria, JIA is divided into seven subtypes: oligoarticular JIA, seropositive polyarticular JIA, seronegative polyarticular JIA, systemic-onset JIA, enthesitis-related arthritis (i.e. ERA), juvenile psoriatic arthritis and undifferentiated JIA [1].

Q3. What subtype of JIA is most likely present in this boy?

A. Systemic JIA
B. Polyarticular JIA
C. Oligoarticular JIA
D. Undifferentiated arthritis
E. Enthesitis-related arthritis

Answer: *The correct* **answer** *is* ***E.***

JIA is a heterogeneous disease group.

A. The patient does not present persistent fever, organomegaly or non-fixed erythematous rush as is with systemic JIA.
B. Polyarticular JIA typically affects ≥5 joints.
C. Our patient apparently had two involved joints, compatible with oligoarticular arthritis. However, enthesitis excludes this diagnosis.
D. The patient had two affected joints. However, he has an enthesopathy and he is HLA-B27 positive that are exclusion criteria for undifferentiated arthritis.
E. ERA is correct.

The boy fulfills the JIA criteria of ERA which are the following ones:

- He presented arthritis and/or enthesitis with the following findings:
  - Positivity of HLA-B27.
  - He is a male and the onset of arthritis was after the age of 6 years.
  - One of first-degree relatives (i.e. father) presented uveitis.
- And following findings are not present or have been excluded:
  - Psoriasis in the patient or a first-degree relative.
  - IgM rheumatoid factor on at least two occasions more than 3 months apart.
  - Systemic arthritis.

JIA is a heterogeneous group of inflammatory joint disease whose common features are duration of at least 6 weeks with an onset before the age of 16.

Q4. Which one of the following conditions is most likely confused with systemic JIA?

A. Antisynthetase syndrome
B. Sjögren's syndrome
C. Adult-onset Still disease
D. Muckle–Wells syndrome
E. Alport syndrome

Answer: *The correct answer is* ***C.***

A. Antisynthetase syndrome is an autoimmune disease characterized by myositis, polyarthritis, interstitial lung disease, thickening and cracking of the hands, and Raynaud phenomenon.

B. Sjögren's syndrome is characterized by the development of a dry mouth and dry eyes and autoimmunity against sweet glands. Patients present muscle and joint pains.
C. Systemic JIA resembles with clinical, laboratory and molecular findings adult-onset Still disease. The ILAR criteria overlap with the Yamaguchi criteria [2].
D. Common characteristics of Muckle–Wells syndrome include chronic, recurrent, urticaria, periodic fevers, joint pain, sensorineural hearing loss and amyloidosis.
E. Alport syndrome results from mutations in type IV collagen leading to glomerulonephritis, hearing loss, and eye diseases.

Chronic inflammation of the joints is limiting the patient's functional ability and productivity in daily life. Thus, the JIA treatment should be prompt and effective.

Q5. In view with these findings, what would be the best treatment option at this time?

A. Corticosteroids
B. Non-steroidal anti-inflammatory drugs (NSAIDs)
C. Leflunomide
D. Methotrexate
E. Sulphasalazine

Answer: *The correct answer is **B.***

Importance of supportive measurements, such as adequate nutrition, calcium and vitamin D supplements, should not be underestimated. Re-evaluation of disease activity should be performed every 3 months, until the goal of treatment is achieved. Compliance of the patient and parent and treatment-related side effects should not be ignored in optimizing the best treatment target.

A. Use of corticosteroids is limited due to numerous side effects and low efficacy in the prevention of joint destruction. Systemic (oral or parenteral) administration of steroids is used in patients with systemic form of the disease. However, intraarticular steroids are the cornerstone of oligoarticular JIA treatment and may represent a valid alternative [3].
B. NSAIDs are traditionally used as initial approach. These drugs are more commonly used in children under 12-years-old. NSAIDs may be used at any time point as needed in addition to other therapies [4].
C. Leflunomide is an inhibitor of pyrimidine synthesis and is administrated orally on a daily basis. It is usually used for patients with mild disease who are intolerant to methotrexate [5].
D. Methotrexate can be used in refractory cases to NSAID. In order to reduce the adverse effects of methotrexate including bone marrow suppression, nausea, oral ulcerations and hair loss, folic acid or folinic acid are used. In addition, clinical response to methotrexate in the first 6 months may predict a more favorable outcome at 5 years [6].
E. Sulphasalazine has been shown to be effective in patients in the oligoarticular- and enthesitis-related forms of JIA and might be an alternative, if NSAIDs are not working [7].

NSAIDs were prescribed initially and relieved the boy's pain. However, he was lost in follow-up and showed up 6 years later at the age of 18. He had been prescribed with NSAIDs through the last years on demand, which have provided sufficient pain relief for his knee and ankle, and muscle pain but unable to relief the new onset left sacroiliac joint pain that had become progressively resistant to NSAIDs. He complained of redness of the eyes, pain, photophobia, and blurred vision since several weeks ago. Eye examination was compatible with bilateral anterior uveitis and MRI revealed a left sacroilitis.

Q6. In view with these findings, which one of the following biologics would be the best treatment option at this time?

A. Tocilizumab
B. Abatacept
C. Rituximab
D. Adalimumab
E. Canakinumab

Answer: *The correct answer is* ***D.***

A. Tocilizumab is a humanized monoclonal antibody against the interleukin-6 receptor. It is used alone or in combination with methotrexate in treatment of unresponsive systemic JIA and in patients with active arthritis that show no improvement or in patients with polyarticular JIA [8].
B. Abatacept is a CTLA4 and IgG Fc fusion protein acting as a T cell co-stimulatory signal blocker through inhibition of the CD80/CD86-CD28. Abatacept down regulates T cell stimulation. Its efficiency and safety has been shown in polyarticular JIA and it is used in cases of unresponsiveness to anti-TNF-α agents [9].
C. Rituximab is an anti-CD20 chimeric murine/human monoclonal antibody that results in complete peripheral B cell apoptosis. Data on the administration of rituximab in JIA patients are limited [10].
D. Adalimumab is a fully humanized monoclonal antibody that binds both soluble and membrane-bound TNF-α. In non-systemic JIA, anti-TNF-α agents are used as first line biologic therapy. Although axial symptoms are rarely seen at onset, up to two-third of patients with ERA develop sacroilitis or similar symptoms over the disease course. Adalimumab is used alone or in combination with methotrexate in the treatment of JIA as a first or second line therapy [11, 12], and in those with JIA-associated uveitis [13].
E. Canakinumab is a fully humanized monoclonal antibody that binds specifically to IL-1β. It has been shown to be efficient in systemic JIA [14].

Practical Points

- Enthesitis-related arthritis (ERA) necessitates presence of arthritis and/or enthesitis for at least 6 weeks in a child under 16 years of age
- In the presence of enthesitis or arthritis alone, at least two of the following should be present to make a diagnosis of ERA: sacroiliac tenderness or

inflammatory spinal pain, HLA-B27 positivity, onset of arthritis in boys aged >6 years, anterior uveitis associated with pain, redness, or photophobia or a family history of HLA-B27-associated disease

- NSAIDs are traditionally used as initial approach in treatment of ERA
- Methotrexate and biologic agents are reserved for patients' refractory to NSAIDS

References

1. Petty RE, Southwood TR, Manners P, Baum J, Glass DN, Goldenberg J, He X, Maldonado-Cocco J, Orozco-Alcala J, Prieur AM, Suarez-Almazor ME, Woo P, International League of Associations for Rheumatology. International League of Associations for Rheumatology classification of juvenile idiopathic arthritis: second revision, Edmonton, 2001. J Rheumatol. 2004;31(2):390–2.
2. Yamaguchi M, Ohta A, Tsunematsu T, Kasukawa R, Mizushima Y, Kashiwagi H, Kashiwazaki S, Tanimoto K, Matsumoto Y, Ota T, et al. Preliminary criteria for classification of adult Still's disease. J Rheumatol. 1992;19(3):424–30.
3. Lanni S, Bertamino M, Consolaro A, Pistorio A, Magni-Manzoni S, Galasso R, Lattanzi B, Calvo-Aranda E, Martini A, Ravelli A. Outcome and predicting factors of single and multiple intra-articular corticosteroid injections in children with juvenile idiopathic arthritis. Rheumatology (Oxford). 2011;50(9):1627–34.
4. Beukelman T, Patkar NM, Saag KG, Tolleson-Rinehart S, Cron RQ, DeWitt EM, Ilowite NT, Kimura Y, Laxer RM, Lovell DJ, Martini A, Rabinovich CE, Ruperto N. 2011 American College of Rheumatology recommendations for the treatment of juvenile idiopathic arthritis: initiation and safety monitoring of therapeutic agents for the treatment of arthritis and systemic features. Arthritis Care Res. 2011;63(4):465–82.
5. Silverman E, Spiegel L, Hawkins D, Petty R, Goldsmith D, Schanberg L, Duffy C, Howard P, Strand V. Long-term open-label preliminary study of the safety and efficacy of leflunomide in patients with polyarticular-course juvenile rheumatoid arthritis. Arthritis Rheum. 2005;52(2):554–62.
6. Bartoli M, Taro M, Magni-Manzoni S, Pistorio A, Traverso F, Viola S, Magnani A, Gasparini C, Martini A, Ravelli A. The magnitude of early response to methotrexate therapy predicts long-term outcome of patients with juvenile idiopathic arthritis. Ann Rheum Dis. 2008;67(3):370–4.
7. Aggarwal A, Misra DP. Enthesitis-related arthritis. Clin Rheumatol. 2015;34(11):1839–46.
8. De Benedetti F, Brunner HI, Ruperto N, Kenwright A, Wright S, Calvo I, Cuttica R, Ravelli A, Schneider R, Woo P, Wouters C, Xavier R, Zemel L, Baildam E, Burgos-Vargas R, Dolezalova P, Garay SM, Merino R, Joos R, Grom A, Wulffraat N, Zuber Z, Zulian F, Lovell D, Martini A, Printo P. Randomized trial of tocilizumab in systemic juvenile idiopathic arthritis. N Engl J Med. 2012;367(25):2385–95.
9. Ruperto N, Lovell DJ, Quartier P, Paz E, Rubio-Perez N, Silva CA, Abud-Mendoza C, Burgos-Vargas R, Gerloni V, Melo-Gomes JA, Saad-Magalhaes C, Chavez-Corrales J, Huemer C, Kivitz A, Blanco FJ, Foeldvari I, Hofer M, Horneff G, Huppertz HI, Job-Deslandre C, Loy A, Minden K, Punaro M, Nunez AF, Sigal LH, Block AJ, Nys M, Martini A, Giannini EH, Paediatric Rheumatology International Trials Organisation, the Pediatric Rheumatology Collaborative Study Group. Long-term safety and efficacy of abatacept in children with juvenile idiopathic arthritis. Arthritis Rheum. 2010;62(6):1792–802.

10. Alexeeva EI, Valieva SI, Bzarova TM, Semikina EL, Isaeva KB, Lisitsyn AO, Denisova RV, Chistyakova EG. Efficacy and safety of repeat courses of rituximab treatment in patients with severe refractory juvenile idiopathic arthritis. Clin Rheumatol. 2011;30(9):1163–72.
11. Schmeling H, Minden K, Foeldvari I, Ganser G, Hospach T, Horneff G. Efficacy and safety of adalimumab as the first and second biologic agent in juvenile idiopathic arthritis: the German Biologics JIA Registry. Arthritis Rheumatol (Hoboken, NJ). 2014;66(9):2580–9.
12. Burgos-Vargas R, Tse SM, Horneff G, Pangan AL, Kalabic J, Goss S, Unnebrink K, Anderson JK. A randomized, double-blind, placebo-controlled multicenter study of adalimumab in pediatric patients with enthesitis-related arthritis. Arthritis Care Res. 2015;67(11):1503–12.
13. Ramanan AV, Dick AD, Jones AP, McKay A, Williamson PR, Compeyrot-Lacassagne S, Hardwick B, Hickey H, Hughes D, Woo P, Benton D, Edelsten C, Beresford MW, Group SS. Adalimumab plus methotrexate for uveitis in juvenile idiopathic arthritis. N Engl J Med. 2017;376(17):1637–46.
14. Ruperto N, Brunner HI, Quartier P, Constantin T, Wulffraat N, Horneff G, Brik R, McCann L, Kasapcopur O, Rutkowska-Sak L, Schneider R, Berkun Y, Calvo I, Erguven M, Goffin L, Hofer M, Kallinich T, Oliveira SK, Uziel Y, Viola S, Nistala K, Wouters C, Cimaz R, Ferrandiz MA, Flato B, Gamir ML, Kone-Paut I, Grom A, Magnusson B, Ozen S, Sztajnbok F, Lheritier K, Abrams K, Kim D, Martini A, Lovell DJ, Printo P. Two randomized trials of canakinumab in systemic juvenile idiopathic arthritis. N Engl J Med. 2012;367(25):2396–406.

Chapter 6
Fever and Urticarial Rash

Mojgan Kianiamin

A 9-year-old well-nourished boy is referred by a physician from a primary care center, with fever of up 39 °C and urticarial rash, presenting 2 weeks after taking amoxicillin for pharyngeal pain and sinusitis. He has a suspicious history of penicillin allergy. His temperature was 38.8 °C on admission, pulse rate: 130/min, RR: 28/min, BP: 100/60 mmHg, and oxygen saturation 94% in room air.

Q1. What is the most probable diagnosis?

A. Serum sickness-like reaction
B. Kawasaki disease
C. Drug allergy
D. Acute rheumatic fever

Answer: *The correct answer is* ***A.***

Serum sickness is an immune complex-mediated hypersensitivity reaction characterized by fever, rash, arthritis, arthralgia, and other systemic symptoms. Serum sickness-like reaction (SSLR) is clinically similar to the classic or primary form described above and has been attributed to many non-protein drugs, including beta-lactam antibiotics, ciprofloxacin, sulfonamides, or metronidazole, developing within several days to weeks after drug administration [1].

Acute rheumatic fever (ARF) is an autoimmune inflammatory process that develops as a sequela of streptococcal infection in form of pharyngitis or less likely skin infection. ARF has extremely variable manifestations ranging from migrating polyarthritis, caritas, erythema marginatum, to chorea and subcutaneous nodules. The most common joints involved in ARF are large joints, usually those that bear weight.

M. Kianiamin (✉)
Chamran Medical Hospital, Tehran, Iran

Clinic of immunology and Allergy, Chamran General Hospital, Army Medical University, Tehran, Iran

© Springer Nature Switzerland AG 2020

F. Rahmani, N. Rezaei (eds.), *Pediatric Autoimmunity and Transplantation*,
https://doi.org/10.1007/978-3-030-26280-8_6

Knees and ankles are most often involved, and elbows and wrists are next. Hip joint arthritis is very uncommon [2, 3].

Next day he complains of mild dyspnea and chest pain with tachycardia and discomfort on right hip while walking.

Q2. Presence of which of the following clinical findings would change your initial suspicions and mandate additional work-up?

A. Wax and waning urticaria
B. Tachycardia and chest pain
C. Hip arthritis
D. Persistent fever

Answer: *The correct answer is* ***B.***

Chest pain and carditis are common problems in rheumatic fever and Kawasaki disease but not in drug allergy or SSLR.

Fever was controlled with ibuprofen, however he still had tachycardia. He did not complain of pruritus despite urticarial rash. In his CBC, he had WBC: 16,700/μL, with 73% PMN and 26% lymphocytes. His ESR was 50 mm/h and platelet count was 445,000/μL. Result of throat culture were negative.

Q3. What other paraclinic evaluation you would request?

A. Anti-streptolysin O titer
B. ECG and echocardiography
C. Total IgE
D. Answers A and B

Answer: *The correct answer is* ***D.***

In this patients with carditis after 2–3 weeks of suspected streptococcal infection, anti-streptolysin O titer (ASOT) is more reliable than throat culture. Chest X-ray and electrocardiogram will help detect cardiac size to rule out acute decompensated heart failure, or severe cardiac involvement with prolonged Q-T interval.

Cardiologist consult revealed mild mitral regurgitation without coronary artery involvement. ASOT was highly positive (=500 IU/L) but throat culture was negative.

Q4. What is the most probable diagnosis at the moment and your treatment of choice?

A. Rheumatic fever → prednisolone followed by high dose aspirin
B. Rheumatic fever → high dose aspirin plus monthly azithromycin
C. Kawasaki disease → prednisolone plus IVIg
D. SSLR → low dose aspirin

Answer: *The correct answer is* ***B.***

Acute carditis of ARF often responds dramatically to high dose salicylate therapy. If the carditis is mild, as in our patient, and the child is asymptomatic from a cardiovascular standpoint, salicylate therapy is usually started as monotherapy. With evidence of severe carditis, corticosteroids are indicated. Severe carditis is manifested by evidence of congestive heart failure, e.g. gallop rhythm, cardiomegaly, or severe myocardial disease as two valve disease or a new or a worsening arrhythmia. Close follow-up and evaluation by the cardiology service is warranted. Repeat echocardiograms will be needed. Prednisone is usually given for 2–3 weeks followed by aspirin while the corticosteroids are tapered [4].

Practical Points

- Serum sickness like reaction, acute rheumatic fever (ARF) and Kawasaki disease are challenging important diagnoses of fever and rash in children
- Acute carditis of ARF often responds dramatically to high dose salicylate therapy
- With evidence of severe carditis, corticosteroids are indicated

References

1. Mathes EF, Gilliam AE. A four-year-old boy with fever, rash, and arthritis. Semin Cutan Med Surg. 2007;26(3):179–87.
2. Bryant P, Robins-Browne R, Carapetis J, Curtis N. Some of the people, some of the time: susceptibility to acute rheumatic fever. Circulation. 2009;119:742–53.
3. Mathur A, Mathes E. Urticaria mimickers in children. Dermatol Ther. 2013;26(6):467–75.
4. Saxena A, Kumar RK, Gera RP, Radhakrishnan S, Mishra S, Ahmed Z. Consensus guidelines on pediatric acute rheumatic fever and rheumatic heart disease. Indian Pediatr. 2008;45(7):565–73.

Chapter 7
Knee Swelling and Rash

Ross Petty and Farhad Salehzadeh

A 10-year-old Turkish boy was admitted to Children's Hospital with a 7 day history of knee swelling and rash particularly on the lower extremity. Four days prior to admission, he developed severe colicky abdominal pain and diarrhea.

Since the age of 5 years, he has had episodes of fever and colicky abdominal pain, lasting 3 days and recurring every 2–3 months. There was no rash with previous episodes. There was no camping or a history of recent travel. His parents were unrelated and there was no family history of a similar disorder. He is taking colchicine very irregularly.

Physical examination revealed an acutely ill child with a temperature of 39.5 °C. His weight was 33 kg and his blood pressure was 100/60 mmHg. He had generalized abdominal tenderness, voluntary guarding of lower abdomen and increased bowel sounds. There were a few petechiae on the calves and ankles. The right knee was swollen, warm and painful on motion.

The boy had leukocytosis with 65% polymorphonuclear cells. His urinalysis showed 2+ protein, 25–35 RBC and 10–20 WBC per high power field. Stool guaiac test was positive.

Serum albumin, globulins, AST, ALT, creatinine, PT and PTT were normal. Antinuclear antibody (ANA) and MONO test (specific antibody testing for Epstein-Barr virus) were negative.

Q1. What is the most likely diagnosis?

A. Serum sickness like disease
B. Hemolytic uremic syndrome

R. Petty
Pediatric Rheumatology, University of British Columbia, Vancouver, BC, Canada

F. Salehzadeh (✉)
Pediatric Rheumatology, Bouali Children's Hospital, ARUMS, Ardabil, Iran

© Springer Nature Switzerland AG 2020
F. Rahmani, N. Rezaei (eds.), *Pediatric Autoimmunity and Transplantation*,
https://doi.org/10.1007/978-3-030-26280-8_7

C. Polyarteritis nodosa
D. Henoch–Schönlein purpura associated with familial Mediterranean fever

Answer: *The correct answer is* ***D.***

On the basis of PRES/EULAR criteria (1) (Table 7.1), and the American College of Rheumatology (ACR) criteria (2) (Table 7.2) this boy has Henoch-Schönlein Purpura (HSP).

HSP occurs most frequently between the ages of 3 and 15 years, is rare in children younger than 2 years, and is more common in boys (1.5:1). Possible triggering events include infection with *β hemolytic streptococcus, Mycoplasma pneumoniae,* or *Helicobacter pylori*, and prior immunizations.

However, there are aspects of this boy's story that do not conform to a diagnosis of HSP. The history of recurrent episodes of fever and severe abdominal pain over the past 5 years without purpura, and his Turkish heritage suggest the possibility of familial Mediterranean fever. The abnormal urinalysis and blood in the stool are not features of FMF, however, but are consistent with HSP. Could this patient have both diseases? Mutations in the familial Mediterranean fever (*MEFV*) gene have been reported to be frequent in patients with HSP [3]. It is probable that this boy has HSP associated with FMF. Biopsy of a cutaneous lesion or of the kidney would reveal the characteristic deposition of IgA in the vessel walls of patients with HSP. Genetic analysis would reveal the presence of a mutation in the *MEFV* gene, thereby confirming the diagnosis of HSP with FMF.

Other diagnoses that might be considered include serum sickness or hypersensitivity vasculitis, an immune complex mediated disease that most commonly occurs as a result of an immune reaction to certain antibiotics (cefaclor, penicillin, trimethoprim-sulfamethoxazole) [4]. The clinical syndrome begins 7–14 days after exposure to the drug and is characterized by fever, arthralgia, and sometimes arthritis, myalgia, lymphadenopathy, and a purpuric, or urticarial rash predominantly

Table 7.1 EULAR/PRINTO/PRES criteria for Henoch-Schönlein Purpura [1]

Purpura or petechiae (mandatory) with lower limb predominance and at least 1 of the 4 following criteria:
• Abdominal pain
• Histopathology
• Arthritis or arthralgia
• Renal involvement

Table 7.2 The American College of Rheumatology 1990 criteria for the classification of Henoch-Schönlein purpura [2]

The presence of two or more of the following criteria has a sensitivity of 87.1% and a specificity of 87.7% for the diagnosis of HSP:
• Palpable purpura
• Age at onset <20 years
• Abdominal pain
• Wall granulocytes on biopsy

over the calves. Michel et al. [5] compared HSP and hypersensitivity vasculitis and found that hematuria, and gastrointestinal bleeding were more frequent in HSP.

Systemic PAN has also been associated with FMF [6]. PAN is characterized by, fever, weight loss, diffuse myalgia, abdominal pain, arthralgia, occasionally arthritis, and cutaneous lesions, particularly livedo reticularis, and tender nodules reflecting inflamed mid-sized arteries. Other clinical features which result from vasculitis include ischemic heart disease, renal involvement, often with hypertension, and central and peripheral neurologic involvement in from of focal defects, hemiplegia, visual loss, mononeuritis multiplex [7]. This patient has none of these characteristics aside from abdominal pain. The immunopathogenesis leading to vascular injury in PAN is probably heterogeneous. Streptococcal infection may be an important trigger, and indirect evidence suggests that bacterial superantigens may play a role in some cases. Hepatitis B virus has been associated with PAN, however, this association has almost disappeared with recent vaccination protocols in children.

HUS is characterized by generalized thrombotic microangiopathy (TMA) and the triad of acute kidney injury (AKI), microangiopathic anemia, and thrombocytopenia [8]. HUS is classified into three categories: (1) typical disease that occurs sporadically or in epidemic outbreaks and that is related to antecedent infection with Shiga toxin-producing strains of *Escherichia coli* (STEC) or other microorganisms that elaborate Shiga toxin; (2) sporadic atypical cases that occur secondary to infections, medication use, systemic disease, or malignancy; and (3) familial atypical cases that are predominantly due to genetic abnormalities in complement regulatory proteins.

HUS usually presents abruptly with pallor and oliguria. STEC–HUS occurs approximately 6–14 days after ingestion of contaminated food or beverage and 2–6 days after the onset of enteritis. Diarrhea occurs in over 90% of cases of STEC enteritis. It is accompanied by severe crampy abdominal pain and stools that change from watery to hemorrhagic [9].

Q2. What is the most common and important long-term morbidity in this patient?

A. Gastrointestinal involvement
B. Renal involvement
C. Joint and articular involvement
D. CNS involvement

Answer: *The correct answer is* ***B.***

The prognosis is excellent for most children with HSP, however significant morbidity or mortality is associated with gastrointestinal tract lesions in the short-term and with nephritis in the long-term. In general the prognosis for children with HSP depends on the extent of renal disease. Approximately 20% of children with HSP develop renal involvement, and 7% develop nephritis or nephrotic syndrome [10]. If the renal biopsy demonstrates crescentic glomerulonephritis in more than 80% of glomeruli, two-thirds will progress to renal failure within a year. If the child presents with nephrotic syndrome of glomerulonephritis, at least one-third will have evidence of chronic renal failure [11].

Abdominal pain occurs in approximately two- thirds of children with HSP, sometimes before the rash, but usually within days after appearance of the rash. Severe gastrointestinal involvement reflects edema and hemorrhage in the gut wall and includes intussusception, gangrene, or perforation.

CNS involvement in HSP is rare (0.65–8%), but poses diagnostic difficulties and sometimes has long-term neurological sequelae. Headache is the most common manifestation.

The clinical signs and symptoms of CNS involvement are altered consciousness (58%), seizures (14%), focal neurological deficit (26%), visual disturbances (24%), and speech disturbances (10%).

CNS vasculitis in HSP may present as edema, ischemia, ischemic infarction, and hemorrhage [12]. Of the patients with HSP who experience CNS involvement, an estimated 20% suffer long-term effects [12].

Arthralgia or arthritis involving only a few large joints occurs in 50–80% of children with HSP. Large joints, such as the knees and ankles, are most commonly affected, but small joints of the fingers, may be involved too. Characteristic findings include periarticular swelling pain, and limitation of movement. The arthritis is transient, and usually resolves completely within a week.

Q3. What is the main initial treatment?

A. Corticosteroids
B. NSAIDs
C. Antibiotic prophylaxis
D. Colchicine

Answer: *The correct answer is* ***D.***

Because of the diagnosis of FMF in this patient colchicine should be prescribed as long-term therapy. With respect to the management of HSP, treatment is supportive with maintenance of good hydration, nutrition and electrolyte balance. Pain control is accomplished with simple analgesics such as acetaminophen or NSAIDs. Control of hypertension is necessary. Although corticosteroids dramatically decrease the severity of joint and cutaneous disease, they are not usually indicated for management of these manifestations. Short-term corticosteroid therapy is effective in relieving the pain of severe orchitis. Prednisone has been advocated in children with severe gastrointestinal disease or hemorrhage. The severity of disease may occasionally prompt the use of intravenous corticosteroids. The use of corticosteroids to treat or prevent renal disease in children with HSP has been demonstrated to be ineffective [13].

HSP is sometimes recurrent, and because of the possible role of upper respiratory tract infection, especially streptococcal pharyngitis, in the etiopathogenesis of HSP some authors recommend prophylactic antibiotics and even tonsillectomy in ecurrent HSP [14].

Practical Points

- The EULAR criteria suggests a diagnosis of Henoch Schonlein purpura (HSP) to be made based on palpable purpura with lower limb predominance and at least one of the symptoms of abdominal pain, arthritis or arthralgia or signs of renal involvement or evidence of vasculitis in histopathology
- The prognosis is excellent for most children with HSP
- Approximately 20% of children with HSP develop renal involvement which could bear significant mortality and morbidity

References

1. Ozen S, Pistorio A, Iusan SM, et al. Paediatric Rheumatology International Trials Organisation (PRINTO). EULAR/PRINTO/PRES criteria for Henoch-Schönlein purpura, childhood polyarteritis nodosa, childhood Wegener granulomatosis and childhood Takayasu arteritis: Ankara 2008. Part II: final classification criteria. Ann Rheum Dis. 2010;69:798–806.
2. Mills JA, Michel BA, Bloch DA, et al. The American College of Rheumatology 1990 criteria for the classification of Henoch-Schonlein purpura. Arthritis Rheum. 1990;33:1114–21.
3. Altug UEC, Sayin DB, Ensari A. MEFV gene mutations in Henoch-Schönlein purpura. Int J Rheum Dis. 2013;16(3):347–51.
4. King B, Goolhoed G. Adverse skin and joint reactions associated with oral antibiotics in children: the role of cefaclor in serum sickness-like reactions. J Paediatr Child Health. 2003;39:677–81.
5. Michel B, Hunder G, Bloch D, Calabrese L. Hypersensitivity vasculitis and Henoch-Schönlein purpura: a comparison between the 2 disorders. J Rheumatol. 1992;19(5):721–8.
6. Ozen S, Ben-Chetrit E, Bakkaloglu A, et al. Semin Arthritis Rheum. 2001;30:281–7. https://doi.org/10.1053/sarh.2001.19958.
7. Eleftheriou D, Dillon MJ, Tullus K, Marks SD, Pilkington CA, Roebuck DJ, Klein NJ, Brogan PA. Systemic polyarteritis nodosa in the young: a single-center experience over thirty-two years. Arthritis Rheum. 2013;65(9):2476–85.
8. Trachtman H. HUS and TTP in children. Pediatr Clin North Am. 2013;60:1513–26.
9. Tarr P, Gordon C, Chandler W. Shiga-toxin-producing Escherichia coli and hemolytic uremic syndrome. Lancet (London, England). 2005;365:1073–86.
10. M. P. Henoch–Schönlein purpura nephritis. Pediatr Nephrol (Berlin Germany). 2015;30:245–52.
11. Ronkainen J, Ala-Houhala M, Huttenen M, et al. Outcome of Henoch-Schonlein nephritis with nephrotic-range proteinuria. Clin Nephrol. 2003;60:80–4.
12. Pacheva IH, Ivanov IS, Stefanova K, Chepisheva E, Chochkova L, Grozeva D, Stoyanova A, Milenkov S, Stefanova P, Petrova A. Central nervous system involvement in Henoch-Schonlein Purpura in children and adolescents. Case Rep Pediatr. 2017;2017:6.
13. Chartapisak W, Opastiraku S, Willis NS. Prevention and treatment of renal disease in Henoch-Schonlein purpura: a systematic review. Arch Dis Child. 2009;94:132–7.
14. Inoue CN, Chiba Y, Morimoto T, Nishio T, Kondo Y, Adachi M, Matsutani S. Tonsillectomy in the treatment of pediatric Henoch-Schönlein nephritis. Clin Nephrol. 2007;67(5):298–305.

Chapter 8
Malaise, Weight Loss and Intermittent Fever

Ross Petty, Farhad Salehzadeh, and Marco Antonio Yamazaki-Nakashimada

A 13-year-old white girl was referred to the Pediatric Rheumatology clinic because of malaise, weight loss, intermittent fever, and painful swelling of her knees, elbow, and wrists for 3 months. She had malar erythema that was exaggerated by sun exposure. Her past medical history was notable for a diagnosis of idiopathic thrombocytopenic purpura 5 years ago.

The family history was notable for a maternal aunt who had glomerulonephritis and died of renal failure. Physical examination revealed blood pressure of 110/70 mmHg, temperature: 37.8 °C, heart rate: 68/min and respiratory rate: 25/min. Height and weight were at the 50th centile. On examination, she appeared unwell, had erythema over the malar eminences and helices of the ears and a shallow painless ragged ulcer on the hard palate. Cardiac and pulmonary examinations were unremarkable and there was no organomegaly or significant lymphadenopathy. Her knees, right elbow and both wrists were swollen, and tender. She has a WBC count of 3500/μL with 40% PMN and 3% eosinophils, hemoglobin was 10.6 g/dL, platelet count: 95,000/μL and ESR: 65 mm/h. In her urinalysis she had 2+ protein and 20–25 RBCs/hpf.

Q1. On the basis of history, physical findings, family history and laboratory studies, you consider a diagnosis of systemic lupus erythematosus. Which of the following investigations would be most helpful to confirm this diagnosis?

A. Imaging studies
B. Bone marrow aspiration

R. Petty
Pediatric Rheumatology, University of British Columbia, Vancouver, BC, Canada

F. Salehzadeh (✉)
Pediatric Rheumatology, Bouali Children's Hospital, ARUMS, Ardabil, Iran

M. A. Yamazaki-Nakashimada
Clinical Immunology Department, Instituto Nacional de Pediatría, Mexico City, Mexico

© Springer Nature Switzerland AG 2020

F. Rahmani, N. Rezaei (eds.), *Pediatric Autoimmunity and Transplantation*,
https://doi.org/10.1007/978-3-030-26280-8_8

C. Skin and kidney biopsy
D. Autoantibody studies

Answer: *The correct answer is* ***D.***

Systemic lupus erythematous (SLE), the prototypic autoimmune disease, is characterized by multiple specific autoantibodies associated with a multi-system illness. The American College of Rheumatology (ACR) modified criteria (1997) with high specificity (93.3%) and sensitivity (76.6%) are the best guide to systemic lupus erythematosus classification [1]. The ACR classification includes six clinical and five laboratory items. A patient is classified as having SLE if any 4 or more of the 11 criteria are present, serially or simultaneously, during any interval of observation.

This patient has at least five criteria: (1) photosensitive skin rash, (2) arthritis, (3) oral ulcer, (4) leukopenia, and (5) thrombocytopenia and a past medical history of idiopathic thrombocytopenic purpura. Importantly, imaging and pathology studies do not have a role in classifying SLE by the ACR criteria. Assessment of serum for the presence of specific autoantibodies will confirm a diagnosis of SLE in our patient.

It is unlikely that a child with SLE would have a negative test for anti-nuclear antibody (ANA). ANA test positivity lacks diagnostic specificity. A positive ANA is associated with other rheumatic diseases, infections, malignancies, and drug exposures, and may be present in relatives of patients with autoimmune disease, and even in a significant number of healthy children. Antibodies against native or anti-double stranded DNA antibody (anti-dsDNA) or extractable nuclear antigens (anti-ENAs) are particularly important. Antibodies against erythrocyte antigens (i.e. Coombs antibodies) detected by differential agglutination test, may be present in children with SLE and hemolytic anemia. Measuring levels of the third and fourth components of complement (C3, C4) or total hemolytic complement with CH50 are important in monitoring disease progression. Anti-phospholipid antibodies (including anticardiolipin antibodies and lupus anticoagulant) and prolonged activated partial thromboplastin time are associated with complications such as thrombosis, acquired bleeding diathesis, central nervous system disease, endocarditis, or Raynaud phenomenon with digital ulceration (Table 8.1).

Table 8.1 Autoantibodies in systemic lupus erythematosus (SLE)

Antibody		% Positive in children with SLE	Clinical utility
Antinuclear antibody (ANA)		98	Screening test; lacks specificity
Anti-double stranded DNA (anti-dsDNA)		75–95	Highly specific for SLE, correlates with disease activity
Anti-extractable nuclear antigens (anti-ENA)			
i	Anti-Smith (anti-Sm)	25	Highly specific for SLE
ii	Anti-ribonucleoprotein (anti-RNP)	40	High titer suggests diagnosis of mixed connective tissue disease
iii	Anti-Ro (SS-A)	30	Associated with subcutaneous lupus, neonatal lupus with congenital heart block, Sjögren syndrome. Associated with decreased risk of nephritis
iv	Anti-La (SS-B)	10	Associated with decreased risk of nephritis, Sjögren syndrome

Q2. In evaluating the characteristics of the renal disease which investigation will yield the most important information necessary for patient's management?

A. 24-hour urine test
B. Renal biopsy
C. Work-up of patients hypertension
D. Measurement of serum C3 and C4

Answer: *The correct answer is **B.***

Although renal biopsy is not routinely required for diagnosis of SLE, the presence of proteinuria, hematuria and hypertension strongly suggest significant renal involvement. A renal biopsy can then provide information that is critical to the management of the patient with SLE. Absolute indications of renal biopsy in SLE patients are: nephrotic syndrome, nephritic syndrome, and renal function tests abnormalities.

Quantitation of proteinuria, including a protein/creatinine ratio, is important in the follow-up of patients with lupus nephritis. Hypertension often accompanies lupus nephritis and may be a complication of therapy with corticosteroids. Management of hypertension is critical to the long-term outcome. Low levels of serum C3 and C4 suggest presence of active disease. A low level of C4, in particular, is associated with active renal disease. Low or undetectable total hemolytic complement might indicate the presence of a genetic deficiency of a complement component [2].

Q3. Renal biopsy result shows the presence of class 3: focal lupus nephritis (Table 8.2)**. Which of the following options is <u>not</u> recommended for this patient right now?**

A. Corticosteroids
B. NSAIDs
C. Hydroxychloroquine
D. Cytotoxic drugs
E. Biologic agents

Answer: *The correct answer is **E.***

Initial therapy should include corticosteroids and hydroxychloroquine. Depending on the disease severity and activity, corticosteroids may be administered as intravenous methylprednisolone (30 mg/kg/day to a maximum of 1 g/day) on 3–5 consecutive days, or given as oral prednisone (1–2 mg/kg/day given in at least 2 doses a day.) Low dose intravenous cyclophosphamide should be administered in

Table 8.2 International Society of Nephrology/Renal Pathology Society 2003 classification of lupus nephritis (abbreviated) [3]

Class 1	Minimal mesangial lupus nephritis
Class 2	Mesangial proliferative lupus nephritis
Class 3	Focal lupus nephritis (involving <50% of all glomeruli)
Class 4	Diffuse lupus nephritis (involving 50% or more of all glomeruli)
Class 5	Membranous lupus nephritis
Class 6	Advanced sclerotic lupus nephritis (90% or more of all glomeruli globally sclerosed)

patients with class III or class IV lupus nephritis according to the Euro-Lupus Nephritis Trial [4]. Alternatively, mycophenolate mofetil could be used for induction therapy. After successful remission induction with cyclophosphamide, maintenance therapy could employ azathioprine or mycophenolate mofetil [5].

Hydroxychloroquine is particularly useful in treating skin disease with benefits for arthritis and systemic inflammation as well. Add on therapy of hydroxychloroquine to corticosteroids reduces the risk of disease flare [6]. NSAIDs can be used to reduce the pain and joint inflammation as necessary.

Biologics, such as rituximab and belimumab, are not indicated in the initial treatment of this patient. Their use is currently recommended for those patients in whom corticosteroids, hydroxychloroquine and one of the cytotoxic drugs have failed to adequately control the disease.

Practical Points

- Antibodies against native or double stranded DNA (anti-dsDNA) or extractable nuclear antigens (anti-ENAs) are specific for systemic lupus erythematosus
- Negative antinuclear antibody (ANA) in children suspected for systemic lupus erythematosus, rules out the diagnosis
- C3, C4 complement level or total hemolytic complement with CH50 give a measure of disease activity

References

1. Hochberg MC. Updating the American College of Rheumatology revised criteria for the classification of systemic lupus erythematosus. Arthritis Rheum. 1997;40(9):1725.
2. Birmingham DJ, Irshaid F, Nagaraja HN, Zou X, Tsao BP, Wu H, Yu CY, Hebert LA, Rovin BH. The complex nature of serum C3 and C4 as biomarkers of lupus renal flare. Lupus. 2010;19(11):1272–80.
3. Weening JJ, D'Agati VD, Schwartz MM, Seshan SV, Alpers CE, Appel GB, Balow JE, Bruijn JA, Cook T, Ferrario F, Fogo AB, Ginzler EM, Hebert L, Hill G, Hill P, Jennette JC, Kong NC, Lesavre P, Lockshin M, Looi LM, Makino H, Moura LA, Nagata M. The classification of glomerulonephritis in systemic lupus erythematosus revisited. J Am Soc Nephrol. 2004;15(2):241–50.
4. Houssiau FA, Vasconcelos C, D'Cruz D, Sebastiani GD, Garrido Ed Ede R, Danieli MG, Abramovicz D, Blockmans D, Mathieu A, Direskeneli H, Galeazzi M, Gul A, Levy Y, Petera P, Popovic R, Petrovic R, Sinico RA, Cattaneo R, Font J, Depresseux G, Cosyns JP, Cervera R. Immunosuppressive therapy in lupus nephritis: the Euro-Lupus Nephritis Trial, a randomized trial of low-dose versus high-dose intravenous cyclophosphamide. Arthritis Rheum. 2002;46(8):2121–31.
5. Henderson L, Masson P, Craig JC, Flanc RS, Roberts MA, Strippoli GF, Webster AC. Treatment for lupus nephritis. Cochrane Database Syst Rev. 2012;12:Cd002922.
6. Pons-Estel GJ, Alarcon GS, McGwin G Jr, Danila MI, Zhang J, Bastian HM, Reveille JD, Vila LM. Protective effect of hydroxychloroquine on renal damage in patients with lupus nephritis: LXV, data from a multiethnic US cohort. Arthritis Rheum. 2009;61(6):830–9.

Chapter 9
Anemia, Microhematuria and Proteinuria

Živanović S. Snežana, Ivana Djuric-Filipovic, and Zorica Živković

A 14-year-old boy was admitted with a complaint of fever and chest discomfort for 2 days preceded by headache and nausea starting from 2 weeks ago. His past medical history revealed recurrent upper respiratory infections from early infancy and episodes of diarrhea. Prodromal phase of these infections was marked by an urticarial vasculitis which resolved without specific treatment. Skin lesions typical for urticaria were seen since he was 3 months old. Mild urticarial attacks occurred a couple of times during infancy. He has also had persistent anemia and microscopic hematuria since 2 years ago. His family history was relevant for maternal benign hematuria, detected 2 years ago. As he has been asymptomatic, and had no hypertension no further investigations were performed for her renal status.

On examination, he was febrile with *T*: 38.2 °C, heart rate: 154 bpm, respiratory rate: 24/min, blood pressure of 123/66 mmHg, and arterial oxygen saturation of 78% in room air. His skin was pale with maculopapular exanthema. He also had cervical lymphadenopathy (<1 cm). Laboratory data revealed WBC: 12,600/μL with 81.1% PMN and 13.3% lymphocytes, RBC: 2,640,000/μL, Hb: 5.1 g/dL, CRP: 4.8 mg/dL. ELISA test for IgM anti-EBV-VCA, IgG anti-VCA, and CMV, were all positive. Chest X-ray showed bilateral symmetric interstitial infiltrates and abdominal ultrasound revealed splenomegaly. Urine analysis showed microhematuria, discrete albuminuria (albumin/creatinine 8.3, reference range < 3) and proteinuria

Ž. S. Snežana
Pediatric Internal Diseases Clinic, Clinical Center of Nis, Faculty of Medicine, University of Nis, Nis, Serbia

I. Djuric-Filipovic
Children's Hospital for Lung Diseases and Tuberculosis, Medical Center "Dr Dragiša Mišović", Belgrade, Serbia

Z. Živković (✉)
Children's Hospital for Lung Diseases and Tuberculosis, Medical Center "Dr Dragiša Mišović", Belgrade, Serbia

Faculty of Pharmacy, University Business Academy in Novi Sad, Novi Sad, Serbia

© Springer Nature Switzerland AG 2020

F. Rahmani, N. Rezaei (eds.), *Pediatric Autoimmunity and Transplantation*,
https://doi.org/10.1007/978-3-030-26280-8_9

(protein/creatinine ratio: 27.3, reference range < 20). These results confirmed moderate glomerular failure.

Q1. Which of the following tests will most probably give you the underlying diagnosis in this patient?

A. Immunoglobulin classes and allergen-specific IgE
B. Anti-tetanus toxoid and anti-diphtheria toxoid antibodies
C. C3, C4, CH50, and AH50 test
D. Nitroblu tetrazolium test

Answer: *The correct answer is **C**.*

Complement deficiencies are relatively rare worldwide, between 1 and 10% of all patients diagnosed with primary immunodeficiencies [1]. Congenital deficiency of early components of the classical pathway (C1q, C1r/s, C2, C4) tends to be linked to autoimmune diseases, whereas deficiency of the C5-C9 components may confer susceptibility to various infections particularly to meningococcal disease [2]. Genes that encode complement components or their isotopes are distributed throughout different chromosomes, with 19 genes comprising three significant complement gene clusters in the human genome [3]. Complement deficiencies predispose patients to infection via two distinct mechanisms: ineffective opsonization and defects in lytic activity of membrane attack complex (MAC). Three major consequences of complement deficiencies are: (1) inadequate opsonization, (2) ineffective pathogen cell membrane lysis, and (3) co-morbid immune complex related disorders [4].

Partial C4 deficiency predisposes to systemic lupus erythematosus (SLE), while complete C4 deficiency is rare. Individuals with genetically determined complement deficiencies have a variety of clinical presentations and no specific physical finding is pathognomonic for complement deficiencies. Importantly, some overlap often exists between increased susceptibility to infection and tendency to develop autoimmune disease, hence both entities need to be addressed simultaneously in any one patient [5, 6].

Q2. Advanced laboratory results return: C3: 0.6 g/L (reference range 0.9–1.8 g/L), C4 0.05 g/L (reference range 0.15–0.55 g/L), negative anti-neutrophil cytoplasmic antibodies (ANCA), anti-nuclear antibody (ANA), and anti-double stranded DNA antibody (anti-dsDNA). What further examination should be performed to make a final diagnosis?

A. Computed tomography of the chest
B. Lung biopsy
C. Renal biopsy

Answer: *The correct answer is **C**.*

Renal biopsy is an essential diagnostic tool for histological diagnosis of glomerular and tubulointerstitial diseases. It allows to classify nephropathies to tailor a therapeutic approach to histopathological lesions and to assess the prognosis of the disease. Nephrotic syndrome is the most common indication of renal biopsy and lupus nephritis is the most common secondary glomerulonephritis [7–9]. Renal biopsy in our patient revealed focal segmental membranoproliferative glomerulonephritis (FS-MPGN), extensively involved blood vessels with hyalinization.

ANA, ANCA and anti-dsDNA were negative. So far, diagnosis of SLE was not confirmed. C3 hypocomplementemia plays a role in initiating glomerular inflammation and injury. Moreover, hypocomplementemia is a consequence of increased catabolism and decreased synthesis [10].

Q3. After confirming the underlying diagnosis in this patient and effectively treating his current infection and anemia, which of the following is the appropriate next step for a patient with FS-MPGN?

A. Initiate antibacterial, antifungal, and antiviral therapy
B. Initiate immunosuppressive therapy
C. Avoid all live virus vaccines
D. Initiate immune-modulators and monoclonal antibodies

Answer: *The correct answer is* ***B.***

The final problem list was: complement deficiency, microscopic polyangiitis, anemia and FS-MPGN. Treatment in our patient consisted of immunosuppressive therapy with mycophenolate mofetil. Importantly, anemia is often disproportional to the degree of renal insufficiency and relates to complement-mediated lysis of red cells, hence requiring aggressive therapy and often administration of recombinant erythropoietin.

Practical Points

- Three major consequences of complement deficiencies are: (1) inadequate opsonization, (2) ineffective pathogen cell membrane lysis, and (3) comorbid immune complex related disorders
- Partial C4 deficiency predisposes to systemic lupus erythematosus (SLE), while complete C4 deficiency is rare

References

1. Grumach AS, Kirschfink M. Are complement deficiencies really rare? Overview on prevalence, clinical importance and modern diagnostic approach. Mol Immunol. 2014;61(2):110–7.
2. Bryan AR, Wu EY. Complement deficiencies in systemic lupus erythematosus. Curr Allergy Asthma Rep. 2014;14(7):448.
3. Mayilyan KR. Complement genetics, deficiencies, and disease associations. Protein Cell. 2012;3(7):487–96.

4. Degn SE, Jensenius JC, Thiel S. Disease-causing mutations in genes of the complement system. Am J Hum Genet. 2011;88(6):689–705.
5. Complement: Deficiency Diseases. In: eLS. https://doi.org/10.1002/9780470015902.a0002154.pub3
6. Kliegman R, Behrman R, Jenson H, Stanton B. Disorders of the complement system. In: Nelson textbook of pediatrics, 16th ed. Philadelphia: WB Saunders; 2000. p. 628–34.
7. Souilmi FZ, Houssaini TS, Alaoui H, Harmouch T, Atmani S, Hida M. Indications and results of renal biopsy in children: a single-center experience from Morocco. Saudi J Kidney Dis Transplant. 2015;26(4):810–5.
8. Paripovic D, Kostic M, Kruscic D, Spasojevic B, Lomic G, Markovic-Lipkovski J, Basta-Jovanovic G, Smoljanic Z, Peco-Antic A. Indications and results of renal biopsy in children: a 10-year review from a single center in Serbia. J Nephrol. 2012;25(6):1054–9.
9. Yin XL, Zou MS, Zhang Y, Wang J, Liu TL, Tang JH, Qiu LR, Chen Y, Yuan HQ, Zhou JH. Twenty-three-year review of disease patterns from renal biopsies: an experience from a pediatric renal center. J Nephrol. 2013;26(4):699–707.
10. Sethi S, Nester CM, Smith RJ. Membranoproliferative glomerulonephritis and C3 glomerulopathy: resolving the confusion. Kidney Int. 2012;81(5):434–41.

Chapter 10
Fever, Anasarca and Arthralgia

Erika Sifuentes-Rodriguez, Francisco Rivas-Larrauri, and Marco Antonio Yamazaki-Nakashimada

A 16-year-old boy with an unremarkable past medical history, presented with a 1 month history of odynophagia, weight loss of 2 kg, dizziness, fever of 40 °C, orthopnea, general edema and arthralgia of the elbows, wrists, hips, knees and ankles. He consulted a general practitioner who diagnosed him with pharyngitis and prescribed amoxicillin/clavulanate and ibuprofen without improvement. The fever and general edema persisted, which brought him to the Emergency Department. The physical examination revealed facial edema, malar rash, cracked lips with hematic crust, oral ulcers on soft palate and maxillary vestibule. He had a prominent left anterior cervical node, which was non-tender and 1.5 cm in diameter, edema of the legs, with arthritis in both knees and erythema in palms and soles.

In his laboratory examination he had: WBC: 3700/μL, ANC: 3100/μL, lymphocytes 400/μL, platelet count 105,000/μL, creatinine: 1.34 mg/dL, BUN: 48.7 mg/dL, total bilirubin: 1.23 mg/dL with direct bilirubin: 0.63 mg/dL, and positive direct coombs test.Additional laboratory evaluation revealed AST: 549 IU/L, ALT: 244 IU/L, GGT: 209 IU/L, ESR: 45 mm/h and ferritin of 35,456 ng/mL. To approach his anasarca we measured serum total protein which was normal, and proteinuria which returned 0.6 g/day. He also had normal serum immunoglobulin levels (IgG: 1740 mg/dL, IgA: 262 mg/dL, and IgM: 221 mg/dL). Echocardiogram showed pericardial effusion. Finally, C3 and C4 levels were low and anti-nuclear antibody (ANA) was positive with a titer of 1:320.

Q1. What is the most likely diagnosis?

A. Juvenile dermatomyositis
B. Systemic juvenile idiopathic arthritis
C. Systemic lupus erythematosus
D. Polyarteritis nodosa

E. Sifuentes-Rodriguez · F. Rivas-Larrauri · M. A. Yamazaki-Nakashimada (✉)
Clinical Immunology Department, Instituto Nacional de Pediatría, Mexico City, Mexico

© Springer Nature Switzerland AG 2020

F. Rahmani, N. Rezaei (eds.), *Pediatric Autoimmunity and Transplantation*,
https://doi.org/10.1007/978-3-030-26280-8_10

Answer: *The correct answer is* ***C.***

The diagnosis of systemic lupus erythematosus (SLE) is established with the presence of malar rash, positive ANA, hypocomplementemia, autoimmune hemolytic anemia and proteinuria. Although the patient also had some characteristics of Kawasaki disease (e.g. fissured lips, edema and erythema of hand and feet, cervical lymphadenopathy), his age, and the prolonged disease argue against the diagnosis. Cheek skin biopsy was performed and revealed lymphocyte exocytosis and basement membrane vacuolization. Loss of focal pigmentation underneath the epidermis, perivascular accumulation of lymphocytes involving mainly the superficial layer of the dermis and a few necrotic keratinocytes, all compatible with SLE.

Q2. Which statement is true comparing adult form with juvenile SLE?

A. Adult SLE is more severe than juvenile SLE
B. Juvenile SLE does not present osteoporosis
C. Juvenile SLE is more frequent than adult SLE
D. Premature atherosclerosis is present in juvenile SLE

Answer: *The correct answer is* ***D.***

Juvenile SLE represents 10–20% of all SLE cases. Juvenile SLE shows a more aggressive clinical presentation. The majority of patient with juvenile SLE will develop systemic complications within 5–10 years of disease onset. Premature atherosclerosis and osteoporosis have become increasingly prevalent pediatric SLE patients [1, 2].

Q3. Which molecular defect is associated with the development of SLE?

A. *DNASE1L3* mutation
B. *IFIH1* mutation
C. C1q deficiency
D. All of the above

Answer: *The correct answer is* ***D.***

Lupus can be secondary to single gene mutations. Primary complement defects can lead to increased susceptibility to SLE. However, less than 1% of SLE cases are associated with complement deficiencies. Complete C1q, C1s and C1r deficiencies are associated with a high risk to of juvenile SLE.

Protein kinase C-delta (PKCδ), deficiency represents a novel genetic defect of apoptosis leading to SLE. Abnormal clearance of DNA in apoptosis plays a role in pathogenesis, as DNA is an important autoantigen in lupus.

Heterozygous null mutations in DNASE1 have been found in SLE patients with high titer anti-DNA antibodies. A familial form of SLE was described in patients with homozygous mutations in DNASE1L3, which encodes for an endonuclease with close homology to DNase 1 protein. Monogenic disorders have been associated with a lupus-like phenotype with overproduction of type 1 IFN. Mutations in genes encoding cytosolic nucleic sensors or their regulators (*TREX1, RNASEH2A,*

RNASEH2B, RNASEH2C, SAMHD1, ADAR or *IFIH1*) all are associated with this phenotype [3–5].

Q4. With persistent fever, cytopenia, elevated liver enzymes and high serum ferritin levels, which of the following diagnoses must be considered?

A. Fanconi anemia
B. Myeloid sarcoma
C. Toxicity of heavy metals
D. Macrophage activation syndrome

Answer: *The correct answer is* ***D.***

Macrophage activation syndrome (MAS) is a known complication of pediatric rheumatic disorders. It has been suggested that MAS is the same disorder as the secondary/reactive form of hemophagocytic lymphohistiocytosis (HLH), and in the case of autoimmune diseases it is also known autoimmune-associated hemophagocytic syndrome. MAS is characterized by proliferation of macrophages and T-lymphocytes resulting in continuous fever, hepatosplenomegaly, mental status changes, purpura, pancytopenia, elevated liver enzymes and hypofibrinogenemia. In SLE, MAS can mimic an acute exacerbation of the underlying disease because both entities share common features, such as fever, lymphadenopathy, splenomegaly and cytopenias. This overlap in clinical presentations can hinder the recognition of incipient MAS. There are limited reports of MAS in SLE. It has been suggested that MAS is not recognized as readily in children with SLE compared with children with other rheumatic disorders. Children with comorbid SLE and MAS have more organ system dysfunction and longer hospital stays for MAS than children with JIA and MAS [6–8].

Q5. What is the ideal treatment in patients with MAS in the context of rheumatological disorders?

A. Cyclosporine
B. Intravenous immunoglobulin
C. Etoposide
D. Corticosteroids
E. All of the above

Answer: *The correct answer is* ***E.***

Diagnostic and treatment approaches for children with HLH are generally based on HLH-04, a protocol that includes treatment with dexamethasone, cyclosporine and etoposide. This protocol was designed for the primary/familial HLH, that are a group of rare autosomal-recessive immune disorders linked to genetic defects affecting cytolytic pathway. The treatment protocol has been used by some as a surrogate for the treatment of MAS given its similar disease manifestation. Significant comorbidities associate with the HLH-protocol treatment regimen, and it has been predominantly studied in primary HLH syndromes, which have a different pathogenesis. Treatment in MAS/sHLH should be personalized and based on the underlying disease. Rituximab instead of etoposide, and also anakinra have been used successfully in MAS complicating SLE [7, 9–11].

Practical Points

- Less than 1% of systemic lupus erythematosus (SLE) cases are associated with complement deficiencies
- Complete C1q, C1s and C1r deficiencies are associated with a high risk to of juvenile SLE
- Macrophage activation syndrome (MAS), is a known complication of pediatric rheumatic disorders and a secondary/reactive form of hemophagocytic lymphohistiocytosis
- In SLE, MAS can mimic an acute exacerbation of the underlying disease with fever, lymphadenopathy, splenomegaly and cytopenia

References

1. Tarr T, Dérfalvi B, Győri N, Szántó A, Siminszky Z, Malik A, Szabó AJ, Szegedi G, Zeher M. Similarities and differences between pediatric and adult patients with systemic lupus erythematosus. Lupus. 2015;24(8):796–803.
2. Kamphuis S, Silverman ED. Prevalence and burden of pediatric-onset systemic lupus erythematosus. Nat Rev Rheumatol. 2010;6:538–46.
3. Costa-Reis P, Sullivan KE. Monogenic lupus: it's all new! Curr Opin Immunol. 2017;49:87–95.
4. Hiraki LT, Silverman ED. Genomics of systemic lupus erythematosus: insights gained by studying monogenic young-onset systemic lupus erythematosus. Rheum Dis Clin North Am. 2017;43(3):415–34.
5. Lo MS. Monogenic Lupus. Curr Rheumatol Rep. 2016;18(12):71.
6. Bennett TD, Fluchel M, Hersh AO, Hayward KN, Hersh AL, Brogan TV, Srivastava R, Stone BL, Korgenski EK, Mundorff MB, Casper TC, Bratton SL. Macrophage activation syndrome in children with systemic lupus erythematosus and children with juvenile idiopathic arthritis. Arthritis Rheum. 2012;64(12):4135–42.
7. Aytaç S, Batu ED, Ünal Ş, Bilginer Y, Çetin M, Tuncer M, Gümrük F, Özen S. Macrophage activation syndrome in children with systemic juvenile idiopathic arthritis and systemic lupus erythematosus. Rheumatol Int. 2016;36(10):1421–9.
8. Liu AC, Yang Y, Li MT, Jia Y, Chen S, Ye S, Zeng XZ, Wang Z, Zhao JX, Liu XY, Zhu J, Zhao Y, Zeng XF, Li ZG. Macrophage activation syndrome in systemic lupus erythematosus: a multicenter, case-control study in China. Clin Rheumatol. 2018;37(1):93–100.
9. Grom AA. Primary hemophagocytic lymphohistiocytosis and macrophage activation syndrome: the importance of timely clinical differentiation. J Pediatr. 2017;189:19–21.e1.
10. Tayer-Shifman OE, Ben-Chetrit E. Refractory macrophage activation syndrome in a patient with SLE and APLA syndrome—successful use of PET- CT and Anakinra in its diagnosis and treatment. Mod Rheumatol. 2015;25(6):954–7.
11. Junga Z, Stitt R, Tracy C, Keith M. Novel use of rituximab in macrophage activation syndrome secondary to systemic lupus erythematosus. BMJ Case Rep. 2017;2017. pii: bcr-2017-221347. https://doi.org/10.1136/bcr-2017-221347

Chapter 11
Bradycardia in a Neonate

Ross Petty and Farhad Salehzadeh

You have been asked to evaluate a 1-day-old Caucasian baby girl who was noted to have bradycardia since 30 weeks of gestation until delivery at term. Her prenatal course and delivery were otherwise uncomplicated. Her Apgar score was 8.

She was the product of the first pregnancy of her 29-year-old mother, whose health status was good except for a history of recurrent bilateral parotid swelling, dry eyes and mouth beginning 4 months prior to delivery. On physical examination, the baby weighed 3300 g, her head circumference was 34 cm, heart rate: 75/bpm, RR: 35/min, and temperature was 36.5 °C axillary. She was not distressed or cyanotic, but was icteric. General physical examination was otherwise normal.

In the primary lab workup her WBC was 8100/μL with 15% PMN, platelet count of 60,000/μL and hemoglobin of 10.3 g/dL. Reticulocytes count was low (1%). Both Mother's and baby's blood group were O+, direct coombs test was negative and finally, total bilirubin was 10 mg/dL, with 8 mg/dL being of direct type. His live enzymes were within normal range.

Q1. What is your initial diagnosis?

A. Congenital hypothyroidism
B. Neonatal congenital long QT syndrome
C. Early-onset sepsis
D. Neonatal lupus erythematosus

Answer: *The correct answer is **D**.*

This baby's weight is appropriate for gestational age, and she appears healthy aside from bradycardia and icter which is not readily explained on the basis of blood

R. Petty
Pediatric Rheumatology, University of British Columbia, Vancouver, BC, Canada

F. Salehzadeh (✉)
Pediatric Rheumatology, Bouali Children's Hospital, ARUMS, Ardabil, Iran

© Springer Nature Switzerland AG 2020
F. Rahmani, N. Rezaei (eds.), *Pediatric Autoimmunity and Transplantation*,
https://doi.org/10.1007/978-3-030-26280-8_11

group incompatibility or autoimmune hemolysis. The maternal history of recurrent bilateral parotid swelling and dry eyes and mouth suggests the possibility of Sjögren syndrome. History of fetal bradycardia suggests the possibility of congenital heart block (CHB) of some degree. Moderate thrombocytopenia and anemia are present. The picture is consistent with a diagnosis of neonatal lupus [1].

Neonatal lupus erythematosus (NLE) has variable clinical manifestations, the most important of which is congenital heart block. Infants with NLE are born to mothers who have antibodies to the Ro (SSA) (especially Ro 52) and/or La (SSB) antigens, although the mother may be completely asymptomatic. Transplacental passage of these autoantibodies results in inflammation, fibrosis and calcification of the atrioventricular node and ensuing heart block. In addition to cardiac damage, dermatologic (15–25%), hematologic (thrombocytopenia, anemia) (25–30%),) and hepatic abnormalities (25%) are other common manifestations of NLE.

Many cases of CHB occur in fetuses of mothers without a diagnosed autoimmune disease (25%). In other cases, mothers have systemic lupus erythematosus (30%), isolated Sjögren syndrome (15%), undifferentiated connective tissue disease (25%) or rheumatoid arthritis (1%) [1]. Asymptomatic mothers might first notice autoantibodies after relevant workup of when the baby is diagnosed as having NLE. In a prospective study of pregnant women with anti-Ro antibodies and an autoimmune disease, the incidence of fetal CHB was approximately 1% [2].

CHB is estimated to occur once in 14,000 live births, 90% of which are secondary to transplacental passage of autoantibodies [3]. First-, second-, or third-degree block is possible, which may or may not be associated with structural cardiac lesions such as ventricular septal defect or patent ductus arteriosus. Myocarditis and endocardial fibroelastosis (EFE) associated with NLE may occur in the absence of conduction abnormalities.

An association of NLE with stippled epiphysis consistent with chondrodysplasia punctate has been reported [3]. These cases have been associated with anti-Ro/La antibodies and with anti-RNP antibodies. The characteristic epiphyseal changes may be isolated or associated with bone dysplasia.

Multiple neurological manifestations have been described in association with NLE [3, 4]. A prospective study of infants born to mothers with anti-Ro/La antibodies found a rate of macrocephaly and hydrocephalus of 8% [5]. It is suggested that head circumferences measurements should be part of the follow-up of children of mothers with these autoantibodies.

Ultrasound abnormalities include subependymal cysts, increased echogenicity of the white matter, and echogenic lenticulostriate vessels.

The rash, which may be present at birth, most often appears by 6 weeks of age, and may be sun-sensitive. The face (especially the periocular area) and scalp are the most commonly involved areas but the rash may occur at any site, including the palms and soles, where it may be bullous.

New lesions may appear for several months, but they rarely develop beyond 6 months of age, at which age, maternal autoantibody levels are minimal. The rash usually resolves without residual scar, although some mild atrophy may remain. Cutaneous telangiectasia may occur later [1].

Alteration in the established feeding behavior is an early and common, although nonspecific symptom in sepsis. Other symptoms are hypothermia, which is more common in low birth weight babies, fever, lethargy, poor cry, poor perfusion, i.e. capillary refill time >2 s, hypotonic or absent neonatal reflexes, bradycardia or tachycardia, respiratory distress, i.e. apnea or gasping respiration, hypoglycemia or hyperglycemia, and metabolic acidosis [6]. This baby had none of the usual manifestations of neonatal sepsis, and appeared well, although icterus and thrombocytopenia might raise this question.

NLE may be mistaken for the effect of intrauterine viral infections (e.g. rubella, cytomegalovirus) which present in the neonatal period with cutaneous, hematologic (thrombocytopenia, neutropenia, anemia) and hepatic abnormalities (hyperbilirubinemia, elevated liver enzymes), and cardiac defects, although heart block does not occur in these infections. Fetal bradycardia may also occur in infants with congenital hypothyroidism [7] and in prolonged QT syndrome [8, 9].

Neonatal symptoms of congenital hypothyroidism are non-specific. The gestation period extends beyond 42 weeks in 20% and up to one third have a birth weight greater than the ninetieth percentile. The infant is often quiet and sleeps through the night. A hoarse cry and constipation may be noted. The most common abnormalities noted on physical examination are umbilical hernia, macroglossia, hypotonia, icterus and cool or mottled skin. The posterior fontanelle might be open [7].

Congenital long QT syndrome (LQTS) is a rare potentially lethal disease caused by mutations in specific cardiac ion channels. The most common prenatal finding of fetal LQTS is sinus bradycardia. Whereas 71% of the fetuses with LQTS in one study showed moderate antenatal sinus bradycardia, intermittent episodes of ventricular tachycardia and second-degree atrioventricular block, were also observed. Both newborns died on the first day of life [8, 9].

Q2. At the time of detection of fetal bradycardia are there any useful therapeutic interventions that can be performed in the antenatal period?

A. Administration of dexamethasone to mother
B. Administration of intravenous immunoglobulin to mother
C. Administration of hydroxychloroquine to the mother
D. Administration of beta agonist to the mother

Answer: *The correct answer is* ***A***.

The efficacy of treating the mother of a fetus with heart block is uncertain. Early studies suggested a benefit from the use of fluorinated corticosteroids [10], but subsequent studies demonstrated only little benefit [11]. The practice in a large NLE cohort in Toronto is to give dexamethasone starting at 28–30 weeks gestation. The addition of intravenous immunoglobulin is indicated if EFE is present [12]. There is some evidence that treating the mother with hydroxychloroquine may decrease the risk of NLE in subsequent pregnancies.

There are a few case report about the efficacy of β-agonists administered to mothers [13]. Although, there are no comprehensive published data about the efficacy of beta agonist drugs in this condition, they have been used to increase fetal heart rates in utero. Duration of beta agonist effect and its impact on mortality are in question, but when used in combination with other therapies, it may provide benefit [14].

Q3. If the mother does not receive any preventive treatments, what is the risk of having a baby with cardiac involvement of NLE in her subsequent pregnancies?

A. Similar to first pregnancy
B. 15–20%
C. Up to 50%
D. Almost 100%

Answer: *The correct answer is* ***B.***

The risk of having a second baby with CHB is within the range of 15–20% [15]. Presence of autoantibodies alone, confers a risk of congenital heart block of 2% [16].

Q4. Which risk factor(s) is/are associated with intrauterine or perinatal death in an infant with NLE?

A. Dilated cardiomyopathy
B. Endocardial fibroelastosis
C. Hydrops fetalis
D. Early onset of bradycardia
E. All of the above

Answer: *The correct answer is* ***E.***

Risk factors that are associated with perinatal death in NLE include non-immune fetal hydrops, secondary to cardiac failure, ventricular rates lower than 50–55 beats per minute, EFE and/or cardiomyopathy and CHB at earlier gestational ages. Most children with CHB require a permanent pacemaker during childhood and thus will carry lifelong risks for pacemaker-related morbidity and mortality. In addition, approximately 5–10% of children with CHB and normal cardiac function at birth will develop a fatal dilated cardiomyopathy and/or EFE during childhood [1, 17].

Practical Points

- The most important complication of neonatal lupus erythematosus (NLE) is congenital heart block (CHB)
- Infants with NLE are born to mothers who have antibodies against Ro (SSA) and/or La (SSB) antigens, although the mother may be completely asymptomatic
- Most children with CHB require a permanent pacemaker during childhood and thus will carry lifelong risks for pacemaker-related morbidity and mortality
- The risk of having a second baby with congenital heart block is within the range of 15–20%

References

1. Vanoni F, Lava SAG, Fossali EF, Cavalli R, Simonetti GD, Bianchetti MG, Bozzini MA, Agostoni C, Milani GP. Neonatal systemic lupus erythematosus syndrome: a comprehensive review. Clin Rev Allergy Immunol. 2017;53(3):469–76.
2. Costedoat-Chalumeau N, Amoura Z, Lupoglazoff JM, Huong DL, Denjoy I, Vauthier D, Sebbouh D, Fain O, Georgin-Lavialle S, Ghillani P, Musset L, Wechsler B, Duhaut P, Piette JC. Outcome of pregnancies in patients with anti-SSA/Ro antibodies: a study of 165 pregnancies, with special focus on electrocardiographic variations in the children and comparison with a control group. Arthritis Rheum. 2004;50(10):3187–94.
3. Silverman E, Jaeggi E. Non-cardiac manifestations of neonatal lupus erythematosus. Scand J Immunol. 2010;72(3):223–5.
4. Prendiville JS, Cabral DA, Poskitt KJ, Au S, Sargent MA. Central nervous system involvement in neonatal lupus erythematosus. Pediatr Dermatol. 2003;20(1):60–7.
5. Boros CA, Spence D, Blaser S, Silverman ED. Hydrocephalus and macrocephaly: new manifestations of neonatal lupus erythematosus. Arthritis Rheum. 2007;57(2):261–6.
6. Kale A, Jaybhaye D, Bonde V. Neonatal sepsis: an update. Iran J Neonatol. 2014;4(4):39–51.
7. Rastogi MV, LaFranchi SH. Congenital hypothyroidism. Orphanet J Rare Dis. 2010;5:17.
8. Anuwutnavin S, Wanitpongpan P, Chungsomprasong P, Soongswang J, Srisantiroj N, Wataganara T. Fetal long QT syndrome manifested as atrioventricular block and ventricular tachycardia: a case report and a review of the literature. Pediatr Cardiol. 2013;34(8):1955–62.
9. Beinder E, Grancay T, Menendez T, Singer H, Hofbeck M. Fetal sinus bradycardia and the long QT syndrome. Am J Obstet Gynecol. 2001;185(3):743–7.
10. Saleeb S, Copel J, Friedman D, Buyon JP. Comparison of treatment with fluorinated glucocorticoids to the natural history of autoantibody-associated congenital heart block: retrospective review of the research registry for neonatal lupus. Arthritis Rheum. 1999;42(11):2335–45.
11. Izmirly PM, Saxena A, Sahl SK, Shah U, Friedman DM, Kim MY, Buyon JP. Assessment of fluorinated steroids to avert progression and mortality in anti-SSA/Ro-associated cardiac injury limited to the fetal conduction system. Ann Rheum Dis. 2016;75(6):1161–5.
12. Jaeggi ET, Fouron JC, Silverman ED, Ryan G, Smallhorn J, Hornberger LK. Transplacental fetal treatment improves the outcome of prenatally diagnosed complete atrioventricular block without structural heart disease. Circulation. 2004;110(12):1542–8.
13. Yoshida H, Iwamoto M, Sakakibara H, Shigeta H, Hirahara F, Sato K. Treatment of fetal congenital complete heart block with maternal administration of beta-sympathomimetics (terbutaline): a case report. Gynecol Obstet Investig. 2001;52(2):142–4.
14. Saxena A, Izmirly PM, Mendez B, Buyon JP, Friedman DM. Prevention and treatment in utero of autoimmune-associated congenital heart block. Cardiol Rev. 2014;22(6):263–7.
15. Llanos C, Izmirly PM, Katholi M, Clancy RM, Friedman DM, Kim MY, Buyon JP. Recurrence rates of cardiac manifestations associated with neonatal lupus and maternal/fetal risk factors. Arthritis Rheum. 2009;60(10):3091–7.
16. Brucato A, Frassi M, Franceschini F, Cimaz R, Faden D, Pisoni MP, Muscara M, Vignati G, Stramba-Badiale M, Catelli L, Lojacono A, Cavazzana I, Ghirardello A, Vescovi F, Gambari PF, Doria A, Meroni PL, Tincani A. Risk of congenital complete heart block in newborns of mothers with anti-Ro/SSA antibodies detected by counterimmunoelectrophoresis: a prospective study of 100 women. Arthritis Rheum. 2001;44(8):1832–5.
17. Eliasson H, Sonesson SE, Sharland G, Granath F, Simpson JM, Carvalho JS, Jicinska H, Tomek V, Dangel J, Zielinsky P, Respondek-Liberska M, Freund MW, Mellander M, Bartrons J, Gardiner HM. Isolated atrioventricular block in the fetus: a retrospective, multinational, multicenter study of 175 patients. Circulation. 2011;124(18):1919–26.

Chapter 12
Annular Rash in a Neonate

Yan Ling Kong and Emily Yiping Gan

A 1-month-old boy presented with annular erythematous plaques on his face, scalp and trunk (Fig. 12.1). The lesions were not present at birth. The antenatal history was otherwise uneventful and the patient was born healthy at term with a birth weight of 3.2 kg. His mother has a history of systemic lupus erythematosus for the past 6 years, on treatment with oral hydroxychloroquine 200 mg daily. Laboratory data revealed WBC: 23,820/μL (neutrophils: 74%, lymphocytes 15%, monocytes: 6%, eosinophils 1%, basophils 1%), hemoglobin: 16.1 g/dL and platelets: 292,000/μL. Anti-La/SSB was positive, and anti-Ro/SSA had an intermediate titer. Anti-U1RNP and anti-smith were negative. Additional laboratory test included; total protein: 5.2 g/dL, albumin 34 g/L, total bilirubin 0.8 mg/dL, alkaline phosphatase 224 IU/L, alanine transaminase 86 IU/L, gamma-glutamyl transferase 223 U/L. Electrocardiogram revealed a normal sinus rhythm.

Q1. What is the most likely diagnosis?

A. Chronic urticaria
B. Neonatal lupus erythematosus
C. Annular erythema of infancy
D. Psoriatic skin lesions

Answer: *The correct answer is* ***B****.*

Neonatal lupus erythematosus (NLE) is a passively acquired autoimmune disease, due to transplacental passage of maternal antibodies. This condition was first described by McCuiston and Schoch in 1954, with a case report of an infant with transient lupus skin lesions and whose mother had positive anti-nuclear antibody

Y. L. Kong
National Skin Centre, Singapore, Singapore

E. Y. Gan (✉)
Dermatology Service, KK Women's and Children's Hospital, Singapore, Singapore

© Springer Nature Switzerland AG 2020
F. Rahmani, N. Rezaei (eds.), *Pediatric Autoimmunity and Transplantation*,
https://doi.org/10.1007/978-3-030-26280-8_12

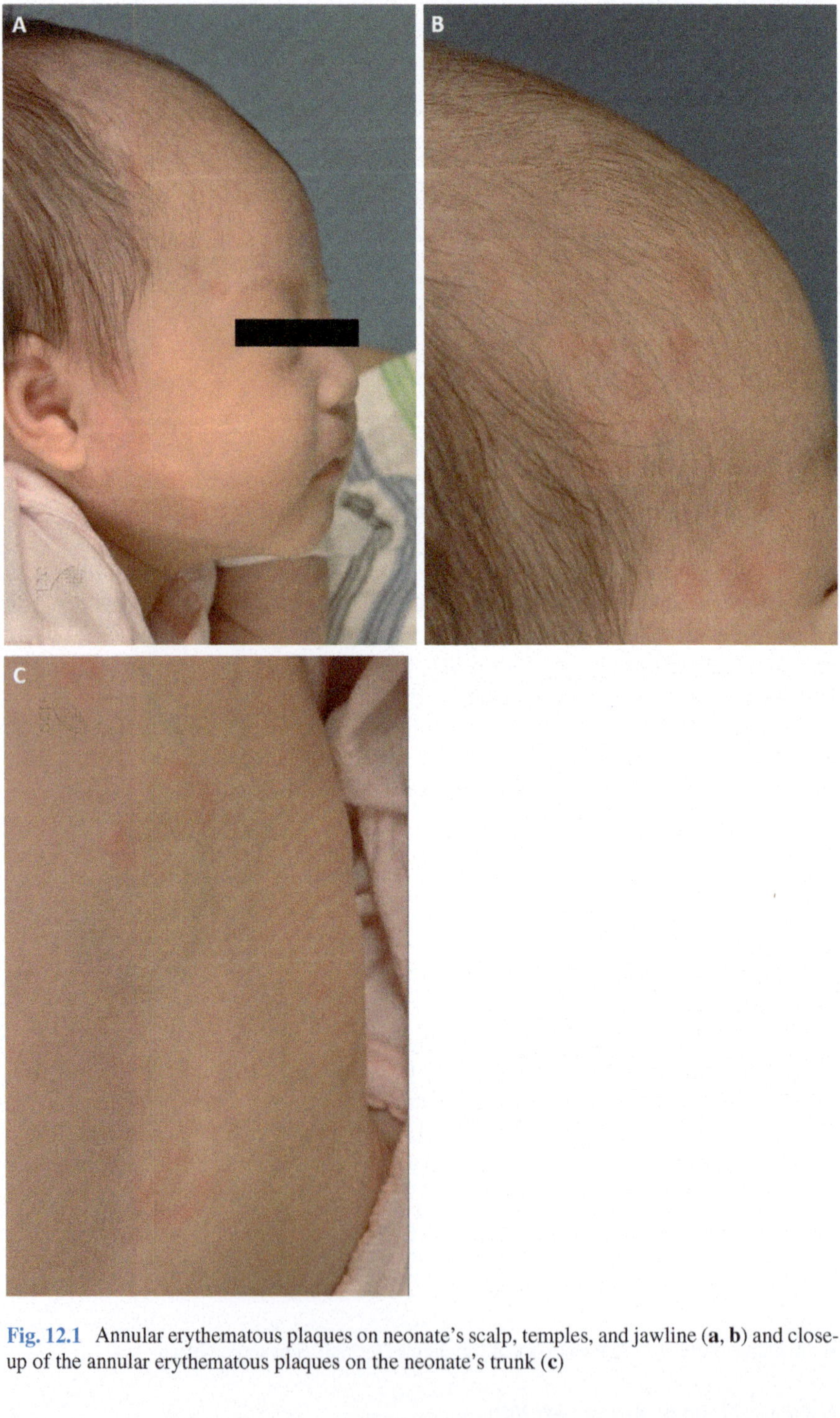

Fig. 12.1 Annular erythematous plaques on neonate's scalp, temples, and jawline (**a**, **b**) and close-up of the annular erythematous plaques on the neonate's trunk (**c**)

(ANA) [1]. Cutaneous lesions of NLE may be present at birth, but more commonly develop during the first few weeks of life. Patients typically present with annular erythematous plaques that predominate on the scalp, neck, or face, especially in a periorbital fashion [2]. The rash resembles subacute cutaneous lupus erythematosus [3], and is transient and self-limited, resolving in a few weeks or months usually without any residual scarring [4]. The diagnosis is usually established in the presence of typical features of NLE in the neonate and the demonstration of NLE-associated antibodies in the serum of the mother.

Q2. What is the most common auto-antibody associated with NLE?

A. Anti-Ro/SSA
B. Anti-La/SSB
C. Anti-double stranded DNA (anti-dsDNA)
D. Anti-U1 ribonucleoprotein antibody (anti-U1RNP)

Answer: *The correct answer is* ***A***.

Anti-Ro/SSA antibody in found in more than 90% of patients with NLE [5], and 16% of all children born to mothers with anti-Ro/SSA antibodies, with or without anti-La/SSB, antibodies develop cutaneous features of NLE [6]. Other associated antibodies include anti-La/SSB, and to a lesser extent, anti-U1RNP antibodies [2, 7]. Although some mothers may have a history of systemic lupus erythematosus (SLE) or Sjögren syndrome, most of them are asymptomatic at the time of the baby's birth, with no evidence or history of autoimmune disease [8]. Antibody screening of infants suspected of having NLE and their mothers, regardless of the presence or absence of symptoms, is recommended. Many asymptomatic mothers will eventually develop SLE, or more commonly, Sjögren syndrome [2, 8].

Q3. After confirming the diagnosis of NLE, what is the most important initial investigation in the evaluation of this patient?

A. Complete blood count
B. Electrocardiogram
C. Skin biopsy
D. Liver function test

Answer: *The correct answer is* ***B***.

The most common cardiac manifestation of neonatal lupus is conduction defects. Patients may develop first-, second-, or third-degree/complete heart block, which typically begins in utero between 18 to 24 weeks of gestation [2, 9]. Older women with higher parity are at an increased risk of giving birth to neonates with second-degree or complete heart block (i.e. CHB) [10]. Conduction block might begin as first- or second-degree block and then progress to CHB [2].

CHB is the most serious manifestation of NLE, in which there is loss of atrioventricular (AV) conduction, resulting in complete dissociation of the atrial and ventricular rates. Once established, CHB is irreversible, and requires insertion of a cardiac pacemaker [4, 11]. Due to the risk of postnatal progression to CHB, infants with first- or second-degree heart block should be observed closely. Unlike babies born with normal AV conduction or with first-degree heart block, those with second-degree or CHB, present with bradycardia and tend to suffer from low birth weights and growth retardation [10]. Other cardiac manifestations include structural valvular malformations, endocardial fibroelastosis, EFE, and cardiomyopathy [12]. Mortality rate approaches 20–30%, in neonates with NLE and cardiac involvement, and this is especially high in cases of CHB with concomitant cardiomyopathy [7].

Apart from an electocardiogram, a complete blood count and liver function test should be performed, as hepatobiliary disease and hematologic cytopenias are well-established, although less common manifestations of NLE [2, 13]. However, due to the significant morbidity associated with cardiac conduction defects, an electrocardiogram is the foremost diagnostic utility. It is unnecessary to perform a skin biopsy unless the diagnosis remains in doubt.

Q4. The patient's mother is worried that the she will develop liver failure in view of his deranged liver function tests. What would you tell her?

A. Liver failure affects 90% of neonates with NLE and is very likely in this boy
B. The deranged liver function tests is due to liver congestion secondary to decompensated heart failure
C. The deranged liver function tests is usually transient, and will resolve spontaneously
D. The deranged liver function tests is unrelated to NLE, and is likely due to a separate etiology

Answer: *The correct answer is* ***C****.*

About 10% of patients with NLE develop hepatic involvement, presenting with asymptomatic elevation of liver enzymes, cholestatic hepatitis or hepatosplenomegaly [2–4]. Liver failure rarely develops. Derangement in liver function tests is usually transient, with spontaneous resolution within 4–6 months [7].

Q5. The patient's mother is worried about recurrence of NLE in her future offspring. Which statement is correct?

A. She should use prenatal diagnosis and avoid further natural conceptions
B. Administration of hydroxychloroquine during pregnancy may reduce the risk of NLE complications
C. Administration of glucocorticoids during pregnancy may reduce the risk of NLE complications
D. Administration of intravenous immune globulin during the pregnancy may reduce the risk of NLE complications

Answer: *The correct answer is* ***B****.*

Mothers of babies with NLE have a two- to three-fold increased risk of having affected offspring in subsequent pregnancies. The risk is higher for future siblings of neonates with CHB [7]. Close monitoring of subsequent pregnancies with regular ultrasonography and echocardiography is advised, especially between the 16th and 24th weeks of gestations. Use of hydroxychloroquine has been shown to reduce the risk of cardiac NLE in subsequent pregnancies of mothers who are anti-Ro/SSA positive with an affected child [13]. In contrast, the risk of developing non-cardiac manifestations of NLE does not diminish with the use of hydroxychloroquine [11]. If initiated before 16 weeks' gestation, prenatal maintenance therapy with oral steroids may be effective in reducing the risk of cardiac NLE in the offspring [14, 15].

Mothers with anti-Ro/SSA and/or anti-La/SSB may continue to breastfeed their infants diagnosed with NLE. Although the maternal milk may contain autoantigen-specific antibodies, serum levels of these remain low in breastfed infants [16].

Practical Points

- Neonatal lupus erythematosus (NLE) is an acquired autoimmune disease resulting from the transplacental passage of maternal antibodies
- NLE is characterized by the presence of annular erythematous plaques seen predominantly on the face and scalp
- Anti-Ro/SSA antibody in the most common auto-antibody found in patients with NLE
- Other associated antibodies include anti-La/SSB and anti-U1RNP antibodies
- Life-threatening cardiac conduction defects commonly occurs in NLE
- Pacemaker insertion is usually required for patients with NLE and congenital heart block
- Use of hydroxychloroquine decreases the risk of cardiac NLE in subsequent offspring, but not the non-cardiac manifestations of NLE

References

1. Mccuistion CH. Possible discoid lupus erythematosus in newborn infant. Report of a case with subsequent development of acute systemic lupus erythematosus in mother. Arch Dermatol. 1983;119(7):615–8.
2. Lee LA. Neonatal lupus: clinical features and management. Pediatr Drugs. 2004;6(2):71–8.
3. Silverman E, Jaeggi E. Non-cardiac manifestations of neonatal lupus erythematosus. Scand J Immunol. 2010;14(72):3.
4. Lee LA. The clinical spectrum of neonatal lupus. Arch Dermatol Res. 2008;301(1):107–10.
5. Eftekhari P, Salle L, Lezoualc'h F, Mialet J, Gastineau M, Briand JP, Isenberg DA, Fournie GJ, Argibay J, Fischmeister R, Muller S, Hoebeke J. Anti-SSA/Ro52 autoantibodies blocking the cardiac 5-HT4 serotoninergic receptor could explain neonatal lupus congenital heart block. Eur J Immunol. 2000;30(10):2782–90.
6. Cimaz R, Spence DL, Hornberg L, Silverman ED. Incidence and spectrum of neonatal lupus erythematosus: a prospective study of infants born to mothers with anti-Ro autoantibodies. J Pediatr. 2003;142(6):678–83.
7. Hon KL, Leung AKC. Neonatal lupus erythematosus. Autoimmune Dis. 2012;2012:301274.

8. Rivera TLI, Izmirly PM, Birnbaum BK, Byrne P, Brauth JB, Katholi M, Kim MY, Fischer J, Clancy RM, Buyon JP. Disease progression in mothers of children enrolled in the Research Registry for Neonatal Lupus. Ann Rheum Dis. 2009;68(6):828–35.
9. Friedman DM, Kim MY, Copel JA, Davis C, Phoon CK, Glickstein JS, Buyon JP. Utility of cardiac monitoring in fetuses at risk for congenital heart block: the PR Interval and Dexamethasone Evaluation (PRIDE) prospective study. Circulation. 2008;117(4):485–93.
10. Skog A, Wahren-Herlenius M, Sundstrom B, Bremme K, Sonesson SE. Outcome and growth of infants fetally exposed to heart block-associated maternal anti-Ro52/SSA autoantibodies. Pediatrics. 2008;121(4):e803–9.
11. Lee L. Cutaneous lupus in infancy and childhood. Lupus. 2010;19(9):1112–7.
12. Guettrot-Imbert G, Cohen L, Fermont L, Villain E, Frances C, Thiebaugeorges O, Foliguet B, Leroux G, Cacoub P, Amoura Z, Piette JC, Costedoat-Chalumeau N. A new presentation of neonatal lupus: 5 cases of isolated mild endocardial fibroelastosis associated with maternal Anti-SSA/Ro and Anti-SSB/La antibodies. J Rheumatol. 2011;38(2):378–86.
13. Barsalou J, Jaeggi E, Laskin CA, Brown P, Tian SY, Hamilton RM, Silverman ED. Prenatal exposure to antimalarials decreases the risk of cardiac but not non-cardiac neonatal lupus: a single-centre cohort study. Rheumatology (Oxford). 2017;56(9):1552–9.
14. Shinohara K. Neonatal lupus erythematosus: results of maternal corticosteroid therapy. Obstet Gynecol. 1999;93(6):952–7.
15. Saleeb S, Copel J, Friedman D, Buyon JP. Comparison of treatment with fluorinated glucocorticoids to the natural history of autoantibody-associated congenital heart block: retrospective review of the research registry for neonatal lupus. Arthritis Rheum. 1999;42(11):2335–45.
16. Klauninger R, Skog A, Horvath L, Winqvist O, Edner A, Bremme K, Sonesson SE, Wahren-Herlenius M. Serologic follow-up of children born to mothers with Ro/SSA autoantibodies. Lupus. 2009;18(9):792–8.

Chapter 13
Itchy Facial Rash

Yan Ling Kong and Emily Yiping Gan

A 7-year-old girl presented with a 1-year history of rashes on her face and hands (Fig. 13.1). The rash began on her face and was occasionally itchy. There was no history of contact with irritants. She had no complain of weakness, malaise, gastrointestinal, pulmonary or joint symptoms or any systemic symptoms. On examination, there were violaceous patches on her face, with periorbital accentuation. Erythematous papules were noted on her knuckles, and there were fine telangiectasia over her nail folds (Figs. 13.2 and 13.3). The rest of her examination was unremarkable. Laboratory data revealed WBC: 8000/IU (neutrophils: 55%, lymphocytes: 38%, monocytes: 5%, eosinophils: 2%), hematocrit: 36%, hemoglobin: 11.9 g/dL, platelet: 343,000/UL; ESR: 12 mm/h. Creatine kinase was normal (132 U/L), but both lactate dehydrogenase (328 U/L) and aldolase (13.6 U/L) were marginally elevated. Anti-nuclear antibody (ANA), extractable nuclear antigen (ENA) and anti-double-stranded DNA autoantibodies (anti-dsDNA) were negative. Serum level of C3 (77 G/L) and C4 (16 G/L) were not elevated. A skin biopsy was performed and her treatment was initiated with a combination of immunosuppressive agents.

Q1. What is your diagnosis, and what is the HLA subtype associated with increased risk of this condition?

A. Systemic lupus erythematosus; HLA-DQA1∗0501
B. Juvenile dermatomyositis; HLA-DQA1∗0501
C. Systemic lupus erythematosus; DRB1∗03:01
D. Juvenile dermatomyositis; DRB1∗03:01

Y. L. Kong
National Skin Centre, Singapore, Singapore

E. Y. Gan (✉)
Dermatology Service, KK Women's and Children's Hospital, Singapore, Singapore

© Springer Nature Switzerland AG 2020

F. Rahmani, N. Rezaei (eds.), *Pediatric Autoimmunity and Transplantation*,
https://doi.org/10.1007/978-3-030-26280-8_13

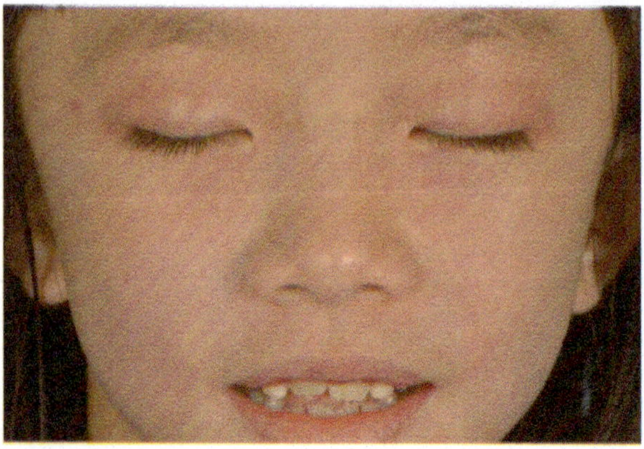

Fig. 13.1 Violaceous patches on the patient's cheeks and periorbital region ("Heliotrope eruption")

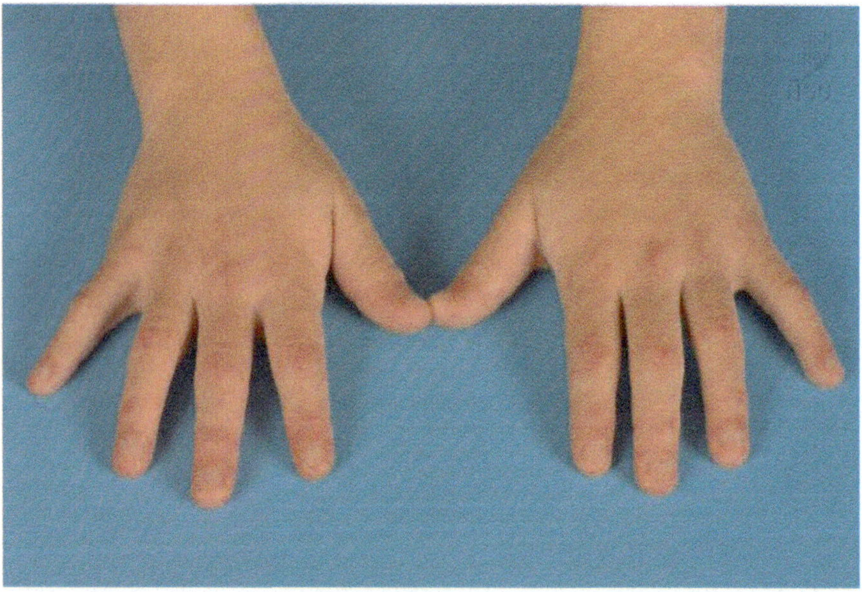

Fig. 13.2 Gottron's papules seen symmetrically over the dorsal aspects of the metacarpal and interphalangeal joints

***Answer:** The correct answer is **B**.*

Juvenile dermatomyositis (JDM) is a rare multisystem disorder that affects children younger than 18-years-old. Although the etiology remains unclear, it has been proposed that JDM is caused by an autoimmune reaction in genetically susceptible individuals, possibly in response to infection or environmental triggers such as prenatal exposure to tobacco smoke and particulate inhalants [1].

The disease most frequently manifests with skin and muscle involvement, but may also affect the joints, and other organs such as the lungs, esophagus and less

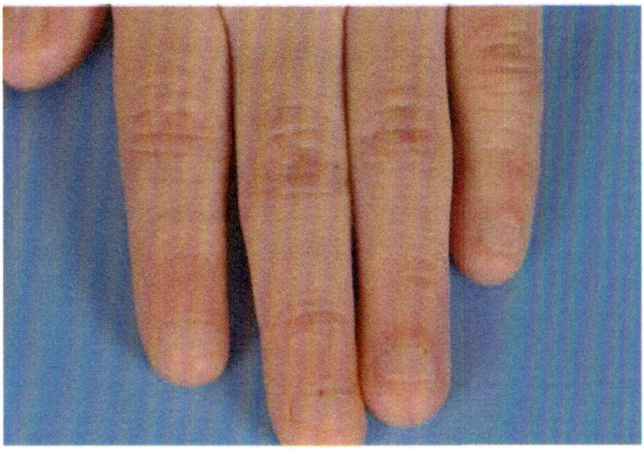

Fig. 13.3 "Ragged cuticles", periungual erythema and prominent nail fold capillary loops

Table 13.1 Cutaneous features of juvenile dermatomyositis [3–5]

Cutaneous feature	Description
Gottron's papules	Erythematous papules that occur symmetrically over the dorsal aspects of the metacarpophalangeal and interphalangeal joints
Heliotrope eruption	Periorbital violaceous erythema which may be associated with edema
Gottron's sign	Erythematous macules, patches, or papules on the extensor surfaces of joints in sites other than the hands, particularly the elbows, knees, or ankles
Photodistributed poikiloderma	Violaceous erythema on sun-exposed areas of face, 'V' of neck and upper chest, upper back (shawl sign)
Periungual changes	Erythema, telangiectasia and ragged cuticles
Holster sign	Poikiloderma on the lateral aspects of the thighs
Calcinosis cutis	Deposition of calcium in the skin. This is more prevalent in JDM.
Mechanic's hands	Hyperkeratotic, fissured skin on palmar and lateral aspects of fingers
Ulceration	May affect the skin and mucous membranes

commonly, the heart [2]. Some of the characteristic cutaneous features of JDM are delineated in Table 13.1 [3–5]. The presence of cutaneous and mucosal ulcerations reflect vasculopathy in the skin, and portends a poorer prognosis [4]. Muscle weakness is present in most patients, and commonly involves the proximal muscle groups. However, up to 5% of patients have amyopathic JDM, with cutaneous features as the sole clinical manifestation of their disease [5]. Approximately 25% of children with amyopathic JDM evolve to classic disease after years of follow-up, but 75% of children remain free from muscle disease [6].

Patients with human leukocyte antigen (HLA) DQA1*0501 have increased susceptibility to JDM [7]. Although similar in many aspects to adult-onset dermatomyositis with characteristic skin findings and muscle weakness, JDM has not been clearly associated with malignancy. Routine malignancy screen is therefore not recommended in children with JDM [8].

Q2. What are the expected histological findings in the skin biopsy of this patient? Would you expect the direct immunofluorescence to be positive or negative?

A. Interface dermatitis with dermal mucin, dermal edema, superficial and deep perivascular infiltrates, and sometimes dermal or subcutaneous calcification → direct immunofluorescence positive
B. Interface dermatitis with dermal mucin, dermal edema, superficial and deep perivascular infiltrates, and sometimes dermal or subcutaneous calcification → direct immunofluorescence negative
C. Atrophic epidermis, interface dermatitis and a thickened dermis composed of abundant collagen bundles, no increase in dermal mucin → direct immunofluorescence positive
D. Atrophic epidermis, interface dermatitis and a thickened dermis composed of abundant collagen bundles, no increase in dermal mucin → direct immunofluorescence negative

Answer: *The correct answer is* ***B***.

The histological features of dermatomyositis include the presence of interface dermatitis, thickened basement membrane, perivascular lymphocytic infiltrate and increased mucin in the dermis. It may be histologically indistinguishable from lupus erythematosus. Direct immunofluorescence allows us to differentiate these conditions: lupus erythematosus lesions are characterized by granular band-like immune deposits in multiple classes of C3, IgG, IgM and/or C1q at the dermal-epidermal junction (lupus band). Direct immunofluorescence is on the other hand often negative in dermatomyositis [9].

Q3. Which antibody is associated with pulmonary involvement in patients with JDM?

A. Anti-double stranded DNA antibody
B. Anti-melanoma differentiation-associated gene 5 antibody
C. Anti Mi-2 antibody
D. Anti-p155/140 antibody

Answer: *The correct answer is* ***B***.

Myositis-specific autoantibodies (MSAs) are a heterogeneous group of autoantibodies found in dermatomyositis. MSAs target either nuclear or cytoplasmic components involved in gene transcription or protein translocation. They are associated with a variety of clinical phenotypes, and may allow for classification of patients into clinico-serological syndromes [10]. The most common MSA present in JDM are the anti-p155/140 autoantibodies, which is associated with more extensive skin disease. Anti-melanoma differentiation-associated gene 5 (MDA5) antibodies are associated with interstitial lung disease [11]. Antisynthetase antibodies are associated with interstitial lung disease, mechanic's hand and arthritis, and are more commonly found in adult-onset dermatomyositis than in JDM. Anti-Mi-2 antibodies are associated with the presence of classical cutaneous features of dermatomyositis, and patients generally have milder muscle disease and respond well to treatment [10].

Q4. The child now complains of severe abdominal pain associated with bilious vomiting and high fever of 40 °C. On examination, the child was toxic and unwell. Her abdomen was distended and exquisitely tender on palpation. Bowel sounds were diminished. What is the most likely cause of the condition described above?

A. Intestinal obstruction
B. Colonic malignancy
C. Intussusception
D. Intestinal perforation

Answer: *The correct answer is **D**.*

Gastrointestinal tract involvement is relatively rare in patients with JDM and manifestations include dysphagia, esophageal reflux, bowel dysmotility, and malabsorption. Vasculopathy affecting the gastrointestinal tract, which is associated with JDM rather than adult-onset DM, may result in ulceration and intestinal perforation [12, 13]. Patients typically present with severe and persistent abdominal pain, and a high index of suspicion can lead to diagnosis. Abdominal radiographs and stool tests for occult blood may be normal. Once diagnosed, surgical intervention is inevitable and patients often require partial excision of the bowel [14].

Q5. Which of the following immunosuppressive agents is most commonly used as a steroid-sparing agent in treatment of this condition?

A. Azathioprine
B. Mycophenolate mofetil
C. Cyclophosphamide
D. Methotrexate

Answer: *The correct answer is **D**.*

There is minimal data from randomized, controlled trials to guide treatment in JDM. Oral corticosteroids are the mainstay of treatment but second-line immunosuppressive agents are routinely added for their steroid-sparing effects and also in the treatment of refractory disease. Methotrexate has been the most widely accepted second-line agent in JDM. This is administered weekly at doses ranging from 10–20 mg/m^2 (mean starting dose: 15 mg/m^2), and may be given orally or subcutaneously [14]. The use of methotrexate in conjunction with a tapering course of glucocorticoids is effective in reducing the cumulative dose of corticosteroids [13]. Methotrexate is effective in treatment of both the cutaneous manifestations and myopathy in patients with JDM [14, 15].

Less commonly used adjunctive immunosuppressants include cyclosporine, intravenous immunoglobulin, mycophenolate mofetil, azathioprine and cyclophosphamide [16, 17]. In particular, a combination of intravenous cyclophosphamide and high-dose glucocorticoids is effective in the treatment of patients with ulcerative skin disease or life-threatening major organ involvement such as interstitial lung disease and gastrointestinal vasculopathy [16].

Practical Points

- Juvenile dermatomyositis (JDM) is a multisystemic disorder affecting children younger than 18 years old
- Patients frequently present with skin and muscle involvement, but other organs such as the lungs, esophagus and heart may also be affected
- Dermatomyositis is histologically indistinguishable from lupus erythematosus, and characterized by the presence of interface dermatitis, thickened basement membrane, perivascular lymphocytic infiltrate and increased mucin in the dermis
- Direct immunofluorescence is often negative in dermatomyositis
- Myositis-specific autoantibodies (MSA) are associated with a variety of clinical phenotypes in dermatomyositis
- The most common MSA present in JDM are the anti-p155/140 autoantibodies
- Methotrexate is the most common steroid-sparing oral immunosuppressant used in the treatment of juvenile dermatomyositis

References

1. Orione M, Silva C, Sallum A, Campos L, Omori C, Braga A, Farhat S. Risk factors for juvenile dermatomyositis: exposure to tobacco and air pollutants during pregnancy. Arthritis Care Res. 2014;66(10):1571–5.
2. Callen JP, Wortmann RL. Dermatomyositis. Clin Dermatol. 2006;24(5):363–73.
3. Callen JP. Cutaneous manifestations of dermatomyositis and their management. Curr Rheumatol Rep. 2010;12(3):192–7.
4. Singh S, Suri D, Aulakh R, Gupta A, Rawat A, Kumar RM. Mortality in children with juvenile dermatomyositis: two decades of experience from a single tertiary care centre in North India. Clin Rheumatol. 2014;33(11):1675–9.
5. Ramanan AV, Feldman BM. Clinical features and outcomes of juvenile dermatomyositis and other childhood onset myositis syndromes. Rheum Dis Clin N Am. 2002;28(4):833–57.
6. Walling HW, Gerami P, Sontheimer RD. Juvenile-onset clinically amyopathic dermatomyositis: an overview of recent progress in diagnosis and management. Paediatr Drugs. 2010;12(1):23–34.
7. Reed AM, Pachman L, Ober C. Molecular genetic studies of major histocompatibility complex genes in children with juvenile dermatomyositis: increased risk associated with HLA-DQA1 *0501. Hum Immunol. 1991;32(4):235–40.
8. Stockton D, Doherty VR, Brewster DH. Risk of cancer in patients with dermatomyositis or polymyositis, and follow-up implications: a Scottish population-based cohort study. Br J Cancer. 2001;85(1):41–5.
9. Burg G, Kempf W, Kutzner H, Feit J, Karai L. Atlas of dermatopathology. New York: Taylor & Francis Inc.; 2015.

10. Gunawardena H, Betteridge ZE, McHugh NJ. Myositis-specific autoantibodies: their clinical and pathogenic significance in disease expression. Rheumatology (Oxford). 2009;48(6):607–12.
11. Kobayashi N, Takezaki S, Kobayashi I, Iwata N, Mori M, Nagai K, Nakano N, Miyoshi M, Kinjo N, Murata T, Masunaga K, Umebayashi H, Imagawa T, Agematsu K, Sato S, Kuwana M, Yamada M, Takei S, Yokota S, Koike K, Ariga T. Clinical and laboratory features of fatal rapidly progressive interstitial lung disease associated with juvenile dermatomyositis. Rheumatology (Oxford). 2015;54(5):784–91.
12. Laskin BL, Choyke P, Keenan GF, Miller FW, Rider LG. Novel gastrointestinal tract manifestations in juvenile dermatomyositis. J Pediatr. 1999;135(3):371–4.
13. Crowe W, Bove K, Levinson J, Hilton P. Clinical and pathogenetic implications of histopathology in childhood polydermatomyositis. Arthritis Rheum. 1982;25(2):126–39.
14. Ramanan AV, Campbell-Webster N, Ota S, Parker S, Tran D, Tyrrell PN, Cameron B, Spiegel L, Schneider R, Laxer RM, Silverman ED, Feldman BM. The effectiveness of treating juvenile dermatomyositis with methotrexate and aggressively tapered corticosteroids. Arthritis Rheum. 2005;52(11):3570–8.
15. Zieglschmid-Adams ME, Pandya AG, Cohen SB, Sontheimer RD. Treatment of dermatomyositis with methotrexate. J Am Acad Dermatol. 1995;32(5 Pt 1):754–7.
16. Al-Mayouf SM, Laxer RM, Schneider R, Silverman ED, Feldman BM. Intravenous immunoglobulin therapy for juvenile dermatomyositis: efficacy and safety. J Rheumatol. 2000;27(10):2498–503.
17. Stringer E, Feldman BM. Advances in the treatment of juvenile dermatomyositis. Curr Opin Rheumatol. 2006;18(5):503–6.

Chapter 14
Muscle Weakness and Fever

Piyush Kumar and Anupam Das

An 11-year-old girl presented with a 3-month history of muscle weakness and pain principally affecting the proximal muscles of both arms and legs. There was associated fever, dysphagia, and dysphonia noticed by the mother. There was no joint pain, joint stiffness, oral sores, hair loss or thickening of the skin and the rest of the medical history was unremarkable.

Physical examination showed an ill-looking, febrile child with a temperature of 40.1 °C. There was a dusky erythematous rash around both eyes with swelling. Multiple atrophic lichenoid papules were noted on the dorsum of both hands, principally over knuckles (Fig. 14.1). Musculoskeletal examination revealed minimal tenderness of the thigh and proximal arm muscles with marked difficulty in raising her arms above the head. Proximal muscles' power was observed at a grade of 2–3, while the distal muscles had normal force. There was no joint tenderness. Examination of other systems did not reveal any abnormality. Laboratory investigations showed elevation of muscle enzymes: creatine phosphokinase: 1639 μg/L (26–140 μg/L), myoglobin: 219 ng/mL, aldolase: IU/L (1.5–8.1 IU/L), alanine aminotransferase: 53 μ/L (10–40 μ/L), aspartate aminotransferase: 162 μ/L (10–42 μ/L), along with ESR: 60 mm/h (0–20 mm/h), and CRP 8.6 mg/dL (0–0.1 mg/dL). Nerve conduction study was normal. Serology for antinuclear antibody was positive, but serology for anti-Jo-I, and rheumatoid factor were negative. Serology for HIV was non-reactive.

Q1. What is the best initial diagnosis?

A. Juvenile dermatomyositis
B. Systemic lupus erythematosus

P. Kumar (✉)
Department of Dermatology, Katihar Medical College, Katihar, Bihar, India

A. Das
Department of Dermatology, KPC Medical College, Kolkata, West Bengal, India

© Springer Nature Switzerland AG 2020

F. Rahmani, N. Rezaei (eds.), *Pediatric Autoimmunity and Transplantation*,
https://doi.org/10.1007/978-3-030-26280-8_14

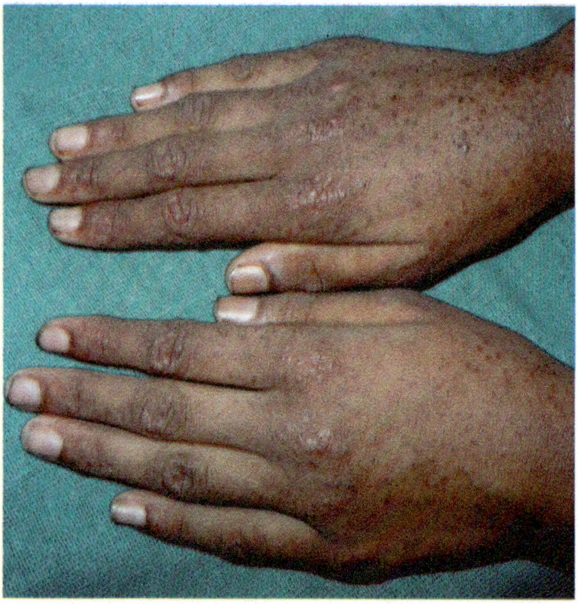

Fig. 14.1 Gottron papules in an 11-year-old girl with muscle weakness and pain

C. Mixed connective-tissue disease
D. Polymyositis

Answer: *The correct answer is* ***A***.

The definitive diagnosis of juvenile dermatomyositis (JDM) is made based on criteria proposed by Bohan and Peter, when **characteristic skin lesion** plus any 3 of the following criteria are present:

- Proximal muscle weakness
- Elevated muscle enzymes
- Myopathic changes on electromyography
- Abnormal muscle biopsy findings

JDM is a systemic, autoimmune condition affecting skin and muscles of children younger than 18 years. JDM appears to be more common in females than in males, and median age of onset of JDM is 6.8 years in girls and 7.3 years in boys [1].

Q2. Which one is a characteristic rash in juvenile dermatomyositis?

A. Heliotrope rash
B. Erythematous violaceous rash on extensors of extremities
C. Gottron papules
D. All of the above

Answer: *The correct answer is* ***D***.

Juvenile dermatomyositis primarily affects skin and muscle. Heliotrope rash results from inflammation of periorbital muscles and is characterized by edematous eyelids having a purple or dusky mauve color and an overlying scale. Similar confluent macular violaceous erythema may affect face, V area of chest, upper trunk and shoulders, i.e. shawl sign, lateral aspects of the hips and thighs, i.e. holster sign, extensor aspects of the arms and forearms and over dorsal aspect of the interphalangeal/metacarpophalangeal joints, olecranon processes, patellae, and medial malleoli, i.e. Gottron sign.

Gottron papules are violaceous papules with atrophic centers, seen typically overlying the dorsal-lateral aspect of interphalangeal and/or metacarpophalangeal joints and are considered pathognomonic. Other classical mucocutaneous findings include nail fold telangiectasia, periungual erythema, hypertrophic ragged cuticles, calcinosis cutis and vasomotor instability manifesting as Raynaud phenomenon, and livedo reticularis.

Symmetrical proximal muscle weakness involving the deltoids, or/and quadriceps is the hallmark of JDM. Like adults dermatomyositis, amyopathic dermatomyositis may be observed in JDM too and is defined as cases having biopsy-confirmed hallmark cutaneous lesions of classical dermatomyositis occurring for 6 months or longer, without any clinical or biochemical evidence of proximal muscle disease [2].

Q3. All of the following are common features of juvenile dermatomyositis, as compared to adult dermatomyositis, except:

A. Calcinosis cutis
B. Underlying malignancy
C. Less frequent lung disease
D. Better overall prognosis

Answer: *The correct answer is **B**.*

The two subsets of dermatomyositis, JDM and dermatomyositis, have classic skin rash and proximal muscles myopathy in common. Their difference lies in frequency of involvement of other systems. Symptomatic lung diseases are much more common in adult dermatomyositis and contribute to patients' mortality. In a recent study, pulmonary damage was reported in 49% cases of adult patients with dermatomyositis. On the other hand, only 3.5% of cases of JDM showed pulmonary damage on long-term follow up [3]. On the other hand, asymptomatic lung involvement documented as abnormal pulmonary function tests, lung volume or HRCT is more common in JDM in contrast to previous reports [4]. Similarly, association with underlying malignancy is strong with adult dermatomyositis and some authors consider adult dermatomyositis a paraneoplastic syndrome, as patients show improvement with treatment of the associated cancer and patients with recurrence of muscle weakness after relapse of malignant disease. In contrast, JDM has not shown to be clearly associated with malignancy and cases of malignancy in children with JDM are limited to case reports [4]. Long-term follow-up for malignancies is warranted in these patients during adulthood [4].

Calcinosis cutis and subsequent cutaneous ulcerations may be seen in up to 30% cases of JDM and typically occurs 1–3 years after diagnosis. Calcinosis usually affects pressure areas such as the elbows, knees, buttocks and digits and is associated with chronic course of an active disease [5].

JDM may have a rapid onset and may cause considerable morbidity and even mortality in some cases. Aggressive treatment warrants recovery of muscular force and more desirable prognosis of JDM compared to adult [4].

Q4. All of the following are used to assess disease activity in juvenile dermatomyositis, except:

A. Erythrocyte sedimentation rate
B. Magnetic resonance imaging of muscles
C. Childhood myositis assessment scale
D. Creatine kinase levels

Answer: *The correct answer is **A**.*

ESR is commonly elevated in patients with JDM, but this finding is non-specific and hence, not a reliable indicator of disease activity.

Muscle involvement can be assessed by MRI, which reveals edema and inflammation, thus helping to localize the potential muscle biopsy area. Muscle biopsy is rarely needed these days [5]. MRI may also show areas of calcinosis.

Muscle enzymes like aspartate aminotransferase, lactate dehydrogenase, creatine kinase, and aldolase are elevated early in disease course and thus, serve as a useful indicator of disease activity [6]. Of note, levels of creatine kinase can be within the reference range in a significant proportion of patients with JDM, unlike adult dermatomyositis, hence mandating simultaneous measurement of other muscle enzymes levels such as aldolase, lactate dehydrogenase and transaminases [6].

Various scales have been developed and validated to assess disease activity of JDM. Cutaneous assessment tool (CAT, to assess cutaneous involvement), Childhood Myositis Assessment Scale (CMAS, measures muscle strength, and endurance), Childhood Health Assessment Questionnaire (CHAQ, measures proximal muscle strength) and Disease Activity Scale (assesses skin and muscle involvement) have found extensive usage in patient management and studies [5].

Q5. Which of the following drugs is considered a standard treatment for juvenile dermatomyositis?

A. Corticosteroids
B. Intravenous immunoglobulin
C. Mycophenolate mofetil
D. All of the above

Answer: *The correct answer is **D**.*

Corticosteroids, both oral prednisolone and intravenous methylprednisolone, are corner stones of induction of JDM resolution. Early aggressive treatment has been found to be associated with better outcomes [7]. Some authors have suggested to start methotrexate along with corticosteroids irrespective of severity of disease. Methotrexate add-on therapy allows shorter duration of steroids treatment and hence result in less steroid related adverse-effects [7].

Intravenous immunoglobulin, cyclophosphamide, and mycophenolate mofetil have been used by some reports as first-line therapy with favorable outcome. Recently, infliximab, a tumor necrosis factor- α antagonist, has been successfully to treat refractory JDM [6, 7].

In addition to drug therapy, intensive physiotherapy has been found to be safe and useful. Physiotherapy helps in maintaining and restoring muscle strength. Strict photoprotection must be emphasized. Specialist skin care is needed to take care of skin lesions of JDM. European League Against Rheumatism (EULAR) guideline recommends topical tacrolimus (0.1%) or topical steroids for skin lesions, especially for symptomatic patients.

Practical Points

- Presence of the characteristic heliotrope rash on eyelids, violaceus rash in sun exposed areas and the Gottron papules on knuckles, is necessary for the diagnosis of juvenile dermatomyositis
- Symptomatic lung diseases and association with underlying malignancy are more common in adult dermatomyositis compared to juvenile dermatomyositis
- Calcinosis cutis and cutaneous ulcerations is seen up to 30% cases of juvenile dermatomyositis
- Intravenous immunoglobulin, cyclophosphamide, and mycophenolate mofetil are first-line immunosuppressive therapy in juvenile dermatomyositis
- Intensive physiotherapy and strict photoprotection should be started along with systemic therapy

References

1. Pachman LM, Lipton R, Ramsey-Goldman R, Shamiyeh E, Abbott K, Mendez EP, Dyer A, Curdy DM, Vogler L, Reed A, Cawkwell G, Zemel L, Sandborg C, Rivas-Chacon R, Hom C, Ilowite N, Gedalia A, Gitlin J, Borzy M. History of infection before the onset of juvenile dermatomyositis: results from the National Institute of Arthritis and Musculoskeletal and Skin Diseases Research Registry. Arthritis Rheum. 2005;53(2):166–72.
2. Boccaletti V, Di Nuzzo S, Feliciani C, Fabrizi G, Pagliarello C. An update on juvenile dermatomyositis. G Ital Dermatol Venereol. 2014;149(5):519–24.
3. Rider LG, Lachenbruch PA, Monroe JB, Ravelli A, Cabalar I, Feldman BM, Villalba ML, Myones BL, Pachman LM, Rennebohm RM, Reed AM, Miller FW. Damage extent and predictors in adult and juvenile dermatomyositis and polymyositis as determined with the myositis damage index. Arthritis Rheum. 2009;60(11):3425–35.

4. Tansley SL, McHugh NJ, Wedderburn LR. Adult and juvenile dermatomyositis: are the distinct clinical features explained by our current understanding of serological subgroups and pathogenic mechanisms? Arthritis Res Ther. 2013;15(2):211.
5. Ravelli A, Trail L, Ferrari C, Ruperto N, Pistorio A, Pilkington C, Maillard S, Oliveira SK, Sztajnbok F, Cuttica R, Beltramelli M, Corona F, Katsicas MM, Russo R, Ferriani V, Burgos-Vargas R, Magni-Manzoni S, Solis-Valleoj E, Bandeira M, Zulian F, Baca V, Cortis E, Falcini F, Alessio M, Alpigiani MG, Gerloni V, Saad-Magalhaes C, Podda R, Silva CA, Lepore L, Felici E, Rossi F, Sala E, Martini A. Long-term outcome and prognostic factors of juvenile dermatomyositis: a multinational, multicenter study of 490 patients. Arthritis Care Res. 2010;62(1):63–72.
6. Martin N, Li CK, Wedderburn LR. Juvenile dermatomyositis: new insights and new treatment strategies. Ther Adv Musculoskelet Dis. 2012;4(1):41–50.
7. Enders FB, Bader-Meunier B, Baildam E, Constantin T, Dolezalova P, Feldman BM, Lahdenne P, Magnusson B, Nistala K, Ozen S, Pilkington C, Ravelli A, Russo R, Uziel Y, van Brussel M, van der Net J, Vastert S, Wedderburn LR, Wulffraat N, McCann LJ, van Royen-Kerkhof A. Consensus-based recommendations for the management of juvenile dermatomyositis. Ann Rheum Dis. 2017;76(2):329–40.

Chapter 15
Pruritic Erythematous Rashes on Face and Eyelids

Selcen Kundak and Malik Ergin

A 13-year-old girl presented with erythematous, violaceous rash with poikiloderma of the face and eyelids, as well as violaceous papules of the hands overlying the joints and the proximal nail fold (Fig. 15.1a, b), starting some 8-years ago. Myalgia and muscle weakness had associated these lesions since the past 2 years. Her personal and family histories were unremarkable. Skin examination revealed lilac erythema of the upper eyelids which were also edematous. Closer examination revealed violaceous poikiloderma of the cheek and forehead and lichenoid papules on the skin overlying interphalangeal and metacarpophalangeal joints and proximal nail folds, along with cuticular dystrophy and nail fold telangiectasia (Fig. 15.1a, b). No muscle weakness was found in systematically performed neurological examinations and her muscle strength was 5 out of 5. The rest of her physical examinations were unremarkable. Complete blood count, hepatic and renal function tests, complement levels (C3, C4), and serum creatine kinase were within the normal range. ESR was elevated to 34 mm/h and anti-nuclear antibodies was positive. Skin biopsy demonstrated basal vacuolar degeneration and minimal interstitial mucin accumulation in epidermis, along with homogenization and chronic band-like lichenoid lymphohistiocytic inflammation in papillary dermis (Fig. 15.2). Direct immunofluorescence (DIF) showed fibrinogen deposition in papillary dermis.

Q1. What is the most likely diagnosis?

A. Clinically amyopathic juvenile dermatomyositis
B. Subacute cutaneous lupus erythematosus
C. Lichen planus
D. Systemic lupus erythematosus

Answer: *The correct answer is* ***A.***

S. Kundak (✉)
Department of Dermatology, Dr. Behçet Uz Children's Hospital, İzmir, Turkey

M. Ergin
Department of Pathology, Dr. Behçet Uz Children's Hospital, İzmir, Turkey

© Springer Nature Switzerland AG 2020

F. Rahmani, N. Rezaei (eds.), *Pediatric Autoimmunity and Transplantation*,
https://doi.org/10.1007/978-3-030-26280-8_15

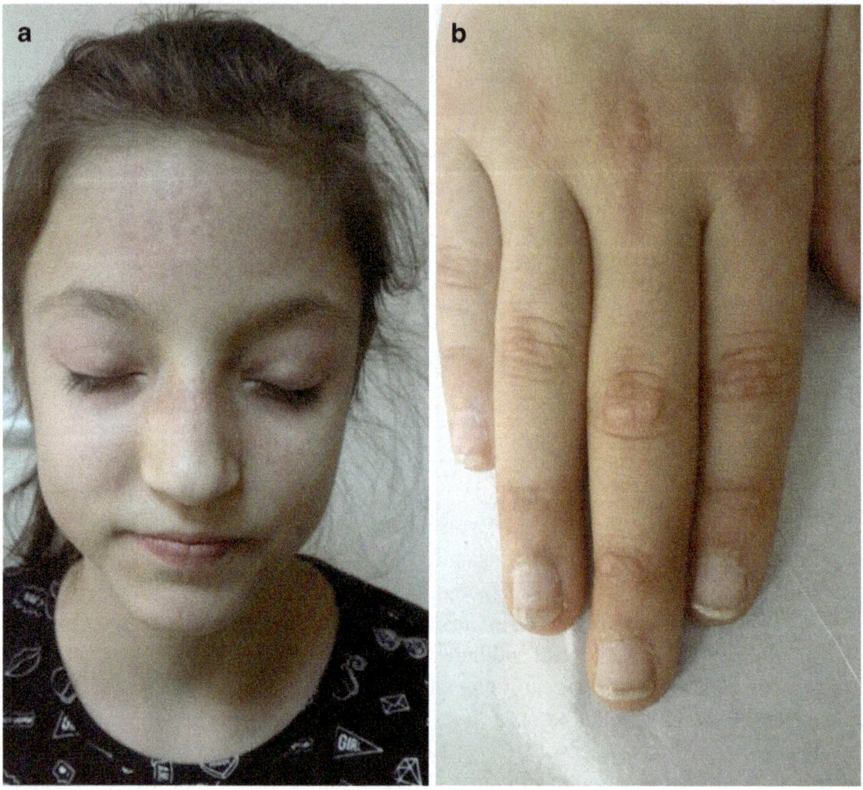

Fig. 15.1 (**a**) poikiloderma of the face (hyperpigmentation, hypopigmentation, telangiectasia and epidermal atrophy) and (**b**) violaceous, flat-topped papules on the skin overlying the interphalangeal and metacarpophalangeal joints, cuticular dystrophy and nail fold telangiectasia

Juvenile dermatomyositis (JDM) is rare autoimmune disease in pediatric population, but account for the most common inflammatory myopathy in childhood [1–6]. Typical clinical findings include proximal muscle weakness, heliotrope rash, Gottron's papules, nail fold capillary changes, skin calcifications and swallowing difficulties [2, 4, 7]. Clinically amyopathic dermatomyositis was first defined by Sontheimer as a subset of dermatomyositis characterized by the absence of clinical signs of muscle involvement and presence of only biopsy-confirmed cutaneous manifestations of dermatomyositis [3, 4]. This patient had complaints of myalgia and weakness but no muscle weakness was found in neurological examinations. Based on the clinical and histological findings and lack of myositis, the patient was diagnosed with clinically amyopathic juvenile dermatomyositis (CAJDM).

Subacute cutaneous lupus erythematosus (SCLE) is characterized by non-scarring papulosquamous skin lesions or annular polycyclic lesions. Lesions usually involve upper trunk and neck and occur along Blaschko lines. Skin biopsy in SCLE is more compatible with epidermal atrophy and less hyperkeratosis. Colloid

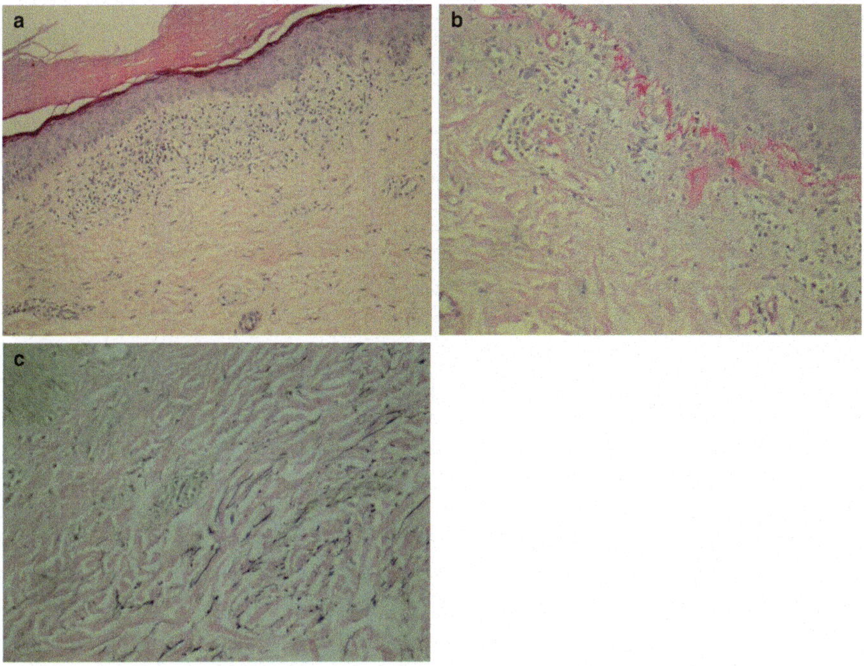

Fig. 15.2 (**a**) Epidermal atrophy, basal vacuolar degeneration and chronic band-like lichenoid lymphohistiocytic inflammation in papillary dermis (H&E, ×100), and (**b**) basement membrane irregularity and minimal interstitial mucin accumulation (PAS-AB, ×200), and (**c**) presence of elastic fibers in the usual appearance of the elastic Von Gieson stain in the dermis (Elastic, ×200)

bodies and epidermal necrosis are also present. Intercellular and intracellular IgG in the basal membrane of the epidermis may be a specific feature for SCLE [2, 4].

Q2. Which one of the following is an appropriate long term follow-up test for this patient?

A. Elevation of serum skeletal muscle enzymes
B. Periodic proximal muscle strength test
C. Periodic electromyography
D. All of the above

Answer: *The correct answer is* ***D.***

CAJDM is by description a functional designation used to refer to either amyopathic dermatomyositis or hypomyopathic dermatomyositis. Subclinical myositis or myopathy may emerge after the onset of skin signs and the onset of weakness can be quite undisclosed [2, 4]. Therefore, all patients with CAJDM should be followed to look for the emergence of myopathy. Proximal muscle strength test, elevation in serum skeletal muscle enzymes, and electromyography should be periodically performed to evaluate myositis.

Q3. What is the most pathognomonic skin sign of dermatomyositis?

A. Lilac erythema and edema of the upper eyelids
B. Nail fold capillary changes
C. Gottron's papules
D. Poikiloderma

Answer: *The correct answer is* ***A.***

Eyelid involvement in dermatomyositis is characteristic, even pathognomonic. Lilac erythema of the upper eyelids which are also edematous is called heliotrope rash. The rest of the facial skin is normal. This feature distinguishes dermatomyositis from lupus erythematosus [2, 4, 8].

Cuticular dystrophy and nail fold telangiectasia are important characteristics of JDM. Nail fold telangiectasia are not included in dermatomyositis classification criteria, as it might reflect a systemic vasculopathy [1, 2, 4, 8]. Secondary lichenoid lesions might develop on extensor surfaces of the hands including the knuckles, elbows and/or knees. These lesions are termed Gottron's papules [2].

Poikiloderma refers to the condition in which hyperpigmentation, hypopigmentation, telangiectasia and epidermal atrophy are all found together. Poikiloderma occurs both in patients with dermatomyositis and in patients with lupus erythematosus, where in the former has violaceous color and in lupus erythematosus poikiloderma is usually red [2, 4]. Of all the above the most pathognomonic and distinctive sign of the dermatomyositis is heliotrope rash.

Q4. Which of the following assessments in necessary in patients with CAJDM?

A. Regular evaluation for the onset of myositis
B. Regular assessment for interstitial lung disease
C. Regular assessment for malignancy
D. All of the above

Answer: *The correct answer is* ***D.***

Although JDM is not associated with increased risk of malignancy, patients with CAJDM appear to be at risk for developing cancers [2, 4, 9].

Interstitial lung disease (ILD) occurs in about 15–30% of patients with DM. A recent study suggested that lung disease is present in about 65% of patients with dermatomyositis [2]. Anti-MDA-5 antibodies have been detected at a significantly higher frequency in CAJDM patients, compared to other patients with dermatomyositis. CAJDM patients with positive anti-MDA-5 antibodies, are at increased risk for developing ILD [2, 4, 9].

Q5. What is the next best step in treatment of this patient?

A. Topical corticosteroid, including potent steroid as monotherapy
B. Oral corticosteroids as monotherapy
C. Low-dose weekly methotrexate in combination with hydroxychloroquine
D. Hydroxychloroquine plus quinacrine

Answer: *The correct answer is* ***C.***

Topical corticosteroid is often insufficient to control CAJDM. Aggressive systemic immunosuppressive treatment is controversial [10]. Oral corticosteroid treatment in combination with hydroxychloroquine or low-dose weekly methotrexate, are as effective in clearing the cutaneous signs. Methotrexate as monotherapy can also be beneficial in controlling skin disease. Due to the high risk of ILD in CAJDM, hydroxychloroquine in combination with low-dose weekly methotrexate treatment seems to be the most appropriate and nonaggressive approach in CAJDM patients. A moderate dose of corticosteroid therapy may also be added to this combination [8]. It should be noted that early severe skin disease in JDM or persistent skin disease at 6 months after diagnosis may predict cardiac dysfunction, worse muscle disease and worse outcomes [8].

Practical Points

- Clinically amyopathic juvenile dermatomyositis (CAJDM) is defined as cases having biopsy-confirmed hallmark cutaneous lesions of classical dermatomyositis occurring for 6 months or longer, without any clinical or biochemical evidence of proximal muscle disease
- Anti-MDA-5 antibodies are associated with CAJDM
- Interstitial lung disease occurs in about 15–30% of patients with dermatomyositis

References

1. Campos LMA, Sallum AME, Camargo CZ, Andrade LEC, Kayser C. Improvement of nailfold capillary microangiopathy after immunosuppressant therapy in a child with clinically amyopathic juvenile dermatomyositis. Rev Bras Reumatol Engl Ed. 2017;57(5):487–90.
2. Jorizzo JL, Sangueza OP. Dermatomyositis. In: Bolognia JL, Jorizzo JL, Rapini RP, editors. Dermatology. Barcelona: Elsevier; 2008. p. 594–603.
3. Okong'o LO, Esser M, Wilmshurst J, Scott C. Characteristics and outcome of children with juvenile dermatomyositis in Cape Town: a cross-sectional study. Pediatr Rheumatol Online J. 2016;14(1):60.
4. Patrick Gordon DC. Dermatomyositis. In: Griffiths CEM, Nickoloff BJ, editors. Rook's textbook of dermatology. 9th ed. Hoboken: Wiley Blackwell; 2016. p. 1496–509.
5. Wakiguchi H, Takei S, Kawano Y. Axillary skin ulcers in infants with juvenile dermatomyositis. Pediatr Neonatol. 2017;58(3):287–8.
6. Orandi AB, Baszis KW, Dharnidharka VR, Huber AM, Hoeltzel MF. Assessment, classification and treatment of calcinosis as a complication of juvenile dermatomyositis: a survey of pediatric rheumatologists by the childhood arthritis and rheumatology research alliance (CARRA). Pediatr Rheumatol Online J. 2017;15(1):71.
7. Khera R, Khare S, Singh SK. Acute presentation of juvenile dermatomyositis with subclinical cardiac involvement: a rare case. J Clin Diagn Res. 2016;10(12):SD01–SD3.
8. Kim S, Kahn P, Robinson AB, Lang B, Shulman A, Oberle EJ, Schikler K, Curran ML, Barillas-Arias L, Spencer CH, Rider LG, Huber AM. Childhood arthritis and rheumatology research alliance consensus clinical treatment plans for juvenile dermatomyositis with skin predominant disease. Pediatr Rheumatol Online J. 2017;15(1):1.
9. Deakin CT, Yasin SA, Simou S, Arnold KA, Tansley SL, Betteridge ZE, McHugh NJ, Varsani H, Holton JL, Jacques TS, Pilkington CA, Nistala K, Wedderburn LR. Muscle biopsy findings

in combination with myositis-specific autoantibodies aid prediction of outcomes in juvenile dermatomyositis. Arthritis Rheumatol (Hoboken NJ). 2016;68(11):2806–16.

10. Spencer CH, Rouster-Stevens K, Gewanter H, Syverson G, Modica R, Schmidt K, Emery H, Wallace C, Grevich S, Nanda K, Zhao YD, Shenoi S, Tarvin S, Hong S, Lindsley C, Weiss JE, Passo M, Ede K, Brown A, Ardalan K, Bernal W, Stoll ML, Lang B, Carrasco R, Agaiar C, Feller L, Bukulmez H, Vehe R, Kim H, Schmeling H, Gerstbacher D, Hoeltzel M, Eberhard B, Sundel R, Kim S, Huber AM, Patwardhan A. Biologic therapies for refractory juvenile dermatomyositis: five years of experience of the Childhood Arthritis and Rheumatology Research Alliance in North America. Pediatr Rheumatol Online J. 2017;15(1):50.

Chapter 16
Edema of Hands and Hypopigmented Lesions on Her Neck and Cheeks

Ana Luisa Rodríguez-Lozano and Marco Yamazaki-Nakashimada

A previously healthy 9-year-old girl noted purplish discoloration and edema on her hands since 8 months ago, along with arthralgia in both wrists and knees, and conjunctival hyperemia starting a few days ago. Her parents had also noted a 6-kg weight loss during the past 1 month. She also complained of dysphagia predominantly with solid meals, bloating, early satiety, and weakness climbing stairs. She was referred to the hospital with a presumptive diagnosis of juvenile arthritis.

On examination she had thickened and lustrous facial skin appearance, with hypopigmented areas with salt and pepper appearance on her neck and cheeks with limited oral aperture (Fig. 16.1a). Raynaud's phenomenon was observed on her distal phalanxes in both hands, and the skin was thickened and hardened over the extensor surfaces of metacarpophalangeal and interphalangeal joints. Salt-and-pepper appearance was also noted on her upper arm and she had experienced pain and difficulty grasping objects since appearance of the lesions (Figs. 16.1b, c).

Laboratory evaluation showed hemoglobin: 13.3 g/dL, WBC: 7600/μL, ANC: 5300/μL, lymphocyte count: 1300/μL, and platelet count: 368,000/μL. Urinalysis, serum urea, creatinine, glucose and liver enzymes were normal with a creatine kinase: 680 IU/mL (reference <150 IU/mL). Immunologic tests reported of a negative rheumatoid factor and anti-double-stranded DNA antibodies (anti-dsDNA), while anti-nuclear antibody (ANA) was positive with homogeneous pattern and a titer of 1:320. She also had hypergammaglobulinemia.

A barium swallow demonstrated a spastic peristaltic wave in the esophagus with no other abnormalities. However a manometry showed an esophageal dysmotility with 100% of failed peristalsis, absent contractility and hypotonic inferior sphincter. Simple thorax radiography demonstrated interstitial pattern and air trapping was shown on the plethysmography, with normal carbon monoxide diffusion capacity on spirometry. Echocardiography reported left ventricle ejection fraction as 66%.

A. L. Rodríguez-Lozano · M. Yamazaki-Nakashimada (✉)
Clinical Immunology Department, Instituto Nacional de Pediatria, Mexico City, Mexico

© Springer Nature Switzerland AG 2020

F. Rahmani, N. Rezaei (eds.), *Pediatric Autoimmunity and Transplantation*,
https://doi.org/10.1007/978-3-030-26280-8_16

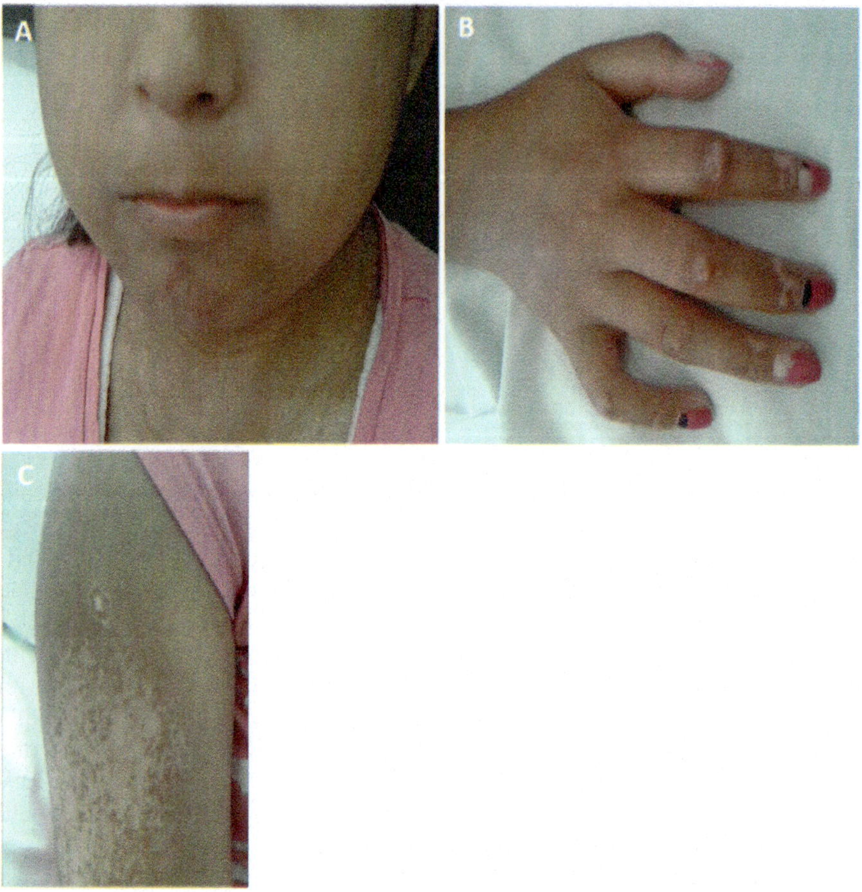

Fig. 16.1 Thickened facial skin appearance with hypopigmented areas with salt and pepper areas and limited oral aperture (**a**). Thickened skin over the extensor surfaces of metacarpophalangeal and interphalangeal joints (**b**), and salt-and-pepper appearance on upper arm (**c**), in a 9-year-old girl

Treatment with corticosteroids and mycophenolate mofetil was started. Four months later the patient presented with progression of her symptoms and complained of dyspnea and increased limitation in hands motility mainly on the interphalangeal joints. On examination, she grumbled of nocturnal reflux, microstomia associated with sharp nose was noted and a decrease in carbon monoxide diffusion capacity to 71% was reported. She has been asymptomatic since 2017, but joint stiffness and skin lesions have continued to progress.

Q1. What is the most likely in this patient?

A. Juvenile idiopathic arthritis
B. Systemic sclerosis
C. Systemic lupus erythematosus
D. Mixed connective tissue disease

Answer: *The correct answer is* ***B.***

Raynaud's phenomenon (RP) is common between different autoimmune diseases, as in systemic lupus erythematosus, mixed connective tissue disease and systemic sclerosis [1, 2]. Raynaud's phenomenon is seen in up to 70% of patients with systemic sclerosis (SSc) on initial presentation [3]. In adults, Raynaud's, confirmed by nail fold capillaroscopy with capillary enlargement or capillary loss, is a strong and independent predictor for development of SSc. Other important predictor is the presence of anti-topoisomerase I, anti-Th/to, anti-SENP-B and anti-RNA polymerase III antibodies in serum [4]. SSc specific antibodies, i.e. anti-Scl-70, anti-centromere, anti-Th/To, anti-RNA polymerase, anti-double stranded-DNA and extractable nuclear antigens, as well as nail bed capillaroscopy is recommended in all patients with Raynaud's phenomenon [1, 5].

Q2. Which set of the following finding are most likely in patients with the aforementioned diagnosis?

A. Raynaud's phenomenon and digital ulcers
B. Arthritis and dysphagia
C. Arthritis and dyspnea
D. Raynaud's phenomenon and proximal skin induration

Answer: *The correct answer is **D**.*

The presence of RP and proximal skin induration are the first and second most frequent signs at the onset in children with SSc [4, 6]. Sclerodactyly, digital pitting, arthralgia, hand's edema, calcinosis, weight loss, dysphagia, arthritis, muscle weakness and dyspnea are among other frequent symptom [6].

Q3. All of the following belong to the American College of Rheumatology (ACR)/European League Against Rheumatism (EULAR) 2013 Classification Criteria for this condition, except?

A. Skin thickening of the fingers of both hands extending proximal to the metacarpophalangeal joints
B. Digital tip ulcers or fingertip pitting scars
C. Normal nail fold capillaries
D. Raynaud's phenomenon
E. Pulmonary arterial hypertension and interstitial lung disease

Answer: *The correct answer is **C**.*

Nail fold capillaroscopy is the most useful clinical tool to discriminate primary from secondary Raynaud's phenomenon [5]. Main indications to perform a capillaroscopy are (1) evaluation and monitoring the transition from primary to secondary Raynaud's phenomenon, (2) early diagnosis of SSc, (3) differential diagnosis of SSc-related conditions, or (4) detection of severe microangiopathy and prognostic evaluation in SSc. Children with SSc present a wide range of abnormalities in capillaroscopy, commonly with dilated loops, avascular areas, followed by irregular loops, hemorrhages, megacapillaries, tortuosity and arborization [6]. The PRES, ACR and EULAR joint efforts led to release of provisional classification criteria for juvenile systemic sclerosis in 2007 [7]. This guideline comprises one major criteria: proximal skin sclerosis/induration of the skin, and multiple minor criteria: sclerodactyly, Raynaud's phenomenon, nail fold capillary abnormalities, digital tip ulcers, gastroesophageal abnormalities, cardiac manifestations, renal crisis, pulmonary abnormalities, neuropathy, musculoskeletal alterations, ANA, and SSc-selective autoantibodies (anti-centromere, anti-toposiomerase I (Scl-70), antifibrillarin, including anti-nucleolar antibodies and anti- Th/To, anti-PM/Scl or anti-RNA polymerase I or III). To classify a patient as having SSc one major criteria plus at least two minor criteria, yields a sensitivity of 90% and specificity of 96% [7].

Q4. Which of the following autoantibodies are most frequent in children with SSc?

A. ANA and anti-topoisomerase I
B. ANA and anti-centromere
C. ANA and anti-dsDNA
D. Anti-neutrophil cytoplasmic antibodies and rheumatoid factor
E. ANA and anti-fibrillarin

Answer: *The correct answer is* ***A.***

It has been noted that the profile of autoantibodies differ between children and adults [8, 9]. Children with SSc show a higher prevalence of ANA and anti-Scl-70 antibodies [4, 6, 10, 11], but not anti-centromere autoantibodies as is frequent in adults [12].

Q5. Which autoantibody is present in myositis and SSc overlap syndrome?

A. Anti-dsDNA antibody
B. Anti-Ro antibody
C. Anti-cardiolipin antibody
D. Anti-PM/Scl antibody

Answer: *The correct answer is* ***D.***

Overlap syndromes in SSc/myositis are rare and have been described mostly in adults (42.6%). However, SSc is the most common connective tissue disease associated with idiopathic inflammatory myopathy [13]. Positive anti-PM/Scl has been reported in this presentation and strongly correlates with this syndrome [14]. Contrary to children, myopathy is associated with poor prognosis in adults with SSc [13, 14].

Q6. Which of the following is the usual first-line immunosuppressant for treatment of SSc children with lung, cardiovascular or gastrointestinal involvement?

A. Steroids and cyclophosphamide or mycophenolate mofetil
B. Steroids and bosentan
C. Steroids and rituximab
D. Bosentan and azathioprine

Answer: *The correct answer is* ***A.***

The management of children with systemic sclerosis has been and still is a challenge. Development of tools, such as the severity score for juvenile systemic sclerosis [15], helps clinicians to better classify a patient from mild to end-stage disease and therefore opt the best treatment option. Methotrexate, prednisone and prostanoids are all recommended for skin, muscle, articular or vascular involvement [16], as seen in this patient. If the patient presents lung, cardiovascular or gastrointestinal involvement, the treatment option should step up to cyclophosphamide, mycophenolate mofetil along with methotrexate [17, 18]. Fortunately, there is a growing interest in the development of targeted therapies base on the pathogenesis of the disease [19–23].

Practical Points

- Raynaud's phenomenon is frequently a prodromal manifestation of systemic sclerosis
- Arthralgia, weight loss, Raynaud's phenomenon and dysphagia are red flags to consider the diagnosis of systemic sclerosis and refer the patient to the specialist
- Myositis is frequently present as an overlapping disease with systemic sclerosis
- Aggressive immunosuppressive therapy is indicated to prevent pulmonary, cardiovascular and gastrointestinal disease in systemic sclerosis

References

1. Pain CE, Constantin T, Toplak N, Moll M, Iking-Konert C, Piotto DP, Aktay Ayaz N, Nemcova D, Hoeger PH, Cutolo M, Smith V, Foeldvari I. Raynaud's syndrome in children: systematic review and development of recommendations for assessment and monitoring. Clin Exp Rheumatol. 2016;34(Suppl 100):200–6.
2. Tellier S, Bader-Meunier B, Quartier P, Belot A, Deslandre C, Kone-Paut I, Tiriau S, Jurquet AL, Rosellini D, Dheu-Bentz C, Mestrallet G, Decramer S. Initial presentation and outcome of pediatric-onset mixed connective tissue disease: a French multicenter retrospective study. Joint Bone Spine. 2016;83(3):369–71.
3. Martini G, Foeldvari I, Russo R, Cuttica R, Eberhard A, Ravelli A, Lehman TJ, de Oliveira SK, Susic G, Lyskina G, Nemcova D, Sundel R, Falcini F, Girschick H, Lotito AP, Buoncompagni A, Sztajnbok F, Al-Mayouf SM, Orbàn I, Ferri C, Athreya BH, Woo P, Zulian F. Juvenile Scleroderma Working Group of the Pediatric Rheumatology European Society. Systemic sclerosis in childhood: clinical and immunologic features of 153 patients in an international database. Arthritis Rheum. 2006;54(12):3971–8.
4. Martini G, Foeldvari I, Russo R, Cuttica R, Eberhard A, Ravelli A, Lehman TJ, de Oliveira SK, Susic G, Lyskina G, Nemcova D, Sundel R, Falcini F, Girschick H, Lotito AP, Buoncompagni A, Sztajnbok F, Al-Mayouf SM, Orban I, Ferri C, Athreya BH, Woo P, Zulian F. Systemic sclerosis in childhood: clinical and immunologic features of 153 patients in an international database. Arthritis Rheum. 54(12):3971–8.
5. Souza EJ, Kayser C. [Nailfold capillaroscopy: relevance to the practice of rheumatology]. Rev Bras Reumatol. 2015;55(3):264–71.

6. Russo RA, Katsicas MM. Clinical characteristics of children with juvenile systemic sclerosis: follow-up of 23 patients in a single tertiary center. Pediatr Rheumatol Online J. 2007;5:6.
7. Zulian FWP, Athreya BH, Laxer RM, Medsger TA, Lehman TJA, et al. The Pediatric Rheumatology European Society/American College of Rheumatology/European League against rheumatism provisional classification criteria for juvenile systemic sclerosis. In: Arthritis Care Res, vol. 57; 2007. p. 203–12.
8. Hatta Y, Hasegawa M, Matsushita T, Hamaguchi Y, Fujimoto M, Takehara K. The clinical characteristics of juvenile-onset systemic sclerosis in Japanese patients. Mod Rheumatol. 2014;24(2):377–9.
9. Alba MA, Velasco C, Simeon CP, Fonollosa V, Trapiella L, Egurbide MV, Saez L, Castillo MJ, Callejas JL, Camps MT, Tolosa C, Rios JJ, Freire M, Vargas JA, Espinosa G. Early- versus late-onset systemic sclerosis: differences in clinical presentation and outcome in 1037 patients. Medicine. 2014;93(2):73–81.
10. Scalapino K, Arkachaisri T, Lucas M, Fertig N, Helfrich DJ, Londino AV Jr, Steen VD, Medsger TA Jr. Childhood onset systemic sclerosis: classification, clinical and serologic features, and survival in comparison with adult onset disease. J Rheumatol. 2006;33(5):1004–13.
11. Györgyi Z, Foeldvari I, Weiser P, Szabó A, Constantin T. Recent advances in systemc scleroderma in childhood. Ann Paediatr Rheum. 2014;3:146–57.
12. Domsic RT. Scleroderma: the role of serum autoantibodies in defining specific clinical phenotypes and organ system involvement. Curr Opin Rheumatol. 2014;26(6):646–52.
13. Paik JJ. Myopathy in scleroderma and in other connective tissue diseases. Curr Opin Rheumatol. 2016;28(6):631–5.
14. Fotis L, Baszis KW, White AJ, French AR. Four cases of anti-PM/Scl antibody-positive juvenile overlap syndrome with features of myositis and systemic sclerosis. J Rheumatol. 2016;43(9):1768–9.
15. La Torre F, Martini G, Russo R, Katsicas MM, Corona F, Calcagno G, Falcini F, Vittadello F, Zulian F. A preliminary disease severity score for juvenile systemic sclerosis. Arthritis Rheum. 2012;64(12):4143–50.
16. Zulian F, Balzarin M, Birolo C. Recent advances in the management of juvenile systemic sclerosis. Expert Rev Clin Immunol. 2017;13(4):361–9.
17. Foeldvari I. Update on juvenile systemic sclerosis. Curr Rheumatol Rep. 2015;17(3):18.
18. Kowal-Bielecka O, Fransen J, Avouac J, Becker M, Kulak A, Allanore Y, Distler O, Clements P, Cutolo M, Czirjak L, Damjanov N, Del Galdo F, Denton CP, Distler JHW, Foeldvari I, Figelstone K, Frerix M, Furst DE, Guiducci S, Hunzelmann N, Khanna D, Matucci-Cerinic M, Herrick AL, van den Hoogen F, van Laar JM, Riemekasten G, Silver R, Smith V, Sulli A, Tarner I, Tyndall A, Welling J, Wigley F, Valentini G, Walker UA, Zulian F, Muller-Ladner U. Update of EULAR recommendations for the treatment of systemic sclerosis. Ann Rheum Dis. 2017;76(8):1327–39.
19. Russell M, Sofat N. Translating autoimmune pathogenesis into targeted therapies for systemic sclerosis. In: Immunopathogenesis and immune-based therapy for selected autoimmune disorders. London: InTech; 2017. p. 97–130.
20. Sakkas LI, Bogdanos DP. Systemic sclerosis: new evidence re-enforces the role of B cells. Autoimmun Rev. 2016;15(2):155–61.
21. Denton CP. Advances in pathogenesis and treatment of systemic sclerosis. Clin Med (Lond). 2015;15(Suppl 6):s58–63.
22. Bruni C, Praino E, Allanore Y, Distler O, Gabrielli A, Iannone F, Matucci-Cerinic M. Use of biologics and other novel therapies for the treatment of systemic sclerosis. Expert Rev Clin Immunol. 2017;13(5):469–82.
23. Reiff A. New insights into the pathogenesis and management of juvenile systemic sclerosis. Int J Clin Rheumatol. 2015;10:97–110.

Chapter 17
Asymptomatic Atrophic Plaque on the Face

Yan Ling Kong and Emily Yiping Gan

A 10-year-old girl presented with a 3-year history of asymptomatic skin changes on the right side of her face, together with partial loss of her right eyebrow. There had been no further progression in the past 1 year. Her vision was unaffected and she denied any neurological symptoms. On examination, she had facial asymmetry with elevation of the right upper eyelid, and a poorly developed right nasal rim. There was an atrophic, sclerotic, shiny brown plaque extending from the right parietal scalp, through the right forehead, to the right nasal bridge (Fig. 17.1). There was no atrophy of the right side of her face and there were no similar lesions elsewhere. Anti-nuclear antibody (ANA) and anti-extractable nuclear antigen (ENA) were negative. ESR was normal at 13 mm/h. The patient declined a skin biopsy.

Q1. What is the most likely diagnosis?

A. *En coup de sabre*
B. Lichen sclerosus et atrophicus
C. Lupus panniculitis
D. Lipodystrophy

Answer: *The correct answer is* ***A***.

Scleroderma may occur as a localized or a systemic disease. Localized scleroderma (LSc), also known as morphea, is a fibrosing condition characterized by thickening and hardening of the skin due to overproduction of collagen. Linear morphea is the most common subtype of LSc in children, and patients present with sclerotic linear or curvilinear plaques with variable associated localized atrophy [1]. When the lesion involves the face or scalp, it is referred to as "*en coup de sabre*"

Y. L. Kong
National Skin Centre, Singapore, Singapore

E. Y. Gan (✉)
Dermatology Service, KK Women's and Children's Hospital, Singapore, Singapore

© Springer Nature Switzerland AG 2020
F. Rahmani, N. Rezaei (eds.), *Pediatric Autoimmunity and Transplantation*,
https://doi.org/10.1007/978-3-030-26280-8_17

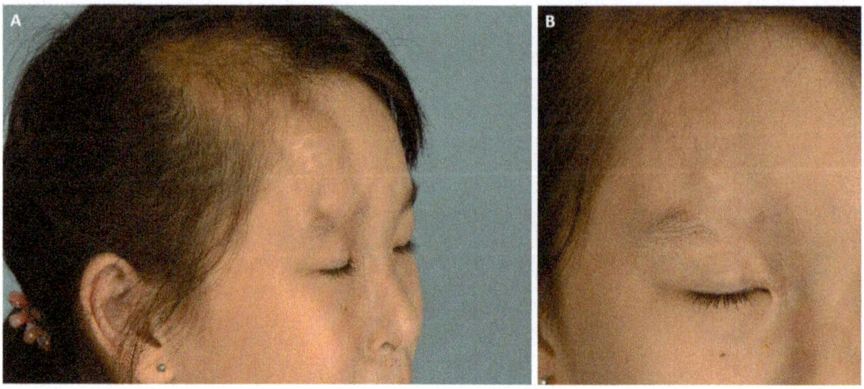

Fig. 17.1 Frontal (**a**) and side (**b**) views of an atrophic, sclerotic, brown plaque extending from the right parietal scalp, through the right forehead, to the right nasal bridge in a 10-year-old girl

(ECDS), as it resembles the strike of a sword. The skin lesions of ECDS undergo an initial inflammatory stage, where patients present with erythematous to violaceous, shiny and indurated plaques. Once the active phase resolves, the skin lesion turns into a nearly complete white sclerotic plaque often with subsequent post-inflammatory hyperpigmentation. Excessive deposition of collagen destroys hair follicles and adnexal structures, resulting in a hairless, anhidrotic plaque. ECDS is a pediatric disease, with a median age of onset of 10 years old [2]. Some authors have postulated that ECDS lie on the same disease spectrum as Parry-Romberg syndrome (PRS), which is a form of progressive hemifacial atrophy that is considered a more severe variant. In PRS, the disease process extends more deeply, often involving the underlying muscle and bone. In contrast to ECDS, the mid- to lower face is frequently affected in PRS [3]. Remission typically occurs after 3–5 years in ECDS, but the disease recurs in about 7% of patients [4].

Q2. What is the most common neurologic symptom associated with this condition?

A. Behavioral changes
B. Movement disorders
C. Intellectual deficit
D. Epilepsy

Answer: *The correct answer is* ***D.***

Central nervous system involvement in ECDS is not rare, and may affect up to 18% of patients [5]. Neurologic symptoms are usually preceded by the cutaneous manifestations, but may also occur concurrently with or after the onset of the skin lesions [6]. Associated neurological manifestations are varied and include seizures, migraines, focal neurological deficits, behavioral changes, movement disorders and progressive intellectual deterioration. Epilepsy, particularly complex partial seizures, remains the most common neurologic symptom associated with ECDS [7]. Classic neuroimaging findings, which are typically found ipsilateral to the skin lesions, include brain parenchyma atrophy, white matter lesions, vascular malformations and calcifications. Calcifications may occur in the basal ganglia, thalami, dentate nuclei and also in the subcortical white matter [8]. Asymptomatic patients are rarely found to have abnormal neuroimaging studies [9].

Q3. If the patient presents with right eye pain, redness and increased sensitivity to light, what is the mostly likely cause of her symptoms?

A. Conjunctivitis
B. Optic neuritis
C. Anterior uveitis
D. Posterior uveitis

Answer: *The correct answer is* ***C****.*

Ocular abnormalities are present in approximately 3% of pediatric patients with LSc, and are more prevalent in those with ECDS [10]. Adnexal abnormalities involving the eyelid and/or eyelashes are the most frequent findings. Anterior uveitis can occur, and patients present with a painful red eye. This condition may be complicated by secondary glaucoma [10]. Ocular symptoms should be actively sought for at every clinical review, and if present, referral to an ophthalmologist is mandatory.

Q4. Assuming the patient agreed to skin biopsy, what would you expect to find in her biopsy?

A. Atrophic epidermis, interface dermatitis and a thickened dermis composed of abundant collagen bundles
B. Atrophic epidermis, homogenized and edematous collagen in the superficial dermis with a band-like lichenoid lymphocytic infiltrate in the mid-dermis
C. Lobular panniculitis, with a lymphoplasmacytic infiltrate and formation of lymphoid follicles
D. Fat necrosis with foamy lipophages, small lipocytes, and a mixed inflammatory infiltrate consisting predominantly of plasma cells and lymphocytes

Answer: *The correct answer is* ***A****.*

Histological features of LSc vary according to the stage and activity of the lesion. Early in the disease, inflammatory lesions are characterized by tissue edema, thickened collaged bundles and a dense interstitial and perivascular inflammatory infiltrate composed primarily of lymphocytes. Biopsies of burnt-out lesions demonstrate a squared-off appearance, with hyalinization of the dermis and thickened collagen bundles. There is also atrophy of the eccrine and pilosebaceus glands, and loss of intradermal fat [11]. Interestingly, the presence of interface dermatitis is a characteristic feature of ECDS, regardless of disease activity [12]. Direct immunofluorescence studies are usually negative.

Q5. Which phototherapy modality is most effective in treatment of the active phase of LSc?

A. Psolaren + ultraviolet A (PUVA)
B. Broadband ultraviolet B (BB-UVB)
C. Narrowband ultraviolet B (NB-UVB)
D. Ultraviolet A (UVA-1)

Answer: *The correct answer is* ***D.***

Various phototherapeutic modalities including, PUVA, NB-UVB, BB-UVA and UVA-1, have been used for the treatment of sclerotic skin diseases, which include ECDS [13–15]. Amongst them, UVA-1 phototherapy has been found to be the most efficacious. This is a specific form of UVA phototherapy that comprises UVA radiation between 340 and 400 nm. The mechanisms through which UVA-1 irradiation improves sclerotic skin disease remain poorly understood. One theory postulates that UVA-1 decreases cellular responsiveness to TGF-beta-1, which is a fibrogenic cytokine [16]. The optimum dose for UVA-1 phototherapy has yet to be determined, but low and medium-dose irradiation were found to be equally efficacious in a randomized trial of 64 patients [13]. Treatments are usually administered three to five times per week [13, 15, 16].

Q6. Which oral immunosuppressive agent is most effective in treatment of the active phase of LSc?

A. Cyclosporine
B. Mycophenolate mofetil
C. Methotrexate
D. Azathioprine

Answer: *The correct answer is* ***C.***

Due to the significant risk of disfigurement and its associated psychosocial consequences, ECDS usually requires more aggressive therapy. Early intervention with immunosuppressive agents during the active, inflammatory phase of the disease is most beneficial. Use of methotrexate alone or with corticosteroids administered either orally or intravenously have been found to be efficacious in the treatment of juvenile LSc, including ECDS [17–19]. The recommended dose of methotrexate is 1 mg/kg/week, and the maximum acceptable weekly dose is 25 mg. Supplementation with folic acid (0.4–1 mg per day) or folinic acid (5 mg weekly) is advised while on treatment with methotrexate [19]. To minimize the risk of relapse, the recommended treatment duration of MTX is at least 2 years [20]. For patients with stable, burnt-out lesions, cosmetic correction of the deformities may be performed. The residual defect may be treated with injectable fillers or autologous fat grafting. Resection of the lesion has also proved to be successful [21]. However, the patient should be warned that the surgical treatment does not prevent a relapse to the active, inflammatory phase.

Practical Points

- Linear morphea is the most common subtype of localized scleroderma in children
- When linear morphea affects the face or scalp it is termed as "En coup de sabre" (ECDS)
- ECDS is commonly associated with neurological complications, with the most common being epilepsy
- Active inflammatory lesions in ECDS require aggressive management with phototherapy or oral immunosuppressive agents
- UVA-1 is the preferred phototherapeutic modality and methotrexate is the oral immunosuppressant of choice

References

1. Miller K, Lehrhoff S, Fischer M, Meehan S, Latkowski J. Linear morphea of the forehead (en coup de sabre). Dermatol Online J. 2012;18(12):22.
2. Blaszczyk M, Królicki L, Krasu M, Glinska O, Jablonska S. Progressive facial hemiatrophy: central nervous system involvement and relationship with scleroderma en coup de sabre. J Rheumatol. 2003;30(9):1997–2004.
3. Polcari I, Moon A, Mathes EF, Gilmore ES, Paller AS. Headaches as a presenting symptom of linear morphea en coup de sabre. Pediatrics. 2014;134(6):e1715–9.
4. Mertens JS, Seyger MM, Kievit W, Hoppenreijs EP, Jansen TL, van de Kerkhof PC, Radstake TR, de Jong EM. Disease recurrence in localized scleroderma: a retrospective analysis of 344 patients with paediatric- or adult-onset disease. Br J Dermatol. 2015;172(3):722–8.
5. Zulian F. Juvenile localized scleroderma: clinical and epidemiological features in 750 children. An international study. Rheumatology. 2006;45(5):614–20.
6. Sartori S, Martini G, Calderone M, Patrizi A, Gobbi G, Zulian F. Severe epilepsy preceding by four months the onset of scleroderma en coup de sabre. Clin Exp Rheumatol. 2009;27:64–7.
7. Chiang KL, Chang KP, Wong TT, Hsu TR. Linear scleroderma "En coup De sabre": initial presentation as intractable partial seizures in a child. Pediatr Neonatol. 2009;50(6):294–8.
8. Kister I, Inglese M, Laxer RM, Herbert J. Neurologic manifestations of localized scleroderma: a case report and literature review. Neurology. 2008;71(19):1538–45.
9. Doolittle DA, Lehman VT, Schwartz KM, Wong-Kisiel LC, Lehman JS, Tollefson MM. CNS imaging findings associated with Parry–Romberg syndrome and en coup de sabre: correlation to dermatologic and neurologic abnormalities. Neuroradiology. 2014;57(1):21–34.
10. Zannin ME, Martini G, Athreya BH, Russo R, Higgins G, Vittadello F, Alpigiani MG, Alessio M, Paradisi M, Woo P, Zulian F. Ocular involvement in children with localised scleroderma: a multi-centre study. Br J Ophthalmol. 2007;91(10):1311–4.
11. Fett N, Werth VP. Update on morphea. J Am Acad Dermatol. 2011;64(2):217–28.
12. Taniguchi T, Asano Y, Tamaki Z, Akamata K, Aozasa N, Noda S, Takahashi T, Ichimura Y, Toyama T, Sugita M, Sumida H, Kuwano Y, Miyazaki M, Yanaba K, Sato S. Histological features of localized scleroderma 'en coup de sabre': a study of 16 cases. J Eur Acad Dermatol Venereol. 2014;28(12):1805–10.

13. Kreuter A, Hyun J, Stücker M, Sommer A, Altmeyer P, Gambichler T. A randomized controlled study of low-dose UVA1, medium-dose UVA1, and narrowband UVB phototherapy in the treatment of localized scleroderma. J Am Acad Dermatol. 2006;54(3):440–7.
14. Kerscher M. PUVA bath photochemotherapy for localized scleroderma. Evaluation of 17 consecutive patients. Arch Dermatol. 1996;132(11):1280–2.
15. El-Mofty M, Mostafa W, El-Darouty M, Bosseila M, Nada H, Yousef R, Esmat S, El-Lawindy M, Assaf M, El-Enani G. Different low doses of broad-band UVA in the treatment of morphea and systemic sclerosis. Photodermatol Photoimmunol Photomed. 2004;20(3):148–56.
16. El-Mofty M, Mostafa W, Esmat S, Youssef R, Bousseila M, Nagi N, Shaker O, Abouzeid A. Suggested mechanisms of action of UVA phototherapy in morphea: a molecular study. Photodermatol Photoimmunol Photomed. 2004;20(2):93–100.
17. Rattanakaemakorn P, Jorizzo JL. The efficacy of methotrexate in the treatment of en coup de sabre (linear morphea subtype). J Dermatolog Treat. 2018;29(2):197–9.
18. Torok KS, Arkachaisri T. Methotrexate and corticosteroids in the treatment of localized scleroderma: a standardized prospective longitudinal single-center study. J Rheumatol. 2012;39(2):286–94.
19. Li SC, Torok KS, Pope E, Dedeoglu F, Hong S, Jacobe HT, Rabinovich CE, Laxer RM, Higgins GC, Ferguson PJ, Lasky A, Baszis K, Becker M, Campillo S, Cartwright V, Cidon M, Inman CJ, Jerath R, O'Neil KM, Vora S, Zeft A, Wallace CA, Ilowite NT, Fuhlbrigge RC. Development of consensus treatment plans for juvenile localized scleroderma: a roadmap toward comparative effectiveness studies in juvenile localized scleroderma. Arthritis Care Res (Hoboken). 2012;64(8):1175–85.
20. Zulian F, Vallongo C, Patrizi A, Belloni-Fortina A, Cutrone M, Alessio M, Martino S, Gerloni V, Vittadello F, Martini G. A long-term follow-up study of methotrexate in juvenile localized scleroderma (morphea). J Am Acad Dermatol. 2012;67(6):1151–6.
21. Franco JPDA, Serra MM, Lima RB, D'Acri AM, Martins CJ. Scleroderma en coup de sabre treated with polymethylmethacrylate—case report. An Bras Dermatol. 2016;91(2):209–11.

Chapter 18
Morbiliform Rash and Fever

Luciana Paula Samorano, João Avancini, and Marcella Soares Pincelli

A 16-year-old girl presented to the pediatric emergency department with a pruriginous morbiliform eruption, fever and diffuse abdominal pain for 5 days (Fig. 18.1). Her physical exam also revealed bilateral cervical and inguinal lymphadenopathy, edema of the face and hands (Fig. 18.2), and fever (101.3 °F/38.5 °C). Examination of the upper respiratory tract had no abnormalities. Abdominal palpation revealed no organomegaly.

Past medical history revealed absence seizures due to vanishing white matter disease, and leukoencephalopathy, and she had started to take carbamazepine 1 month earlier. Patient was admitted to the hospital ward for investigation and treatment.

Main laboratory data revealed leukocytosis with marked eosinophilia, eosinophils: 3160/μL (22.1%), gamma-glutamyl transferase: 1074 U/L (reference range: 5–36), ALP: 654 U/L (reference range: 50–117), AST: 341 IU/L (reference <31), ALT: 288 IU/L (reference <31). Meanwhile, HIV, HBV and HBC, toxoplasmosis, rubella, cytomegalovirus, and Epstein-Barr virus serologies were negative. Chest radiograph was normal. Skin biopsy showed epidermal spongiosis and a moderate perivascular lymphocytic infiltrate associated with eosinophils on superficial dermis.

Q1. What is the most probable diagnosis?

A. Hypereosinophilic syndrome
B. Toxic epidermal necrolysis
C. Drug reaction with eosinophilia and systemic symptoms
D. Leukemia cutis

Answer: *The correct answer is **C**.*

L. P. Samorano (✉) · J. Avancini · M. S. Pincelli
Department of Dermatology, Hospital das Clínicas of the University of São Paulo Medical School, São Paulo, Brazil

© Springer Nature Switzerland AG 2020
F. Rahmani, N. Rezaei (eds.), *Pediatric Autoimmunity and Transplantation*,
https://doi.org/10.1007/978-3-030-26280-8_18

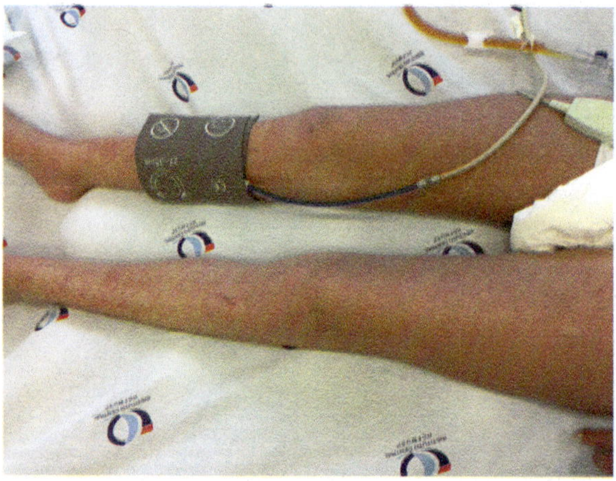

Fig. 18.1 A 16-year-old girl with an acute morbiliform eruption

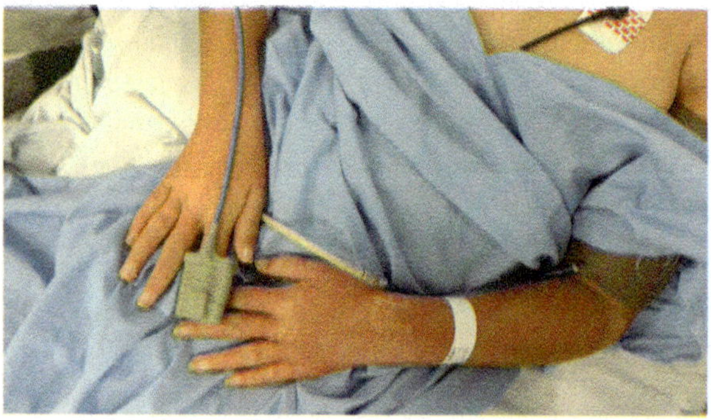

Fig. 18.2 Associated edema on hands of the girl with DRESS

Drug reaction with eosinophilia and systemic symptoms (DRESS) or drug induced hypersensitivity syndrome (DIHS) is characterized by an extensive maculopapular rash, fever and multi-visceral involvement, such as lymphadenopathy, hepatic and hematologic abnormalities as eosinophilia and atypical lymphocytes [1]. Periorbital and facial edema are hallmarks of this syndrome [2].

Exposure to aromatic anticonvulsants such as phenytoin, carbamazepine, and phenobarbital, or allopurinol comprise the majority of patients presenting with DRESS. There are several other drugs described in literature, including antidepressants, sulfonamides and sulfones, nonsteroidal anti-inflammatory drugs, antibiotics, angiotensin-converting enzyme inhibitors, beta blockers, ranitidine, diltiazem, gold salts and azathioprine. Symptoms may appear from 3 weeks to 3 months after the introduction of the drug [3]. Carbamazepine is responsible for 27% of the cases of DRESS/DIHS described in literature [4].

RegiSCAR inclusion criteria for possible cases of DRESS/DIHS can be used in suspect patients, and include: fever above 38 °C or 100.4 °F, acute skin rash, involvement of at least one internal organ such as liver, kidneys, heart and pancreas, lymphopenia or lymphocytosis, eosinophilia, thrombocytopenia, swollen lymph nodes in at least two sites, need for hospitalization, and reaction possibly related to drug [5]. A scoring system also described by the RegiSCAR can be used for the definite diagnosis [5].

Findings of the skin biopsy are not specific and are varied, and can include mild to dense perivascular lymphocytic infiltrate associated with eosinophils on superficial dermis, interface dermatitis and atypical lymphocytes in dermal infiltrate [6]. DRESS/DIHS is a life threatening disease that should be diagnosed with no delay.

Q2. Which of the following microorganisms might be playing a role in the pathogenesis of this disease?

A. Human T cell lymphotropic virus 1
B. *Staphylococcus aureus*
C. *Borrelia burgdorferi*
D. Human herpesvirus 6

Answer: *The correct answer is* ***D.***

Human herpesvirus 6 (HHV-6) reactivation can be seen in patients with clinical manifestations consistent with DRESS/DIHS. HHV-6 reactivation also heralds a worse prognosis for DRESS [7, 8].

A Japanese group included HHV-6 reactivation as a criterion for the diagnosis of DRESS/DIHS in 2007 [9]. Besides HHV-6 reactivation, cytomegalovirus, Epstein-Barr virus and HHV-7 have also been described in association with DRESS/DIHS. It is hypothesized that herpesvirus reactivation in DRESS syndrome may be related to ability of some drug components to stimulate T cells that harbour latent herpesviruses [10, 11].

Q3. Which of the following drugs would be the safest to replace carbamazepine?

A. Phenobarbital
B. Clobazam
C. Lamotrigine
D. Phenytoin

Answer: *The correct answer is* ***B.***

Aromatic anticonvulsants, especially phenytoin, carbamazepine and phenobarbital are the most common causes of DRESS.

This group of drugs is metabolized by the cytochrome P450 system and the product is normally detoxified by the enzymes epoxide hydroxylase or glutathione transferase. Genetic mutations involving the epoxide hydroxylase result in accumulation of toxic metabolites that can affect function of the P450 and lead to immunological responses involving skin or hepatocytes, and also reactivation of viral infections [12].

Although lamotrigine is not considered an aromatic anticonvulsant, it also contains aromatic structure. As cross-reactivity between the various aromatic anticonvulsant drugs is well described, varying between 40 and 80%, lamotrigine should be avoided [3].

Q4. Which of the following medications can be used to treat this patient?

A. Methylprednisolone and ganciclovir
B. Chemotherapy
C. Hydroxychloroquine and methotrexate
D. Radiation therapy

Answer: *The correct answer is* ***A****.*

Systemic corticosteroid is the first choice in the treatment of DRESS/DIHS, usually with 1.0–1.5 mg/kg of prednisone or equivalent as starting dose. Clinical and laboratorial improvement is generally noticed several days after the withdrawal of the culprit drug and introduction of steroid therapy [3, 13, 14]. Anti-herpesvirus medications (ganciclovir, valganciclovir) can be used as add one therapy in severe cases of DRESS/DIHS in which HHV-6 reactivation is detected.

Other drugs described to treat DRESS are high dose IVIG, plasmapharesis and immunosuppressive drugs, such as cyclophosphamide, cyclosporine, interferons, muromonab-CD3, mycophenolate mofetil, and rituximab [15]. Use of N-acetylcysteine may be useful in drug detoxification [16].

Q5. What is the most common cause of death in patients with DRESS?

A. Hyperkalemia and cardiac arrest
B. Hepatic necrosis and liver failure
C. Interstitial pneumonia and respiratory failure
D. Hemophagocytic syndrome

Answer: *The correct answer is* ***B****.*

DRESS syndrome is a potentially life-threatening drug reaction, with an estimated mortality of 10%, primarily because of hepatic necrosis and liver failure [1, 3].

Practical Points

- Drug reaction with eosinophilia and systemic symptoms (DRESS) or drug induced hypersensitivity syndrome (DIHS) is a potentially fatal disease and can be associated with reactivation of herpesvirus, mainly HHV-6
- The main causative drugs are aromatic anticonvulsants and allopurinol
- The prompt withdrawal of the suspect drug is imperative in order to prevent complications, such as skin necrosis and hepatic failure

References

1. Bocquet H, Bagot M, Roujeau JC. Drug-induced pseudolymphoma and drug hypersensitivity syndrome (Drug Rash with Eosinophilia and Systemic Symptoms: DRESS). Semin Cutan Med Surg. 1996;15(4):250–7.
2. Ganeva M, Gancheva T, Lazarova R, Troeva J, Baldaranov I, Vassilev I, Hristakieva E, Tzaneva V. Carbamazepine-induced drug reaction with eosinophilia and systemic symptoms (DRESS) syndrome: report of four cases and brief review. Int J Dermatol. 2008;47(8):853–60.

3. Criado PR, Criado RF, Avancini JM, Santi CG. Drug reaction with Eosinophilia and Systemic Symptoms (DRESS)/Drug-induced Hypersensitivity Syndrome (DIHS): a review of current concepts. An Bras Dermatol. 2012;87(3):435–49.
4. Hagiya H, Iwamuro M, Tanaka T, Hasegawa K, Hanayama Y, Kimura M, Otsuka F. Reactivation of human herpes virus-6 in the renal tissue of a patient with drug-induced hypersensitivity syndrome/drug rash with eosinophilia and systemic symptoms (DIHS/DRESS). Intern Med. 2016;55(13):1769–74.
5. Kardaun SH, Sidoroff A, Valeyrie-Allanore L, Halevy S, Davidovici BB, Mockenhaupt M, Roujeau JC. Variability in the clinical pattern of cutaneous side-effects of drugs with systemic symptoms: does a DRESS syndrome really exist? Br J Dermatol. 2006;155(2):422–8. https://doi.org/10.1111/j.1365-2133.2006.07704.x.
6. Ortonne N, Valeyrie-Allanore L, Bastuji-Garin S, Wechsler J, de Feraudy S, Duong TA, Delfau-Larue MH, Chosidow O, Wolkenstein P, Roujeau JC. Histopathology of drug rash with eosinophilia and systemic symptoms syndrome: a morphological and phenotypical study. Br J Dermatol. 2015;173(1):50–8.
7. Tohyama M, Hashimoto K, Yasukawa M, Kimura H, Horikawa T, Nakajima K, Urano Y, Matsumoto K, Iijima M, Shear NH. Association of human herpesvirus 6 reactivation with the flaring and severity of drug-induced hypersensitivity syndrome. Br J Dermatol. 2007;157(5):934–40.
8. Shiohara T, Kano Y. Drug reaction with eosinophilia and systemic symptoms (DRESS): incidence, pathogenesis and management. Expert Opin Drug Saf. 2017;16(2):139–47.
9. Shiohara T, Iijima M, Ikezawa Z, Hashimoto K. The diagnosis of a DRESS syndrome has been sufficiently established on the basis of typical clinical features and viral reactivations. Br J Dermatol. 2007;156(5):1083–4. https://doi.org/10.1111/j.1365-2133.2007.07807.x.
10. Oskay T, Karademir A, Erturk OI. Association of anticonvulsant hypersensitivity syndrome with Herpesvirus 6, 7. Epilepsy Res. 2006;70(1):27–40.
11. Seishima M, Yamanaka S, Fujisawa T, Tohyama M, Hashimoto K. Reactivation of human herpesvirus (HHV) family members other than HHV-6 in drug-induced hypersensitivity syndrome. Br J Dermatol. 2006;155(2):344–9.
12. Husain Z, Reddy BY, Schwartz RA. DRESS syndrome: Part I. Clinical perspectives. J Am Acad Dermatol. 2013;68(5):693.e691–14; quiz 698–706
13. Chiou CC, Yang LC, Hung SI, Chang YC, Kuo TT, Ho HC, Hu S, Hong HS, Chung WH. Clinicopathological features and prognosis of drug rash with eosinophilia and systemic symptoms: a study of 30 cases in Taiwan. J Eur Acad Dermatol Venereol. 2008;22(9):1044–9.
14. Avancini J, Maragno L, Santi CG, Criado PR. Drug reaction with eosinophilia and systemic symptoms/drug-induced hypersensitivity syndrome: clinical features of 27 patients. Clin Exp Dermatol. 2015;40(8):851–9.
15. Husain Z, Reddy BY, Schwartz RA. DRESS syndrome: Part II. Management and therapeutics. J Am Acad Dermatol. 2013;68(5):709.e701–9; quiz 718–720
16. Tas S, Simonart T. Management of drug rash with eosinophilia and systemic symptoms (DRESS syndrome): an update. Dermatology. 2003;206(4):353–6.

Chapter 19
Recurrent Interstitial Keratitis and Audiovestibular Dysfunction

Kristina A. Dzhuma, Oleg B. Iaremenko, and Maksym I. Situkho

A 17-year-old girl presented to the department of otorhinolaryngology with severe vertigo, vestibular ataxia, feeling of fullness in the ear, nausea, and vomiting. She had experienced progressive hearing loss on the left ear, partial hearing loss on the right one, and tinnitus in both ears all in 1 week. Current symptoms started 2 weeks ago and were considered and treated as Meniere's disease, however, the hearing deficit had aggravated despite low doses of prednisolone and diuretics.

She had a history of influenza and recurrent interstitial keratitis since 2 months ago. Ulcerous interstitial inflammation of the left cornea was noted on current visit. Her physical examination findings were unremarkable, with no signs of other neurological disorders.

The patient was admitted to the hospital for further evaluation. Head and internal ear MRI were insignificant. Laboratory studies were negative for herpes or borreliosis and syphilis. CBC revealed WBC count elevated up to 17 cells/μL with 80% neutrophils in differential count. She had elevated ESR (22 mm/h). ENT examination showed no signs of middle ear inflammation. Pure-tone audiograms documented left-sided moderate-to-severe sensorineural hearing loss and right-sided mild sensorineural hearing loss. No systemic manifestations were found.

Q1. What is the most likely diagnosis?

A. Congenital Rubella
B. Acute otitis media
C. Otosclerosis

K. A. Dzhuma (✉)
Bogomolets National Medical University, National Specialized Children's Hospital, Kyiv, Ukraine

O. B. Iaremenko
Department of Internal Medicine, Bogomolets National Medical University, Kyiv, Ukraine

M. I. Situkho
O. Kolomijchenko Otolaryngology Institute, Kyiv, Ukraine

© Springer Nature Switzerland AG 2020

F. Rahmani, N. Rezaei (eds.), *Pediatric Autoimmunity and Transplantation*,
https://doi.org/10.1007/978-3-030-26280-8_19

D. Electrolyte imbalance with prednisolone use
E. Cogan's syndrome

Answer: *The correct answer is* ***E.***

Cogan's syndrome (CS) is a rare presumed autoimmune disorder characterized by non-syphilitic interstitial keratitis and Meniere's syndrome-like audiovestibular dysfunction [1]. Congenital rubella is among differential diagnoses of sensorineural hearing loss, with direct chochlear damage and relative sparing of vestibular system. In this patients however, her age, history of vaccination and vestibular symptoms ruled out this diagnosis. Otosclerosis yields to predominantly conductive hearing loss and cannot justify patients high ESR. Electrolyte imbalance rarely happens with low dose prednisolone. In this patient her symptoms started before taking prednisolone, and her hearing loss could not be justified by this diagnosis. Otitis media does not involve internal ear, nor does yield to cochlear or vestibular symptoms.

Haynes et al. proposed in 1980 diagnostic criteria for patients, differentiating two forms of clinical presentation: typical and atypical CS. The real incidence of CS is not known [2]. Since CS was first described in 1945, 300 cases have been reported in the literature, although this is likely an underrepresentation of its prevalence as it can easily go undiagnosed [3]. CS occurs primarily in young adults in the third decade, with no apparent gender or racial specific prevalence [4–6]. CS may also occur in children and the elderly [7].

CS is believed not to be hereditary. Its etiology and pathogenesis are still unknown, but it has currently been assumed to be an immune-mediated disorder with vasculitis [8, 9]. Autoimmunologic mechanism has been suggested based on the demonstration of antibodies against corneal tissue, inner ear and endothelial antigens. A viral infection can set-off autoimmunologic phenomena via a number of mechanisms, i.e. antigenic mimicry, self-perpetuating inflammation by cytokine release and unveiling hidden epitopes. Additionally to the clinical similar features some of the autoantigens have been identified, mainly against CD148 and connexine 26 as well as the other serum antibodies such as antineutrophil cytoplasmatic autoantibodies or rheumatoid factor have been identified that support to the autoimmune nature of the disease [10, 11]. Nevertheless, they are not consistently demonstrated in all CS patients and do not always correlate with clinical signs of activity.

Q2. Which of the following pathomechanisms is <u>unlikely</u> involved in this patient?

A. Neurolabyrinthitis
B. Fibrous tissue in Cochlea and Labyrinth
C. Endolymphatic hydrops
D. Occlusion of the Cochlear duct with cholesteamatous debri

Answer: *The correct answer is* ***D.***

Temporal bone histological analysis has shown atrophy of the organ de Corti, fibrous tissue and bone proliferation that involves the cochlea and vestibular labyrinths, demyelination of the eighth cranial nerve, degeneration of the sensory receptors and endolymphatic hydrops [1, 9]. Cytopathologic studies have demonstrated that polymorphonuclear cells arrive first in the sites of inflammation, followed by T cells and B cells, with secretion of specific antibodies as a relatively late event. Concomitant is the formation of a dense extracellular matrix, which ultimately results in ossification of the inner ear [12]. These histopathologic findings suggest that the pathogenesis of sensorineural hearing loss in CS may be related to an immunologic mechanism secondary to an inflammatory attack on the membranous labyrinth [1, 9].

Q3. Which of the following diagnostic modalities would be unnecessary in a patient with progressive hearing loss and vestibular symptoms?

A. MRI study of the cerebellopontine angle
B. Antibody testing for TORCH
C. Audiometry
D. Serology for autoimmune encephalopathies
E. Checking systemic inflammation markers

Answer: *The correct answer is* ***B.***

Diagnosis of CS is often missed or delayed because it is a rare disease, there is no confirmatory test and its clinical sings at the onset are not specific [13]. CS should be suspected whenever there is a close temporal association between ocular abnormalities and cochleovestibular symptoms [5]. Lab results are usually non-diagnostic and non-specific. Patients may have leukocytosis, anemia, thrombocytosis or raised inflammatory markers although none of these are discriminatory. Autoantibodies are usually negative [14]. Only in 15% of cases low titters of rheumatoid factor, antinuclear antibodies and cryoglobulins may be detected [12]. Patients exhibiting hearing loss should undergo imaging studies as part of their initial evaluation [10]. MRI and CT scan may look for enhancement of inner ear structures as well as the absence of eighth nerve tumors [14]. Based on all these reasons, the diagnosis of CS is a challenge and based upon a good response to corticosteroid treatment.

Q4. All of the following should be considered in the differential diagnoses of a patient with Cogan's syndrome?

A. Wegener's granulomatosis
B. Polyarthritis nodosa
C. Giant cell arteritis
D. Takayasu arteritis
E. Sarcoidosis

Answer: *The correct answer is* ***B.***

A wide spectrum of infectious and immunologic conditions that cause ocular manifestations associated with audiovestibular dysfunction and hearing loss should be consider in the differential diagnosis, such as Wegener's granulomatosis, giant cell arteritis, Takayasu arteritis, sarcoidosis, rheumatoid arthritis, Ménière's disease with ocular inflammation or coincident unrelated eye and ear disease [10].

Q5. What is the most appropriate long-term management for this patient?

A. Systemic corticosteroid
B. External endolymphatic drainage
C. Cyclophosphamide
D. Diuretics
E. Cochlear replacement

Answer: *The correct answer is* ***A.***

Treatment of CS is difficult, and the information found in the literature is based upon clinical case reports, there are no randomized clinical trials to guide decisions [7, 15]. Due to the possible autoimmune pathogenesis of this disease, the first choice in immunosuppressive therapy is glucocorticoids [15, 16]. High dose systemic corticosteroid treatment should be initiated with a favourable response expected in 82% [14]. When no improvement is achieved, this treatment should be stopped rapidly after 2 weeks. On the other hand, when improvement is seen, the prednisone dose can be tapered gradually within 2–6 months based upon responses on the audiogram test [17]. In case of corticosteroid treatment failure or for patients requiring high doses or prolonged treatment courses, immunosuppressive agents such as cyclophosphamide, methotrexate or cyclosporine A are added, with various levels of reported success [7, 17]. TNF-alpha blockers like etanercept, infliximab or rituximab are a category of immunosuppressive agents representing a novel therapeutic option in CS [8]. Cochlear implantation is an excellent treatment modality for the profound hearing loss in CS [7].

Q6. All of the following conditions are associated with poor prognosis in this patient, <u>except</u>:

A. Delay in onset of treatment
B. High serum ESR levels
C. Lack of clinical response to prednisolone
D. History of keratitis since childhood
E. Involvement of coronary and renal vessels and the aorta

Answer: *The correct answer is* ***D.***

Systemic manifestations such as vasculitis of medium and large size vessels which are more frequent for the atypical forms have worse prognosis with the mortality rate 10% depending the organ effected [18]. In addition to ocular and vestibuloauditory dysfunctions, 70% of patients have underlying systemic disease associated with vasculitis. Vasculitis usually affects medium-sized vessels, although any sized vessel may be affected [19]. The prognosis for hearing loss is poor in long-term especially when there is long interval between the onset of ocular manifestations and hearing loss or ataxia, as in this patient. Furthermore, a long delay between the onset of symptoms and the initiation of treatment can issue irreversible atrophy and degeneration in the inner ear structures [2]. The early use, within 2 weeks of onset of high-dose oral corticosteroids can reduce the severity of hearing loss to mild or moderate, but not reverse it all together [5].

Practical Points

- Cogan's syndrome is a rare presumed autoimmune disorder characterized by non-syphilitic interstitial keratitis and Meniere's syndrome-like audiovestibular dysfunction
- Patients exhibiting hearing loss should undergo imaging studies as part of their initial evaluation
- Important differential diagnoses include: Wegener's granulomatosis, giant cell arteritis, Takayasu arteritis, sarcoidosis, rheumatoid arthritis, and Ménière's disease with ocular inflammation or coincident unrelated eye and ear disease
- High dose systemic corticosteroid treatment should be initiated with a favourable response expected in 82%

References

1. Cogan DS. Syndrome of nonsyphilitic interstitial keratitis and vestibuloauditory symptoms. Arch Ophtalmol. 1945;33:144–9.
2. Haynes BF, Kaiser-Kupfer MI, Mason P, Fauci AS. Cogan syndrome: studies in thirteen patients, long-term follow-up and a review of the literature. Medicine. 1980;59(6):426–41.
3. Grasland A, Pouchot J, Hachulla E, Blétry O, Papo T, Vinceneux P. Typical and atypical Cogan's syndrome: 32 cases and review of the literature. Rheumatology. 2004;43:1007–15.
4. Tayer-Shifman IO, Tovi H. Cogan's syndrome—clinical guidelines and novel therapeutic approaches. Clin Rev Allergy Immunol. 2014;47:65–72.
5. Jung DH, Nadol JB, Folkerth RD, Merola JF. Histopathology of the inner ear in a case with recent onset of Cogan's syndrome: evidence for vasculitis. Ann Otol Rhinol Laryngol. 2016;125:20–4.
6. Bovo R, Ciorba A, Trevisi P, Aimoni C, Cappiello L, Castiglione A, Govoni M, Martini A. Cochlear implant in Cogan syndrome. Acta Otolaryngol. 2011;131:494–7.
7. Greco A, Gallo A, Fusconi M, Magliulo G, Turchetta R, Marinelli C, Macri GF, De Virgilio A, De Vincentiis M. Cogan's syndrome: an autoinmune inner ear disease. Autoimmun Rev. 2013;12:396–400.
8. Jung HH. Side selection for cochlear implantation in a case of Cogan's syndrome. J Lanryngol Otol. 2008;122:310–3.
9. Espinoza GM, Prost A. Cogan's syndrome and other vasculitides. Curr Rheumatol Rep. 2015;17:24–8.
10. Bacciu A, Pasanisi E, Di Lella F, Guida M, Bacciu S, Vicenti V. Cochlear implantation in patients with Cogan's syndrome: long-term results. Eur Arch Otorhinolaryngol. 2015;272:3201–7.
11. Cundiff J, Kansal S, Kumar A, Goldstein DA, Howard H. Tessler, Cogan's syndrome: a cause of progressive hearing deafness. Am J Otolaryngol Head Neck Med Surg. 2006;27:68–70.
12. Wang JR, Yueng HW, Shipp DB, Stewart S, Lin VY, Chen JM, Nedzelski JM. Cochlear implantation in patients with autoimmune inner ear diseases including Cogan syndrome: a comparison with age- and sex-matched controls. The Lanryngoscope. 2010;120:2478–83.

13. Lee LY, Majid Akhtar M, Kirresh O, Giibson T. Interstitial keratitis and sensorineural hearing loss as a manifestation of rheumatoid arthritis: clinical lessons from a rare complication. BMJ Case Rep. 2012;2012:2.
14. Vasileiadis I, Stratoudaki R, Karakostas E. Complete restoration of auditory impairment in a pediatric case of Cogan's syndrome: report of a rare case with long-term follow-up and literature review. Int J Pediatr Otorhinolaryngol. 2012;76(4):601–5.
15. Gluth MB, Baratz KH, Matteson EL, Driscolli CL. Cogan syndrome: a retrospective review of 60 patients throughout a half century. Mayo Clin Proc. 2006;81:483–8.
16. Teece KH, Olund AP. Audiological Management of Cogan's syndrome. Semin Hear. 2011;32:308–20.
17. Migliori G, Battisti E, Pari M, Vitelli N, Cingolani C. A shifty diagnosis: Cogan's syndrome. A case report and review of the literature. Acta Otorhinolayngol Ital. 2009;29(2):108–13.
18. Baumann A, Helbling A, Oertle S, Häusler R. Cogan's syndrome: clinical evolution of deafness and vertigo in three patients. Eur Arch Otorhinolaryngol. 2005;262:45–9.
19. Ghadban R, Couret M, Zenone T. Efficacy of infliximab in Cogan's syndrome. J Rheumatol. 2008;35:2456–8.

Chapter 20
Breathlessness and Weight Loss

Sowmya Shashidhara, H. Koushik, and Sangita Trivedi

A 15-year-old Asian girl is seen for fever and breathlessness since 5 days ago. She reports no complaint of weight loss, night sweats or wheeze, cyanosis or syncopal episodes. She was vaccinated according to national guidelines and the mother, who is currently at 30 weeks of gestation, has received no prenatal care during any of her deliveries. Her medical history at birth is therefore unavailable. She has a younger brother who is apparently well. She has a history of recurrent episodes of cough and cold since 3 years of age and underwent tonsillectomy for the same reason. On examination, her temperature was 37 °C and she was tachypneic and tachycardic with a blood pressure of 94/60 mmHg. Her BMI was 15.7 kg/m^2. Auscultation of her lungs revealed fine bilateral crepitation with decreased air entry in all lung fields. Laboratory examination revealed leukocytosis (neutrophils: 46% and lymphocytes: 31%). A chest X-ray is as shown in Fig. 20.1.

She was started on cephalosporins and aminoglycosides to which she showed no response. Five days into her antibiotic regimen, her breathlessness worsened with increasing lung shadows on X-ray. Arterial blood gas was obtained due to progressive dyspnea, revealing pO_2: 36 mmHg, pCO_2: 43 mmHg, pH: 7.34, and HCO_3:

S. Shashidhara (✉)
Department of Pediatrics, Kasturba Medical College, Manipal University, Manipal, Karnataka, India

Network of Immunity in Infection, Malignancy and Autoimmunity (NIIMA), Universal Scientific Education and Research Network (USERN), Manipal, Karnataka, India
e-mail: sowmya.s@manipal.edu

H. Koushik
Department of Pediatrics, Kasturba Medical College, Manipal University, Manipal, Karnataka, India

S. Trivedi
Department of Pediatrics, Government Medical College, Veer Narmad South Gujarat University, Surat, Gujarat, India

© Springer Nature Switzerland AG 2020

F. Rahmani, N. Rezaei (eds.), *Pediatric Autoimmunity and Transplantation*,
https://doi.org/10.1007/978-3-030-26280-8_20

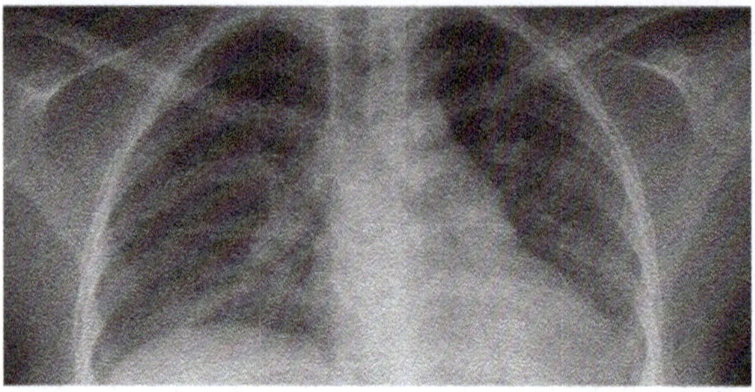

Fig. 20.1 Chest X-ray of a girl with breathlessness

22 meq/L. She was sexually inactive and has not received any blood products. Due to high index of suspicion, a resident performs an ELISA antibody test against human immunodeficiency virus (HIV) which is positive, and her $CD4^+$ levels are found to be as low as 4 cells/μL.

Q1. Which of the following conditions is suggestive for stage 4 of HIV infection in the described case?

A. Unexplained severe wasting, stunting or severe malnutrition not responding to standard therapy
B. Acute necrotizing ulcerative gingivitis/periodontitis
C. Extensive molluscum contagiosum
D. Persistent generalized lymphadenopathy
E. Symptomatic lymphoid interstitial pneumonitis
F. Unexplained persistent parotid enlargement

Answer: *The correct answer is* ***A***.

Pneumocystis pneumonia is an AIDS-defining illness and categorized as suggestive for stage 4 of HIV according to WHO classification of pediatric HIV. Unexplained severe wasting, stunting or severe malnutrition not responding to standard therapy is also an indication of stage 4 HIV infection in infants and children according to WHO classification revised in 2010. On the contrary, unexplained moderate malnutrition not responding to standard therapy, symptomatic lymphoid interstitial pneumonitis, and acute necrotizing ulcerative gingivitis/periodontitis are defined in stage 3 HIV. Unexplained persistent parotid enlargement and extensive molluscum contagiosum are features of stage 2 HIV. Finally, persistent generalized lymphadenopathy is usually asymptomatic and accompanies stage 1 HIV.

In the above-described case, patient's respiratory distress discordant with arterial blood oxygenation levels led to suspicion of *Pneumocystis jirovecii* pneumonia. Severe grade 3 malnutrition is an additional finding suggesting a clinical diagnosis of stage 4 HIV. Treatment with oxygen, high-dose co-trimoxazole, and dexamethasone is warranted in these cases. Initiation of anti-retroviral therapy (ART) is recommended after standard treatment course of PCP pneumonia for 3 weeks, or any other AIDS defining opportunistic infection [1].

Q2. Which of the following receptors is most likely the mediator for HIV transmission responsible for this patient's contamination?

A. Toll-like receptors
B. CD195
C. CXCR4
D. MHC class I receptors

Answer: *The correct answer is* ***B****.*

CCR5 and CXCR4 are structurally related chemokine receptors belonging to the superfamily of the seven-transmembrane G-protein coupled receptors present on $CD4^+$ T cells. The vast majority of vertically transmitted HIV-strains are R5-tropic and therefore depend on CCR5 also known as CD195, as a co-receptor to infect $CD4^+$ T cells as well as macrophages. In human infants, $CCR5^+$ $CD4^+$ T cells are virtually absent in cord blood [2], but abundant in the intestinal mucosa and are highly susceptible to HIV infection [3]. Toll-like receptors are implicated in persistent immune activation in chronically infected HIV individuals and do not play a role in primary HIV infection [4]. CXCR4/CD184 is a chemokine receptor specific to $CD4^+$ cells that HIV utilizes to infect $CD4^+$ T cells. These isolates are thus traditionally known as T cell tropic isolates. Typically, T cell tropic isolates are found late in infection and are suspected to be responsible for $CD4^+$ count decline in late disease. HIV Nef protein reduces the level of cell surface MHC class I protein expression and thus protects the HIV-infected cells from recognition by cytotoxic T lymphocyte [5].

Q3. Which of the following cells in the placenta mediates transmission of HIV from the mother to the fetus?

A. Hofbauer cells
B. T cells
C. B cells
D. NK cells
E. Neutrophils

Answer: *The correct answer is* ***A****.*

Placental macrophages (Hofbauer cells) are principal mediators in the in-utero transmission of HIV-1. Hofbauer cells express elevated concentrations of regulatory cytokines, which inhibit HIV-1 replication in vitro and possess inherent antiviral properties. Hofbauer cells harbor HIV-1 in intracellular compartments and allow its replication. The placenta shows a variety of mechanisms to limit HIV-1 replication. It has been suggested that de novo activaiton of placental Hofbauer cells by cytomegalovirus may overcome this protection and enable in-utero transmission of HIV-1 [6].

At follow-up visit after 6 months, she complained of diarrhea lasting for more than 1 month, weight loss of 12% and was significantly dehydrated. Stool microscopy with modified acid-fast staining showed parasite oocysts (4–6 μm) having distinct walls appearing light pink to bright red.

Q4. Which of the following drugs is least likely to be used to treat this condition?

A. Zinc supplementation
B. ORS supplementation
C. Nitazoxanide
D. Highly active ART (HAART) therapy
E. Co-trimoxazole
F. Vitamin A supplementation

Answer: *The correct answer is* ***C.***

Diarrhea in HIV-infected children may be either acute (<7 days), or chronic (i.e. three or more loose stools daily for >14 days). Cryptosporidiosis is caused by a protozoan that infects the lining of the small intestine and results in severe chronic diarrhea and malabsorption. Patients with $CD4^+$ counts <100 cells/μL are at greatest risk. Watery diarrhea, abdominal pain, nausea, vomiting, weight loss, loss of appetite and dehydration are common manifestations of cryptosporidiosis. There is presently no WHO endorsement for managing Cryptosporidium infection, and treatment of HIV-infected children with cryptosporidiosis has proved particularly challenging because of low efficacy of the existing drugs. Evidence on superiority of nitazoxanide over supportive care for chronic diarhhea in HIV is of low quality, and no significant developments in oocyst clearance or mortality is found after 8 days in immunocompromised children and adults [7]. Vitamin A supplementation is suggested for all HIV-infected and HIV-exposed infants and generally for children aged 6 months to 5 years. Recommended dose for HIV supplementation is 100,000 IU every 6 months for infants between 6 and 12 months, and 200,000 IU for those aged >12 months [8]. Elemental zinc supplementation for 10–14 days is acclaimed, to be combined with increased fluids and continued feeding, for all HIV-infected and HIV-exposed children with diarrhea. The recommended dose is 10 mg/day for infants under 6 months of age and 20 mg/day for infants and children more than 6 months [8].

With further enquiring, the father was revealed to be a truck driver, and her mother tested subsequently, to be found positive for anti-retroviral infection.

Q5. If a mother with HIV infections choses to breastfeed her child, which condition excludes any chances for perinatal transmission in this child? (NAT: nucleic acid testing)

A. Negative NAT at 6 weeks of age
B. Negative antibody testing at 6 weeks of age
C. Negative antibody testing at 18 months while not on breastfeeding for the last 3 months
D. Negative NAT testing at 18 months while not on breastfeeding for the last 3 months

Answer: *The correct answer is* ***C.***

According to WHO guidelines for diagnosis and treatment of HIV in children, all HIV-exposed infants should have HIV virological analysis at 4–6 weeks or at the earliest opportunity after that [9]. HIV infection in infants is only entirely established with virological measurement using nucleic acid testing (NAT) technology due to presence of maternal anti-HIV antibody in child's blood by up to 18 months of age [9]. Hence, a negative NAT at 6 weeks of age, performed on a breastfeed infant does not exclude HIV infection altogether. In developing countries, infants HIV positive mothers are advised to continue breastfeeding if there are financial constraints for alternate feeds as the risk of infection is higher in mixed breastfed/formula infants. Infants who are still breastfed remain at risk for HIV acquisition. These patients will require an age-appropriate testing strategy at the end of the breastfeeding period to either definitively exclude HIV infection or determine final HIV status [9]. Serological testing is recommended to assess HIV infection, providing best results 3 months after cessation of breastfeeding. A negative antibody test after 3 months of termination of breastfeeding is considered as the exclusion of the infection and does not require NAT confirmation [1].

Patients' mother delivers the child, and the child is given recommended postnatal care. At follow-up at 6 weeks, NAT is positive for p24 antigen and treatment is initiated according to the current WHO recommendations for ART in children <3 years.

Q6. Which of the following drug: side-effect pairs are more likely to occur during ART regimen in a newborn?

A. Hypercytemia due to zidovudine
B. Pancreatitis, fat redistribution due to stavudine
C. Acute kidney injury due to tenofovir
D. Hepatotoxicity secondary to efavirenz
E. Dyslipidemia due to lopinavir
F. IRIS secondary to emtricitabine

Answer: *The correct answer is* ***E****.*

ART should be introduced to all children living with confirmed HIV, regardless of WHO clinical stage or at any CD4$^+$ cell count. As a priority, ART should be started in all children ≤2 years of age diagnosed as being infected or children younger than 5 years old with WHO clinical stage 3 or 4 or CD4$^+$ count ≤750 cells/μL or CD4 percentage (1, 2). For infants and children younger than 3 years, the nucleoside reverse transcriptase inhibitors (NRTI) backbone for an ART regimen should be abacavir (ABC) or zidovudine (AZT) + lamivudine (3TC). An lopinavir (LPV)/ritonavir-based regimen must be used as first-line ART for all children infected with HIV younger than 3 years (36 months) of age, irrespective of non-NRTI exposure. If lopinavir/ritonavir is not feasible, treatment should be initiated with an nevirapine (NPV)-based regimen. Considering above discussed treatment regimens, as this child is aged <3 years is likely to have received ABC or AZT / 3TC / LPV or NVP. Therefore, stavudine, tenofovir, emtricitabine, efavirenz are not the possible options. Zidovudine and lopinavir are part of the regimen. As AZT is known to cause anemia and lopinavir (protease inhibitors), tenofovir, lamivudine cause dyslipidemia, we would anticipate problems related to those drugs. So, 1 and 5 are appropriate answers [1, 10].

Practical Points

- Patients presenting with disproportionate hypoxia and pneumonia unresponsive to conventional antibiotics have a high index of suspicion for Pneumocystis pneumonia
- *Pneumocystis jirovecii* pneumonia is an AIDS-defining infection
- Placental macrophages and CD195 receptors are implicated in the pathogenesis of HIV
- Prompt initiation of highly active anti-retroviral therapy (HAART) therapy can resolve cryptosporidiosis infection in patients with HIV, even with no antibiotic therapy
- Exclusion of HIV infection is possible with antibody testing after at least 3 months of cessation of breastfeeding
- Evaluation of anti-retroviral therapy side effects at of is necessary during follow-ups

References

1. World Health Organization. Consolidated guidelines on the use of antiretroviral drugs for treating and preventing HIV infection. 2nd ed. Geneva: World Health Organization; 2016.
2. Muenchhoff M, Prendergast AJ, Goulder PJR. Immunity to HIV in early life. Front Immunol. 2014;5:1–13.
3. Bunders MJ, van der Loos CM, Klarenbeek PL, van Hamme JL, Boer K, Wilde JC, de Vries N, van Lier RA, Kootstra N, Pals ST, Kuijpers TW. Memory CD4(+)CCR5(+) T cells are abundantly present in the gut of newborn infants to facilitate mother-to-child transmission of HIV-1. Blood. 2012;120(22):4383–90.
4. Chang JJ, Altfeld M. TLR-mediated immune activation in HIV. Blood. 2009;113(2):269–70.
5. Swann SA, Williams M, Story CM, Bobbitt KR, Fleis R, Collins KL. HIV-1 Nef blocks transport of MHC class I molecules to the cell surface via a PI 3-kinase-dependent pathway. Virology. 2001;282(2):267–77.
6. Johnson EL, Chakraborty R. HIV-1 at the placenta: immune correlates of protection and infection. Curr Opin Infect Dis. 2016;29(3):248–55.
7. Abubakar I, Aliyu SH, Arumugam C, Usman NK, Hunter PR. Treatment of cryptosporidiosis in immunocompromised individuals: systematic review and meta-analysis. Br J Clin Pharmacol. 2007;63(4):387–93.
8. World Health Organization. WHO recommendations on the management of diarrhoea and pneumonia in HIV-infected infants and children. 1st ed. Geneva: WHO Press, World Health Organization; 2010.
9. World Health Organisation. WHAT'S new in infant diagnosis. Geneva: World Health Organisation; 2015.
10. World Health Organisation. WH Guidelines on the Treatment of Skin and Oral HIV-Associated Conditions in Children and Adults. Geneva: World Health Organization; 2014. Annex 1, ART recommendations. https://www.ncbi.nlm.nih.gov/books/NBK305414/. Accessed 09/18/2016.

Chapter 21
Neck Swelling and Fever

Sowmya Shashidhara, H. Koushik, and Sangita Trivedi

A 9-year-old pale-looking boy presents to the outpatient with a complaint of fever since 2 months ago along with swellings in the neck noticed by the mother since the past 10 days. The swelling appear to enlarge in size and become tender. He also had a weight loss of 3 kg during this period as confirmed by hospital records. His family and perinatal history were unremarkable. His weight was below the third percentile and height was at the third percentile. His pulse was 108/min, respiratory rate: 32/min, BP: 90/52 mmHg and T: 36.7 °C. On examination, axillary, inguinal and cervical lymph nodes were enlarged (5.5 ∗ 6.5 cm), palpable and tender. Abdominal examination showed firm hepatomegaly of 6 cm and an enlarged spleen up to 7 cm along its axis. Laboratory parameters are as given below: Hb: 5.4 g/dL, hematocrit: 16.0%, RBC: 1,970,000/μL, MCV: 81.3 fL, platelets: 5000/μL, WBC: 3000/μL, and ANC: 20/μL.

Q1. Which of the following disorders is least likely to explain for this patient's presentation according to history and clinical evidence?

A. Aplastic Anemia
B. Acute lymphoblastic leukemia

S. Shashidhara (✉)
Department of Pediatrics, Kasturba Medical College, Manipal University, Manipal, India

Network of Immunity in Infection, Malignancy and Autoimmunity (NIIMA), Universal Scientific Education and Research Network (USERN), Manipal, India
e-mail: sowmya.s@manipal.edu

H. Koushik
Department of Pediatrics, Kasturba Medical College, Manipal University, Manipal, India

S. Trivedi
Department of Pediatrics, Government Medical College, Surat, Veer Narmad South Gujarat University, Surat, India

© Springer Nature Switzerland AG 2020

F. Rahmani, N. Rezaei (eds.), *Pediatric Autoimmunity and Transplantation*,
https://doi.org/10.1007/978-3-030-26280-8_21

C. Hemophagocytic syndrome
D. Myelodysplastic syndrome
E. Megaloblastic anemia

Answer: *The correct answer is **E**.*

In a child presenting with prolonged fever, weight loss and tender, enlarged lymph nodes, the most common differentials are infections, malignancies, and bone marrow failure syndromes. While certain infections like typhoid, leishmaniosis, or malaria, which affect the reticuloendothelial systems, might present with pancytopenia, they do not cause a drastic reduction in the neutrophil counts. Megaloblastic anemia due to vitamin B12 or folate deficiency presents with pancytopenia, fever, and hepatosplenomegaly with less severity, along with neurological manifestations without a significant reduction in neutrophil counts along with hypersegmented neutrophils, which are absent in this case. Aplastic anemia, acute lymphoblastic leukemia, hemophagocytic syndrome and myelodysplastic syndromes comprise the most common origins of pancytopenia with neutropenia in childhood [1].

Q2. Which of the following laboratory/genetic findings would be against the diagnosis of myelodysplastic syndrome in this patient?

A. Pancytopenia with a cellular bone marrow
B. Persistent anemia with ringed sideroblasts
C. Bone marrow blasts >20%
D. Monosomy 7 in cytogenetic studies
E. Bicytopenia, macrocytes in peripheral blood and increased hemoglobin F

Answer: *The correct answer is **C**.*

Patients with MDS may present initially with a monocytopenia, which usually progresses to pancytopenia with anemia, leukopenia, and thrombocytopenia. Morphologic features of MDS include a normo/hypercellular bone marrow with dysplastic changes involving all three-cell lineages [2]. Also, megaloblastoid circulating nucleated RBCs with perinuclear ring-like deposits of iron (i.e., ringed sideroblasts) are frequently detected. Peripheral blood dysgranulopoiesis manifests as circulating myeloblasts, progranulocytes, and Pelger-Huët cells. Peripheral blood may also exhibit increased numbers of monocytes and monoblasts [2]. Few studies have also demonstrated increased levels of hemoglobin F in MDS although it is more consistently found in myelofibrosis [3]. Bone marrow blasts >20% are usually suggestive of leukemia.

Q3. A detailed review of his hospital records also revealed that he was diagnosed with neuroblastoma when he was 2 years old and received chemotherapy with etoposide, cyclophosphamide, and vincristine. Oncogenic aberrtions in all <u>except</u> which of the following gene/s are associated with acquired myelodysplastic syndrome?

A. Del(7q)
B. *Tp53*

C. *KRAS2*
D. Del(5q)
E. GATA2 deficiency

Answer: *The correct answer is* ***E***.

Monosomy 7/del(7q), as well as monosomy 5/del(5q) , characterize the most common cytogenetic aberrations in therapy-related myelodysplastic syndromes, and alkylating agents and etoposide are commonly implicated in these instances [4]. *Tp53* and *KRAS2* mutations are also associated with acquired genetic abnormalities causing myelodysplastic syndromes [5, 6]. GATA2 is a zinc finger transcription factor essential for embryonic and definitive hematopoiesis as well as lymphatic angiogenesis. GATA2 deficiency is a germline disease which causes a full spectrum of phenotypes including viral and bacterial infections, cytopenia, myelodysplasia, myeloid leukemias, pulmonary alveolar proteinosis, and lymphedema [7].

Q4. Which of the following modalities of treatment is the only proven curative therapy for myelodysplastic syndrome?

A. Hematopoietic stem cell transplantation
B. AML-based chemotherapy without hematopoietic stem cell transplantation
C. AML-based chemotherapy with hematopoietic stem cell transplantation
D. All-trans retinoic acid
E. Gene therapy

Answer: *The correct answer is* ***A***.

The only proven curative treatment for MDS is allogeneic hematopoietic stem cell transplantation (HSCT). AML-based chemotherapy without HSCT reduces 5-year survival by 30% [8] Noncytotoxic therapies like all-trans retinoic acid have been shown to add minimal benefits [2]. HSCT is the treatment of choice and results in cure rates of around 60%. Intensive chemotherapy before HSCT provides no survival benefits and is not recommended. Intensive chemotherapy before HSCT should be considered in patients with myelodysplasia-related-AML (MDR-AML).

Q5. Which of the following features can better predict survival in childhood myelodysplastic syndromes?

A. Cytopenia
B. Cytogenetics
C. Bone marrow blasts >5%
D. Age of presentation
E. Platelet counts >100,000/μL
F. Answers C and E are correct

Answer: *The correct answer is* ***F***.

The clinical characteristics and prognostic factors predicting survival or progression in adults with MDS are of little value in children. According to The International Prognostic Scoring System (IPSS) for childhood myelodysplastic syndrome (MDS), the bone marrow blast count and thrombocytopenia are the only factors associated with outcome in childhood MDS [9]. Neither hemoglobin <10 g/dL, neutrophil count <1500/μL, nor the number of cytopenic lineages are associated with survival, while platelet counts less than or equal to 100,000/μL, is a poor prognostic factor [9].

Practical Points

- Clinical suspicion of bone marrow failure syndrome should be raised in any child presenting with fever, weight loss, organomegaly with neutropenia and peripheral blood pancytopenia
- A cellular bone marrow with dysplastic cells and peripheral blood dysgranulopoiesis in the above clinical setting is suggestive of myelodysplastic syndrome (MDS)
- GATA2 deficiency results from a genetic aberration found in congenital types of myelodysplastic syndrome
- Acquired myelodysplastic syndrome is associated with previous chemotherapy with cyclophosphamide and etoposide which leads to activation of proto-oncogenes
- Hematopoietic stem cell transplantation is the definitive treatment for MDS
- Bone marrow blast count and thrombocytopenia are the factors associated with outcome in childhood MDS

References

1. Wu J, Cheng YF, Zhang LP, Liu GL, Lu AD, Jia YP, Wang B. [Clinical features and etiological spectrum in children with pancytopenia]. Zhongguo dang dai er ke za zhi = Chin J Contem Pediatr. 2011;13(9):718–21.
2. Jason N, Berman ATL. Pediatric myeloid leukemia, myelodysplasia, and myeloproliferative disease. In: Orkin SH, editor. Nathan and Oski's hematology and oncology of infancy and childhood. Philadelphia, PA: Elsevier; 2015. p. 1555–613.
3. Mendek-Czajkowska E, Slomkowski M, Zdebska E, Mokras U, Sikorska A, Maryniak R, Gorski T, Zych-Mordzinska J, Bielecka B. Hemoglobin F in primary myelofibrosis and in myelodysplasia. Clin Lab Haematol. 2003;25(5):289–92.
4. Side LE, Curtiss NP, Teel K, Kratz C, Wang PW, Larson RA, Le Beau MM, Shannon KM. RAS, FLT3, and TP53 mutations in therapy-related myeloid malignancies with abnormalities of chromosomes 5 and 7. Genes Chromosomes Cancer. 2004;39(3):217–23.
5. Takahashi K, Patel K, Bueso-Ramos C, Zhang J, Gumbs C, Jabbour E, Kadia T, Andreff M, Konopleva M, DiNardo C, Daver N, Cortes J, Estrov Z, Futreal A, Kantarjian H, Garcia-Manero G. Clinical implications of TP53 mutations in myelodysplastic syndromes treated with hypomethylating agents. Oncotarget. 2016;7(12):14172–87.
6. Lindsley RC, Ebert BL. Molecular pathophysiology of myelodysplastic syndromes. Annu Rev Pathol. 2013;8:21–47.
7. Hsu AP, McReynolds LJ, Holland SM. GATA2 deficiency. Curr Opin Allergy Clin Immunol. 2015;15(1):104–9.

8. Strahm B, Nollke P, Zecca M, Korthof ET, Bierings M, Furlan I, Sedlacek P, Chybicka A, Schmugge M, Bordon V, Peters C, O'Marcaigh A, de Heredia CD, Bergstraesser E, Moerloose BD, van den Heuvel-Eibrink MM, Stary J, Trebo M, Wojcik D, Niemeyer CM, Locatelli F. Hematopoietic stem cell transplantation for advanced myelodysplastic syndrome in children: results of the EWOG-MDS 98 study. Leukemia. 2011;25(3):455–62.
9. Hasle H, Baumann I, Bergstrasser E, Fenu S, Fischer A, Kardos G, Kerndrup G, Locatelli F, Rogge T, Schultz KR, Stary J, Trebo M, van den Heuvel-Eibrink MM, Harbott J, Nollke P, Niemeyer CM. The International Prognostic Scoring System (IPSS) for childhood myelodysplastic syndrome (MDS) and juvenile myelomonocytic leukemia (JMML). Leukemia. 2004;18(12):2008–14.

Chapter 22
Puffy Face and Abdominal Distension

Sowmya Shashidhara, H. Koushik, and Sangita Trivedi

An 11-year-old boy presents to the emergency department with edema, facial puffiness, and abdominal distension since 5 days ago. He was diagnosed with nephrotic syndrome and started on oral prednisolone (2 mg/kg/day). Despite 6 weeks of steroids and good compliance he failed to achieve remission and repeat 24-h urinary protein was 5 g/day. He was given a repeat course of steroids for 2 weeks, but proteinuria was still persistent. Therefore, he underwent a renal biopsy which showed focal segmental glomerulosclerosis.

Q1. Which of the following groups of vaccines are contraindicated in this patient?

A. DtaP, BCG, OPV, measles
B. IPV, MMR, BCG, yellow fever
C. BCG, OPV, MMR, yellow fever
D. BCG, hepatitis B, yellow fever, measles

Answer: *The correct answer is* ***C***.

S. Shashidhara (✉)
Department of Pediatrics, Kasturba Medical College, Manipal University, Manipal, India

Network of Immunity in Infection, Malignancy and Autoimmunity (NIIMA), Universal Scientific Education and Research Network (USERN), Manipal, India
e-mail: sowmya.s@manipal.edu

H. Koushik
Department of Pediatrics, Kasturba Medical College, Manipal University, Manipal, India

S. Trivedi
Department of Pediatrics, Government Medical College, Surat, Veer Narmad South Gujarat University, Surat, India

© Springer Nature Switzerland AG 2020
F. Rahmani, N. Rezaei (eds.), *Pediatric Autoimmunity and Transplantation*,
https://doi.org/10.1007/978-3-030-26280-8_22

The case described in this scenario is suggestive of immunosuppression due to nephrotic syndrome in which loss of immunoglobulins through urine and prolonged steroid therapy are implicated. According to CDC, children with immunosuppression should not receive live vaccines like MMR, varicella, MMRV, live attenuated influenza virus, herpes zoster, yellow fever, Ty21a oral typhoid, BCG, smallpox, or rotavirus. OPV is no longer offered in the United States, but is absolutely contraindicated in primary or acquired immunosuppression. Vaccines containing killed or toxoid components can be used in these individuals. Hepatitis B is recommended even in immunosuppressed patients, as it contains a recombinant form of viral antigen [1].

Q2. Since he does not respond to 6 weeks of steroid therapy, he is diagnosed with steroid-resistant nephrotic syndrome and is started on immunosuppressive agent. His physician explains that the drug used for this condition binds to a cytosolic protein of T cells called cyclophilin, responsible for activating transcription of IL-2. What is that drug?

A. Azathioprine
B. Mycophenolate mofetil
C. Rituximab
D. Cyclosporine
E. Sirolimus
F. Trastuzumab

Answer: *The correct answer is* ***D***.

Tacrolimus and cyclosporine are the preferred initial treatments for children with steroid-resistant nephrotic syndrome. Mycophenolate mofetil may be another option for these patients [2]. Calcineurin inhibitors (CNIs) have revolutionized treatment of resistant nephrotic syndrome and remain the standard of therapy 40 years after the discovery of cyclosporine. These drugs bind to intracellular proteins called immunophilins, i.e., cyclophilins in the case of cyclosporine A (CsA), or the FK-binding proteins, as does tacrolimus (also known as FK506). This complex then binds to an intracellular molecule called calcineurin, leading to an inhibition of IL-2 production, and hence inhibiting T cell activation [3]. Sirolimus inhibits IL-2 and other cytokines receptor-dependent signal transduction mechanisms, via its action on mTOR, and thereby blocks activation of T and B cells. Azathioprine is converted to 6-mercaptopurine and antagonizes purine metabolism inhibiting synthesis of DNA, RNA, and proteins. Mycophenolate mofetil acts as a prodrug of mycophenolic acid, an inhibitor of inosine-5′-monophosphate dehydrogenase. Rituximab is an anti-CD20 monoclonal antibody and mediates antibody-dependent cellular cytotoxicity (ADCC) and complement-dependent cytotoxicity (CDC) of $CD20^+$ B cells. Herceptin or trastuzumab, is a monoclonal antibody precisely intended to target HER2 receptors implicated in breast cancer.

Following cyclosporine therapy, 6 months later, he developed decreased urine output with worsening of edema. His pulse was 142 bpm and his BP was 160/110 mmHg with a respiratory rate of 22/min. He became drowsy with GCS: 9/15. Pallor, pedal edema, and facial puffiness were present. His serum creatinine was 12 mg/dL, serum potassium: 8 mEq/L. He underwent renal transplantation after which he was started on azathioprine and tacrolimus therapy using standard doses and pharmacogenetic testing for thiopurine S-methyltransferase (TPMT) alleles, which showed decreased enzyme activity.

Q3. Which significant modification in therapy is appropriate in this patient considering his TPMT deficiency?

A. Alkalinisation of urine
B. Decrease the dose of azathioprine
C. Substitute azathioprine with 6-mercaptopurine
D. Substitute azathioprine with 6-thioguanine

Answer: *The correct answer is **B**.*

The thiopurine methyltransferase (TPMT) enzyme metabolizes thiopurine drugs which are extensively used in numerous chemotherapy disciplines such as leukemia. Specific enzyme activity varies depending on the genetic polymorphisms of TPMT gene. TPMT-deficient patients can efficiently be treated with decreased thiopurine doses if enzyme status is documented by the previous testing. TPMT status documentation is a pioneering experience in an application of pharmacogenetic testing in clinical settings [4]. Alkalinization of urine is used in recipients with high dose methotrexate to promote renal excretion and to avoid nephrotoxicity. 6-mercaptopurine and 6-thioguanine belong to thiopurine group of drugs and require similar metabolic alterations as azathioprine during chemotherapy.

One year after successful transplantation, he developed fever, chest pain, cough, malaise, weight loss, and dyspnea, for 2 weeks duration. He was started on antibacterial therapy with no response, and a chest CT showed widespread and massive bilateral infiltrates. A lung biopsy is taken and shows regular, relatively slender (3–6 μ) hypha which dichotomously branch at 45° and have distinct septae.

Q4. Based on the morphological characteristics in the biopsy, which of the following options would <u>not</u> help to the diagnosis of this condition?

A. A positive CT scan with characteristics findings
B. Culture and microscopic evidence of disease
C. Detection of specific antigens in the serum
D. Clinical symptoms of fever, chest pain and cough.

Answer: *The correct answer is **D**.*

Aspergillus fumigatus has become the most prevalent airborne fungal pathogen, causing severe and usually fatal invasive infections in immunocompromised host. The above description suggests the diagnosis of invasive aspergillosis. Features currently considered in the diagnosis of invasive aspergillosis include: (1) a positive CT scan, (2) culture and microscopic evidence of disease, and (3) detection of *Aspergillus* antigen(s) in serum. Clinical symptoms are usually too nonspecific to be helpful in narrowing the focus down to IA [5]. General signs of invasive aspergillosis, primarily fever, chest pain, cough, malaise, weight loss, and dyspnea, are nonspecific. A core body temperature of >38.5 °C that is unresponsive to antibacterial therapy, previously recognized as the hallmark for initiating antifungal treatment, is no longer applicable since corticosteroid-treated patients are afebrile. Radiographic appearances of pulmonary invasive aspergillosis are very heterogeneous and can vary from single or multifocal nodules, with and without cavitation, to widespread and massive infiltrates which are often bilateral [5]. Enzyme-linked immunosorbent assay (ELISA) which measures the presence of serum antigens is both sensitive and specific for the diagnosis of invasive aspergillosis.

Q5. Following Tacrolimus therapy, he remains asymptomatic for 4 years after which he develops fever, pallor, hepatosplenomegaly and multiple petechiae. Laboratory examination shows pancytopenia with blasts >20% and a bone marrow examination reveals acute lymphoblastic leukemia. His oral temperature is 38.5 °C on two occasions within next 48 h with an ANC of 400 cells/μL. He is started with appropriate empirical antibiotics pending culture reports. After 72 h of initiation of empirical antibiotics, he remains febrile. Which of the following statements is correct regarding treatment of this condition?

A. Initially, the treating team is justified in starting empirical dual antibiotic therapy including antipseudomonal beta-lactam with an aminoglycoside
B. In case of febrile neutropenia with low risk, empirical mono antibiotic therapy is justifiable
C. Vancomycin is routinely part of febrile neutropenia empirical antibiotic therapy
D. With persistent fever spikes, broadening the antibiotic spectrum and antifungal therapy is considered

Answer: *The correct answer is* ***B****.*

Systemic tacrolimus therapy predisposes to cancers and blood dyscrasia. This child fits into the definition of febrile neutropenia. A bone marrow showing >20% blasts also supports the diagnosis of an underlying acute lymphoblastic leukemia. In the beginning, being a case of renal transplant with neutropenia <7 days and stable hemodynamic parameters fits this situation into low-risk febrile neutropenia. It was found that monotherapy is similar in efficacy and safety in comparison with aminoglycoside-containing combination regimens in empirical therapy of low risk pediatric febrile neutropenia. However, the study does not serve to identify an optimal monotherapy regimen in these cases [6]. A patients with ALL and low-risk neutropenia should be therefore started on monoantibiotic therapy. Vancomycin is not routinely part of empirical treatment and is indicated only during severe pneumonia, respiratory distress, shock, mucositis, skin breakdown, or colonization with MRSA. Persisting fever spikes with negative culture is an indication to initiate empirical antifungals with azoles or echinocandins like caspofungin.

Q6. Which of the following statements is false regarding usage of granulocyte, monocyte colony stimulating factor (GM-CSF)?

A. GM-CSF can be used in children with post-transplant drug-induced myelosuppression

B. GM-CSF is indicated as supportive treatment in high-risk febrile neutropenia like sepsis, hypotension, pneumonia, prolonged neutropenia
C. Myelosuppressive therapy with only colony stimulating factors has not shown benefit in infection-related mortality
D. Potency of intravenous and subcutaneous administration of CSF are same

Answer: *The correct answer is* ***D***.

FDA has approved GM-CSF only in post-transplant recipients whereas G-CSF can be used in chemotherapy-induced myelosuppression as well. Though pediatric data are limited, following are indications for GM-CSF administration: (1) children expected to have a ≥20% risk of chemotherapy-induced neutropenia, (2) Children who have previously suffered chemotherapy-induced febrile neutropenia which may affect treatment outcome. GM-CSF is administered as supportive treatment in high-risk febrile neutropenia, variably defined as >7–10 days of neutropenia with uncontrolled primary disease, hypotension, profound neutropenia (i.e., ANC <100/μL), sepsis, pneumonia, or fungal infection. The optimal dose of G-CSF in pediatric patients is 5 μg/kg of filgrastim, and the subcutaneous route is more efficacious than intravenous though the latter is more comfortable to administer [7].

Practical Points

- All live vaccines are contraindicated in children who are immunosuppressed secondary to disease or immunosuppressive therapy
- Calcineurin inhibitors are commonly used immunosuppressive agents and act via cyclophilin and inhibit IL-2 production
- The thiopurine S-methyltransferase pharmacogenetic testing is recommended before using thiopurine drugs for immunosuppression
- Tacrolimus therapy is associated with subsequent cancer risk
- Febrile neutropenia in low risk patients is treated with empirical antibiotics
- Colony-stimulating factors are used to treat prolonged immunosuppression due to therapy

References

1. (ACIP) ACoIP. General best practice guidelines for immunization: best practices guidance of the Advisory Committee on Immunization Practices (ACIP). Atlanta, GA: Advisory Committee on Immunization Practices; 2017.
2. Li S, Yang H, Guo P, Ao X, Wan J, Li Q, Tan L. Efficacy and safety of immunosuppressive medications for steroid-resistant nephrotic syndrome in children: a systematic review and network meta-analysis. Oncotarget. 2017;8(42):73050–62.
3. Azzi JR, Sayegh MH, Mallat SG. Calcineurin inhibitors: 40 years later, can't live without. J Immunol. 2013;191(12):5785–91.

4. Asadov C, Aliyeva G, Mustafayeva K. Thiopurine S-methyltransferase as a pharmacogenetic biomarker: significance of testing and review of major methods. Cardiovasc Hematol Agents Med Chem. 2017;15:23–30.
5. Latge JP. Aspergillus fumigatus and aspergillosis. Clin Microbiol Rev. 1999;12(2):310–50.
6. Robinson PD, Lehrnbecher T, Phillips R, Dupuis LL, Sung L. Strategies for empiric management of pediatric fever and neutropenia in patients with cancer and hematopoietic stem-cell transplantation recipients: a systematic review of randomized trials. J Clin Oncol. 2016;34(17):2054–60.
7. Mehta HM, Malandra M, Corey SJ. G-CSF and GM-CSF in neutropenia. J Immunol. 2015;195(4):1341–9.

Chapter 23
Hematuria and Abdominal Mass

Sowmya Shashidhara, H. Koushik, and Sangita Trivedi

A 3-year-old boy is seen in the pediatric emergency room with a complaint of a 1-day history of sudden onset hematuria and abdominal pain. On detailed evaluation, he is found to have an abdominal mass in the right iliac fossa and contrast-enhanced CT scan of abdomen reveals a suprarenal mass with no metastases. A right radical nephrectomy is performed, and histopathology of the mass shows the mass to be a Wilms tumor stage 1. He is started on chemotherapy and is lost to follow up after three cycles for 6 months after which he is reassessed for tumor staging. A repeat CT abdomen shows stage 3 Wilms tumor with metastases to lungs and bone marrow. He is started on neo-adjuvant chemotherapy and radiotherapy as a part of relapse protocol.

Q1. All of the following options are among implicated effects of radiotherapy on mammalian cells, except:

A. Direct interaction of electrons with DNA strands causing breakage
B. Generation of free radicals
C. Generation of chromosomal aberrations
D. Denaturation of proteins and lipids of cellular organelles

Answer: *The correct answer is **D**.*

S. Shashidhara (✉)
Department of Pediatrics, Kasturba Medical College, Manipal University, Manipal, India

Network of Immunity in Infection, Malignancy and Autoimmunity (NIIMA), Universal Scientific Education and Research Network (USERN), Manipal, India
e-mail: sowmya.s@manipal.edu

H. Koushik
Department of Pediatrics, Kasturba Medical College, Manipal University, Manipal, India

S. Trivedi
Department of Pediatrics, Government Medical College, Surat, Veer Narmad South Gujarat University, Surat, India

© Springer Nature Switzerland AG 2020
F. Rahmani, N. Rezaei (eds.), *Pediatric Autoimmunity and Transplantation*,
https://doi.org/10.1007/978-3-030-26280-8_23

The effects of irradiation on immune responses are complex. When irradiation is given in doses that are potentially lethal, the immune mechanisms throughout the body, both humoral and cell-mediated, are affected. This is a direct result of the suppression of the progenitors of plasma cells and lymphocytes by the multiple mechanisms. In direct action during radiotherapy, a secondary electron resulting from absorption of an X-ray photon interacts with the DNA to produce an effect. In indirect action, the secondary electron produces a hydroxyl radical (OH·), which produces secondary damage to the DNA. When cells are irradiated with X-rays, many breaks occur in single DNA strands, which can be observed and scored as a proxy of the radiation dose. Denaturation of proteins and lipids are usually secondary to free radical injury and are not a direct consequence of radiation damage.

Q2. Which of the following procedures requires prior adjunctive total body irradiation, in order to induce therapeutic immunosuppression?

A. Autologous transplant
B. Syngeneic transplant
C. Allogenic transplant
D. Xenogenic transplant

Answer: *The correct answer is* ***C.***

Targeted irradiation of the bone marrow with radiolabeled monoclonal antibodies, i.e. radioimmunotherapy, represents a novel therapeutic approach with both myeloablative and antileukemic potential [1]. In autologous transplants, where the donor is also the recipient, stem cells are harvested from the patient and frozen, after which the patient undergoes a conditioning regimen involving ablative chemotherapy. Syngeneic transplantation takes place between genetically identical twins and does not require prior conditioning with radiation. Xenogenic transplant requires tissue harvested from species other than humans and is rarely performed.

Q3. All of the following measures are indicated to reduce side-effects of radiotherapy in children, except?

A. Omitting or delaying radiotherapy in the young
B. Usage of chemotherapy to lower radiotherapy dose and volume
C. Elimination of radiotherapy in favorable subset of patients
D. Hypofractionation of dose of radiotherapy

Answer: *The correct answer is* ***D.***

Hypofractionated radiation treatment is a subtype, in which the entire dose of radiation is divided into large doses and treatments are given once a day or less often. Hyperfractionation delivers a lower dose per fraction, which is given more than once a day. As late appearing side-effects of radiotherapy are directly related to the fraction size, lowering the dose per fraction, in theory, should reduce these complications [2]. The younger the child while receiving radiotherapy, the more severe is the damage to growing tissues. Hence, radiation oncologists might choose to delay radiotherapy till the child is older. In certain brain tumors, chemotherapy has been used to decrease radiotherapy volume and dose as it shrinks the field of irradiation, hence reducing toxicity of RT. Treatment strategies are evolving to evaluate whether RT can be eliminated in the treatment regimen or not. Examples of cancers where this approach is used are stage 2 Wilms tumor with favorable histology and Hodgkins lymphoma [2]. Genetic testing and hippocampal sparing radiotherapy are newer modalities to minimize radiation toxicity in children.

Q4. Which of the following radiotherapy side-effects are unique to pediatric age group?

A. Hepatotoxicity
B. Renal failure
C. Neuropsychiatric disturbances
D. Growth and mental retardation
E. Options C and D

Answer: *The correct answers is* ***E.***

It is incumbent on the radiation oncology community to recognize the functional consequences of childhood cancer and its therapies. Growth disturbances are seen only in pediatric patients undergoing radiotherapy in growing children, appearing in approximately 40% of long-term survivors. Vertebral growth changes, muscle hypoplasia, reduction in bone length as a consequence of radiation therapy have all been described [3]. Alterations in growth also occur because of radiation-related endocrine dysfunction. Growth hormone deficiency has been identified in more than 50% of children who have undergone irradiation of the pituitary-hypothalamic region [4]. Neuropsychiatric disturbances and intellectual disability have been described only in children with ALL who have received radiotherapy [5, 6] while hepatotoxicity, and renal failure are therapy-related side effects in both children and adults.

Practical Points

- Radiotherapy affects the immune system by direct interaction with DNA strands and by generation of free radicals causing chromosomal aberrations
- Total body irradiation before allogenic transplant induces therapeutic immunosuppression and provides higher success rates
- Hyperfractionation of radiation dose reduces dose-related side effects related to radiotherapy
- Growth retardation, as a side effect of radiotherapy is of particular concern in young children, compared to adults

References

1. Schulz AS, Glatting G, Hoenig M, Schuetz C, Gatz SA, Grewendorf S, Sparber-Sauer M, Muche R, Blumstein N, Kropshofer G, Suttorp M, Bunjes D, Debatin KM, Reske SN, Friedrich W. Radioimmunotherapy-based conditioning for hematopoietic cell transplantation in children with malignant and nonmalignant diseases. Blood. 2011;117(17):4642–50.

2. Paulino AC. Treatment strategies to reduce radiotherapy late effects in children. J Radiat Oncol. 2013;2(2):121–8.
3. Probert JC, Parker BR. The effects of radiation therapy on bone growth. Radiology. 1975;114(1):155–62.
4. Shalet SM, Morris-Jones PH, Beardwell CG, Pearson D. Pituitary function after treatment of intracranial tumours in children. Lancet. 1975;306(7925):104–7.
5. Eiser C. Intellectual abilities among survivors of childhood leukaemia as a function of CNS irradiation. Arch Dis Child. 1978;53(5):391–5.
6. Meadows A, Massari D, Fergusson J, Gordon J, Littman P, Moss K. Declines in IQ scores and cognitive dysfunctions in children with acute lymphocytic leukaemia treated with cranial irradiation. Lancet. 1981;318(8254):1015–8.

Chapter 24
Pitting Edema and Desquamation

Sowmya Shashidhara, H. Koushik, and Sangita Trivedi

A 2-year-old girl was brought to the pediatric emergency unit with gradually worsening edema which was initially observed over both her lower limbs. A rash starting over both legs and spread to her abdomen, and arms followed the edema. The rash was described as being blackish in color occurring in large plaques looking like a "pavement" over the affected areas. On examination, there was pallor, pitting type of edema over legs, abdomen, and face, cracked lips, and angular stomatitis. The characteristic rash was present over legs, trunk, and arms, with serous discharge and desquamation of skin from feet and hands. Her weight was 8.7 kg on the third centile for age (recumbent with edema), her height was 67 cm; less than third centile for age; and mid upper arm circumference (MUAC) was 113 mm. Her pulse was 132 bpm and BP: 96/60 mmHg. Lung examination showed dull on percussion and auscultation showed reduced air entry bilaterally. The abdominal study revealed distension with fluid thrill and shifting dullness without any organomegaly.

Q1. What is the most likely diagnosis?

A. Dengue shock syndrome
B. Severe acute malnutrition

S. Shashidhara (✉)
Department of Pediatrics, Kasturba Medical College, Manipal University, Manipal, India

Network of Immunity in Infection, Malignancy and Autoimmunity (NIIMA), Universal Scientific Education and Research Network (USERN), Manipal, India
e-mail: sowmya.s@manipal.edu

H. Koushik
Department of Pediatrics, Kasturba Medical College, Manipal University, Manipal, India

S. Trivedi
Department of Pediatrics, Government Medical College, Surat, Veer Narmad South Gujarat University, Surat, India

© Springer Nature Switzerland AG 2020

F. Rahmani, N. Rezaei (eds.), *Pediatric Autoimmunity and Transplantation*,
https://doi.org/10.1007/978-3-030-26280-8_24

C. Nephrotic syndrome
D. Congestive cardiac failure
E. Hepatic failure

Answer: *The correct answer is* ***B***.

According to the WHO, severe acute malnutrition is defined as infants and children who are 6–59 months of age and have a MUAC <115 mm or a weight-for-height/length <3 Z-scores of the WHO growth standards, or have bilateral edema. Therefore, this child fitting into the diagnostic criteria is diagnosed to have severe acute malnutrition even though her weight is on the third centile and the weight for height is above third centile. Additionally, when "flaky paint" dermatosis is seen in a malnourished child with edema, it is pathognomonic of the disease kwashiorkor. The diagnosis of illnesses like dengue shock syndrome requires evidence of bleeding with shock and supporting laboratory evidence and hence is unlikely. Nephrotic syndrome and congestive cardiac failure mimic severe malnutrition and can be misdiagnosed, but the characteristic rash is absent in these conditions. Hepatic failure is accompanied by other signs of liver failure like icterus, a flapping tremor and altered sensorium which are not present in this patient and hence ruled out [1].

Q2. All of the following statements are correct according to WHO recommendations for management of severe acute malnutrition (SAM), except:

A. A child satisfying the definition of severe acute malnutrition with good appetite and without edema or medical complication can be treated on an out-patient basis
B. After initial inpatient treatment, the child can be transferred to outpatient care when specific anthropometric outcomes are met
C. Percentage of weight gain compared to baselien should not be used as discharge criteria
D. Children admitted with only bilateral pitting edema should be discharged from treatment based on whichever anthropometric indicator, MUAC or weight-for-height, routinely used in their health care program

Answer: *The correct answer is* ***B***.

In the treatment of severe acute malnutrition, children with good appetite who are clinically well and alert should be treated as outpatients. Children who have medical complications, severe edema (about 3+), or reduced appetite or who present with one or more danger signs should be treated as inpatients. After initial inpatient treatment, the decision to transfer children from inpatient to outpatient care should be determined by their clinical condition and not based on specific anthropometric outcomes. To be eligible for discharge, the child should have weight-for-height/length is ≥2 Z-score and they should have had no edema for at least 2 weeks, or alternatively; their MUAC should be above ≥125 mm, and they should have had no edema for at least 2 weeks [1].

Q3. If the same child develops acute gastroenteritis with severe dehydration, which of the following statements are correct regarding the management of this condition?

A. The fluid of choice for SAM children with shock is ringer's lactate solution with 5% dextrose or 0.45% saline +5% dextrose
B. WHO low-osmolarity oral rehydration solution (75 mmol/L sodium) can be used for oral or nasogastric rehydration in children with severe acute malnutrition who present with some dehydration or severe dehydration
C. ReSoMol (rehydration solution for malnutrition) is rich in sodium compared to low osmolarity WHO oral rehydration solution
D. Once children are stabilized, have an appetite and reduced edema and are therefore ready to move into the rehabilitation phase, they should transition from F-75 to ready-to-use therapeutic food over 2–3 days, as tolerated
E. Answers A and D are correct

Answer: *The correct answers is* ***E****.*

Shock is the only compelling indication for intravenous fluids in SAM management. As SAM is a state of relative sodium overload and potassium depletion, intravenous fluids and rehydration solution are modified accordingly. Full-strength, standard WHO low-osmolarity oral rehydration solution with 75 mmol/L of sodium should not be used for oral or nasogastric rehydration in children with severe acute malnutrition who present with some dehydration or severe dehydration. Either ReSoMal or half-strength standard WHO low-osmolarity oral rehydration solution should be given, with added potassium and glucose. Same way half-strength Darrow's solution with 5% dextrose or Ringer's lactate solution with 5% dextrose or 0.45% saline +5% dextrose should be used as intravenous fluid whenever indicated. After initial stabilization, once child tolerates F75 shift to F100 or ready to use therapeutic food should be done gradually over 2–3 days [1].

Q4. Which of the following is a consequence of malnutrition?

A. The liver produces more albumin, transferrin, and other transport proteins. It can cope with excess dietary protein and to excrete toxins
B. The kidneys are unable to excrete excess fluid and sodium, and fluid readily accumulates in the circulation, increasing the risk of fluid overload
C. The heart enlarged and has increased output, and fluid overload readily leads to death from cardiac failure
D. The gut produces more gastric acid and enzymes. Motility is increased, and bacteria may colonize the stomach and small intestine. Digestion and absorption are impaired

Answer: *The correct answer is* ***B****.*

Physiologic and metabolic changes, which take place when a child has reduced intake of calories, is called reductive adaptation. In this process, all organs are involved in concert and make a joint effort to conserve energy. The liver makes glucose less readily, causing the child more prone to hypoglycemia, produces less albumin, transferrin, and other transport proteins and is less able to cope with excess dietary protein and excrete toxins such as urea. The heart is smaller and weaker and has a reduced output, and fluid overload readily leads to death from cardiac failure. The gut produces less gastric acid and enzymes. Motility is reduced, and bacteria may colonize the stomach and small intestine, damaging the mucosa and deconjugating bile salts. Immune function is impaired, especially cell-mediated immunity. Usual responses to infection may be absent, even in severe illness, increasing the risk of undiagnosed disease. Red cell mass is reduced, releasing iron which requires glucose and amino acids to be converted to ferritin, increasing the risk of hypoglycemia and amino acid imbalances. If conversion to ferritin is incomplete, unbound iron promotes pathogen growth and formation of free radicals [2].

Q5. All of the following statements are correct regarding the immune status of children with severe malnutrition, except:

A. Acute phase reactant response is blunted but complement levels are unaltered
B. Leukocyte and lymphocyte counts are unaffected, and levels of immunoglobulins, particularly immunoglobulin A, are high
C. Reduced Barrier function leads to easy invasion of organisms
D. Thymus undergoes atrophy with reduced delayed-type hypersensitivity responses.

Answer: *The correct answer is* ***A***.

Malnutrition is associated with impaired gut-barrier function, reduced exocrine secretion of protective substances, and low levels of plasma complement. Lymphatic tissue, particularly the thymus, undergoes atrophy, and delayed-type hypersensitivity responses are reduced. Levels of antibodies produced after vaccination are reduced in severely malnourished children, but intact in moderate malnutrition. Cytokine patterns are skewed towards a Th2-response. Other immune parameters seem intact or elevated: leukocyte and lymphocyte counts are unaffected, and levels of immunoglobulins, particularly immunoglobulin A, are high. The acute phase response appears intact, and sometimes elevated in the absence of clinical infection. The immunological alterations associated with malnutrition in children may contribute to increased mortality [3].

Q6. Which of the following micronutrients plays an immunomodulatory role and its deficiency is frequently seen in malnourishment?

A. Copper
B. Sodium
C. Potassium
D. Vitamin A
E. Vitamin K

Answer: *The correct answer is* ***D***.

Vitamin A–deficient children have significantly lower numbers of T cells in circulation with a proportionate decrease in $CD4^{+}$ and $CD8^{+}$ subsets. Contrary to observations in experimental animals, vitamin A deficiency in children appears to have no significant effects on humoral immune mechanisms in human. The effect of vitamin A deficiency on innate immune mechanisms is also variable. Copper, sodium, and potassium are deficient in malnutrition but do not play a significant role in immunomodulation. Vitamin K also plays a minimal role in immunomodulation and is associated with malnutrition secondary to malabsorption or liver disease [4].

Practical Points

- Generalized edema with dermatosis in a malnourished child should raise clinical suspicion of kwashiorkor
- The clinical presentation of kwashiorkor may mimic features of sepsis, heart and kidney disease
- A child satisfying WHO criteria for severe acute malnutrition (SAM) with good appetite in the absence of medical complications can be treated on an outpatient basis
- In the management of shock or severe dehydration in children with SAM, cautious use of fluids must be done as it is a state of relative sodium excess in the body
- Reductive adaptation is a compensatory response to chronic malnutrition, which simply means limitation of functioning of multiple organs
- Chronic malnutrition is an immunosuppressed state, affecting both cell-mediated and humoral immunity
- Micronutrient deficiency contributes to immunosuppression in chronic malnutrition

References

1. World Health Organisation. Updates on the management of severe acute malnutrition in infants and children. Geneva: World Health Organisation; 2013.
2. Ashworth A. Nutrition, food security, and health. In: Kliegman RM, St Geme JW, Schor NF, editors. Nelson's textbook of pediatrics, vol. 1. Philadelphia, PA: Elsevier; 2016. p. 295–306. e291.
3. Rytter MJ, Kolte L, Briend A, Friis H, Christensen VB. The immune system in children with malnutrition—a systematic review. PLoS One. 2014;9(8):e105017.
4. Bhaskaram P. Micronutrient malnutrition, infection, and immunity: an overview. Nutr Rev. 2002;60(5 Pt 2):S40–5.

Chapter 25
Fever and Cutaneous Nodules

Sowmya Shashidhara, H. Koushik, and Sangita Trivedi

A 6-year-old girl was presented by her mother to the pediatric outpatient clinic complaining of fever for last 4 days and becoming pale, as described by her mother. The fever had an insidious onset and associated with development of multiple small swellings over her neck which were painful. There was no associated rash. The mother noticed similar episodes over last 2 years occurring transiently and resolving with a blood transfusion. There was no history of consanguinity. Her development and immunization were appropriate. On examination, her weight was 20.3 kg, height: 123.5 cm, BMI: 13 kg/m^2 (less than third centile). Pallor and icter were present. Submandibular, submental and cervical lymph nodes were palpable and tender. Her pulse was 122 bpm, blood pressure was 102/70 mmHg and respiratory rate was 24/min. On abdominal examination, the spleen was enlarged up to 4 cm along its axis, and the liver up to 5 cm below the costal margin along the midclavicular line with a span of 12 cm. A hemoglobin electrophoresis showed elevated HbS and reduced HbA.

The physician attending the patient during rounds explains to his students that the causative organism is most likely a non-enveloped icosahedral particle 18–26 nm

S. Shashidhara (✉)
Department of Pediatrics, Kasturba Medical College, Manipal University, Manipal, India

Network of Immunity in Infection, Malignancy and Autoimmunity (NIIMA), Universal Scientific Education and Research Network (USERN), Manipal, India
e-mail: sowmya.s@manipal.edu

H. Koushik
Department of Pediatrics, Kasturba Medical College, Manipal University, Manipal, India

S. Trivedi
Department of Pediatrics, Government Medical College, Surat, Veer Narmad South Gujarat University, Surat, India

© Springer Nature Switzerland AG 2020
F. Rahmani, N. Rezaei (eds.), *Pediatric Autoimmunity and Transplantation*,
https://doi.org/10.1007/978-3-030-26280-8_25

in diameter, with two capsid proteins and a linear single-stranded DNA and supportive laboratory evidence shows a positive IgM and PCR for the same organism.

Q1. Which of the following pathogens is the most likely cause of this condition?

A. Epstein-Barr virus
B. Cytomegalovirus
C. Parvovirus B19
D. Rhinovirus
E. Herpes Simplex 1

Answer: *The correct answer is* ***C****.*

Parvoviruses are known to be pathogenic to humans. Immunocompromised hosts suffer from severe aplastic crises when infected. The B19 virion has a simple structure composed of only two proteins and a linear, single-strand DNA molecule. The non-enveloped viral particles are ~18–26 nm in diameter and show icosahedral symmetry [1]. Epstein-Barr virus is approximately 122–180 nm in diameter and is composed of a double helix of DNA surrounded by a nucleocapsid. In immunocompetent hosts, EBV causes infectious mononucleosis a self-limiting illness, but in immunosuppressed hosts, it plays an etiological role in cancers like Burkitt lymphoma and nasopharyngeal carcinoma. Cytomegalovirus, also causing infectious mononucleosis with a negative Paul-Bunnell test, has an enveloped genome with double-stranded DNA and a capsid. The herpes simplex virus has a similar morphology to CMV. Rhinovirus has a single-stranded RNA genome and is non-enveloped.

Q2. Which statement is correct regarding parvovirus infection in sickle cell disease?

A. As the child grows older the chances of aplasia increase
B. At least one other cell line is involved apart from red blood cells
C. Apart from viruses, streptococcal/staphylococci infection can also lead to this situation
D. It is a transient phenomenon, invariably recovering in 1–2 weeks
E. Answers C and D are correct

Answer: *The correct answer is* ***E****.*

In a child with a known sickle cell anemia, a short history of viral prodrome followed by sudden and severe anemia happens secondary to the aplastic crisis. Though Parvovirus B19 is most common organism involved, EBV, streptococci, and staphylococci can lead to RBC aplasia. As protective antibody titer raises with advancing age, the incidence of aplasia decreases. The rapidly proliferating erythroblast lineage is most commonly affected, yet other cell lines might undergo transient aplastic episodes, with no apparent sign in peripheral blood. This transient response may require a blood transfusion, and usually remits by 1–2 weeks [2].

Q3. All of the following are among the causes of immunosuppression in sickle cell disease, except:

A. Aplastic crises due to Parvovirus infections.
B. Functional asplenia due to microvascular occlusion.
C. Inability to utilize alternate pathway for C3 fixation.
D. Devitalization of gut and bone due to repetitive vasoocclusive crises.
E. Impaired cell-mediated immunity.

Answer: *The correct answer is **E**.*

Sickle cell disease is a substantial cause of morbidity and mortality in tertiary care centers, and a state of immunosuppression. Repeated episodes of sickling and ischemic damage with progressive sclerosis of arterioles lead to multiple infarcts of spleen tissue. Unable to regenerate, the spleen becomes scarred and atrophied, culminating in "autosplenectomy", where the organ shrinks to a small remnant, and the individual is efficiently rendered asplenic. Reduced functional activity of the alternative pathway, with lower levels of the active form of factor B, has been demonstrated by several studies in patients with sickle cell disease [3]. Repeated vasoocclusive episodes predispose these individuals to osteomyelitis and reduction local mucosal defence [4]. However, no mechanism has been described by which cell-mediated immunity is affected by sickle cell disease.

Q4. Invasive infections by encapsulated organisms is a life-threatening condition in children with sickle cell anemia. Which of the following anticipatory guidelines is recommended to prevent infections by these organisms?

A. For <5-year-old children prophylactic penicillin therapy has shown benefit to reduce sepsis.
B. Pneumococcal polysaccharide vaccine should be administered concomitantly with conjugate vaccine.
C. No routine booster recommended for PPSV.
D. All patients having a history of pneumococcal sepsis should remain on penicillin prophylaxis indefinitely.
E. Answers A and D are correct.

Answer: *The correct answer is **E**.*

Children should be immunized against *Streptococcus pneumonia*, *Haemophilus influenzae*, hepatitis B, and influenza. Vaccination schedules recommend inoculation with pneumococcal conjugate vaccine at 2 months followed by two more doses 6–8 weeks apart, primary series, and a booster at 12 months. This is followed by pneumococcal polysaccharide vaccine (PPSV) at 2 and 5 years. For children younger than 5 years old, prophylactic penicillin recommendations are 125 mg penicillin V orally twice daily until age 2–3 years and 250 mg after that. No established guideline exists for penicillin prophylaxis beyond 5 years of age. Penicillin prophylaxis should be continued beyond 5 years of age in children with a history of pneumococcal infection because of the increased risk of recurrence. An alternative for children who are allergic to penicillin is erythromycin ethyl succinate 10 mg/kg twice a day [5].

Practical Points

- Parvovirus is a single-stranded DNA virus which causes aplastic crises in children with sickle cell disease or other forms of anemia
- Younger children are more susceptible to parvovirus infection, primarily affecting red cell lineages transiently
- Although sickle cell disease is a state of chronic immunosuppression, cell-mediated immunity remains relatively intact
- Penicillin prophylaxis is a part of routine care to prevent infection with encapsulated organisms up to 5 years of age and indefinitely in sickle cell patients who have suffered a previous pneumococcal disease

References

1. Heegaard ED, Brown KE. Human Parvovirus B19. Clin Microbiol Rev. 2002;15(3):485–505.
2. Rao SP, Miller ST, Cohen BJ. Transient aplastic crisis in patients with sickle cell disease. B19 parvovirus studies during a 7-year period. Am J Dis Child. 1992;146(11):1328–30.
3. Booth C, Inusa B, Obaro SK. Infection in sickle cell disease: a review. Int J Infect Dis. 2010;1:e2–e12.
4. Onwubalili JK. Sickle cell disease and infection. J Infect. 1983;7(1):2–20.
5. DeBaun MR. Hemoglobinopathies. In: Kliegman RM, St Geme JWS, Schor NF, editors. Nelson's textbook of pediatrics, vol. 2. 20th ed. Philadelphia, PA: Elsevier; 2016. p. 2336–53.

Chapter 26
Neck Stiffness and Fever

Tangie Ngek Larry and Derrick Tembi Efie

An 8-year-old HIV-positive boy is brought to the health facility with a 2-week history of headache, vomiting, fever and neck stiffness. His mother died of tuberculosis (TB) 6 months ago and he is currently taken care of by his grandmother. Physical examination revealed an irritable and febrile child, with neck stiffness and a positive Brudzinski's sign. There is no motor deficit or sensory loss. Pupils are symmetrical and reactive to light.

Q1. What is the most likely diagnosis?

A. Meningitis
B. Severe malaria
C. Space occupying lesion
D. Cerebrovascular accident

Answer: *The correct answer is* ***A***.

Q2. What test will you do to confirm the diagnosis?

A. CT-scan
B. Lumber puncture
C. CD4 count
D. All of the above

Answer: *The correct answer is* ***D***.

T. N. Larry (✉)
Faculty of Medicine and Biomedical Sciences, University of Yaounde 1, Yaounde, Cameroon

D. T. Efie
Tokombere District Hospital, Tokombere, Cameroon

Health and Human Development Research Network, Douala, Cameroon

© Springer Nature Switzerland AG 2020

F. Rahmani, N. Rezaei (eds.), *Pediatric Autoimmunity and Transplantation*,
https://doi.org/10.1007/978-3-030-26280-8_26

Your requested laboratory investigations above come with the following results: CD4⁺: 300 cells/μL. His lumbar puncture results return with WBC of 100 cells/μL (almost all lymphocytes), protein of 150 mg/dL, glucose of 15 mg/dL, negative Ziehl-Neelsen stain for acid-fast bacili, but positive gene Xpert MTB/RIF and finally negative gram and Indian ink staining.

Q3. What is the most probable diagnosis at this stage?

A. Cryptococcal meningitis
B. Tuberculous meningitis
C. Acute bacterial meningitis
D. Viral meningitis

Answer: *The correct answer is* ***B***.

Q4. What is the best treatment option for this patient? (R: rifampicin; H: isoniazid; E: etambutol; Z: pirazineamide)

A. 2 months RHEZ plus 10 months RH plus steroids
B. 2 months RHEZ plus 4 months RH plus steroids
C. 2 months RHEZS plus 1 month RHEZ plus 5 months RH
D. 2 months RHEZ plus 9 months RH

Answer: *The correct answer is* ***A***.

TB meningitis (TBM) is an infection of the meninges of the brain caused by the bacteria *Mycobacterium tuberculosis* [1]. It usually presents initially with fever and headache, with coma and confusion in the later stages. Patients may or may not have focal neurological deficits and up to a fifth of patients do not exhibit signs and symptoms of meningismus [2]. The diagnosis of TB meningitis is based on a lumber puncture and subsequent analysis of the cerebrospinal fluid [1]. The CSF usually has a high protein, low glucose and a raised number of lymphocytes. Acid-fast bacilli are sometimes seen on a CSF smear, but more commonly, *M. tuberculosis* is grown in culture. Xpert gene MTB/RIF is a rapid and sensitive way of detecting microbiologically proven TBM with a sensitivity of 62% as opposed to 12% with microscopy [3]. The treatment of TB meningitis is isoniazid (H), rifampicin (R), pyrazinamide (Z) and ethambutol (E) for 2 months, followed by isoniazid and rifampicin alone for a further 10 months [1].

Practical Points

- Tuberculosis (TB) meningitis is an infection of the meninges of the brain caused by the bacteria *Mycobacterium tuberculosis*
- Up to 20% of patients with TB meningitis have no meningismus signs
- Xpert gene MTB/RIF is a rapid and sensitive way of detecting microbiologically proven TBM with a sensitivity

References

1. Chin JH. Tuberculous meningitis. Neurol Clin Pract. 2004;4(3):199–205.
2. Harman R. Handbook of pharmacy healthcare: diseases and patient advice. 2nd ed. London: Pharmaceutical Press; 2002.
3. Patel VB, Theron G, Lenders L, Matinyena B, Connolly C, Singh R, Coovadia Y, Ndung'u T, Dheda K. Diagnostic accuracy of quantitative PCR (Xpert MTB/RIF) for tuberculous meningitis in a high burden setting: a prospective study. PLoS Med. 2013;10(10):e1001536.

Chapter 27
Rash and Generalized Body Pains

Tangie Ngek Larry and Derrick Tembi Efie

A 16-year-old girl, presents with a 1-week history of a rash and complains of generalized body pains. On examination, we notice pruritic vesicular rash on an erythematous base, following the T4 dermatome, associated with tenderness of the skin in an afebrile context (Fig. 27.1).

Q1. What is the most likely diagnosis?

A. Contact dermatitis
B. Shingles
C. Varicella zoster
D. Staphylococcal skin infection

Answer: *The correct answer is **B**.*

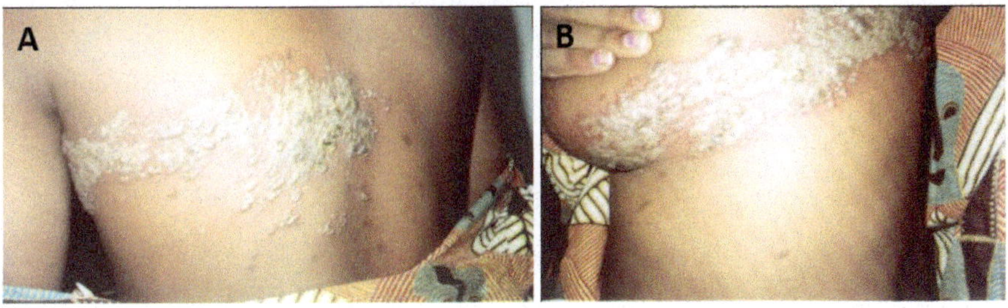

Fig. 27.1 Pruritic vesicular rash in a 16-year-old girl. (**a**) vesicular rash on an erythematous base on the posterior trunk T4 dermatome. (**b**) vesicular rash on an erythematous base on the anterior trunk T4 dermatome

T. N. Larry (✉)
Faculty of Medicine and Biomedical Sciences, University of Yaounde 1, Yaounde, Cameroon

D. T. Efie
Tokombere District Hospital, Tokombere, Cameroon

Health and Human Development Research Network, Douala, Cameroon

© Springer Nature Switzerland AG 2020

F. Rahmani, N. Rezaei (eds.), *Pediatric Autoimmunity and Transplantation*,
https://doi.org/10.1007/978-3-030-26280-8_27

Q2. You request an HIV test which comes back positive. What is the next best step?

A. Do CD4⁺ count, wait for CD4 count to choose appropriate antiviral treatment
B. Do CD4⁺ count and initiate antiretroviral treatment
C. Do CD4⁺ count, give acyclovir and prepare for antiretroviral therapy initiation
D. Initiate on antiretroviral therapy

Answer: *The correct answer is* ***C****.*

Q3. Treatment of Shingles for a patient in her condition is best achieved by:

A. Acyclovir 200 mg 5 times a days
B. Acyclovir 800 mg 5 times a day for 10 days
C. Acyclovir 400 mg 2 times a day
D. Acyclovir 500 mg 2 times a day for 10 days

Answer: *The correct answer is* ***B****.*

Herpes zoster is a viral disease characterized by a painful skin rash with blisters in a localized area particularly among HIV patients and patients above 50 years old [1]. Shingles occurs due to reactivation of varicella zoster virus in an immunocompromised patient, potentially due to HIV or malignancy. Risk factors include age, poor immune function and first exposure to chicken pox virus before 18 months of age [2]. Herpes zoster reactivation is commonly associated with low CD4⁺ count [3]. Clinical manifestations of herpes zoster can be divided into three phases namely pre-eruptive, acute eruptive and post-eruptive [4]. Cardinal symptoms of the pre-eruptive phase is pain or less commonly itching or paresthesia, involving one or more skin dermatomes [4]. Classic findings in the acute eruptive phase are grouped vesicles on an erythematous base also following a skin dermatomal distribution [5]. Diagnosis is primarily clinical though PCR and direct fluorescent antibody testing (DFA) of vesicular fluid could be done [6]. Treatment options include analgesics, antivirals including acyclovir over a period of 10 days which may reduce the severity and duration of shingles [1].

Practical Points

- Herpes zoster infection in form of Shingles is a characteristic of stage 2 HIV infection
- Shingles usually appears in CD4⁺ counts between 350–400/μL
- Diagnosis of Shingles is primarily clinical though PCR and direct fluorescent antibody testing (DFA) of vesicular fluid could be done

References

1. Bader M. Herpes zoster: diagnostic, therapeutic, and preventive approaches. Postgrad Med. 2013;125(5):78–91.
2. Lidhoo P, Unemori P, Leslie K, Maurer T. Disseminated herpes zoster with increased CD4 counts in 3 HIV-infected patients. J Am Acad Dermatol. 2009;61(2):345–7.
3. Engels E, Rosenberg P, Biggar R. Zoster incidence in human immunodeficiency virus-infected hemophiliacs and homosexual men, 1984–1997. J Infect Dis. 1999;180(6):1784–9.
4. Goh C, Khoo L. A retrospective study of the clinical presentation and outcome of herpes zoster in a tertiary dermatology outpatient referral clinic. Int J Dermatol. 1997;36(9):667–72.
5. Pasqualucci A, Pasqualucci V, Galla F, De Angelis V, Marzocchi V, Colussi R, Paoletti F, Girardis M, Lugano M, Del Sindaco F. Prevention of post-herpetic neuralgia: acyclovir and prednisolone versus epidural local anesthetic and methylprednisolone. Acta Anaesthesiol Scand. 2000;44(8):910–8.
6. Beards G, Graham C, Pillay D. Investigation of vesicular rashes for HSV and VZV by PCR. J Med Virol. 1998;54(3):155–7.

Chapter 28
Positive HIV and Violet Macular Rash

Tangie Ngek Larry and Derrick Tembi Efie

A 15-year-old HIV-positive male presented with non-tender nodular lesion on the left lower limb and violet macular rash as shown on the image below (Fig. 28.1).

Q1. What is the most likely diagnosis?

A. Onchocerciasis
B. Cutaneous Kaposi sarcoma
C. Cutaneous TB
D. Prurigo nodularis

Answer: *The correct answer is* ***B***.

Q2. What is the name of the microorganism responsible for this disease?

A. HHV8
B. Onchocerca volvulus
C. HHV6
D. *Mycobacterium tuberculosis*

Answer: *The correct answer is* ***A***.

Q3. Cutaneous Kaposi sarcoma can present in all of the following forms, except:

A. Nodular
B. Macular

T. N. Larry (✉)
Faculty of Medicine and Biomedical Sciences, University of Yaounde 1, Yaounde, Cameroon

D. T. Efie
Tokombere District Hospital, Tokombere, Cameroon

Health and Human Development Research Network, Douala, Cameroon

© Springer Nature Switzerland AG 2020
F. Rahmani, N. Rezaei (eds.), *Pediatric Autoimmunity and Transplantation*,
https://doi.org/10.1007/978-3-030-26280-8_28

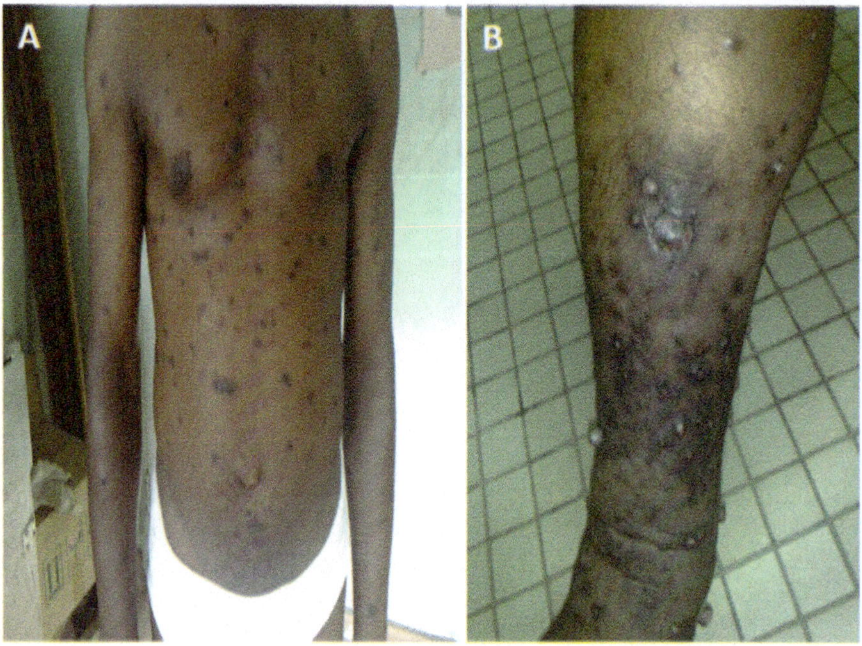

Fig. 28.1 (**a**) Violet macular rash on abdomen and trunk, (**b**) Nodular rash on left lower limb

C. Visceral
D. Lymphedema
E. Ulcerating lesion

Answer: *The correct answer is* ***E***.

Q4. What is the best treatment for this patient's condition?

A. HAART
B. Chemotherapy
C. Neomycine cream
D. Cryotherapy

Answer: *The correct answer is* ***A***.

Kaposi sarcoma (KS) is a malignant disease caused by the human herpes virus 8 [1]. There are four main subtypes of KS: Classic KS, African endemic KS, KS in iatrogenically immunosuppressed patients and AIDS-related KS, with the AIDS-related type being common among HIV patients. KS usually presents as popular/nodular lesions or blotches that may be red, purple, brown, or black. In a majority of patients, these lesions are found on the skin, but could also involve the mouth, gastrointestinal tract and respiratory tract [2]. KS could be suspected from the history, although definitive diagnosis can be made only by biopsy and microscopic examination. Detection of the KSHV protein LANA in tumor cells confirms the diagnosis. HHV8 is present in almost 100% of Kaposi sarcoma lesions [3]. KS has no cure, but can be treated and limited. The modality of treatment depends on the subtype of KS. Initiating highly active antiretroviral therapy (i.e. HAART) will shrink the KS lesions in about 40% of patients with AIDS-associated KS. Other treatment modalities include local surgery, radiotherapy and chemotherapy [4, 5].

Practical Points

- Kaposi sarcoma is an AIDS defining, benign tumor of poorly differentiated cell of endothelial origin
- Kaposi sarcoma is the most common malignancy in patients with HIV
- Kaposi sarcoma typically appears in skin or oropharynx with persistent initially flat, patches of redish-purpulish color and involutes to nodules
- HHV8 is present in almost 100% of Kaposi sarcoma lesions
- HAART therapy limits or resolves Kaposi sarcoma

References

1. Stanescu L, Foarfa C, Georgescu AC, Georgescu I. Kaposi's sarcoma associated with AIDS. Roman J Morphol Embryol. 2007;48(2):181–7.
2. Dezube BJ. Clinical presentation and natural history of AIDS-related Kaposi's sarcoma. Hematol Oncol Clin North Am. 1996;10(5):1023–9.
3. Cavallin LE, Goldschmidt-Clermont P, Mesri EA. Molecular and cellular mechanisms of KSHV oncogenesis of Kaposi's sarcoma associated with HIV/AIDS. PLoS Pathog. 2014;10(7):e1004154.
4. Tappero JW, Berger TG, Kaplan LD, Volberding PA, Kahn JO. Cryotherapy for cutaneous Kaposi's sarcoma (KS) associated with acquired immune deficiency syndrome (AIDS): a phase II trial. J Acquir Immune Defic Syndr. 1991;4(9):839–46.
5. Anglemyer A, Agrawal AK, Rutherford GW. Treatment of Kaposi sarcoma in children with HIV-1 infection. Cochrane Database Syst Rev. 2014;(1):CD009826.

Chapter 29
Weight Loss and Tuberculin Skin Test Anergy

Léila Dangou, Medeton Grâce Hounkpe, Josephiel Fortunato, and Crescent Darius Cossou-Gbeto

An 18-month-old girl was referred for consultation by her parents due to weight faltering and deteriorating general condition. There are precarious family socio-economic conditions. The child has only received her BCG vaccine and the vaccination schedule not up-to-date. Physical examination was remarkable for cachexia with height: 79.4 cm, weight: 8.4 kg and mean upper arm circumference (MUAC) of 118 mm.

She was afebrile and had positive appetite test and no other signs.

Q1. Which of the parameters below are the best indices to assess the child's nutritional status?

1. Brachial perimeter
2. Weight and size index
3. Size and weight index
4. Weight and age index

A. 1, 2
B. 3, 4
C. 1, 3
D. 2, 4

Answer: *The correct answer is* ***A***.

L. Dangou
Pediatric Department, Bethesda Hospital in Cotonou, Cotonou, Benin

M. G. Hounkpe
ENT Department, University Hospital Hubert Koutoucou Maga of Cotonou, Cotonou, Benin

J. Fortunato
Pediatric Department, Goho Hospital Center of Abomey, Abomey, Benin

C. D. Cossou-Gbeto (✉)
Internal Medicine, Hematology and Oncology Department, Aix-en-Provence Hospital Center, Aix-en-Provence, France

© Springer Nature Switzerland AG 2020

F. Rahmani, N. Rezaei (eds.), *Pediatric Autoimmunity and Transplantation*,
https://doi.org/10.1007/978-3-030-26280-8_29

The MUAC is used in children between 6 months and 5 years for rapid screening of acute malnutrition and allows to measure the thickness of subcutaneous fat. The weight/height index reflects a recent loss or weight gain, i.e. acute malnutrition. The weight for age index best reflects child's status as being under/overweight. The size-for-age index is an indicator of stunting.

Q2. The girl's weight-for-height index is reported as:

A. As standard deviation
B. As a percentage of the reference median

Answer: *The correct answer is **A**.*

The weight for height index is expressed in standard deviation if the height is less than 120 cm and as a percentage of the reference median if the height is greater than or equal to 120 cm.

Q3. The weight-for-height index for this girl can be calculated as:

A. Below −3 standard deviation
B. Between −3 and −2 standard deviation
C. Less than −4 standard deviation

Answer: *The correct answer is **B**.*

The weight-for-height index compares weight versus average weight for child size. A low weight-for-age index indicates being underweight for a given age. This index makes it possible to identify children suffering from current or acute undernutrition. Children whose weight/height ratio is less than two standard deviations from the median weight/height of the reference population suffer from acute malnutrition (i.e. emaciation or wasting). Those who are less than 3 standard deviations suffer from severe acute malnutrition [1].

Q4. Based on her weight-for-height index, the girl can be categorized as:

A. Moderate acute malnutrition
B. Severe acute malnutrition without complications
C. Severe acute malnutrition with complications

Answer: *The correct answer is **A**.*

Moderate acute malnutrition is identified as moderate wasting if the weight-for-height index is less than −2 Z score and greater than −3 Z score, for children less than 5 years old, or MUAC less than 125 mm and greater than or equal to 115 mm for children 6 to 59 months old [2].

During her hospitalization she presented a dry cough. Her pulmonary examination was normal. The tuberculin skin test showed anergy. Gastric lavage culture did not reveal Bacillus of Koch. HIV serology was negative.

Q5. What could this reaction translate to about the over condition of the patients and the test?

1. An impairment of cell-mediated immunity
2. An impairment of humoral mediated immunity
3. Improper vaccination
4. Failure to exert standards of tuberculin skin test
5. Answers A and D are correct

A. 1, 2
B. 3, 4
C. 1, 4
D. 2, 3

Answers: *The correct answer is* ***C***.

Alteration of cell-mediated immunity is the most common immunological abnormality in malnutrition. A predominant global lymphopenia is observed in T cells. The lymphocyte typing of the T subpopulations shows a significant decrease of $CD4^+$ T cells. On the other hand, the cytotoxic suppressor $CD8^+$ T cells remain stable, thus causing a drop in the $CD4^+/CD8^+$ ratio. This immunological situation is almost identical to that seen in HIV infection. The functional consequence of this lymphopenia is reduced production of interferon and interleukin-2 responsible for cutaneous anergy in tuberculin skin test [3, 4].

Practical Points

- The mid upper arm circumference (MUAC) is a rapid screening test for malnutrition
- The weight/height index reflects a recent loss or weight gain
- The weight-for-age index best reflects child's status as being under/overweight
- The size-for-age index is an indicator of stunting

References

1. World Health Organization, United Nations Children's Fund. WHO growth standards and identification of severe acute malnutrition in children. Geneva: World Health Organization; 2009.
2. World Health Organization. Moderate malnutrition. http://www.who.int/nutrition/topics/moderate_malnutrition/en/.
3. Ibrahim M, Zambruni M, Melby C, Melby P. Impact of childhood malnutrition on host defense and infection. Clin Microbiol Rev. 2017;30(4):919–71.
4. Chandrasekaran P, Saravanan N, Bethunaickan R, Tripathy S. Malnutrition: modulator of immune responses in tuberculosis. Front Immunol. 2017;8:1316.

Chapter 30
Edema on Lower Limbs

Medeton Grâce Hounkpe, Léila Dangou, Josephiel Fortunato, and Crescent Darius Cossou-Gbeto

A 15-month-old baby girl, is referred by her grandmother due to appearance of bilateral edema of the lower limbs. Her vaccination record was not available, as her mother had passed away shortly after her birth and her grandmother did not honor the immunization appointments. Quick nutritional survey shows a lack of nutriment intake adapted to her age.

Physical examination highlighted her weight: 8 kg and height at 79.6 cm.

She was febrile, temperature: 39.8 °C, and she was tachycardic and tachypenic. She also had evidence of respiratory distress, with flaring of nares and appearance of xiphoidal funnel, i.e. subcostal retraction. She had small eyes and skin folds were fading due to undernutrition. Fungal lesions were found in the oral cavity.

Q1. The infants' weight-for-height index is reported as:

A. As standard deviation
B. As a percentage of the reference median

Answer: *The correct answer is* ***A***.

The weight for height index is expressed in standard deviation for a size less than 120 cm.

M. G. Hounkpe
ENT Department, University Hospital Hubert Koutoucou Maga of Cotonou, Cotonou, Benin

L. Dangou
Pediatric Department, Bethesda Hospital in Cotonou, Cotonou, Benin

J. Fortunato
Pediatric Department, Goho Hospital Center of Abomey, Abomey, Benin

C. D. Cossou-Gbeto (✉)
Internal Medicine, Hematology and Oncology Department, Aix-en-Provence Hospital Center, Aix-en-Provence, France

© Springer Nature Switzerland AG 2020

F. Rahmani, N. Rezaei (eds.), *Pediatric Autoimmunity and Transplantation*,
https://doi.org/10.1007/978-3-030-26280-8_30

Q2. The weight-for-height index for this infant can be estimated as:

A. Below −3 standard deviation
B. Between −3 and −2 standard deviation
C. Less than −4 standard deviation

Answer: *The correct answer is* ***A***.

Q3. Based on her weight-for-height index, the infant is categorized as having:

A. Moderate acute malnutrition
B. Severe acute malnutrition without complications
C. Severe acute malnutrition with complications

Answer: *The correct answer is* ***C***.

Severe acute malnutrition is diagnosed in a child having symmetrical edema or a weight-for-height index of less than −3 standard deviations or a weight-for-height index of less than 70% of the reference median or a mean upper arm circumference (MUAC) of less than 115 mm [1].

Malnutrition is "complicated" when it is accompanied by signs that are life-threatening such as respiratory distress, dehydration, infections, etc.

Q4. Which of the answers below give the best of care for this patient?

1. Transfer to pediatric intensive care unit
2. Nutritional management with commercial milk
3. Nutritional management with therapeutic milks (F75 and F100), and ready-to-use therapeutic food (RUTF)
4. Systematic treatment of infections and comorbidities

A. 1, 2
B. 3, 4
C. 1, 3
D. 2, 4

Answer: *The correct answer is* ***B***.

WHO recommendation for severe malnutrition entails giving a protein and energy-poor mixture of F75 that is used during the treatment of infections and as long as anorexia persists. Another mixture, the F100 which is used in a second phase, i.e. nutritional recovery phase, when the child is infectious free and has regained his appetite. It has a higher protein and energy content and allows for greater weight gains. The F100 should be gradually replaced by solid foods that have the advantage of being used as part of a nutritional rehabilitation after discharge of the patient at home [2].

Practical Points

- Severe acute malnutrition presents with the child having a weight-for-height index of less than −3 standard deviations or a weight-for-height index of less than 70% of the reference median or a mean upper arm circumference of less than 115 mm
- WHO recommend to start a giving a protein and energy-poor mixture of F75 that is used during the treatment of infections and as long as anorexia persists
- This can be graded up to F100 in the nutritional recovery phase, when the child is infectious free and has regained his appetite

References

1. National protocol for the management of malnutrition. Available at: www.sante.gouv.bj/.../PROTOCOLE_NATIONALE_PEC_MALNUTRITION.pdf.
2. World Health Organization. WHO Management of severe malnutrition: a manual for use by doctors and other health personnel in managerial positions. Geneva: World Health Organization; 2000.

Chapter 31
Asthenia and Fatigue

Dominique M. A. Bullens and Isabelle Meyts

A 5-year-old boy with a history of IgE-mediated multiple food allergy, is seen at the outpatient clinic for extreme fatigue since 2 weeks ago. He complains of having the need for 13 h of sleep a day to maintain normal daily activities.

His parents had results of his routine laboratory examination from a month and several days ago, with elevated liver enzymes (AST: 106–123 U/L (reference range ≤37 U/L), ALT: 119–213 U/L (reference range ≤41 U/L)), and mild leukopenia and neutropenia (2900/μL WBC and 998/μL ANC respectively). Recent EBV serology was negative, CMV IgG was negative and CMV IgM was detected within "grey zone". Recent cortisol, ACTH and IGF-1 level were within normal range for age.

His past medical history was positive for skin rash following initial breast feedings, after which introduction of hypo-allergenic cow's milk based formula. The new formula had resulted in vomiting and failure to thrive. Specific IgE for cow's milk and hen's egg at the age of 9 months were 3.78 UA/L (reference range <0.10) and 77.1 UA/L (reference range <0.10) respectively (Phadia Immunocap). He received an amino acid formula (Neocate®) and gained weight, but parallel introduction of fruit and vegetables, especially potato's, induced vomiting and diarrhea. Specific IgE and skin prick test for potato yielded to inconclusive results: 0.57 UA/L (reference range <0.10 UA/L) and 2 mm respectively. Specific IgE for banana and pear were 32.2 UA/L (reference range <0.10) and 13.8 UA/L (reference range <0.10) respectively at the age of 18 months. Total IgE remained above detection limit at all time points (>5000 IU/L). Specific IgE levels to pan-allergens were tested to explain potential food reactions: lipid transfer protein and rBet v 1 (PR-10) specific IgE levels were low (0.15 and 0.20 aU/L) as was cross-reactive carbohydrate determinant (bromelain) specific IgE (1.34 aU/L).

D. M. A. Bullens (✉)
Allergy and Clinical Immunology Research Group, KU Leuven, Leuven, Belgium
e-mail: Dominique.Bullens@uzleuven.be

I. Meyts
Inborn Errors of Immunity, KU Leuven, Leuven, Belgium

© Springer Nature Switzerland AG 2020

F. Rahmani, N. Rezaei (eds.), *Pediatric Autoimmunity and Transplantation*,
https://doi.org/10.1007/978-3-030-26280-8_31

The boy's diet remained free of cow's milk, hen's egg, potato, soy, and fruits, with exception of heated melon, spinach, mammal and poultry meat, with exception of duck meat, tree nuts and peanuts, based on micro-array (Immunocap ISAC) testing at the age of 3 years old. He passed a provocation test with extensive cow's milk hydrolysate at the age of three, but still received amino-acid formula, 2 or 3 times a day, due to its better taste. Wheat, rice, corn, sweet potato, salmon and several vegetables were furthermore introduced by the age of three without any problem. He has been since regularly followed by a dietician with growth charts remaining within normal ranges, around 25th percentile, for his age. His weight had remained steady since the onset of current symptoms over the last month.

Also, Gilbert's syndrome had been diagnosed postnatally (A(TA)7TAA/A(TA)7TAA homozygote), *FOXP3* Sanger sequencing had showed no mutations and anti-harmonin and anti-villin antibodies were absent.

Q1. Which one of the following should be the initial step in the management of this patient?

A. No further steps are needed. The boy has normal daily activities and the need for 13 h sleep at this age is not unusual
B. Referral to a specialized dietician
C. Repeat CMV testing and search for CMV excretion in urine
D. Peripheral blood testing for viral and autoimmune hepatitis with new transaminase detection and thyroid function

Answer: *The correct answer is* ***D****.*

Although the boy has normal daily activities, the sudden increase in sleeping hours as well as and the fact that he did not gain any weight during the last month, are suspicious. Moreover, he was seen on a regular basis by a dietician; it would rather make sense to demand the specific findings of her/his previous consults than to refer him to a new dietician without apparent reason. He received an amino-acid based formula with several essential nutrients, reducing the chance that his condition was related to his severe food allergy by omission of necessary nutrients. Although repeating CMV testing could be useful, it is rather necessary to study whether the transaminases are still rising which might point to hepatitis, than to prove CMV diagnosis.

Peripheral blood testing excluded HAV, HCV, CMV and HBV infection and status was immune after immunization. Liver transaminases had slightly declined, while still being above laboratory limits (AST 90 IU/L, ALT 167 IU/L), and thyroid function was normal.

Q2. What test would you demand to help make the most common diagnosis?

A. Abdominal ultrasound
B. Abdominal CT-scan
C. Liver puncture biopsy
D. Repeat CMV testing and search for CMV excretion in urine

Answer: *The correct answer is* ***A****.*

Given the still risen transaminase levels, it is of utmost importance to rule out malignancies and/or hepatosplenomegaly, which is most easily done by ultrasound. Although CT abdomen would reveal similar information, but the radiation burden of the test is in its disadvantage when compared to ultrasound. Liver biopsy is not indicated as transaminase levels are spontaneously decreasing. Finally, CMV IgM was first within grey zone and upon repeat tested negative. There is no good reason to suspect that the second test was wrong.

Ultrasound sonography revealed normal liver span, homogenous liver parenchyma and normal sharp liver angle, normal spleen, kidneys and gall bladder. Multiple small peritoneal lymph nodes, with the largest one measuring 1 cm, were also demonstrated.

Q3. Which of the following laboratory investigations is more likely to give you the most probable diagnosis?

A. Benzodiazepine dosage on urine sample
B. Arterial pO_2 measurement
C. Tissue transglutaminase IgA antibodies on venous blood
D. Sodium chloride measurement on sweat sample

Answer: *The correct answer is* ***C***.

Incidental benzodiazepine intake should have been administered by the boy's parents, which is arguable given his normal daily function. The case does not orient towards severe cardiac or respiratory dysfunction, and arterial pO_2 measurement would not help establish or rule out any of the above diagnoses. Given the severe food allergy, increased chance to find Celiac disease can be suspected, moreover: other signs pointed towards this potential diagnosis especially the lack of weight gain. Diagnosis of cystic fibrosis would be relevant if the failure to thrive (FTT) would remain present for a longer period or when other signs would orient towards CF, which are not in this case.

IgA anti-tissue transglutaminase (anti-tTG) antibodies levels was above 4965.5 CU (reference range ≤20). A duodenal biopsy afterwards revealed subtotal villus atrophy with increased intra-epithelial lymphocytosis, Marsh grade 3a.

Q4. Which statement is correct considering the above clinical and laboratory findings?

A. Diagnosis of celiac disease is highly unlikely
B. Diagnosis of celiac disease is proven
C. Diagnosis of IgE mediated wheat allergy is likely
D. Diagnosis of IgE mediated gluten allergy is proven

Answer: *The correct answer is* ***B***.

Marsh is a clinical classification of celiac disease. Marsh 3a and high tissue transglutaminase IgA levels are sufficient to diagnose celiac disease [1]. The positive predictive value of diagnosis of celiac disease reaches 100% when anti-tTG ab titer is 14-fold higher over the cutoff value [2].

Q5. Which of the following statements is correct regarding long-term management of this condition?

A. The chance to become tolerant for wheat/gluten is 80% within the next 5 years
B. Gluten has to be eliminated from the diet for a life-long term
C. Gluten-free wheat based products should be eliminated life-long
D. Wheat should be temporary substituted by spelt

Answer: *The correct answer is* ***B****.*

Spontaneous induction of tolerance is possible in IgE-mediated wheat allergy, not in celiac disease. In order for complete control of symptoms to be achieved, gluten should be eliminated life-long. Also, gluten-free wheat based products can be used in this child without overt wheat IgE-mediated allergy. Spelt is an inappropriate substitution for wheat, as Spelt and wheat are 95% identical, in protein content and their gluten content is similar.

Q6. Which statement is true regarding co-morbid celiac disease in this boy with multiple IgE-mediated food allergy?

A. Is just a coincidental finding of two unrelated diseases in one patient
B. Decreases the risk to develop new food allergen sensitizations in the boy
C. Increases the chance to detect autoimmune polyendocrine syndrome type 1 (APS-1) or autoimmune polyendocrinopathy candidiasis ectodermal dystrophy (APECED)
D. Is consistent with a five-fold higher risk of developing celiac disease in children with severe food allergy

Answer: *The correct answer is* ***D****.*

Incidence of pediatric celiac disease in Europe is 1%. It is plausible that celiac disease and villous atrophy might increase incidence of food allergy due to disrupted gut barrier. The old Th1/Th2 dichotomy is not correct. The diagnosis of APECED is more suspected with other co-morbid autoimmune pathologies while malabsorption is not an uncommon (18%) finding in APECED. The diagnostic triad of hypoparathyroidism, Addison's disease and candidiasis is not present in all patients and symptoms do not necessarily manifest in early childhood.

The prevalence of the most common disease components of APECED, as reported in Finnish patients were for nonendocrine manifestations candidiasis (100%), enamel hypoplasia (77%), alopecia (72%), nail dystrophy (52%) and keratopathy (35%), and for endocrine manifestations hypoparathyroidism (79%), Addison's disease (72%), ovarian failure (60% of postpubertal patients), and diabetes mellitus (12%) [3, 4].

Another differential diagnosis would be immune dysregulation, polyendocrinopathy, enteropathy-X-linked (IPEX) syndrome, in this boy. However, main diagnostic criteria: Foxp3 and autoimmune antibodies are negative [3].

Practical Points

- The chance to develop celiac disease is five-folds higher in children with severe food allergy than in general population
- Concomitant autoimmunity and severe IgE-mediated allergy are not uncommon and should alert the physician to exclude more complex diagnoses such as IPEX-syndrome, APECED or even celiac disease
- Asthenia in a well-nourished allergic child should be taken seriously and deserves a thorough workup

References

1. Fasano A, Catassi C. Current approaches to diagnosis and treatment of celiac disease: an evolving spectrum. Gastroenterology. 2001;120(3):636–51.
2. Singh P, Kurray L, Agnihotri A, Das P, Verma AK, Sreenivas V, Dattagupta S, Makharia GK. Titers of anti-tissue transglutaminase antibody correlate well with severity of villous abnormalities in celiac disease. J Clin Gastroenterol. 2015;49(3):212–7.
3. Lampasona V, Passerini L, Barzaghi F, Lombardoni C, Bazzigaluppi E, Brigatti C, Bacchetta R, Bosi E. Autoantibodies to harmonin and villin are diagnostic markers in children with IPEX syndrome. PLoS One. 2013;8(11):e78664.
4. Pillon R, Ziberna F, Badina L, Ventura A, Longo G, Quaglia S, De Leo L, Vatta S, Martelossi S, Patano G, Not T, Berti I. Prevalence of celiac disease in patients with severe food allergy. Allergy. 2015;70(10):1346–9.

Chapter 32
Infections, Whitish Skin Papules and Subcutaneous Nodules

Delara Babaei

A 2-year-old girl was admitted to the hospital with a history of recurrent infections and recently developed skin papules. There were whitish pearly papules on her face and neck and subcutaneous nodules around her mouth, nose, and perianal regions (Fig. 32.1). Her mother also complained of joint contracture and limited range of motion in her shoulders, knees, and hips appearing since a year ago, and that she suffered from gingival hypertrophy and rectal prolapse. The patient had been admitted because of upper respiratory infection at the age of 6 and 9 months and due to severe diarrhea at the age of 8 and 11 months. Immunologic workup was performed. CBC was normal. Her serum immunoglobulin levels were within normal range, except for low serum IgG. NBT was normal and there was no abnormality in peripheral blood flow cytometry.

Then after, intravenous immunoglobulin (IVIG) was started due to low level of IgG with the suspicion of humoral immunodeficiency. She was receiving monthly IVIG and her symptoms such as respiratory infections and diarrhea were controlled. Her parents reported excessive crying while changing her cloths. The shoulder X-ray was unremarkable.

IVIG was discontinued so that we were able to perform immunologic evaluations. The level of serum immunoglobulins 1 month after receiving IVIG was as following: IgM: 35 mg/dL, IgA: 58 mg/dL, IgG: 680 mg/dL. Anti-tetanus antibody titers was 1.2 IU/mL (>1 IU/mL protective), and anti-diphtheria antibody titers were 3.4 IU/mL (>1 IU/mL protective). At that time peripheral blood flow cytometry was unremarkable. The lymphocyte transformation test (LTT) response to antigens and mitogens was performed and returned within normal ranges.

D. Babaei (✉)
Department of Allergy and Clinical Immunology, Mofid Children's Hospital, Shahid Beheshti University of Medical Sciences, Tehran, Iran
e-mail: dbabaie@sbmu.ac.ir

© Springer Nature Switzerland AG 2020

F. Rahmani, N. Rezaei (eds.), *Pediatric Autoimmunity and Transplantation*,
https://doi.org/10.1007/978-3-030-26280-8_32

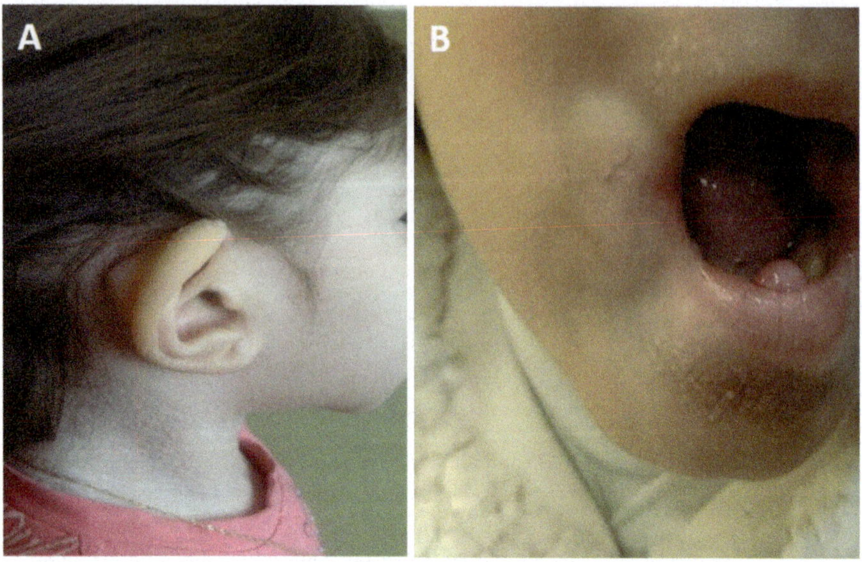

Fig. 32.1 (**a**) Whitish papules on neck, face, and ears, and (**b**) subcutaneous nodules and gingival hypertrophy in a 2-year-old girl with recurrent infections

Skin manifestations are common in primary immunodeficiency disorders (PID). These could be infectious skin lesions or noninfectious including eczematous lesions, erythroderma, cutaneous granulomas, dysplasia of skin, hair, and nails, autoimmune conditions, or frank vasculitis [1]. Cutaneous manifestations of PID diseases are often early findings of the underlying syndrome. Therefore, awareness of these associations may lead to early detection of some immunodeficiency syndromes. Dental and periodontal abnormalities may accompany immunodeficiency and require awareness directed toward diagnosis of hidden disease of the immune system [2]. Some skeletal abnormalities have been reported with immunodeficiency syndromes like Schimkeimmunoosseous dysplasia, cartilage-hair hypoplasia or hyper IgE syndrome [3]. Rectal prolapse is not a common feature in any of the PIDs.

Q1. Which of the following is the most appropriate next step in the evaluation and management of this patient?

A. Continuing regular immunoglobulin infusions
B. Excisional biopsy of subcutaneous nodule
C. Colonoscopy
D. Shoulder MRI

Answer: *The correct answer is* ***B***.

Excisional biopsy of subcutaneous nodule around her mouth was performed, to reveal fibrosis and hyalinization cells with abundant granular cytoplasm, spindle-shaped cells spread in the hyaline material which was suggestive of

Table 32.1 Immunohistochemistry results of subcutaneous nodule of the patient

SMA	Weakly positive in few dispersed cells
Desmin	Negative
CD34	Negative
CD117	Negative (cytoplasmic staining in few dispersed cells)
Ki-67	Positive in rare dispersed cell
S-100	Positive

hyaline fibromatosis syndrome. Immunohistochemistry (IHC) panel was compatible with fibromatosis (Table 32.1).

Hyaline fibromatosis syndrome (HFS) is a rare autosomal recessive disease [4]. It is characterized by abnormal deposition of amorphous hyaline material into dermis and several other tissues [4]. HFS usually presents with pearly papules or fleshy nodules on the face, neck, ears, scalp, hands, feet and perianal regions [4, 5]. Additional features may include progressive joint contracture resulting in mobility limitation, severe pain with movement, skeletal muscle atrophy, gingival hypertrophy, thickened skin, coarse facial features, osteopenia and osteoporosis [6, 7]. The severity is variable: individuals with severe form present in infancy and die in early childhood, previously called infantile systemic hyalinosis, while other patients who have later onset of milder form of disease survive into adulthood, previously called juvenile hyaline fibromatosis [8, 9]. Histopathology of skin lesions demonstrate hyaline material as an amorphous eosinophilic substance in the dermis and spindle-shaped fibroblasts spread in it [10].

Q2. What is the most likely cause of the patient's recurrent infections and severe diarrhea?

A. Transient hypogammaglubinemia of infancy
B. Nonfunctional immunoglubolines
C. Protein losing enteropathy
D. Common variable immunodeficiency

Answer: *The correct answer is* ***C***.

Failure to thrive and protein losing enteropathy (PLE) are important complications in infants with HFS resulting decreased levels of immunoglobulins and some cellular and humoral deficiency which lead to infection susceptibility and affect survival [11]. Common variable immunodeficiency is a heterogeneous group of PIDs described by low level of immunoglobulins, and poor or lack of specific antibody responses to vaccination [3]. Low level of IgG (≤2 SD the mean of the age-adjusted normal range), with low levels of either IgA or IgM is found in CVID patients [12, 13]. Over 90% of adult patients with CVID have IgA levels under the normal range [14]. Serum levels of IgM is more variable but it is reduced in more than 50% of CVID patients [14]. In this patient, low level of IgG and IgA and recurrent infections and optimal response to IVIG primarily lead to the diagnosis of CVID. Although antibody response is not reliable at the age of 11 months, it could distinguish transient hypogammaglobulinemia of infancy (THI) from CVID.

Meanwhile, some findings like reduced range of motions, rectal prolapse that emerged later in the course of disease, are not compatible with neither THI nor CVID. PLE can be considered as a differential diagnosis, and could predispose patient to recurrent infection, and is a common cause of profound hypogammaglobulinemia [15], on the other hand other hand low serum levels of IgA can be justified by incomplete synthesis due to the patient's age. Indeed, levels of specific antibody response and isohemagglutinin titers are helpful in discrimination of THI and PLE from CVID. In this case normal level of immunoglobulins and antibody response is in favor of PLE and against CVID or THI.

Q3. All of the following can be used as treatment options in this patient, except?

A. Regular intravenous immunoglobulin
B. Physical therapy
C. Surgical debulking of rectal prolaps
D. Partial gingivectomy

Answer: *The correct answer is* ***A***.

There is no specific treatment for the hyalinoses. Some modalities like early surgical excision are recommended but recurrences are quite common [16]. Spontaneous regression has been reported in some cases [17]. Intra-lesional steroid injection could be efficient in early stages [18]. Capsulotomy of joint contractures might have temporary benefit [18]. Gingival overgrowth may be treated with partial gingivectomy and shall be repeated if necessary [19].

In this patient excision of hypertrophied gingiva was performed and repeated four other times.

Q4. Which of the following would be the best confirmatory diagnostic option?

A. Excisional study
B. Immunohistochemistry
C. Skin biopsy
D. Molecular study

Answer: *The correct answer is* ***D***.

Molecular genetic testing revealed mutations in the capillary morphogenesis gene 2 (*CMG2*) gene being responsible for this autosomal recessive condition [20]. Expression of CMG2 as a transmembrane protein is mandatory during capillary formation. CMG2 binds to collagen IV through its Von-Willebrand factor type A (VWA) domain [21].

Practical Points

- Hyaline fibromatosis syndrome (HFS) is an autosomal recessive condition featured by abnormal hyaline deposition in the body tissues, primarily skin and mucous membranes

- Joint contractures, gingival hypertrophy, osteopenia, osteoporosis, failure to thrive, and protein losing enteropathy are additional features of HFS
- Protein losing enteropathy might lead to infection susceptibility and secondary immunodeficiency

References

1. Lehman H. Skin manifestations of primary immune deficiency. Clin Rev Allergy Immunol. 2014;46(2):112–9.
2. Szczawinska-Poplonyk A, Gerreth K, Breborowicz A, Borysewicz-Lewicka M. Oral manifestations of primary immune deficiencies in children. Oral Surg Oral Med Oral Pathol Oral Radiol Endod. 2009;108(3):e9–20.
3. Rezaei N, de Vries E, Gambineri E, Haddad E. Common presentations and diagnostic approaches. In: Sullivan KE, Stiehm ER, editors. Stiehm's immune deficiencies. London: Elsevier; 2014. p. 29.
4. Shieh JTC, Hoyme HE, Arbour LT. Hyalinosis, inherited systemic. GeneReviews, 11 Apr 2013.
5. Momin YA, Bharambe BM, D'Costa G. Juvenile hyaline fibromatosis: a rare lesion. Indian J Pathol Microbiol. 2011;54(4):838–9.
6. Aghighi Y, Bahremand S, Nematollahi LR. Infantile systemic hyalinosis: report of three Iranian children and review of the literature. Clin Rheumatol. 2007;26(1):128–30.
7. Lindvall LE, Kormeili T, Chen E, Ramirez MCM, Grum-Tokars V, Glucksman MJ, et al. Infantile systemic hyalinosis: case report and review of the literature. J Am Acad Dermatol. 2008;58(2):303–7.
8. Nofal A, Sanad M, Assaf M, Nofal E, Nassar A, Almokadem S, et al. Juvenile hyaline fibromatosis and infantile systemic hyalinosis: a unifying term and a proposed grading system. J Am Acad Dermatol. 2009;61(4):695–700.
9. Glover MT, Lake BD, Atherton DJ. Infantile systemic hyalinosis: newly recognized disorder of collagen? Pediatrics. 1991;87(2):228–34.
10. Urbina F, Sazunic I, Murray G. Infantile systemic hyalinosis or juvenile hyaline fibromatosis? Pediatr Dermatol. 2004;21(2):154–9.
11. Klebanov Y, Schwindt C. Infantile systemic hyalinosis: a case report of compromised cellular and humoral branches of the immune system leading to infections. Pediatr Asthma Allergy Immunol. 2009;22(3):127–30.
12. Conley ME, Notarangelo LD, Etzioni A. Diagnostic criteria for primary immunodeficiencies. Representing PAGID (Pan-American Group for Immunodeficiency) and ESID (European Society for Immunodeficiencies). Clin Immunol. 1999;93(3):190–7.
13. Al-Herz W, Bousfiha A, Casanova JL, Chapel H, Conley ME, Cunningham-Rundles C, et al. Primary immunodeficiency diseases: an update on the classification from the International Union of Immunological Societies Expert Committee for Primary Immunodeficiency. Front Immunol. 2015;35(8):696–726.
14. Cunningham-Rundles C, Warnatz K. Hypogammaglobulinemia and common variable immunodeficiency. In: Sullivan KE, Stiehm ER, editors. Stiehm's immune deficiencies. London: Elsevier; 2014. p. 347–61.
15. Onigbanjo MT, Orange JS, Perez EE, Sullivan KE. Hypogammaglobulinemia in a pediatric tertiary care setting. Clin Immunol. 2007;125(1):52–9.
16. Woyke S, Domagala W, Markiewicz C. A 19-year follow-up of multiple juvenile hyaline fibromatosis. J Pediatr Surg. 1984;19:302–4.

17. Remberger K, Krieg T, Kunze D, Weinmann H-M, Hübner G. Fibromatosis hyalinica multiplex (juvenile hyalin fibromatosis). Light microscopic, electron microscopic, immunohistochemical, and biochemical findings. Cancer. 1985;56:614–24.
18. Kitano Y. Juvenile hyaline fibromatosis. Arch Dermatol. 1976;112:86–8.
19. Aldred MJ, Crawford PJ. Juvenile hyaline fibromatosis. Oral Surg Oral Med Oral Pathol. 1987;63:71–7.
20. Dowling O, Difeo A, Ramirez MC, Tukel T, Narla G, Bonafe L, et al. Mutations in capillary morphogenesis gene-2 result in the allelic disorders juvenile hyaline fibromatosis and infantile systemic hyalinosis. Am J Hum Genet. 2003;73(4):957–66.
21. Deuquet J, Lausch E, Superti-Furga A, Van Der Goot FG. The dark sides of capillary morphogenesis gene 2. EMBO J. 2012;31(1):3–13.

Chapter 33
Recurrent Pneumonia and History of Transplantation

Sonia de Arriba-Méndez, Eva Macías, and Ignacio Dávila

Our patient is a 5-year-old girl who has been suffering from recurrent respiratory infections for a year and a half. She has been diagnosed on numerous occasions with pneumonia in different lobes and otitis media, such that, she is prescribed oral antibiotic treatment at least once a month. She was referred to our clinic for further evaluation and workup.

From her medical history, we highlight that she was diagnosed with a Hurler syndrome a few months after her birth and received a bone marrow transplant at 23 months old. One hundred and seventy days after the transplant she suffered from autoimmune thrombocytopenia, which triggered an intracranial hemorrhage. She was treated with several courses of intravenous gammaglobulin, romiplostim (N-plate), rituximab (8 courses), vincristine and mesenchymal stem cell therapy. Following this last treatment, she fully recovered. Three months later she had a bone marrow failure caused by parvovirus. She fully recovered from this complication as well.

She was doing well until the aforementioned respiratory infections appeared a year and a half before the present consultation.

S. de Arriba-Méndez (✉)
Pediatric Service, University Hospital of Salamanca, Salamanca, Spain

Faculty of Medicine, Department of Biologic and Diagnostics Sciences, University of Salamanca, Salamanca, Spain
e-mail: sdearriba@usal.es

E. Macías · I. Dávila
Faculty of Medicine, Department of Biologic and Diagnostics Sciences, University of Salamanca, Salamanca, Spain

Allergy Service, University Hospital of Salamanca, Salamanca, Spain

© Springer Nature Switzerland AG 2020

F. Rahmani, N. Rezaei (eds.), *Pediatric Autoimmunity and Transplantation*,
https://doi.org/10.1007/978-3-030-26280-8_33

Q1. According to clinical presentation and history above, what is the first diagnostic suspicion?

A. Combined immunodeficiency
B. Predominantly antibody deficiency
C. Hyper-IgE syndrome
D. Chronic granulomatous disease

Answer: *The correct answer is* ***B****.*

The most common infections in predominantly antibody deficiency are respiratory tract infections caused by encapsulated pyogenic bacteria, such as *Streptococcus pneumonia* and *Haemophilus influenza*, often leading to bronchiectasis. Viral infections are often well tolerated, except for enteroviruses, as immunoglobulins are quite important in antibody mediated opsonization of this type of viruses [1, 2].

Patients with combined immunodeficiencies usually present with infections and lymph node hypoplasia during the first months of life. These infections are usually severe and prolonged, and are caused by gram-negative bacteria, opportunistic organisms, fungal infections like persistent candidiasis or invasive infections by *Aspergillus* spp. [1]

Recurrent cutaneous and systemic infections in hyper-IgE syndrome are caused mainly by *S. aureus*. Pulmonary infections are severe and complications like pneumatocele are frequent. Mucocutaneous candidiasis and other fungal infections are typical manifestations of this disorder. Opportunistic infections are also reported [1, 3].

Patients with chronic granulomatous disease are susceptible to catalase-positive bacteria such as *Staphylococcus aureus* and Burkholderia, or fungi like Aspergillus or Nocardia. Typical infections in these patients include purulent bacterial infections, such as pneumonia, sinusitis, suppurative lymphadenitis or liver abscess. Necrotizing fungal infections, osteomyelitis, and sepsis are also among frequently observed complications [4, 5].

Q2. What are the primary tests that you would order?

A. Complete blood count and quantitation of serum immunoglobulin concentrations
B. Lymphocyte proliferation tests in response to PHA, Con-A, and PMA/I
C. Dihydrorhadamine and nitroblu-tetrazolium tests
D. Thoracic computed tomography

Answer: *The correct answer is* ***A****.*

Given the suspicion of predominantly antibody deficiency, initial step would be CBC and quantification of serum immunoglobulin concentrations [6, 7].

The patient's complete blood count was normal, but she had hypogammaglobulinemia. We found low serum IgG level (42.3 mg/dL; reference range: 400–1100), low IgA level (<6.25 mg/dL; reference range: 10–160), and normal IgM (37.9 mg/dL; normal range: 40–180).

The cytometry showed a decrease in memory B cells, 96% of which were unswitched $IgM^{+}IgD^{+}$ cells and a decrease in plasma cells, but no alteration in $CD4^{+}$ or $CD8^{+}$ T cell count. Regulatory T cells were normal, and $CD3^{+}CD4^{-}CD8^{-}$ (i.e. double negative) T cells were not increased.

Q3. Which of the following is the most probable cause of hypogammaglobulinemia in this patient?

A. Common variable immunodeficiency
B. Antibody deficiency secondary to vincristine
C. Antibody deficiency secondary to rituximab
D. Autosomal recessive agammaglobulinemia

Answer: *The correct answer is* ***C****.*

Rituximab is an anti-CD20 monoclonal antibody used for the treatment of autoimmune diseases, like rheumatoid arthritis or anti-neutrophil cytoplasm antibody-associated vasculitis. It is increasingly used to treat idiopathic thrombocytopenic purpura [8]. Rituximab depletes pre-plasma B cell repertoire and alters B cell signaling hence impairing the production of anti-pathogen autoantibody [9].

Normal IgG levels are usually resumed after this treatment, yet prolonged post-rituximab hypogammaglobulinemia and associated infections have been reported [9, 10]. Rituximab might block humoral responses to immunization for several months [9–11].

Q4. What is the best treatment option for this patient?

A. Immunoglobulin replacement
B. Sulfamethoxazole-trimethoprim prophylaxis
C. Monthly antibiotic treatment courses
D. Bone marrow transplant

Answer: *The correct answer is* ***A****.*

There are no guidelines for the initiation of the IgG replacement in secondary humoral immunodeficiency. Most authors start IgG replacement when hypogammaglobulinemia is moderate (IgG <500 mg/dL) or severe (IgG <200 mg/dL). Severity of hypogammaglobulinemia, IgG antibody titers, frequency of infections and other risk factors should be considered when considering to put a patients in immunoglobulin replacement therapy [9, 11].

Our patient had severe hypogammaglobulinemia and recurrent infections, justifying to start immunoglobulin replacement therapy.

Practical Points

- Predominantly antibody deficiencies are characterized by respiratory tract infections caused by encapsulated pyogenic bacteria
- Prolonged hypogammaglobulinemia and associated infections have been reported post-rituximab therapy
- Most authors recommend to start IgG replacement when post-rituximab hypogammaglobulinemia is moderate or severe, although IgG antibody titers, infections, and other patient risk factors should be considered

References

1. Stiehm ER, Ochs HD, Winkelstein JA. Immunodeficiency disorders: general considerations. In: Stiehm ER, Ochs HD, Winkelstein JA, editors. Immunologic disorders in infants and children. 5th ed. Philadelphia, PA: Saunders/Elsevier; 2004.
2. Seymour B, Miles J, Haeney M. Primary antibody deficiency and diagnostic delay. J Clin Pathol. 2005;58(5):546–7.
3. Erlewyn-Lajeunesse MD. Hyperimmunoglobulin-E syndrome with recurrent infection: a review of current opinion and treatment. Pediatr Allergy Immunol. 2000;11(3):133–41.
4. Chiriaco M, Salfa I, Di Matteo G, Rossi P, Finocchi A. Chronic granulomatous disease: Clinical, molecular, and therapeutic aspects. Pediatr Allergy Immunol. 2016;27(3):242–53.
5. Song E, Jaishankar GB, Saleh H, Jithpratuck W, Sahni R, Krishnaswamy G. Chronic granulomatous disease: a review of the infectious and inflammatory complications. Clin Mol Allergy. 2011;9(1):10.
6. Ballow M. Approach to the patient with recurrent infections. Clin Rev Allergy Immunol. 2008;34(2):129–40.
7. Oliveira JB, Fleisher TA. Laboratory evaluation of primary immunodeficiencies. J Allergy Clin Immunol. 2010;125(2 Suppl 2):S297–305.
8. Arnold DM, Dentali F, Crowther MA, Meyer RM, Cook RJ, Sigouin C, Fraser GA, Lim W, Kelton JG. Systematic review: efficacy and safety of rituximab for adults with idiopathic thrombocytopenic purpura. Ann Intern Med. 2007;146(1):25–33.
9. Roberts DM, Jones RB, Smith RM, Alberici F, Kumaratne DS, Burns S, Jayne DR. Rituximab-associated hypogammaglobulinemia: incidence, predictors and outcomes in patients with multi-system autoimmune disease. J Autoimmun. 2015;57:60–5.
10. Nishio M, Fujimoto K, Yamamoto S, Endo T, Sakai T, Obara M, Kumano K, Minauchi K, Yamaguchi K, Takeda Y, Sato N, Koizumi K, Mukai M, Koike T. Hypogammaglobulinemia with a selective delayed recovery in memory B cells and an impaired isotype expression after rituximab administration as an adjuvant to autologous stem cell transplantation for non-Hodgkin lymphoma. Eur J Haematol. 2006;77(3):226–32.
11. Looney RJ, Srinivasan R, Calabrese LH. The effects of rituximab on immunocompetency in patients with autoimmune disease. Arthritis Rheum. 2008;58(1):5–14.

Chapter 34
Painful Skin Nodules, Prolonged Fever and Cervical Lymphadenopathy

Michelle N. G. Ying, Emily Yiping Gan, and Jean Aan Mark Koh

A 16-year-old girl presented with multiple painful skin nodules associated with intermittent high fever. There was a 10-year history of recurrent painful oral ulcers lasting several weeks. Physical examination revealed multiple, deep, tender, erythematous "sweet's-syndrome like" nodules on her trunk, upper and lower limbs (Fig. 34.1). There were several non-tender lymph node swellings in bilateral post-auricular regions, all below 1 cm in diameter. A systemic review of the major organ systems including respiratory and gastrointestinal tract was unremarkable.

Laboratory investigations showed raised inflammatory markers: CRP was 11.6 mg/dL (reference range: 0.0–5.0) and ESR was 59 mm/h (reference range: 3–15). CBC showed hemoglobin 11.9 g/dL, WBC: 10,950/μL and platelet count: 235,000/μL. Punch biopsy of a nodular lesion showed neutrophilic and histiocytic infiltrates extending from the superficial to deep dermis, consistent with a neutrophilic dermatosis. Incisional biopsy of a deep nodule revealed thickening of the subcutaneous septa with involvement of the adjacent fat lobules by a mixed inflammatory infiltrate, consistent with septolobular panniculitis. Infective stains and tissue cultures for fungus and acid fast bacilli (AFB) were negative on both skin biopsies. Clinical and pathological features were consistent with a diagnosis of Sweet's syndrome. Thorough investigations for inflammatory bowel disease, autoimmune diseases and hematologic malignancies returned negative. The skin lesions improved with a tailing course of oral prednisolone and oral colchicine and the disease remained quiescent.

M. N. G. Ying · E. Y. Gan (✉) · J. A. M. Koh
Dermatology Service, KK Women's and Children's Hospital, Singapore, Singapore

© Springer Nature Switzerland AG 2020
F. Rahmani, N. Rezaei (eds.), *Pediatric Autoimmunity and Transplantation*,
https://doi.org/10.1007/978-3-030-26280-8_34

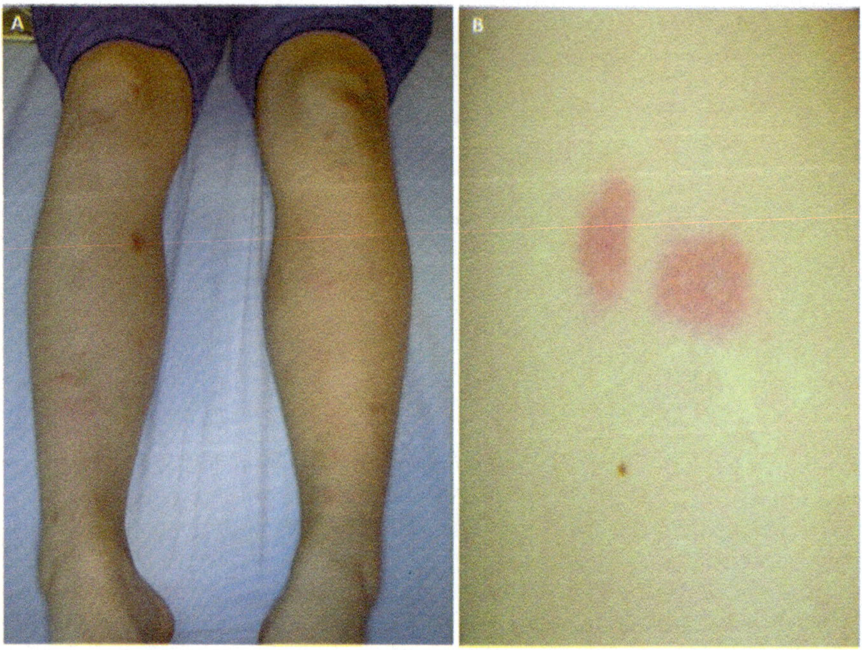

Fig. 34.1 (**a**) Multiple tender erythematous nodules over both lower limbs. (**b**) The size of the lesions vary from less than 1 cm to as large as 2 cm in diameter

She re-presented 1 year later with prolonged fever and multiple bilateral enlarged cervical lymph nodes of a 2 month duration. The WBC count was raised at 23,350/μL, mainly due to neutrophilia. CRP was 17.9 mg/dL and ESR was 92 mm/h. Serology for HIV, hepatitis B and C, cytomegalovirus, bartonella and toxoplasma returned negative. CT scan showed multiple enlarged lymph nodes in the neck, thorax and upper abdomen with no evidence of liquefaction or calcification. In view of the positive CT scan findings, suspicion of TB was raised, as it is endemic in Singapore. TB T-Spot screening test was sent and returned positive. Excision biopsy of an enlarged cervical node showed necrotizing granulomatous inflammation. Tissue culture of the lymph node grew *Mycobacterium abscessus*. At the same time, the patient developed generalized non-pruritic pin-point erythematous-to-brown macules, clinically suggestive of lichen scrofulosorum (Fig. 34.2).

The patient was started empirically on intravenous cefoxitin 12 g daily, intravenous amikacin 500 mg daily, and twice daily oral clarithromycin 500 mg. After 6 weeks of treatment with the initial anti-tuberculous regimen, treatment was changed to a combination of oral linezolid and azithromycin according to culture sensitivities, and this was continued for 6 months. On subsequent outpatient reviews, cervical lymph nodes had reduced dramatically in size with minimal evidence of the initial rash.

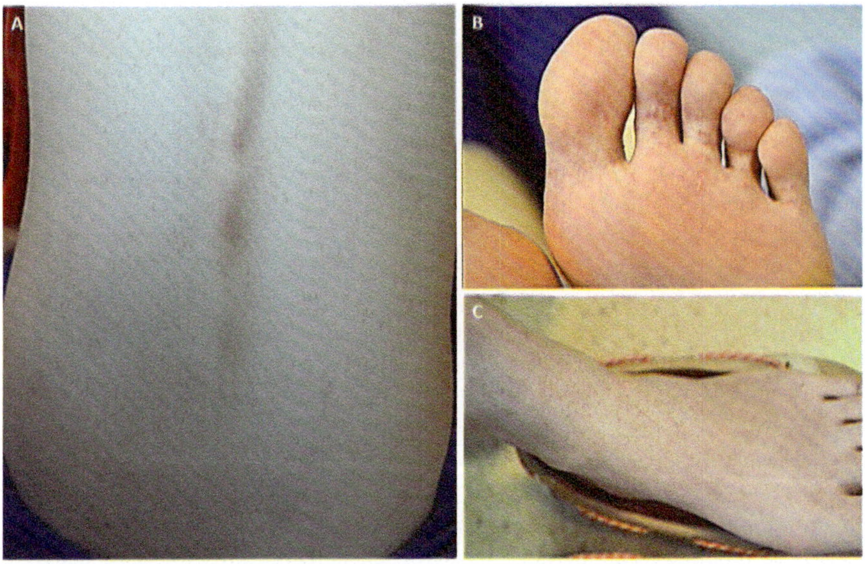

Fig. 34.2 (**a**) Extensive flat erythematous pin-point macules over the entire body and (**b**, **c**) limbs suggestive of lichen scrofulosorum

Q1. Given the overall clinical history and progress, which disease category is most likely present in this patient?

A. Chronic inflammatory disorder
B. Autoimmune disease
C. Primary immunodeficiency
D. Chronic atypical bacterial or fungal infection

Answer: *The correct answer is* ***C***.

Non-tuberculous mycobacterial (NTM) infections are uncommon and characterized as opportunistic infections that typically occur in the setting of an immunocompromised host. Cell-mediated immunity is responsible for defence against intracellular pathogens, especially the NTM species. In particular, IFN-γ is a key cytokine produced predominantly by T helper 1 cells and natural killer cells and plays a crucial role in this immune cascade. Disseminated NTM infections occurring in a young but otherwise healthy immunocompetent host should raise the suspicion of an underlying PID. While a majority of the classic PID cases are disorders of genetic origin, commonly diagnosed in children below the age of one, milder forms may not be recognized until late adolescence, as in our case.

Q2. Which of the following investigations is most appropriate in patients with recurrent *Mycobacterium abscessus* infections?

A. Measurement of complement levels
B. Measurement of serum immunoglobulin levels

C. Bone marrow aspiration and trephine
D. Screen for Mendelian susceptibility to mycobacterial disease (MSMD)

Answer: *The correct answer is* ***D.***

As described in medical literature, children presenting with severe NTM infections should be investigated for potential genetic defects in genes encoding components of the IFN-γ/IL-12 axis, a condition termed Mendelian susceptibility to mycobacterial disease (MSMD) [1]. First-line investigation, before considering other non-genetic reasons, would therefore be screening for MSMD.

As many as 13 genetic mutations involving the *IFNGR1*, *IFNGR2*, *STAT1*, *IL12RB1* and *IL12B* genes have been identified, and disease severity correlates with the amount of residual functional signalling between IFN-γ and IL-12 [1]. Mean age at onset of mycobacterial infection is 13.4 years old (ranging from 1.5 to 57 years old). Mutations that cause complete receptor deficiencies typically result in a very severe disseminated infection of an early onset with a very poor prognosis. These children are mostly infected by BCG and NTM, notably rapid growers like *M. fortuitum, M. chelonae, M. smegmatis* and *M. peregrinum*. Salmonellosis has also been reported to be the next most frequent infectious disease particularly in patients with IL-12β1 (*IL12B* gene) deficiency [1].

Most PIDs are of genetic origin and manifest early in life. Secondary immunodeficiencies and a small proportion of PIDs might present later during adulthood. This was demonstrated in our case, in which a screen for MSMD in the child returned as negative. This warranted a search for non-genetic, acquired defects that could disrupt the IFN-γ-associated immune pathway displaying a similar immunodeficiency picture.

The MSMD screening test highlights the crucial role of the IFN-γ/IL-12 in the phagocyte respiratory burst axis. Screening is performed by analysing peripheral blood mononuclear cell's response to Bacillus Calmette–Guérin (BCG) stimulation with or without IFN-γ and IL-12. If the cells are able to demonstrate detectable response to BCG ± IFN-γ/IL-12 stimulation, as shown in our patient, it means that the cytokine production profile is normal, i.e. there are no genetic defects.

Q3. What is the most likely underlying cause of immunodeficiency in this child?

A. Production of anti-IFN-γ autoantibodies
B. IFN-γ hypofunctional receptor mutation
C. Deficiency in serum IL-12 levels
D. Loss of cell surface expression of IL-12 receptors

Answer: *The correct answer is* ***A.***

A screen for anti-IFN-γ autoantibodies in our child returned positive (as shown in Table 34.1). First described in 2004 [2, 3], an acquired defect of the IFN-γ pathway signalling renders susceptibility to multiple opportunistic infections caused by dimorphic fungi, parasites, bacteria and mycobacteria including tuberculosis and

Table 34.1 Comparative assays demonstrating inhibition in the detection of IFN-γ by ELISA

Sample number	Date of sample extraction	Plasma dilution for 50% inhibition of input IFN-γ	Interpretation	Conclusion
1	15/02/17	1:16,129	There was a ~2 times reduction in plasma dilution between first and second blood samples to achieve 50% inhibition for assay.	Upon anti-NTM treatment initiation, there is a consistent trend in reduction of IFN-γ autoantibody titers in both assays tested respectively, taken at subsequent outpatient follow up visits.
2	28/03/17	1:7472		
1	15/02/17	1:6758	There was a 34% reduction in plasma dilution between first and second blood samples to achieve 50% inhibition for assay.	
2	10/07/17	1:4444		

IFN-γ interferon gamma, *NTM* non-tuberculosis mycobacteria

more commonly, NTM species [2, 4]. The distinctive role of IFN-γ in the control of NTM-specific infection has been well documented in the literature [1–3, 5–7].

In our patient, the pathological anti-IFN-γ autoantibodies with neutralizing capacity impaired the killing of intracellular organisms by macrophages, and led to severe disseminated NTM infection.

This syndrome is uncommon and has been reported to affect only adults, mostly females, of predominantly East Asian origin, with presentation between 30 to 50 years of age [2, 4, 5, 8, 9]. Exceptionally, two recent case reports have described the disease in Caucasians [10, 11]. To our knowledge, there have so far been no reports of this condition occurring in children or adolescents.

In healthy persons, low-titers of naturally-occurring anti-cytokine autoantibodies may be part of an immune regulatory response to inflammation and infection [5, 12]. It is unclear, however, what causes an overproduction of autoantibodies that exhibit inhibitory effects at high-titers, nor do we understand their causal role in the disease [2]. A genetic origin is strongly suspected given the racial predisposition in adults of East Asian origin [13, 14]. There may be a stronger role for a genetic predisposition as we now know that the disease can occur early in childhood. One putative hypothesis to explain this condition is that certain infections are capable of stimulating production of these high-titer neutralizing IFN-γ autoantibodies [5]. A screening study of 41 anti-cytokine autoantibodies performed on a group of patients in Thailand and Taiwan, demonstrated that only autoantibodies against IFN-γ correlated with disseminated opportunistic infection, with a large proportion (88%) caused by NTM species [4].

Our case has shown that in children and adolescents who present with severe NTM infections with no obvious genetic defects found in the IFN-γ/IL-12 axis, and with no apparent iatrogenic cause, a screen for serum neutralizing anti-IFN-γ autoantibodies needs to be undertaken.

Q4. What is the first step in treatment of disseminated NTM infection in this patient?

A. Monoclonal antibodies such as rituximab
B. Start intravenous anti-NTM treatment
C. One dose of intravenous methylprednisolone, followed by intravenous anti-NTM treatment
D. Plasmapheresis and activated factor VII injection

Answer: *The correct answer is* ***B****.*

Primary step in treatment of immunodeficiency due to anti-IFN-γ autoantibodies, is successful eradication of NTM disease by targeted combination antibiotic therapy for at least 4–6 months duration. Our patient showed a good response to anti-NTM treatment as reflected by a reduction of IFN-γ autoantibody titers on subsequent follow-up visits (Table 34.1). Skin and subcutaneous infections, such as cervical lymphadenitis as seen in our case, are typically caused by rapid NTM growers such as *M. abscessus, M. fortuitum* and *M. chelonae*. The most effective antibiotic choices include amikacin, cefoxitin, imipenem and clarithromycin, with multidrug clarithromycin-based therapy offering the best chance of cure.

Many patients however, remain actively infected despite antimicrobial therapy [2, 15, 16]. Cautious use of rituximab, a monoclonal anti-CD20 antibody therapy has been used with success in some patients [17, 18].

Q5. What is the most important prognostic factor in this patient?

A. Type of NTM infection
B. Age of onset
C. Serum level of anti-IFN-γ autoantibodies
D. Onset of treatment

Answer: *The correct answer is* ***C****.*

The prognosis of the disease is largely dependent on the amount of IFN-γ inhibition, reflecting the level of intact IFN-γ signaling in the individual. High-titers of anti-IFN-γ autoantibodies indicate a more significant inhibitory effect, leading to ineffective eradication of the NTM infection with greater propensity for widespread dissemination and resistance to therapy [1, 5].

Practical Points

- Disseminated non-tuberculous mycobacterial infections occurring in a young patient should raise the suspicion of an underlying primary immunodeficiency
- First line investigations should comprise a search for mendelian susceptibility to mycobacterial disease (MSMD), in particular IL-12:IFN-γ loop defects

- Patients with acquired defects that could disrupt the IFN-γ-associated immune pathway, such as pathological presence of anti-IFN-γ autoantibodies with neutralizing capacity, display a similar immunodeficiency picture to MSMD

References

1. Filipe-Santos O, Bustamante J, Chapgier A, Vogt G, de Beaucoudrey L, Feinberg J, Jouanguy E, Boisson-Dupuis S, Fieschi C, Picard C, Casanova JL. Inborn errors of IL-12/23- and IFN-gamma-mediated immunity: molecular, cellular, and clinical features. Semin Immunol. 2006;18(6):347–61.
2. Doffinger R, Helbert MR, Barcenas-Morales G, Yang K, Dupuis S, Ceron-Gutierrez L, Espitia-Pinzon C, Barnes N, Bothamley G, Casanova JL, Longhurst HJ, Kumararatne DS. Autoantibodies to interferon-gamma in a patient with selective susceptibility to mycobacterial infection and organ-specific autoimmunity. Clin Infect Dis. 2004;38(1):e10–4.
3. Hoflich C, Sabat R, Rosseau S, Temmesfeld B, Slevogt H, Docke WD, Grutz G, Meisel C, Halle E, Gobel UB, Volk HD, Suttorp N. Naturally occurring anti-IFN-gamma autoantibody and severe infections with Mycobacterium cheloneae and Burkholderia cocovenenans. Blood. 2004;103(2):673–5.
4. Browne SK, Burbelo PD, Chetchotisakd P, Suputtamongkol Y, Kiertiburanakul S, Shaw PA, Kirk JL, Jutivorakool K, Zaman R, Ding L, Hsu AP, Patel SY, Olivier KN, Lulitanond V, Mootsikapun P, Anunnatsiri S, Angkasekwinai N, Sathapatayavongs B, Hsueh PR, Shieh CC, Brown MR, Thongnoppakhun W, Claypool R, Sampaio EP, Thepthai C, Waywa D, Dacombe C, Reizes Y, Zelazny AM, Saleeb P, Rosen LB, Mo A, Iadarola M, Holland SM. Adult-onset immunodeficiency in Thailand and Taiwan. N Engl J Med. 2012;367(8):725–34.
5. Patel SY, Ding L, Brown MR, Lantz L, Gay T, Cohen S, Martyak LA, Kubak B, Holland SM. Anti-IFN-gamma autoantibodies in disseminated nontuberculous mycobacterial infections. J Immunol (Baltimore, MD: 1950). 2005;175(7):4769–76.
6. Baerlecken N, Jacobs R, Stoll M, Schmidt R, Witte T. Recurrent, multifocal Mycobacterium avium-intercellulare infection in a patient with interferon-gamma autoantibody. Clin Infect Dis. 2009;49(7):e76–8.
7. Kampmann B, Hemingway C, Stephens A, Davidson R, Goodsall A, Anderson S, Nicol M, Scholvinck E, Relman D, Waddell S, Langford P, Sheehan B, Semple L, Wilkinson KA, Wilkinson RJ, Ress S, Hibberd M, Levin M. Acquired predisposition to mycobacterial disease due to autoantibodies to IFN-gamma. J Clin Invest. 2005;115(9):2480–8.
8. Wongkulab P, Wipasa J, Chaiwarith R, Supparatpinyo K. Autoantibody to interferon-gamma associated with adult-onset immunodeficiency in non-HIV individuals in Northern Thailand. PLoS One. 2013;8(9):e76371.
9. Liu TT, Weng SW, Wang MC, Huang WT. Nontuberculous mycobacterial infection with concurrent IgG4-related lymphadenopathy. APMIS. 2016;124(3):216–20.
10. O'Connell E, Rosen LB, LaRue RW, Fabre V, Melia MT, Auwaerter PG, Holland SM, Browne SK. The first US domestic report of disseminated Mycobacterium avium complex and anti-interferon-gamma autoantibodies. J Clin Immunol. 2014;34(8):928–32.
11. Hanitsch LG, Lobel M, Muller-Redetzky H, Schurmann M, Suttorp N, Unterwalder N, Monnich U, Meisel C, Wittke K, Volk HD, Scheibenbogen C, Kolsch U. Late-onset disseminated Mycobacterium avium intracellulare complex infection (MAC), cerebral toxoplasmosis and salmonella sepsis in a German caucasian patient with unusual anti-interferon-gamma IgG1 autoantibodies. J Clin Immunol. 2015;35(4):361–5.

12. Revoltella RP. Natural and therapeutically-induced antibodies to cytokines. Biotherapy (Dordrecht, Netherlands). 1998;10(4):321–31.
13. Pithukpakorn M, Roothumnong E, Angkasekwinai N, Suktitipat B, Assawamakin A, Luangwedchakarn V, Umrod P, Thongnoppakhun W, Foongladda S, Suputtamongkol Y. HLA-DRB1 and HLA-DQB1 are associated with adult-onset immunodeficiency with acquired anti-interferon-gamma autoantibodies. PLoS One. 2015;10(5):e0128481.
14. Chi CY, Chu CC, Liu JP, Lin CH, Ho MW, Lo WJ, Lin PC, Chen HJ, Chou CH, Feng JY, Fung CP, Sher YP, Li CY, Wang JH, Ku CL. Anti-IFN-gamma autoantibodies in adults with disseminated nontuberculous mycobacterial infections are associated with HLA-DRB1∗16:02 and HLA-DQB1∗05:02 and the reactivation of latent varicella-zoster virus infection. Blood. 2013;121(8):1357–66.
15. C JF, Trendell-Smith N, Chan J, Hung I, Tang B, Cheng V, Yeung C, Yuen K. Reactive and infective dermatoses associated with adult-onset immunodeficiency due to anti-interferon-gamma autoantibody: Sweet's syndrome and beyond. Dermatology. 2013;226(2):157–66.
16. Hase I, Morimoto K, Sakagami T, Kazumi Y, Ishii Y, van Ingen J. Disseminated Mycobacterium gordonae and Mycobacterium mantenii infection with elevated anti-IFN-gamma neutralizing autoantibodies. J Infect Chemother. 2015;21(6):468–72.
17. Browne SK, Zaman R, Sampaio EP, Jutivorakool K, Rosen LB, Ding L, Pancholi MJ, Yang LM, Priel DL, Uzel G, Freeman AF, Hayes CE, Baxter R, Cohen SH, Holland SM. Anti-CD20 (rituximab) therapy for anti-IFN-gamma autoantibody-associated nontuberculous mycobacterial infection. Blood. 2012;119(17):3933–9.
18. Pruetpongpun N, Khawcharoenporn T, Damronglerd P, Suthiwartnarueput W, Apisarnthanarak A, Rujanavej S, Suwantarat N. Disseminated Talaromyces marneffei and Mycobacterium abscessus in a patient with anti-interferon-gamma autoantibodies. Open Forum Infect Dis. 2016;3(2):ofw093.

Chapter 35
Malaise, Laryngitis and Fever

Claus-Philipp Maier and Dominik Schneidawind

An 18-year-old male patient presented to the emergency department of a University Medical Center with malaise, laryngitis and fever lasting for 4 weeks. He had taken ibuprofen (400 mg twice daily) for 3 weeks to soothe his swollen and ulcerated gingiva as well as painful teeth. Moreover, he had lost 6 kg weight without intention within the last month. He had no night sweats.

He was healthy and doing well until his symptoms appeared. He had been on vacation with friends in Southern Florida after graduation from high school 2 months ago. He had no sisters or brothers and his parents were healthy. He lived with his family and had no pets. His past medical history was remarkable for few episodes of benign paroxysmal positional vertigo.

On physical examination, the patient was pale and appeared sick. Oral inspection revealed hyperplastic ulcerating gingivitis as well as two mucosal lesions in his left cheek. Tonsils were enlarged and covered with multiple stipples. Cervical lymph nodes were painful and swollen bilaterally (up to 3 cm in diameter). Further physical examination was normal.

On admission, laboratory data showed: WBC: 125,030/µl, Hb: 10.9 g/dl, platelets: 24,000/µl, AST: 70 U/l, ALT: 160 U/l, LDH: 1652 U/l.

Q1. What is the next best test in your diagnostic workup?

A. Serological testing for EBV and HIV
B. Fluorescence-activated cell sorting (FACS) searching Reed-Sternberg Cells in this patient's blood
C. Peripheral blood smear and differential blood count
D. Biopsy and immunostaining (for CD3/CD4/CD8/CD30) of one tonsil

Answer: *The correct answer is* ***C****.*

C.-P. Maier · D. Schneidawind (✉)
Department of Internal Medicine II, University Hospital Tuebingen, Tuebingen, Germany
e-mail: dominik.schneidawind@uni-tuebingen.de

© Springer Nature Switzerland AG 2020

F. Rahmani, N. Rezaei (eds.), *Pediatric Autoimmunity and Transplantation*,
https://doi.org/10.1007/978-3-030-26280-8_35

In patients presenting with massive leukocytosis (i.e. WBC > 30,000/μl), acute or chronic leukemia is the most important diagnosis to be considered. Thus, as a first step, a peripheral blood smear is done to search for myeloblasts or lymphoblasts, respectively. Besides, complete blood count often reveals anemia and thrombocytopenia, whereas white blood cells may be increased, normal, or even decreased. Importantly, lack of blasts on the peripheral blood smear does not exclude acute leukemia.

This patient's peripheral blood smear was dominated by blasts. Few eosinophils, nearly no granulocytic neutrophils and no platelets were visible. Red blood cells were slightly reduced. Thus, acute leukemia was suspected.

Fluorescence-activated cell sorting (FACS) and immunostaining are additional studies needed to analyze and categorize leukemia more precisely.

Infections due to Epstein-Barr virus (EBV) as well as to human immunodeficiency virus (HIV) do not commonly cause leukocyte counts as high as in this case.

Q2. Which of the following tests are mandatory to perform prior to initiation of chemotherapy? (Which combination of tests fits best?)

A. Blood: anti-CMV-IgM, anti-CMV-IgG, anti-HSV-IgM, anti-HSV-IgG, anti-HBc-IgG, anti-HCV, anti-HIV.
   Gargling water: not necessary.
B. Blood: anti-HBc-IgG, HBsAg, anti-HCV, HCV-PCR, anti-HIV/gp24, anti-CMV-IgG, CMV-PCR, anti-EBV-VCA (*viral capsid antigen*)-IgG, anti-EBV-EBNA (*Epstein-Barr nuclear antigen*), EBV-PCR.
   Gargling water: HSV-/CMV-/EBV-PCR.
C. Blood: anti-HBc-IgG, HBsAg, anti-HCV, anti-HIV/gp24, anti-CMV-IgG, CMV-PCR, anti-HPV-IgG, HHV8-PCR, anti-Chikungunya-IgG, anti-Zika-IgG.
   Gargling water: Adenovirus-PCR, Parvovirus B19-PCR.
D. Blood: Anti-HAV-IgM, anti-HBc-IgG, HBsAg, anti-HCV, anti-HIV/gp24.
   Gargling water: CMV-/HHV6-PCR.

Answer: *The correct answer is* ***B****.*

Reactivation of viruses quite often occurs in immunocompromised patients [1]. Clinical manifestations are often not typical or abortive resulting in delayed diagnosis. Fulminant viral reactivations in non-immunocompetent hosts may be life-threatening. Thus, patients receiving chemotherapy or any other immunosuppressive treatment should be screened in advance at least for HBV, HCV, and HIV [2].

This patient presents with enlarged tonsils and swollen lymph nodes—either due to the underlying hematological disease or because of viral infection. Consequently, testing gargling water for EBV and cytomegalovirus (CMV) is recommended, along with testing for HSV because of the ulcerative buccal lesions.

Serological testing for Chikungunya and Zika is recommended under special circumstances, and for anti-HAV-IgM if acute hepatitis A is assumed. Screening for HHV-8 is only indicated in patients suffering from Kaposi sarcoma, primary effusion lymphoma or Castleman's disease. Human Papilloma Virus (HPV) which may provoke uterine and oral carcinomas as well as HHV-8 are classified as human carcinogenic viruses.

Q3. Which is the next best step to confirm the diagnosis and assess the prognosis?

A. Whole-body-PET-CT or PET-MRI scan and lymph node biopsy (cytological analysis)
B. Whole-body-PET-CT or PET-MRI scan, lymph node extirpation (histology + *myc* rearrangement analysis) and FACS (blood)
C. Bone marrow smear cytology, bone marrow immunostaining, FACS (bone marrow), karyotyping (bone marrow) and molecular genetics (bone marrow)
D. Bone marrow smear cytology, bone marrow immunostaining, FACS (bone marrow) and BCR-ABL-FISH (bone marrow)

Answer: *The correct answer is* ***C***.

Apart from taking a thorough medical and family history, careful physical examination, extensive laboratory studies including a differential microscopic blood count and bone marrow aspiration are essential for morphologic and immunophenotypic assessment and definitive diagnosis of AML. Bone marrow aspirate is further analyzed by metaphase cytogenetics (karyotyping), fluorescence in-situ hybridization (FISH) and molecular genetics that are absolutely indispensable for accurate risk stratification.

Cytogenetically, bone marrow aspirates should be evaluated by classical karyotyping [3]. On a molecular level, bone marrow aspirate should be routinely screened for gene mutations and rearrangements with prognostic relevance: *NPM1, CEBPA, RUNX1, FLT3-ITD, FLT3-TKD, TP53, ASXL1, PML-RARA*/t(15;17), *CBFB-MYH11*/inv(16) or t(16;16), *RUNX1-RUNX1T1*/t(8;21), and *BCR-ABL1*/t(9;22), and, if applicable, *c-KIT* and *WT1* [4;5]. *ASXL1* has been newly added to the risk stratification of the 2017 European LeukemiaNet recommendations for AML [4].

Histology provides further information, e.g. in disorders undergoing fibrosis, and confirms the cytological diagnosis.

DNMT3A, BRAF and *SRSF2* mutations may be found in myeloid leukemia or myelodysplastic syndromes, but are not yet commonly tested with regard to genetic risk stratification [4].

In general, whole-body-PET-CT scan or MRI imaging is not necessary at the time of diagnosis, but patients with AML presenting with extramedullary involvement should receive radiographic imaging of the suspected sites. In contrast to adults, lumbar puncture with cerebrospinal fluid analysis including cytologic examination is a standard procedure in children with newly diagnosed AML [5].

The patient's cytogenetic investigations revealed: "AML with recurrent genetic abnormalities", "AML with inv(16) and normal karyotype (46,XY)".

Q4. What chemotherapeutic regimen should be recommended as first line therapy for this patient?

A. 2 induction cycles (daunorubicin + cytarabine), 3 consolidation cycles (cytarabine high dose)
B. 2 induction cycles (daunorubicin + cytarabine), 3 consolidation cycles (cytarabine high dose + dasatinib)
C. 1 induction cycle (daunorubicin + cytarabine) followed by allogeneic PBSCT
D. 2 induction cycles (daunorubicin + cytarabine) followed by autologous PBSCT

Answer: *The correct answer is* ***A***.

Patients with AML inv(16) have a favorable prognosis with standard chemotherapy [3, 4]. Thus, high dose chemotherapy followed by autologous or allogeneic peripheral blood stem cell transplantation (PBSCT) is not indicated as first line treatment. Treatment with chemotherapy alone results in an overall survival rate of approximately 70–80% in children and adolescents [5].

AML with inv(16) as well as AML with the chromosomal abnormalities t(16;16) and t(8;21) belong to the so-called core binding factor (CBF) AML. At a molecular level, AML with inv(16) results in the fusion gene *CBFB/MYH11* leading to the disruption of the CBF complex, normally needed to control hematopoietic stem cell differentiation.

AML with inv(16) or t(16;16) is generally associated with a more favorable prognosis and a high percentage of complete remission initially, in contrast to those harboring an additional *c-KIT* mutation showing a poorer outcome. Additional treatment of KIT^{mut} inv(16) or t(16;16) AML with dasatinib, a second generation tyrosine kinase inhibitor (TKI) extensively evaluated in the treatment of chronic myeloid leukemia (CML), represents a new promising targeted-directed approach [6]. The main targets inhibited by dasatinib are *BCR-ABL*, the *SRC* family and *c-KIT*. Dasatinib is not yet used in standard first line chemotherapy, but is evaluated in ongoing clinical trials.

Five months after completing chemotherapy AML relapses. Diagnostic workup reveals relapse of the same AML subtype as diagnosed initially, but, in addition, CSF involvement is observed (i.e. leukemic meningeosis). The patient is in good clinical condition, has no concomitant illness and wishes to be treated with curative intention.

Q5. The patient is a candidate for allogeneic hematopoietic stem cell transplantation. Which of the following conditioning regimens is the most effective?

A. Flu (120 mg/m^2)/Bu (6.4 mg/kg) + intrathecal chemotherapy
B. FLAMSA-TBI (4 Gy)/Cy (120 mg/kg) + intrathecal chemotherapy
C. Flu (120 mg/m^2)/TBI (8 Gy) + intrathecal chemotherapy
D. Total lymphoid irradiation + intrathecal chemotherapy

Answer: *The correct answer is* ***B***.

FLAMSA-TBI/Cy in combination with intrathecal chemotherapy offers the best cure rates.

About one third of children with AML experience a relapse [5]. The prognosis for these children is unfortunately poor with only an approximately 30% chance of cure. Among others, survival depends on the duration of complete remission, high-risk cytogenetic or molecular genetic abnormalities.

Reinduction chemotherapy for children and adolescents presenting with relapsed AML usually consists of high-dose cytarabine (HiDAC) with or without an anthracycline [5]. HiDAC may be combined with clofarabine or fludarabine. Before an anthracycline is used, cardiac function as well as the cumulative anthracycline dose have to be checked.

As this patient presents with early relapse of AML after having completed standard induction and consolidation regimen, long-term prognosis is poor. To overcome this dismal prognosis, a sequential regimen of chemotherapy (FLAMSA: fludarabine, cytarabine, amsacrine), reduced-intensity conditioning (RIC: cyclophosphamide and TBI 4 Gy or cyclophosphamide and busulfan) for allogeneic stem cell transplantation, and prophylactic donor lymphocyte infusion (DLI) has been evaluated in adults with high-risk AML including relapsed AML and AML with primary induction failure since the late 1990s [7–9]. DLI are applied prophylactically from day +120 [8], if infections and graft-versus-host disease (GvHD) are absent and if GvHD prophylaxis could be stopped on day +90 at the latest.

Q6. Which of the following factor(s) is associated with a higher risk of CNS involvement in pediatric AML?

A. Hyperleukocytosis
B. Age <2 years
C. Monocytic leukemia (FAB M4 or M5, including M4Eo with inv(16))
D. Answers A, B, and C are correct.

Answer: *The correct answer is* ***D****.*

Risk factors for CNS involvement include high WBC count, younger age and AML with inv(16) [10], as in this case. Intrathecal therapy consists of either cytarabine alone or triple therapy with cytarabine, methotrexate, and cortisone. In general, frequent intrathecal chemotherapy is necessary to maintain blast clearance. A standardized approach in AML patients with CNS involvement is not established [10]. Additional cerebral radiation may not be necessary, particularly not when intrathecal chemotherapy is combined with intensified systemic chemotherapy, e.g. HiDAC.

The global outcome of CNS-positive AML patients does not differ significantly from CNS-negative patients, although relapses in the CNS occur more often in patients with CNS involvement at initial diagnosis [10].

Practical Points

- Acute myeloid leukemia (AML) with inv(16) or t(16;16) is generally associated with a more favorable prognosis and a high percentage of complete remission.
- Risk factors for CNS involvement in pediatric AML include high WBC count, younger age and AML with inv(16).

References

1. European Conference on Infections in Leukaemia (ECIL) guidelines 1–6. www.ecil-leukaemia.com.
2. Firpi R, Nelson D. Management of viral hepatitis in hematologic malignancies. Blood Rev. 2008;22(3):117–26.
3. Grimwade D, Hills RK, Moorman AV, Walker H, Chatters S, Goldstone AH, Wheatley K, Harrison CJ, Group AKBobotNCRIALW. Refinement of cytogenetic classification in acute myeloid leukemia: determination of prognostic significance of rare recurring chromosomal abnormalities among 5876 younger adult patients treated in the United Kingdom Medical Research Council trials. Blood. 2010;116(3):354–65.
4. Döhner H, Estey E, Grimwade D, Amadori S, Appelbaum FR, Büchner T, Dombret H, Ebert BL, Fenaux P, Larson RA, Levine RL, Lo-Coco F, Naoe T, Niederwieser D, Ossenkoppele GJ, Sanz M, Sierra J, Tallman MS, Tien H-F, Wei AH, Löwenberg B, Bloomfield CD. Diagnosis and management of AML in adults: 2017 ELN recommendations from an international expert panel. Blood. 2017;129(4):424–47.
5. Creutzig U, van den Heuvel-Eibrink M, Gibson B, Dworzak MN, Adachi S, de Bont E, Harbott J, Hasle H, Johnston D, Kinoshita A, Lehrnbecher T, Leverger G, Mejstrikova E, Meshinchi S, Pession A, Raimondi S, Sung L, Stary J, Zwaan C, GJL K, Group DRobotACotIBS. Diagnosis and management of acute myeloid leukemia in children and adolescents: recommendation from an international expert panel. Blood. 2012;120(16):3187–205.
6. Boissel N, Renneville A, Leguay T, Lefebvre PC, Recher C, Lecerf T, Delabesse E, Berthon C, Blanchet O, Prebet T, Pautas C, Chevallier P, Leprêtre S, Girault S, Bonmati C, Guièze R, Himberlin C, Randriamalala E, Preudhomme C, Jourdan E, Dombret H, Ifrah N. Dasatinib in high-risk core binding factor acute myeloid leukemia in first complete remission: a French Acute Myeloid Leukemia Intergroup trial. Haematologica. 2015;100(6):780–5.
7. Pfeiffer T, Schleuning M, Mayer J, Haude K-H, Tischer J, Buchholz S, Bunjes D, Bug G, Holler E, Meyer RG, Greinix H, Scheid C, Christopeit M, Schnittger S, Braess J, Schlimok G, Spiekermann K, Ganser A, Kolb H-J, Schmid C. Influence of molecular subgroups on outcome of acute myeloid leukemia with normal karyotype in 141 patients undergoing salvage allogeneic stem cell transplantation in primary induction failure or beyond first relapse. Haematologica. 2013;98(4):518–25.
8. Schmid C, Schleuning M, Ledderose G, Tischer J, Kolb H-J. Sequential regimen of chemotherapy, reduced-intensity conditioning for allogeneic stem-cell transplantation, and prophylactic donor lymphocyte transfusion in high-risk acute myeloid leukemia and myelodysplastic syndrome. J Clin Oncol. 2005;23(24):5675–87.
9. Schmid C, Schleuning M, Schwerdtfeger R, Hertenstein B, Mischak-Weissinger E, Bunjes D, Sv H, Scheid C, Holtick U, Greinix H, Keil F, Schneider B, Sandherr M, Bug G, Tischer J, Ledderose G, Hallek M, Hiddemann W, Kolb H-J. Long term survival in refractory acute myeloid leukemia after sequential treatment with chemotherapy and reduced intensity conditioning for allogeneic stem cell transplantation. Blood. 2006;108(3):1092–9.
10. Creutzig U, Dworzak MN, Zimmermann M, Reinhardt D, Sramkova L, Bourquin JP, Hasle H, Abrahamsson J, Kaspers G. Characteristics and outcome in patients with central nervous system involvement treated in European pediatric acute myeloid leukemia study groups. Pediatr Blood Cancer. 2017;64(12):e26664.

Chapter 36
Acute Myeloid Leukemia Requiring Hematopoietic Stem Cell Transplantation

Soumya Pandey and Terry Harville

Our patient is a 16-year-old Caucasian boy with acute myeloid leukemia (AML) requiring hematopoietic cell transplantation (HCT). As part of the initial pre-transplant work-up, patient underwent HLA typing and anti-HLA antibody screen. The next step requires identifying a suitable donor, which can be a related or unrelated donor. As per the NMDP guidelines, an 8 of 8 HLA matched donor (matched at both HLA-A, -B, -C, and -DRB1 loci) is the minimal preferred, but we prefer using a 10 of 10 HLA matching to include HLA-DPB1.

Q1. True or False: Based on NMDP guidelines, a patient scheduled to receive transplantation from a matched unrelated donor (MUD) should have HLA typing performed on two separate occasions, with two separate specimens.

A. True
B. False

Answer: *The correct answer is* ***A***.

S. Pandey
Department of Pathology and Laboratory Services, University of Arkansas for Medical Sciences, Little Rock, AR, USA

T. Harville (✉)
Department of Pathology and Laboratory Services, University of Arkansas for Medical Sciences, Little Rock, AR, USA

Departments of Pediatrics and Internal Medicine, University of Arkansas for Medical Sciences, Little Rock, AR, USA
e-mail: harvilleterryo@uams.edu

© Springer Nature Switzerland AG 2020

F. Rahmani, N. Rezaei (eds.), *Pediatric Autoimmunity and Transplantation*,
https://doi.org/10.1007/978-3-030-26280-8_36

Q2. Which of the following statements is most accurate? (DSA: donor-specific antibodies)

A. HLA class I typing of the patient is all that is required to initiate a donor search and select the best donor.
B. Determining which anti-HLA antibodies are present in the patient can help with donor selection to exclude a potential mismatched donor if DSA are present, as well as for platelet transfusion support.
C. At the current time, determining HLA class II typing results by a serologic technique is sufficient for donor selection for transplantation.
D. Under most circumstances, HLA-DPB1 typing results can be ignored regarding donor selection.
E. Under most circumstances, HLA-DQB1 matching is required for donor selection, according to the NMDP guidelines.

Answer: *The correct answer is* ***B***.

According to NMDP requirements, the patient is to have two separate HLA typing performed with two separately obtained specimens [1, 2]. A potential donor had to have HLA typing performed to allow for entry into the registry. If that typing appears to provide a match, a specimen is requested and confirmatory typing is performed by the receiving transplantation center, for determining the true extent of matching. Determining which anti-HLA antibodies are present is important for donor selection, if locus mismatching is present. If DSA are present in the patient and directed towards the mismatched type in the donor, then resistance to engraftment may occur. Since platelets express HLA class I, the presence of anti-class I HLA antibodies can result in problems with platelet transfusion support post-chemotherapy and transplantation. Knowing the antibody profile can be used for specific platelet donor selection [3].

This patient had eight siblings; hence, these related potential donors were evaluated to determine a potentially suitable donor prior to initiating an unrelated donor search. Since the cost of HLA typing of all these related donors is substantial, the initial search included only HLA class I typing as a cost containment process.

Q3. True or False: Due to linkage disequilibrium, a sibling donor only requires HLA class I typing for verification of suitability

A. True
B. False

Answer: *The correct answer is* ***B***.

Unfortunately, despite linkage disequilibrium, HLA-DP crossover events are not uncommon. HLA-DP is the most distal of the HLA loci from class I, which sets the situation for possible crossovers during meiosis. Additionally, extended DNA lengths which can include, HLA-DQ and -DP, and HLA-DR, -DQ, and -DP, can undergo crossover events [4, 5].

Based on the HLA class I typing results (Table 36.1), donors 2–8 were shown to be matches in only one haplotype and thus not considered suitable donors. No

Table 36.1 HLA typing results for HCT of a 16-year-old boy with AML

	A	B	C	DRB1	DRB3/4/5	DQB1	DQA1	DPB1	DPA1
Patient	*02:01	*27:05	*01:02	*01	4*01	*05	*01	*02:01	*01:03
	*03:01	*49:01	*07:02	*09	–	*03	*03	*04:01	*01:03
Potential Donor 1	*02	*27	*01	*01	4*01	*05	*01	*02:01	*01:03
	*03	*49	*07	*09	–	*03	*03	*04:01	*01:03
Potential Donor 2	*01	*08	*07	–	–	–	–	–	–
	*03	*49	*07	–	–	–	–	–	–
Potential Donor 3	*01	*08	*07	–	–	–	–	–	–
	*03	*49	*07	–	–	–	–	–	–
Potential Donor 4	*01	*08	*07	–	–	–	–	–	–
	*02	*44	*05	–	–	–	–	–	–
Potential Donor 5	*01	*08	*07	–	–	–	–	–	–
	*02	*44	*05	–	–	–	–	–	–
Potential Donor 6	*01	*08	*07	–	–	–	–	–	–
	*03	*49	*07	–	–	–	–	–	–
Potential Donor 7	*01	*08	*07	–	–	–	–	–	–
	*03	*49	*07	–	–	–	–	–	–
Potential Donor 8	*02	*27	*01	–	–	–	–	–	–
	*02	*44	*05	–	–	–	–	–	–

The patient and potential donors are listed in column 1. The separate HLA locus results are listed in columns 2–10. Note: Donors 2–8 were found to be at the most only one HLA haplotype matched. Donor 1 was matched at both HLA class I alleles and subsequently demonstrated to be matched also at all HLA class II alleles

further testing was performed on these donors. Donor 1 matched 6/6 HLA Class I loci, hence further HLA class II typing was performed that showed that this donor also matched at all other loci.

Q4. As shown here, the potential donors were screened for HLA class I matching using a lower-resolution typing method. Which of the following statements is most accurate?

A. This same approach can be used for screening potential matched-unrelated donors; screen by low-resolution for HLA class I and confirm by high-resolution for HLA class II.
B. Matched-unrelated donors are prescreened to be in the registry; low-medium confirmatory HLA typing is all that is required for final donor selection.
C. Matched-unrelated donors require high-resolution HLA class I and class II typing for final donor selection.
D. Cost-saving measures through screening by lower-resolution HLA typing are required by the NMDP in order to help contain the costs of transplantation.
E. Two separate specimens are sent by the NMDP once a potential MUD is identified. One can be screened by low-resolution HLA typing, but the other must be confirmed by high-resolution typing.

Answer: *The correct answer is* ***C***.

While cost-containing measures, such as screening of related donors by lower-resolution HLA typing is acceptable, this does not apply to NMDP matched-unrelated donors. The NMDP requires the patient to undergo HLA typing with two separate specimens. The potential MUD are placed into the registry based on the HLA type that each has received by whichever resolution level was used. This typing is utilized for the initial potential donor selection screening process. Once a potential MUD has been identified, based on the registry, a specimen is sent by the NMDP for "confirmatory" typing by the transplant center. This latter, high-resolution, HLA class I and class II typing is then used to determine the extent of match with the patient as the final selection process.

Practical Points

- If donor-specific antigen are present in the HSCT recipient and directed towards the mismatched type in the donor, then resistance to engraftment may occur
- The NMDP requires the patient receiving matched-unrelated donor (MUD) transplantation to undergo HLA typing with two separate specimens

References

1. Bray RA, Hurley CK, Kamani NR, Woolfrey A, Muller C, Spellman S, Setterholm M, Confer DL. National marrow donor program HLA matching guidelines for unrelated adult donor hematopoietic cell transplants. Biol Blood Marrow Transpl. 2008;14(9 Suppl):45–53.
2. Spellman S, Setterholm M, Maiers M, Noreen H, Oudshoorn M, Fernandez-Vina M, Petersdorf E, Bray R, Hartzman RJ, Ng J, Hurley CK. Advances in the selection of HLA-compatible donors: refinements in HLA typing and matching over the first 20 years of the National Marrow Donor Program Registry. Biol Blood Marrow Transpl. 2008;14(9 Suppl):37–44.
3. Lee SKJ, Haagenson M, et al. High-resolution donor-recipient HLA matching contributes to the success of unrelated donor marrow transplantation. Blood. 2007;110(13):4576–83.
4. Pidala J, Lee SJ, Ahn KW, Spellman S, Wang HL, Aljurf M, Askar M, Dehn J, Fernandez Vina M, Gratwohl A, Gupta V, Hanna R, Horowitz MM, Hurley CK, Inamoto Y, Kassim AA, Nishihori T, Mueller C, Oudshoorn M, Petersdorf EW, Prasad V, Robinson J, Saber W, Schultz KR, Shaw B, Storek J, Wood WA, Woolfrey AE, Anasetti C. Nonpermissive HLA-DPB1 mismatch increases mortality after myeloablative unrelated allogeneic hematopoietic cell transplantation. Blood. 2014;124(16):2596–606.
5. Petty RE, Southwood TR, Manners P, Baum J, Glass DN, Goldenberg J, He X, Maldonado-Cocco J, Orozco-Alcala J, Prieur AM, Suarez-Almazor ME, Woo P. International League of Associations for Rheumatology classification of juvenile idiopathic arthritis: second revision, Edmonton, 2001. J Rheumatol. 2004;31(2):390–2.

Chapter 37
Discrepant Cytomegalovirus Serology Between Donor and Recipient in Hematopoietic Stem Cell Transplantation

Soumya Pandey and Terry Harville

A 14-year-old Caucasian female, diagnosed with acute myeloid leukemia (AML), was considered for hematopoietic cell transplantation (HCT). She had three siblings, 1 sister and 2 brothers, two of whom were evaluated as potential donors. Complete HLA typing was performed (Table 37.1).

Q1. Based on the HLA typing results above, which of the following statements is most correct? (NIMA: non-inherited maternal antigen)

A. Either donor is suitable due to the NIMA present
B. Either donor is suitable because they are siblings
C. Donor 1 is most suitable since the donor and patient will be gender-matched
D. Donor 2 is most suitable
E. Neither donor is acceptable

Answer: *The correct answer is* ***D****.*

Q2. Inspection of the results in Table 37.1 indicates that a crossover event during meiosis may have occurred in potential donor 1…

A. Between HLA-A and -C
B. Between HLA Class I and Class II

S. Pandey
Department of Pathology and Laboratory Services, University of Arkansas for Medical Sciences, Little Rock, AR, USA

T. Harville (✉)
Department of Pathology and Laboratory Services, University of Arkansas for Medical Sciences, Little Rock, AR, USA

Departments of Pediatrics and Internal Medicine, University of Arkansas for Medical Sciences, Little Rock, AR, USA
e-mail: harvilleterryo@uams.edu

© Springer Nature Switzerland AG 2020

F. Rahmani, N. Rezaei (eds.), *Pediatric Autoimmunity and Transplantation*,
https://doi.org/10.1007/978-3-030-26280-8_37

Table 37.1 HLA typing results for HCT for a 14-year-old boy, candidate of HCT

	A	B	C	DRB1	DRB3/4/5	DQB1	DQA1	DPB1	DPA1
Patient	*31:01	*40:01	*03:04	*13:01	3*01:01	*06:01	*01:03	*04:01	*01:03
	*31:01	*15:01	*03:03	*12:01	3*02:02	*03:01	*05:01	*04:01	*01:03
Donor 1 (sister)	*01:01	*08:01	*07:01	*11:01	3*01:01	*02:01	*05:01	*02:01	*01:03
	*02:01	*15:01	*03:03	*12:01	3*02:02	*03:01	*05:01	*04:01	*01:03
Donor 2 (brother)	*31:01	*40:01	*03:04	*13:01	3*01:01	*06:01	*01:03	*04:01	*01:03
	*31:01	*15:01	*03:03	*12:01	3*02:02	*03:01	*05:01	*04:01	*01:03

The high-resolution (molecular) typing results for the patient and potential donors are listed for each HLA locus

C. Between HLA-A and -B with gene duplication in HLA-DQA1
D. Between HLA-DQ and HLA-DP
E. There is no evidence for a crossover event

Answer: *The correct answer is* ***A***.

Q3. True or False: The concept of linkage disequilibrium indicates that cross-over events, observed in this case are quite common

A. True
B. False

Answer: *The correct answer is* ***B***.

Based on the typing results (Table 37.1), donor 1 (sister) is mismatched in one haplotype and HLA-A locus of the second haplotype, and therefore is not compatible for transplantation. Patient and donor 2 (brother) are fully matched at all loci and thus donor 2 would appear to be a very suitable donor. NIMA cannot be determined without knowing the mother and father HLA types. Since the second haplotype listed in each pair is shared between the patient and the donors, except for the HLA-A locus in potential donor 1, there appears to have been a crossover resulting in an HLA-A*02:01 substituting for an HLA-A*31:01, so that the crossover event may have occurred somewhere between HLA-A and HLA-C (see Fig. 1.1). Linkage disequilibrium is the concept that the HLA genes remain more tightly associated than predicted from the expected crossover rate during meiosis. Thus, having the apparent HLA-A locus crossover as observed here is a rare event.

Considering other variables other that HLA matching, our patient was cytomegalovirus (CMV) negative, while his brother was CMV positive.

Q4. True or False: Since the patient and donor are fully HLA-matched, their CMV status is less relevant, considering availability of good anti-virals

A. True
B. False

Answer: *The correct answer is* ***B***.

The CMV status of patient and donor are very important to "match", regardless of the extent of HLA matching. If the recipient is CMV negative, a CMV negative donor is preferred since this will greatly reduce the risk of subsequent reactivation of CMV and infection with CMV, assuming that the patient receives CMV negative blood products. If the recipient is CMV positive, a CMV positive donor is used with the hope that this will result in a faster restoration of anti-CMV immunity, due to the passive transfer of anti-CMV immunity from the donor to the recipient. It the setting of a CMV positive patient and CMV negative donor, the chemotherapy conditioning removes the patient's immunity and no anti-CMV immunity is passively-acquired. Thus, reactivation of CMV in the patient can result in tremendous morbidity, not only to the infected organs, but also for promoting GVHD. In the situation of a CMV negative patient and CMV positive donor, there will be a likely risk of acquisition of CMV from the donor, considering the immunosuppressed status of the host [1].

Thus, in this case the fully HLA-matched donor brother was not considered as the best option, due to the CMV risks. An NMDP search was performed to identify an HLA- and CMV-matched donor.

Practical Points

- If the recipient is cytomegalovirus (CMV) negative, a CMV negative donor is preferred since this will greatly reduce the risk of subsequent reactivation of CMV and infection with CMV, assuming that the patient receives CMV negative blood products
- If the recipient is CMV positive, a CMV positive donor is used with the hope that this will result in a faster restoration of anti-CMV immunity, due to the passive transfer of anti-CMV immunity from the donor to the recipient

Reference

1. Bray RA, Hurley CK, Kamani NR, Woolfrey A, Muller C, Spellman S, Setterholm M, Confer DL. National marrow donor program HLA matching guidelines for unrelated adult donor hematopoietic cell transplants. Biol Blood Marrow Transpl. 2008;14(9 Suppl):45–53.

Chapter 38
Suspected Immunodeficiency

Soumya Pandey and Terry Harville

Our patients is a 6-month-old African-American male with a history of hypoparathyroidism, suspected diabetic embryopathy, solitary kidney, rash, dysphagia, inguinal hernia, skin infections, profound anemia, and peripheral eosinophilia. Workup for immunodeficiency included a CBC with differential, lymphocyte subset enumeration by immunophenotyping, T lymphocyte proliferative responses to mitogens, and mutational analysis for known causes of severe combined immunodeficiency (SCID), confirming the diagnosis of SCID. We were consulted to perform HLA typing in order to comment on possible maternal engraftment of maternal T lymphocytes acquired transplacentally in utero. Additionally, we were asked to HLA type his parents, for possible haploidentical hematopoietic cell transplantation (HCT) from a parental donor.

Initially, HLA class I typing was performed on the patient and his mother (Table 38.1). The request for only HLA class I was made to reduce the amount of blood sample size from the baby, since many blood samples had already been obtained and it was desired not to have to transfuse the baby.

S. Pandey
Department of Pathology and Laboratory Services, University of Arkansas for Medical Sciences, Little Rock, AR, USA

T. Harville (✉)
Department of Pathology and Laboratory Services, University of Arkansas for Medical Sciences, Little Rock, AR, USA

Departments of Pediatrics and Internal Medicine, University of Arkansas for Medical Sciences, Little Rock, AR, USA
e-mail: harvilleterryo@uams.edu

© Springer Nature Switzerland AG 2020

F. Rahmani, N. Rezaei (eds.), *Pediatric Autoimmunity and Transplantation*,
https://doi.org/10.1007/978-3-030-26280-8_38

Table 38.1 Initial class I HLA typing results for HCT of a 6-month old boy with SCID

	A	B	C
Patient	*02:02	*53:01	*04:01
	*29:02	*35:01	*15:02
Mother	*02:02	*53:01	*04:01
	*29:02	*35:01	*15:02

Both sets of A, B, and C locus alleles were typed and aligned by possible haplotypes. The patient and mother appear to have identical HLA Class I typing results

Q1. Which of the following statements is most correct? (NIMA: non-inherited maternal antigen)

A. Both the baby and the mother share the same HLA class I alleles and therefore, by linkage disequilibrium must share the HLA class II alleles.
B. The apparent homozygosity is a consequence of shared NIMA.
C. This study is sufficient to prove that maternal lymphocytes are present in the baby's blood.
D. HLA class II typing is not required before it can be declared that the cells in the baby are of maternal origin.
E. The baby, the father, and the mother must have complete HLA typing performed before the origin of the cells in the baby can be determined.

Answer: *The correct answer is* ***E***.

Q2. Which of the following statements is most correct?

A. These results are sufficient to identify the mother as the most suitable donor for HCT
B. Since it appears that maternal cells are already in the baby, there will be no need for HCT, but a "booster" transplant of maternal cells may be required to achieve full engraftment
C. There is no further need to type the father as a HCT donor
D. Complete HLA typing of the baby, father, and mother is required for the best donor-selection
E. There is no need to consider the father as a donor because of the presence of NIMA

Answer: *The correct answer is* ***D***.

Complete HLA class I and class II typing is required to determine the identity of cells, as in this case, as well as required for identifying the most suitable donor for HCT. While linkage disequilibrium does indicate that certain HLA haplotypes can be "statistically" predicted from limited known HLA loci, the concept cannot be used for "actual" prediction of class II typing, hence HLA class I and II typing are both required to confirm the actual HLA type present. Further, to understand fully which HLA haplotypes are present in an individual child, it remains very helpful to type both parents [1].

Engraftment with maternal T-cells may be seen in patients with SCID. Indeed, studies have demonstrated that every child has some lymphocytes from maternal origin, and even mothers are demonstrated to have lymphocytes from their previous children. Thus, the transplacental transfer of lymphocytes is bidirectional and more common than originally though. Therefore, finding cells of maternal origin in a patient with SCID would be a relatively common occurrence [2]. Unfortunately, these cells may have a detrimental effect and may affect the outcome of HCT, especially if chemotherapeutic conditioning is not used for the transplant. Further, the presence of maternal lymphocytes may indicate that the mother could be considered as a better donor for haploidentical HCT. Although low, with a paternal donor, there may be a risk for "graft versus graft" reaction, i.e. the transplacental maternal T-lymphocytes against the donated paternal cells. Another reason to use a maternal donor is that she has spent 9 months of "tolerization" with the fetus, which means tolerization to the IPA (i.e. inherited paternal HLA haplotype, see Chap. 1), conferring a reduced risk of GVHD and resistance to engraftment [3].

Complete HLA typing was performed for all three. For the infant, there were sufficient cells to separate into CD2, CD3, CD4, CD8, CD16, and CD19 subpopulations using magnetic microspheres. All of these had identical HLA typing results, and are presented with the parents complete HLA typing results in Table 38.2.

Q3. Which of the following statements is most correct regarding the information in Table 38.2?

A. The father and mother must be related, since they share an identical HLA class I type, as well as, identical HLA class II components (DQA1*01:02/DQB1*06:02 and DPA1*02:01/DPB1*01:01).
B. These results confirm that the infant has engrafted maternal T lymphocytes.
C. The haplotypes as depicted indicate that the infant has inherited one haplotype from the father and one from the mother.
D. In this case, the HLA-DR results are not very helpful for discriminating the origin of the cells in the baby.
E. Based on the identical shared HLA Class I between the father and the mother, and that this is one half of an HLA haplotype, and further on Mendelian genetics, one parent of the father and one parent of the mother are siblings.

Answer: *The correct answer is **C**.*

Table 38.2 Complete HLA typing results for HCT of a 6-month old boy with SCID

	A	B	C	DRB1	DRB3/4/5	DQB1	DQA1	DPB1	DPA1
Patient	*02:02	*53:01	*04:01	*11:02	3*02:02	*03:19	*05:05	*01:01	*02:01
	*29:02	*35:01	*15:02	*08:06	–	*06:02	*01:01	*02:01	*01:03
Mother	*02:02	*53:01	*04:01	*10:01	–	*05:01	*01:02	*17:01	*02:01
	*29:02	*35:01	*15:02	*08:06	–	*06:02	*01:01	*02:01	*01:03
Father	*02:02	*53:01:	*04:01	*11:02	3*02:02	*03:19	*05:05	*01:01	*02:01
	*30:01	*18:01	*02:02	*15:03	5*01:01	*06:02	*01:02	*105:01	*03:01

The infant, mother, and father HLA typing results are shown for each locus, and aligned by the haplotypes identified

Q4. True or False: Based on the fact that the father shares identical HLA-DQB1 type with his son, as well as HLA class I, one HLA-DRB1, and one HLA-DRB3, he is the most suitable donor for haploidentical HCT

A. True
B. False

Answer: *The correct answer is **B**.*

Q5. True or False: Even though the mother provided only one HLA class I haplotype, having a separate identical haplotype with the father and the NIMA, make the mother the most suitable haploidentical HCT donor

A. True
B. False

Answer: *The correct answer is **A**.*

Complete HLA typing allows for identification of the individual haplotypes. The mother and father do share an HLA Class I haplotype, yet this does not prove consanguinity. In this case, simple chance has led to the apparent relationship. When examining the haplotypes, both parents share a HLA-DQB1*06:02. HLA-DQ6 is found in ~37% of the population, so there is about a 1 in 3 chance for anyone to have it present. In this case, the father's HLA-DQB1*06:02 is coupled with HLA-DQA1*01:02, which is commonly found associated with HLA-DRB1*15:03 in people with African origin. Whereas, the mother's HLA-DQB1*06:02 is coupled with HLA-DQA1*01:02, which is commonly associated with HLA-DRB1*08:06 in persons of African origins. Thus, it is probable that the maternal and paternal HLA-DQB1*06:02 are not the same, and actually have polymorphisms which do not affect the two-field typing results [4, 5]. Based on NMDP guidelines, HLA-DQ and HLA-DRB3, -DRB4, and -DRB5 HLA types are not necessary for donor selections, and therefore do not make the father a better HCT donor [6]. The mother is the most suitable haploidentical HCT donor. Fortunately, the mother's NIMA is HLA identical with the IPA, reducing the risk for GVHD and resistance to engraftment, due to in utero tolerization.

Practical Points

- During pregnancy, the fetus is exposed to the non-inherited maternal HLA haplotype (NIMA, non-inherited maternal antigens)
- The fetal exposure to NIMA results in generation of tolerance to those HLA components
- If a related HLA-mismatched donor is all that is available, demonstrating that the mismatched HLA component is a NIMA could result in successful transplantation

References

1. Bray RA, Hurley CK, Kamani NR, Woolfrey A, Muller C, Spellman S, Setterholm M, Confer DL. National marrow donor program HLA matching guidelines for unrelated adult donor hematopoietic cell transplants. Biol Blood Marrow Transpl. 2008;14(9 Suppl):45–53.
2. Buckley R. Transplantation of hematopoietic stem cells in human severe combined immunodeficiency: longterm outcomes. Immunol Res. 2011;49:25–43.
3. Liu C, Duffy B, Bednarski JJ, Calhoun C, Lay L, Rundblad B, Payton JE, Mohanakumar T. Maternal T-cell engraftment interferes with human leukocyte antigen typing in severe combined immunodeficiency. Am J Clin Pathol. 2016;145(2):251–7.
4. Crocchiolo R, Ciceri F, Fleischhauer K, Oneto R, Bruno B, Pollichieni S, Sacchi N, Sormani MP, Fanin R, Bandini G, Bonifazi F, Bosi A, Rambaldi A, Alessandrino PE, Falda M, Bacigalupo A. HLA matching affects clinical outcome of adult patients undergoing haematopoietic SCT from unrelated donors: a study from the Gruppo Italiano Trapianto di Midollo Osseo and Italian Bone Marrow Donor Registry. Bone Marrow Transplant. 2009;44(9):571–7.
5. Lee SJ, Klein J, Haagenson M, Baxter-Lowe LA, Confer DL, Eapen M, Fernandez-Vina M, Flomenberg N, Horowitz M, Hurley CK, Noreen H, Oudshoorn M, Petersdorf E, Setterholm M, Spellman S, Weisdorf D, Williams TM, Anasetti C. High-resolution donor-recipient HLA matching contributes to the success of unrelated donor marrow transplantation. Blood. 2007;110(13):4576–83.
6. Spellman S, Setterholm M, Maiers M, Noreen H, Oudshoorn M, Fernandez-Vina M, Petersdorf E, Bray R, Hartzman RJ, Ng J, Hurley CK. Advances in the selection of HLA-compatible donors: refinements in HLA typing and matching over the first 20 years of the National Marrow Donor Program Registry. Biol Blood Marrow Transpl. 2008;14(9 Suppl):37–44.

Chapter 39
Linkage Disequilibrium Between HLA Alleles in Hematopoietic Stem Cell Transplantation

Soumya Pandey and Terry Harville

Our patients was a 12-year-old Caucasian girl with acute myeloid leukemia (AML) who was considered a candidate for allogeneic transplantation. Patient underwent routine pre-transplant work-up including HLA typing (Table 39.1) and HLA antibody screen, where no significant anti-class I and II HLA antibodies were detected. Patient did not have any related donors, and hence an NMDP search was initiated. Based on the preliminary NMDP donor typing results, multiple donors appeared to be suitable. Specimen were obtained from two donors to perform confirmatory HLA typing.

As noted in Table 39.1, some data from the NMDP registry may be obtained through serologic-based typing results or lower-resolution molecular typing results, which might not match the high-resolution HLA results from the patient. This is a major reason as to why confirmatory HLA typing of the donor is performed by the same HLA Laboratory which typed the patient. During the initial screening of the data, the concept of Common and Well-Documented Alleles (CWD) may be used. For example, HLA-DQA1*04:01 is the only CWD for HLA-DQA1*04, and hence is likely allele present in potential donor 2. Further, HLA-DQA1*04:01/DQB1*04:02 commonly associate with HLA-DRB1*08:01, thus, even though not tested, HLA-DQA1*04:01 is also likely present in potential donor 1.

S. Pandey
Department of Pathology and Laboratory Services, University of Arkansas for Medical Sciences, Little Rock, AR, USA

T. Harville (✉)
Department of Pathology and Laboratory Services, University of Arkansas for Medical Sciences, Little Rock, AR, USA

Departments of Pediatrics and Internal Medicine, University of Arkansas for Medical Sciences, Little Rock, AR, USA
e-mail: harvilleterryo@uams.edu

© Springer Nature Switzerland AG 2020

F. Rahmani, N. Rezaei (eds.), *Pediatric Autoimmunity and Transplantation*,
https://doi.org/10.1007/978-3-030-26280-8_39

Table 39.1 Patient and NMDP HLA typing results in a 12-year-old girl with AML

	A	B	C	DRB1	DRB3/4/5	DQB1	DQA1	DPB1	DPA1
Patient	*02:01	*07:02	*05:01	*08:01	3*02:02	*02:01	*04:01	*03:01	*01:03
	*32:01	*18:01	*07:02	*03:01	–	*04:02	*05:01	*04:01	*01:03
Potential Donor 1	2	7	5	*8:01	52	2			
	*32:01	*18:01	7	17		4			
Potential Donor 2	*02	*07:02	*05:01	*08:01	3*02:02	*02	*04		
	*32:01	*18:01	*07:02	*03:01	–	*04	*05		

The patient had high-resolution HLA typing performed, which was used for the search of the NMDP registry. Several potential donors were identified. These were narrowed to four potential donors based on the completeness of the typing in the registry and CVM match. The two selected for confirmatory typing were younger and female, and cytomegalovirus (CMV)-matched

Q1. True or False: Based on the extent of typing present in the registry, there is a reasonable chance to obtain an HLA-matched suitable donor; considering the concept of linkage disequilibrium and Common and Well-Documented Alleles

A. True
B. False

Answer: *The correct answer is* ***A***.

Linkage disequilibrium is the concept that HLA types are associated into inherited haplotypes more commonly than is expected from DNA crossover events, which occur during normal meiosis. Review of Fig. 1.1 in Chap. 1 indicates that the distal HLA loci HLA-DP and HLA-A may have some of the greatest chances to undergo crossover exchanges, due to their relative isolation from the remaining HLA loci. HLA-B and -C remain tightly associated, as well as HLA-DR and HLA-DQ. Knowing which HLA-B or -C, or -DR or -DQ, is present can allow one to predict the associated component, and vice versa. Yet, HLA-B and HLA-DR remain relatively associated despite the spatial separation by the class III region [1]. Undoubtedly, there are genes in the class III region in association with HLA-B and HLA-DR, which would definitely interact best with these specific associations. Thus, if the HLA-A, -B, -C, and -DR are known, then -DQ can be predicted with reasonable accuracy, and likewise if HLA-A, -B, -C, -DR, and -DQ are known, the -DP may be predicted, albeit with somewhat less accuracy. Further, specific HLA associations and CWD alleles can be utilized to help predict potential donors during the screening process. Even without HLA-DP typing results, the potential donor typing found in the NMDP registry, as depicted in Table 39.1, provide some reassurance to find an HLA-matched donor. Major limitation of this method is considering HLA-DP crossover events, especially in non-related individuals. Potential donor specimen were sent for confirmatory typing (Table 39.2).

Table 39.2 High-resolution HLA typing results for hematopoietic cell transplantation (HCT) of a 12-year-old girl with AML

	A	B	C	DRB1	DRB3/4/5	DQB1	DQA1	DPB1	DPA1
Patient	*02:01	*07:02	*05:01	*08:01	3*02:02	*02:01	*04:01	*03:01	*01:03
	*32:01	*18:01	*07:02	*03:01	–	*04:02	*05:01	*04:01	*01:03
Potential Donor 1	*02:01	*07:02	*05:01	*08:01	3*02:02	*02:01	*04:01	*03:01	*01:03
	*32:01	*18:01	*07:02	*03:01	–	*04:02	*05:01	*20:01	*01:03
Potential Donor 2	*02:01	*07:02	*05:01	*08:01	3*02:02	*02:01	*04:01	*01:01	*01:03
	*32:01	*18:01	*07:02	*03:01	–	*04:02	*05:01	*04:01	*02:01

The high-resolution HLA typing results are listed for each HLA locus

Q2. Which of the following statements is most correct?

A. Due to the HLA identical A, B, C, DR, and DQ loci 10 of 10 matching, either potential donor would be suitable, since the HLA-DP mismatching can be ignored
B. Additional analysis of the HLA-DP mismatching should be performed
C. Even though HLA-DQ mismatching is not considered relevant from the NMDP data, the fact that the two donors match at HLA-DQ indicate that either is a suitable HCT donor
D. The HLA-DRB3 matching adds to the credibility of each potential donor as the candidate for donation, since complete HLA-DR matching is most necessary in HCT
E. There are insufficient data present to select a donor

Answer: *The correct answer is* ***B***.

Q3. Which of the following statements is most correct?

A. Matching at HLA-DQA1 and HLA-DPA1 is considered highly relevant due to their relative associations in the bimolecular three-dimensional constructs for HLA-DQ and HLA-DP, respectively.
B. Slight mismatching in the two-field nomenclature for HLA-C is not considered relevant for HCT considerations, since HLA-C primarily interacts with NK cells.
C. Mismatching at HLA-DP may or may not be relevant for HCT transplantation, depending on which epitopes are present.
D. Since HLA-A and HLA-DP have the greatest chance to undergo crossover during meiosis, these have the least impact on HCT donor selection.
E. One of the positions with highest risk for crossover during meiosis is between HLA-DRB1 and HLA-DRB3/4/5, due to the sequences similarities on different alleles, thus HLA-DRB3/4/5 matching is critical for HCT.

Answer: *The correct answer is* ***C***.

If a transplant center uses 8 of 8 or 10 of 10, then either of the donors in Table 39.2 would be suitable, but there would have been no need to obtain HLA-DP typing data, under those circumstances. According to what discussed above, including HLA-DPB1 in the HCT donor selection criteria is mandatory to maximize the transplant outcomes. The differences between the individual HLA-DPB1 molecules involve specific T cell epitopes (TCE). HLA-DPB1 with different two-field typing names may share the same or similar TCE, and thus become TCE permissive HLA-DPB1 mismatches. Alternatively, if there is TCE mismatch, then the pair is designated as a TCE non-permissive HLA-DPB1 mismatch, which could result in ~10% worse long-term outcome following HCT [2]. The international ImMunoGeneTics information (IMGT) system has created a website with an algorithm to determine the extent of HLA-DPB1 TCE mismatching (http://www.ebi.ac.uk/ipd/imgt/hla/dpb.html), which can be readily utilized to determine suitable donors.

Q4. Which of the following statements is most correct regarding information presented in Table 39.3? (below)

A. Since both potential donors share TCE group 3 with the patient, either should be a compatible HCT donor.
B. Potential donor 2 is the most compatible since they share TCE group 3 and an identical HLA-DPB1*04:01.
C. Potential donor 1 is the most acceptable donor for HCT since both TCE group 2 and 3 are present in accord with the patient.
D. Either donor is equally acceptable since either is haploidentical at HLA-DPB1, either *03:01 or *04:01
E. Based on the lack of exact matching at HLA-DPB1, neither donor is acceptable.

Answer: *The correct answer is* ***C***.

In Table 39.3, potential donor 1 shares HLA-DPB1*03:01 (which carries a TCE group 2 designation) with the donor. While the second allele (HLA-DPB1*20:01) mismatches the patient (HLA-DPB1*04:01) in nomenclature but both share TCE group 3. Thus, this is acceptable, as a "permissive mismatch", with essentially the same long-term outcomes in HCT as an HLA-DPB1 matched situation. Conversely,

Table 39.3 HLA-DPB1 TCE groups for each DPB1 allele in HCT of a 12-year-old girl with AML

	HLA-DPB1 allele	TCE group
Patient	*03:01	2
	*04:01	3
Potential Donor 1	*03:01	2
	*20:01	3
Potential Donor 2	*01:01	3
	*04:01	3

The TCE group for each HLA-DPB1 allele is list for the patient and potential donors

even though potential donor 2 and the patient share HLA-DPB1*04:01, they mismatch by two-field nomenclature in the other allele. Further, potential donor 2 expresses HLA-DPB1*01:01, which is in TCE group 3 and there is no tolerization to TCE group 2. Thus, potential donor 2 has a much higher risk for causing GVHD. In this case, potential donor 1 is a 9 of 10 HLA-A, -B, -C, -DRB1, and -DPB1, match, with one permissive TCE group 3 HLA-DPB1 mismatch, being the most suitable non-related HCT donor for this patient.

Practical Points

- Linkage disequilibrium is the concept that HLA types are associated into inherited haplotypes more commonly than is expected from DNA cross-over events, which occur during normal meiosis
- The distal HLA loci HLA-DP and HLA-A may have some of the greatest chances to undergo crossover exchanges, due to being at the opposite extreme ends of the HLA locus on the short arm of chromosome 6
- If the HLA-A, -B, -C, and -DR are known, then -DQ can be predicted with reasonable accuracy, and likewise if HLA-A, -B, -C, -DR, and -DQ are known, the -DP may be predicted, albeit with somewhat less accuracy, further, HLA-C can be predicted when HLA-B is known

References

1. Spellman S, Setterholm M, Maiers M, Noreen H, Oudshoorn M, Fernandez-Vina M, Petersdorf E, Bray R, Hartzman RJ, Ng J, Hurley CK. Advances in the selection of HLA-compatible donors: refinements in HLA typing and matching over the first 20 years of the National Marrow Donor Program Registry. Biol Blood Marrow Transpl. 2008;14(9 Suppl):37–44.
2. Pidala J, Lee SJ, Ahn KW, Spellman S, Wang HL, Aljurf M, Askar M, Dehn J, Fernandez Vina M, Gratwohl A, Gupta V, Hanna R, Horowitz MM, Hurley CK, Inamoto Y, Kassim AA, Nishihori T, Mueller C, Oudshoorn M, Petersdorf EW, Prasad V, Robinson J, Saber W, Schultz KR, Shaw B, Storek J, Wood WA, Woolfrey AE, Anasetti C. Nonpermissive HLA-DPB1 mismatch increases mortality after myeloablative unrelated allogeneic hematopoietic cell transplantation. Blood. 2014;124(16):2596–606.

Chapter 40
T-Lymphoblastic Lymphoma

Soumya Pandey and Terry Harville

A 13-year-old Caucasian male, diagnosed with T cell lymphoblastic lymphoma, presenting with a mediastinal mass with no bone marrow involvement. He completed 8 cycles of HyperCVAD and AraC/MTX over 6 months. Subsequently, the patient was shown to be in complete remission. Initially there were no plans for HCT due to standard risk of disease in this young patient: age at diagnosis <35, low white count on diagnosis, and Philadelphia chromosome negative disease. Unfortunately, 1 year after remission had been achieved, the patient presented with bilateral testicular enlargement and possible aortocaval nodal involvement. Biopsy findings were consistent with recurrence of T cell lymphoblastic leukemia/lymphoma. The patient underwent orchiectomy and was placed on the LARSON lymphoma treatment protocol. At this point, he was considered a candidate for allogeneic hematopoietic cell transplantation, once he would again achieve clinical remission.

Q1. True or False: HCT should always be considered as first line therapy for any hematologic malignancy during the initial remission

A. True
B. False

Answer: *The correct answer is* ***B****.*

S. Pandey
Department of Pathology and Laboratory Services, University of Arkansas for Medical Sciences, Little Rock, AR, USA

T. Harville (✉)
Department of Pathology and Laboratory Services, University of Arkansas for Medical Sciences, Little Rock, AR, USA

Departments of Pediatrics and Internal Medicine, University of Arkansas for Medical Sciences, Little Rock, AR, USA
e-mail: harvilleterryo@uams.edu

© Springer Nature Switzerland AG 2020

F. Rahmani, N. Rezaei (eds.), *Pediatric Autoimmunity and Transplantation*,
https://doi.org/10.1007/978-3-030-26280-8_40

Q2. True or False: Many subtypes of lymphoma can be well treated using autologous HCT once remission is achieved

A. True
B. False

Answer: *The correct answer is* ***A***.

While it may seem that if a cancer occurs in someone, their "surveillance" immunity may not be functioning at full capacity, and thus, replacement with a "more-effective" immunity would seem logical, the morbidity and mortality associated with HCT has made this assumption less appealing. With improvements in treatment options, many childhood cancers have considerably high 5-year survival rates without HCT (e.g. B cell ALL in children >85% and AML in children >60%). Therefore, for most leukemia, HCT is not a first option, but may be an important component of therapy once the second remission is achieved following a relapse [1].

Lymphoma tends to be more insidious disease than leukemia. While once again, improvements in diagnosis and treatment have overall improved the outcomes, treatment can also adversely impact the patient's hematopoietic system function, especially in chemotherapy with certain types of lymphoma. Using autologous HCT can improve the recovery and reinforce the self-immunity against the cancer, once remission has been achieved. Thus, autologous HCT is used for more rapid recovery of the hematopoietic system after extensive chemotherapy.

The patient's HLA typing results were evaluated and a search was initiated to find potential donors. Based on the NMDP match grade/calculation, three potential donors with possible 10 of 10 match were identified. Samples were received for confirmatory HLA typing (results are listed in Table 40.1).

Q3. Based on the HLA typing results in Table 40.1 HCT, which of the following statements is most correct?

A. None of the potential donors is suitable
B. All of the potential donors are suitable
C. Potential donors 1 and 2 appear to be the best
D. Potential donors 2 and 3 appear to be the best
E. Potential donors 1 and 3 appear to be the best

Answer: *The correct answer is* ***E***.

Table 40.1 HLA typing results in a 13-year-old boy with TLL

	A	B	C	DRB1	DRB3/4/5	DQB1	DQA1	DPB1	DPA1
Patient	*01:01	*08:01	*07:01	*03:01	3*01:01	*02:01	*05:01	*04:01	*01:03
	*01:01	*57:01	*06:02	*07:01	4*01:03 N	*03:03	*02:01	*09:01	*02:01
Potential Donor 1	*01:01	*08:01	*07:01	*03:01	3*01:01	*02:01	*05:01	*04:01	*01:03
	*01:01	*57:01	*06:02	*07:01	4*01:03 N	*03:03	*02:01	*09:01	*02:01
Potential Donor 2	*01:01	*08:01	*07:01	*03:01	3*01:01	*02:01	*05:01	*04:01	*01:03
	*01:01	*57:01	*06:02	*07:01	4*01:03 N	*03:03	*02:01	*10:01	*02:01
Potential Donor 3	*01:01	*08:01	*07:01	*03:01	3*01:01	*02:01	*05:01	*04:01	*01:03
	*01:01	*57:01	*06:02	*07:01	4*01:03 N	*03:03	*02:01	*09:01	*02:01

HLA typing results are listed for both alleles by each locus

Q4. True or False: The fact that all three potential donors share a 10 of 10 match, i.e. HLA-A, -B, -C, -DRB1, and -DQB1, with the patient, makes them equally suitable

A. True
B. False

Answer: *The correct answer is* ***B***.

Q5. True or False: The fact that all three potential donors share the same HLA-DRB1, -DRB3, and -DRB4 with the patient indicates are all three are good matches as potential donors for HCT

A. True
B. False

Answer: *The correct answer is* ***B***.

Q6. Which of the following criteria is important for consideration in the donor selection process for this patient? (CMV: cytomegalovirus)

A. The 10 of 10 HLA-A, -B, -C, -DRB1, and -DQB1 match, alone, with the potential donor gender and CMV match.
B. The 10 of 10 HLA-A, -B, -C, -DRB1, and -DQB1 match, and the matching at HLA-DRB3, -DRB4, and -DQA1.
C. Matching at HLA-A, -B, -C, -DRB1, and -DPB1, including permissive HLA-DPB1 TCE mismatching.
D. Additional information not listed, including donor, age, gender, and blood type.
E. Whether the conditioning for HCT will be myeloablative or non-myeloablative.

Answer: *The correct answer is* ***C***.

Data reported from the NMDP indicate that HLA-DQB1 matching is not as important as HLA-A, -B, -C, and -DRB1 matching [2]. Additional data from the NMDP indicate that non-permissive mismatching of HLA-DPB1 T cell epitope (TCE) does reduce long-term outcome results. In this case, potential donor 2 expresses HLA-DPA1*02:01/DPB1*10:01, rather than HLA-DPA1*02:01/DPB1*09:01, as do the patient and other donors. Therefore, on the initial observation, potential donors 1 and 3 would be better suited, if there is CMV status match (Table 40.2). However, it should be determined whether the HLA-DPB1*10:01 is a permissive or non-permissive HLA-DPB1 TCE mismatch. If potential donors 1 and 3 do not have the correct CMV status match with the patient, then potential donor 2 could be the best option, if there is the correct CMV match, and permissive HLA-DPB1 TCE mismatch. The CMV status of a donor is important for matching CMV+ with CMV+ and CMV− with CMV−, but blood type is not considered relevant and gender is somewhat less relevant. There may be a higher risk of GVHD using a female donor into a male patient. This would have been advantageous for a more difficult to treat cancer, such as high-risk AML, but not so in a situation such as aplastic anemia, where engraftment is needed, but a "graft-versus-leukemia" effect

Table 40.2 HLA-DPB1 TCE groups for HCT in a 13-year-old boy with TLL

Allele	TCE group
DPB1*04:01	3
DPB1*09:01	1
DPB1*04:01	3
DPB1*10:01	1

The HLA-DPB1 TCE groups are listed in the upper rows for the patient (and potential donors 1 and 3, since they share the same HLA type), and bottom two rows for potential donor 2

is not [3, 4]. Overall, HLA-DRB3, -DRB4, and -DRB5 are not considered in the matching process and once again, mismatching HLA-DQB1 is not considered to adversely affect the HCT outcomes.

Q7. True or False: This is likely a permissive HLA DPB1 TCE group 1 mismatch

A. True
B. False

Answer: *The correct answer is* ***A***.

Matching of HLA-DPB1 TCE groups indicates the likelihood of permissive mismatch. Whereas, TCE group mismatches may result in the risk for GVHD or graft rejection, depending on homozygosity of the TCE groups in the donor or patient, respectively.

Practical Points

- Overall, the highest-resolution HLA typing is thought to provide the best opportunity for matching a patient with a donor in order to reduce the risks for graft-versus host disease (GVHD) and graft rejection
- Linkage disequilibrium is an important concept regarding HLA type associations, and can be used to help surmise which HLA alleles may be present, while actual typing is typically necessary for the true confirmation of the results
- The use of "Common and Well-Documented" alleles is also helpful in determination of the HLA types are present
- Currently, the NMDP does not consider matching for HLA-DRB3, -DRB4, -DRB5, or -DQ to be relevant for HCT. Despite this, in clinical practice, many transplanters prefer donors matched for these as well, rather than those not matched
- HLA-DPB1 is now recognized as relevant for HCT

- Matching can occur at two levels; first, the two-field nomenclature match and second, the examination of the TCE groups for permissive versus non-permissive mismatching of HLA-DPB1
- Long-term outcomes are similar to those with the HLA-DPB1 two-field nomenclature match and HLA-DPB1 TCE permissive mismatches
- Cytomegalovirus status match of the patient and donor is a critical factor for successful outcomes
- The NMDP website provides invaluable information regarding HLA typing and HCT outcomes

References

1. Rimsza L, Pittaluga S, Dirnhofer S, Copie-Bergman C, de Leval L, Facchetti F, Pileri S, Rosenwald A, Wotherspoon A, Fend F. The clinicopathologic spectrum of mature aggressive B cell lymphomas. Virchows Archiv. 2017;471(4):453–66.
2. Spellman S, Setterholm M, Maiers M, Noreen H, Oudshoorn M, Fernandez-Vina M, Petersdorf E, Bray R, Hartzman RJ, Ng J, Hurley CK. Advances in the selection of HLA-compatible donors: refinements in HLA typing and matching over the first 20 years of the National Marrow Donor Program Registry. Biol Blood Marrow Transpl. 2008;14(9 Suppl):37–44.
3. Horowitz MM, Gale RP, Sondel PM, Goldman JM, Kersey J, Kolb HJ, Rimm AA, Ringden O, Rozman C, Speck B, et al. Graft-versus-leukemia reactions after bone marrow transplantation. Blood. 1990;75(3):555–62.
4. Kolb HJ, Schattenberg A, Goldman JM, Hertenstein B, Jacobsen N, Arcese W, Ljungman P, Ferrant A, Verdonck L, Niederwieser D, van Rhee F, Mittermueller J, de Witte T, Holler E, Ansari H. Graft-versus-leukemia effect of donor lymphocyte transfusions in marrow grafted patients. Blood. 1995;86(5):2041–50.

Chapter 41
No Lymphocytes in an Infant

Beatriz Morillo-Gutierrez and Mary Slatter

A first child of non-consanguineous parents, presented at 6 months of age with cough, tachypnea and grunting. He had a previous history of severe eczema, failure to thrive and diarrhea with large swellings in the inguinal area since 4 months of age.

He was admitted and started on oral antibiotics, but developed progressive respiratory distress requiring intubation and mechanical ventilation. On examination he also had absent hair and sparse eyebrows with thickened red peeling over his scalp, and enlarged lymph nodes in the neck, axillae and groins. His liver edge was just palpable.

A bronchoalveolar lavage was performed which revealed *Pneumocystis jirovecii*. CBC showed marked lymphopenia with a normal neutrophil count, and normal hemoglobin and platelet values, while immunoglobulin levels showed markedly decreased IgG, IgA and IgM. He was started on high doses of co-trimoxazole and prednisolone treatment for *Pneumocystis jirovecii* pneumonia (PCP).

In his past medical history he was diagnosed with transposition of great arteries that was corrected by surgery on day 2 of life, with secondary total thymectomy. His immunisations were up-to-date, including live rotavirus vaccine. Family history was non-significant.

B. Morillo-Gutierrez
Translational Paediatrics and Infectious Diseases Unit, Santiago de Compostela University Hospital, Santiago de Compostela, Spain

M. Slatter (✉)
Department of Paediatric Immunology, Great North Children's Hospital, Royal Victoria Infirmary, Newcastle upon Tyne, UK

Institute of Cellular Medicine, Newcastle University, Newcastle upon Tyne, UK
e-mail: mary.slatter@nuth.nhs.uk

© Springer Nature Switzerland AG 2020

F. Rahmani, N. Rezaei (eds.), *Pediatric Autoimmunity and Transplantation*, https://doi.org/10.1007/978-3-030-26280-8_41

Q1. What is your initial diagnosis and what investigations would you order?

A. My initial diagnosis is lymphopenia secondary to an ongoing infection. I would look for other infections including viral PCRs in blood and extensive imaging investigations and treat them appropriately.
B. My initial diagnosis is severe combined immunodeficiency. I would complete his immunology work up with extended lymphocyte subsets and functional lymphocyte tests together with screening for other infections.
C. My initial diagnosis is transient hypogammaglobulinemia of infancy. I would manage the acute infection and wait and see with no further investigations.
D. My initial diagnosis is chronic granulomatous disease. I would perform a nitroblue tetrazolium and a dihydrorhodamine test.

Answer: *The correct answer is* ***B.***

Even in the absence of lymphocyte subsets enumeration, the clinical presentation is typical of severe combined immunodeficiency (SCID). In this particular case, the signs of skin rash, lymphadenopathy, sparse hair and the leaky phenotype, makes us think of Omenn's syndrome or materno-fetal engraftment [1, 2].

The laboratory test confirmed subsequently the diagnosis of SCID with materno-fetal engraftment: his lymphocyte subsets showed few activated $CD4^+$ with no $CD8^+$, B or naïve cells, but normal numbers of NK cells. Lymphocytes response to PHA showed absent proliferation and the T cell receptor (TCR) variable beta chain was very skewed. Moreover, his genetics detected a *RAG1* mutation and 10–15% of his additional alleles were shown to be of maternal origin, consistent with a diagnosis of materno-fetal engraftment.

Apart from rotavirus vaccine strain in faeces he did not have any other virus isolated in blood, respiratory or stool samples.

Q2. We are facing a SCID male baby with a known *RAG1* mutation and materno-fetal engraftment, PJP pneumonia and rotavirus vaccine strain diarrhea. What treatment options from the list below are indicated in this step?

1. Treat infections aggressively and start infection control measures: continue treatment for PJP, infection prophylaxis using immunoglobulin replacement, antifungal prophylaxis and avoid exposure to other infections: isolation of the patient, stop breastfeeding until CMV status of the mother is known
2. Start immunosuppression to control the inflammatory reaction secondary to engrafted maternal cells.
3. Start donor search and work up pre-HCT as soon as possible
4. Start enzyme replacement with PEGylated adenosine deaminase
5. Consider the patient a candidate to gene therapy

A. Options 1, 4, 5
B. Options 1, 4
C. Option 1, 2, and 3
D. Options 1, 3, 4, and 5

Correct answers: *The correct answer is* ***C.***

Hematopoietic stem cell transplantation (HSCT) is still the curative treatment of choice for most forms of SCID with an excellent overall survival rate of over 90% when performed promptly in the absence of infection [3, 4]. For some non-SCID primary immunodeficiencies (PIDs), HSCT is also the first option for curative treatment (Table 41.1), and for some other emerging disorders it can be considered depending on the phenotype of the patient [5–7]. The overall survival of other PIDs with HSCT is usually lower than for SCID, but outcomes are rapidly improving. The immunodeficiency will be cured, if the underlying defect lies within the hematopoietic system [8].

The underlying principle is that hematopoietic stem cells from a donor will restore the patient's mature blood cells and progenitors. There are different options for donor, cell sources and medication given for the transplant, such as chemotherapy, that will be explained in the following questions [9–11].

Initially, a donor search must be performed after tissue typing the patient and a pre-HSCT workup must be arranged to assess his/her baseline situation. These include investigations for infection, including CMV, EBV, varicella-zoster virus, herpes simplex virus, adenovirus, hepatitis B, C and HIV. Depending on the type of transplant and the chemotherapy chosen other baseline investigations such as cardiac assessment or audiology may be required. Special care needs to be taken by using leukodepleted or blood-irradiated products for any transfusions due to the risk of transfusion-associated graft-versus host disease (GVHD). Lastly, aggressive management of ongoing infections and antibiotic prophylaxis are paramount, to avoid organ damage that could potentially prohibit a successful outcome [12].

Table 41.1 Indications for HSCT in primary immunodeficiency disorders

SCID
CID
CD40 ligand deficiency
WAS
PNP deficiency
XLP syndrome
MHC class II deficiency
LAD
Osteopetrosis
Haemophagocytic disorders
Undefined T cell disorders
HLH
CHS
Griscelli syndrome
CGD

CGD Chronic granulomatous disease, *CHS* Chédiak–Higashi syndrome, *HLH* hemophagocytic lymphohistiocytosis, *LAD* Leukocyte adhesion deficiency, *MHC* major histocompatibility complex, *PNP* Purine nucleoside phosphorylase, *WAS* Wiskott-Aldrich syndrome, *XLP* X-linked lymphoproliferative, *HSCT* hematopoietic stem cell transplantation

As a brief comment for the last two options, enzyme replacement is only available for adenosine deaminase-SCID and gene therapy is not currently an option for *RAG1* SCID, although there are promising studies in mice for future times [13, 14].

Q3. What donor source would you prefer in an ideal scenario?

A. Matched sibling donor
B. Unrelated matched donor
C. Haploidentical family donor (mother/father) with graft manipulation, such a T cell depletion
D. Unrelated cord

Answer: *The correct answer is* ***A.***

Matching the cells of the donor with the patient is important to avoid both graft rejection and GVHD. In ideal conditions, a matched sibling donor is the first option for a HSCT, with the best-known survival rates.

Fortunately, nowadays, a well matched (9/10 or above) unrelated donor can often be found. In addition there are new techniques for graft manipulation and lower rates of GVHD, such as TCR alpha-beta T cell depletion of a haploidentical graft. With the advent of these techniques a donor should be available for almost all patients [15–18].

Regarding the source, we can procure stem cells from bone marrow, granulocyte-monocyte colony stimulating factor mobilized peripheral blood stem cells, or umbilical cord blood. It is important to deliver maximum amount of $CD34^+$ stem cells to increase the success rate of the graft [9, 12], but not too many T cells, which increases the risk of GVHD.

In our particular case there were some concerns about his thymectomy which means that, in spite of receiving a graft, he may not be able to produce naïve T cells which are dependent on the presence of thymus or thymus-dependent T cell generation. These cells will later proliferate and will be responsible for a sustained long-term immune reconstitution. An 11/12 matched unrelated adult donor was chosen over a cord blood. Even after giving some conditioning, we know that some of the T cells present in this graft will survive, and our hope was that receiving a graft from an adult, a broader T cell repertoire of mature cells would be able to proliferate peripherally and sustain an adequate T cell compartment.

Q4. What would be the best combination of conditioning regimen and GVHD prophylaxis options in our patient?

1. No conditioning regimen is needed
2. High intensity conditioning is mandatory
3. Reduced intensity conditioning
4. No GVHD prophylaxis post-transplant needed
5. GVHD prophylaxis with either mycophenolate mofetil, cyclosporine, tacrolimus etc.

A. Options 1 and 5
B. Options 1 and 4
C. Options 2 and 3
D. Options 3 and 5
E. Options 2 and 4

Answer: *The correct answer is* ***E.***

A combination of chemotherapy is advisable to produce myeloablation and immunosuppression: the first term, myeloablation, refers to ablation of host hematopoiesis and the second term, immunosuppression, is intended to prevent rejection of the incoming donor cells by the host immune cells. It is also postulated that conditioning helps create space in the stem cell niches for new cells to engraft. In case of malignancies, myeloablation helps eradicate disease [19]. These medications have known adverse effects both in the short term, being responsible for lethal veno-occlusive disease (VOD) and in the long term, potentially causing growth retardation, infertility, and malignancy. It is therefore important to find a balance between optimising cell engraftment while avoiding drug toxicity.

In the setting of HSCT for PIDs, achieving full donor chimerism in all cell lineages is not always needed to cure the disease. We can afford to adopt less myeloablative effects of the drugs used, and this is why we use reduced-intensity or reduced-toxicity conditioning regimens, using more "immunoablation" than "myeloablation". This could be achieved with targeted low dose busulfan, treosulfan or fludarabine. Additional immunosuppressive medication might be indicated, directed to decrease the risk of GVHD. These entail monoclonal antibodies to produce *in vivo* lymphodepletion e.g. alemtuzumab or anti-thymocyte globulin (ATG), or lymphocyte inhibitors post-HSCT e.g. cyclosporine, tacrolimus and mycophenolate mofetil, to avoid overstimulation of the engrafted cells.

Although in theory we could be tempted to give unconditioned stem cells in a SCID because of the lack of T cells, several studies described lower rates of engraftment and long term immune reconstitution. Unconditioned transplants are hence used in very restricted situations [9, 19, 20].

To review the recommended regimens, there are periodic guidelines released by recognised societies, such as the "EBMT/ESID" guidelines for HSCT for PIDs.

In our patient in particular, he received a combination of alemtuzumab, treosulfan and fludarabine, with MMF and cyclosporine as post-HSCT GVHD prophylaxis. In addition, he had previously received a 5-day course of ATG to eliminate maternal cells and cyclosporine to control the ongoing inflammation secondary to maternal engraftment as mentioned in Q2.

Our patient became aplastic after the conditioning and received his stem cells on day 0. He had to remain isolated for some weeks initially while his cells engrafted.

Q5. What would you need to be monitoring during the conditioning period and the first few weeks before engrafment?

A. Mucositis
B. Viral, bacterial and fungal infections

C. Acute GVHD
D. Complications of vascular origin, like VOD of the liver, capillary leak syndrome, engraftment syndrome or thrombotic microangiopathy
E. Drug toxicity, such as posterior reversible encephalopathy syndrome (PRES)
F. All of the above

Answer: *The correct answer is* ***F.***

All the above complications are well described following HSCT. Some of them are related to immunosuppression, especially neutropenia, following the conditioning i.e. mucositis or high risk of infections. Other complications are directly caused by drug toxicity, e.g. VOD, and some others have mixed and complex mechanisms, i.e. engraftment and capillary leak syndromes [21]. GVHD and infections are still the main complications seen in the setting of HSCT for PIDs, and fortunately, with the use of less toxic regimen those secondary to drug toxicity like VOD are less and less common [9]. Some of the complications depend on the patient status pre-transplant, such as liver damage or viral infections that could reactivate.

For our patient, his transplant was very smooth. He became fluid overloaded following his conditioning with changes in his chest X-rays, requiring O2 overnight. He was managed with a combination of fluid restriction, diuretics and broad spectrum antibiotics and subsequently improved. He did not show any signs of mucositis, viral reactivation or GVHD.

As mentioned, our patient had a very smooth transplant. His neutrophils engrafted at day +21, meaning that he had an unsupported neutrophil count above 500/μL for 3 consecutive days. His chimerism on day +23 was 95% donor and he was discharged from the HSCT unit after 2 months. He continued receiving co-trimoxazole, acyclovir, intravenous immunoglobulins (IVIG) and cyclosporine.

Q6. What is the best follow up and medication plan for him?

A. He needs to continue on cyclosporine for his entire life to avoid rejection of the transplant.
B. After the transplant he is not immunosuppressed anymore, he should stop all the infection prophylaxis medication as soon as possible to avoid toxicities.
C. His chimerism is 95% donor and it needs to be 100%. This means transplant failure and he will probably need to be retransplanted.
D. He will need regular follow up to check his donor chimerism and signs of immune reconstitution; as this happens, he can stop medications and start re-immunisation. In the long term, his growth and fertility need to be monitored.

Answer: *The correct answer is* ***D.***

He needs to be weaned off cyclosporine between 4 and 6 months after HSCT if there are no signs of GVHD. He could stop the prophylactic medications provided that signs of immune reconstitution appear, monitoring lymphocyte subpopulations and immunoglobulin levels. IgM levels are of particular importance which will show that he is making his own immunoglobulin rather than the IgG which we are giving him in his replacement infusions. Donor chimerism must be stable over time, but not necessarily 100% in all cell lines, to correct the immunodeficiency, as in our patient [22].

In the long term, our patient should be able to have a normal life, off medications, yet being monitored for long-term toxicity from the conditioning regimen, such as growth and infertility.

Practical Points

- Hematopoietic stem cell transplantation (HSCT) is a curative and lifesaving treatment for many primary immunodeficiency disorders, with the best overall survival for severe combined immunodeficiency (>90%)
- Advanced techniques for graft manipulation allow the use of other donor sources than matched sibling donor, still with very good outcomes
- Current regimens with reduced intensity/toxicity conditioning allow better engraftment with less toxicity
- Long-term effects of transplantation need to be monitored over time, particularly growth and infertility

References

1. Fischer A. Severe combined immunodeficiencies (SCID). Clin Exp Immunol. 2000;122:143–9.
2. Burg M, Gennery A. Educational paper. Eur J Pediatr. 2011;170:561–71.
3. Pai S-Y, Logan BR, Griffith LM, Buckley RH, Parrott RE, Dvorak CC, Kapoor N, Hanson IC, Filipovich AH, Jyonouchi S, Sullivan KE, Small TN, Burroughs L, Skoda-Smith S, Haight AE, Grizzle A, Pulsipher MA, Chan KW, Fuleihan RL, Haddad E, Loechelt B, Aquino VM, Gillio A, Davis J, Knutsen A, Smith AR, Moore TB, Schroeder ML, Goldman FD, Connelly JA, Porteus MH, Xiang Q, Shearer WT, Fleisher TA, Kohn DB, Puck JM, Notarangelo LD, Cowan MJ, O'Reilly RJ. Transplantation outcomes for severe combined immunodeficiency, 2000–2009. N Engl J Med. 2014;371:434–46.
4. Brown L, Xu-Bayford J, Allwood Z, Slatter M, Cant A, Davies EG, Veys P, Gennery AR, Gaspar HB. Neonatal diagnosis of severe combined immunodeficiency leads to significantly improved survival outcome: the case for newborn screening. Blood. 2011;117:3243–6.
5. Gennery AR, Slatter MA, Grandin L, Taupin P, Cant AJ, Veys P, Amrolia PJ, Gaspar HB, Davies EG, Friedrich W, Hoenig M, Notarangelo LD, Mazzolari E, Porta F, Bredius RG, Lankester AC, Wulffraat NM, Seger R, Gungor T, Fasth A, Sedlacek P, Neven B, Blanche S, Fischer A, Cavazzana-Calvo M, Landais P. Transplantation of hematopoietic stem cells and long-term survival for primary immunodeficiencies in Europe: entering a new century, do we do better? J Allergy Clin Immunol. 2010;126(3):602–10.e1-11.
6. Slatter MA, Engelhardt KR, Burroughs LM, Arkwright PD, Nademi Z, Skoda-Smith S, Hagin D, Kennedy A, Barge D, Flood T, Abinun M, Wynn RF, Gennery AR, Cant AJ, Sansom D, Hambleton S, Torgerson TR. Hematopoietic stem cell transplantation for CTLA4 deficiency. J Allergy Clin Immunol. 2016;138(2):615–9.e1.
7. Leiding JW, Okada S, Hagin D, Abinun M, Shcherbina A, Balashov DN, Kim VHD, Ovadia A, Guthery SL, Pulsipher M, Lilic D, Devlin LA, Christie S, Depner M, Fuchs S, van Royen-Kerkhof A, Lindemans C, Petrovic A, Sullivan KE, Bunin N, Kilic SS, Arpaci F, Calle-Martin O, Martinez-Martinez L, Aldave JC, Kobayashi M, Ohkawa T, Imai K, Iguchi A, Roifman CM, Gennery AR, Slatter M, Ochs HD, Morio T, Torgerson TR. Hematopoietic stem cell

transplantation in patients with gain-of-function signal transducer and activator of transcription 1 mutations. J Allergy Clin Immunol. 2018;141(2):704–17.e5.
8. Picard C, Bobby Gaspar H, Al-Herz W, Bousfiha A, Casanova JL, Chatila T, Crow YJ, Cunningham-Rundles C, Etzioni A, Franco JL, Holland SM, Klein C, Morio T, Ochs HD, Oksenhendler E, Puck J, Tang MLK, Tangye SG, Torgerson TR, Sullivan KE. International Union of Immunological Societies: 2017 primary immunodeficiency diseases committee report on inborn errors of immunity. J Clin Immunol. 2018;38(1):96–128.
9. Slatter M, Gennery A. Advances in hematopoietic stem cell transplantation for primary immunodeficiency. Expert Rev Clin Immunol. 2013;9:991–9.
10. Booth C, Silva J, Veys P. Stem cell transplantation for the treatment of immunodeficiency in children: current status and hopes for the future. Expert Rev Clin Immunol. 2016;12:713–23.
11. Dvorak C, Cowan M. Hematopoietic stem cell transplantation for primary immunodeficiency disease. Bone Marrow Transplant. 2008;41:119–26.
12. Larghero J, Garcia J, Gluckman E. Sources and procurement of stem cells. Haematop Stem Cell Transplant EBMT Handbook. 2008.
13. Rivers L, Gaspar H. Severe combined immunodeficiency: recent developments and guidance on clinical management. Arch Dis Child. 2015;100:667–72.
14. Ferrua F, Aiuti A. Twenty-five years of gene therapy for ADA-SCID: from bubble babies to an approved drug. Hum Gene Ther. 2017;28:972–81.
15. Shah RM, Elfeky R, Nademi Z, Qasim W, Amrolia P, Chiesa R, Rao K, Lucchini G, Silva JMF, Worth A, Barge D, Ryan D, Conn J, Cant AJ, Skinner R, Abd Hamid IJ, Flood T, Abinun M, Hambleton S, Gennery AR, Veys P, Slatter M. T-cell receptor alphabeta(+) and CD19(+) cell-depleted haploidentical and mismatched hematopoietic stem cell transplantation in primary immune deficiency. J Allergy Clin Immunol. 2018;141(4):1417–26.e1.
16. Balashov D, Shcherbina A, Maschan M, Trakhtman P, Skvortsova Y, Shelikhova L, Laberko A, Livshits A, Novichkova G, Maschan A. Single-Center experience of unrelated and haploidentical stem cell transplantation with TCRalphabeta and CD19 depletion in children with primary immunodeficiency syndromes. Biol Blood Marrow Transplant. 2015;21(11):1955–62.
17. Bertaina A, Merli P, Rutella S, Pagliara D, Bernardo ME, Masetti R, Pende D, Falco M, Handgretinger R, Moretta F, Lucarelli B, Brescia LP, Li Pira G, Testi M, Cancrini C, Kabbara N, Carsetti R, Finocchi A, Moretta A, Moretta L, Locatelli F. HLA-haploidentical stem cell transplantation after removal of alphabeta+ T and B cells in children with nonmalignant disorders. Blood. 2014;124(5):822–6.
18. Slatter MA, Gennery AR. Approaches to the removal of T-lymphocytes to minimize graft-versus-host disease in patients with primary immunodeficiencies who do not have a matched sibling donor. Curr Opin Allergy Clin Immunol. 2017;17(6):414–20.
19. Gratwohl A. Principles of conditioning. ESH-EBMT Handb Haematop Stem Cell Transplant ESH. 2008.
20. Chiesa R, Veys P. Reduced-intensity conditioning for allogeneic stem cell transplant in primary immune deficiencies. Expert Rev Clin Immunol. 2012;8:255–66.
21. Carreras E. Early complications after HSCT. In EBMT Handb Hematop Stem Cell Transplant. 5th ed. 2008.
22. Heimall J, Buckley R, Puck J, Fleisher T, Gennery A, Haddad E, Neven B, Slatter M, Roderick S, Baker K, Dietz A, Duncan C, Griffith L, Notarangelo L, Pulsipher M, Cowan M. Recommendations for screening and management of late effects in patients with severe combined immunodeficiency after allogenic hematopoietic cell transplantation: a consensus statement from the second pediatric blood and marrow transplant consortium international conference on late effects after pediatric HCT. Biol Blood Marrow Transplant. 2017;23:1229–40.

Chapter 42
DOCK8 Deficiency and No Matched Donor

Beatriz Morillo-Gutierrez and Mary Slatter

A 7-year-old boy was referred to the immunology reference unit with the diagnosis of dedicator of cytokinesis (DOCK8) deficiency.

The patient was diagnosed with DOCK8 deficiency in the context of investigations for severe eczema since infancy, asthma and cow's milk protein allergy, and severe, recurrent infections including osteomyelitis, enteritis, repeated pneumonias and plantar warts. His laboratory parameters showed moderate T cell lymphopenia, low serum IgM and high serum IgE levels. He was screened by sequence analysis and was found to have a homozygous deletion of exon 8 on the *DOCK8* gene.

Q1. Which management option is correct? (HSCT: hematopoietic stem cell transplantation)

A. HSCT is not recommended in this disease. I would optimize his skin care and asthma plan, ensure he is on antibiotic prophylaxis and manage his infections aggressively
B. HSCT is recommended but not at this age, the patient is too young. I would start a donor search but wait until the patient is older to go ahead with the procedure
C. HSCT is recommended in DOCK8 deficiency and should be performed promptly. I would start a donor search and pre-transplant workup without delay

Answer: *The correct answer is* ***C.***

B. Morillo-Gutierrez
Translational Paediatrics and Infectious Diseases Unit, Santiago de Compostela University Hospital, Santiago de Compostela, Spain

M. Slatter (✉)
Department of Paediatric Immunology, Great North Children's Hospital, Royal Victoria Infirmary, Newcastle upon Tyne, UK

Institute of Cellular Medicine, Newcastle University, Newcastle upon Tyne, UK
e-mail: mary.slatter@nuth.nhs.uk

© Springer Nature Switzerland AG 2020

F. Rahmani, N. Rezaei (eds.), *Pediatric Autoimmunity and Transplantation*,
https://doi.org/10.1007/978-3-030-26280-8_42

DOCK8 deficiency is a condition with high morbidity and mortality, and the only curative treatment is HSCT [1, 2]. Our patient was the first born child to his parents, who were first cousins and were both well. He had a younger brother who was asymptomatic.

In spite of extensive family, community and registry searches including cords, a suitably matched donor was not found.

Q2. What is the best management decision at this point?

A. Postpone the HSCT, focus on management of infection and allergies, and repeat periodic donor searches
B. Use an unrelated donor, even if it is not matched. Using a conventional myeloablative conditioning
C. Use a haploidentical donor with graft manipulation

Answer:** The correct answer is **C.

Option A was reasonable many years ago when graft manipulation was not available. In that time, unrelated or haploidentical donor transplants were associated with high risks of severe graft-versus-host disease (GVHD) and graft rejection [3], and these risks favoured a more conservative approach. Advent of new methods for in vivo and in vitro graft manipulation have changed this balance [4, 5].

The first approach was to use a positive selection of only $CD34^+$ hematopoietic stem cells, but this was shown to have poor rates of engraftment in non-SCID PIDs [4]. Later a negative selection of $CD3^+$ T-lymphocytes, ± $CD19^+$ B cells, was adopted, leaving the $CD34^+$ compartment together with other cell types that might enhance engraftment [6]. The rationale behind the latter was that graft $CD3^+$ cells were the main cells responsible for GVHD. The major limitation to this selection was that there was a significantly slower immune reconstitution of the T cell compartment, leaving the patient immunosuppressed for a longer period and thus highly susceptible to viral infections. Subsequently, other approaches have been developed, trying to optimise engraftment and immune reconstitution while decreasing the risk of graft rejection and GVHD. The ultimate choice for anti-GVHD graft preparation, is selective depletion of $TCR\alpha\beta^+$ T cells, which are known to be the major effectors of GVHD, while the remaining $TCR\gamma\delta^+$ T cells, which do not cause GVHD, promote an early immune reconstitution and have anti-viral effects [7–9].

We chose a haploidentical parental (father) donor and administered a conditioning regimen that included anti-GVHD medication, both pre and post-transplant, as it is known than the depletion of $TCR\alpha\beta^+$ T cells is not complete even after the graft manipulation [9]. He had a mild transplant course, and although he had intermittent viral reactivations, these were controlled with antivirals and were not clinically significant. 18 months after transplant, he was engrafted, with full immune reconstitution, no signs of acute or chronic GVHD and off antimicrobial prophylaxis.

Although a mismatched unrelated donor transplant could be used equally with this technique, we recommend the choice of a haploidentical parental donor due to availability, less risk of GVHD and reduced costs [9].

Finally, it is worth mentioning other T lymphocyte depletion approaches have developed and are currently in use, such as post-transplant cyclophosphamide, with the benefit of being less expensive than in vitro depletions [10], enabling specific depletion of alloreactive T cells [4], or naïve T cell depletion [11]. There are additional techniques being studied, such as the addition of "inducible caspase-9 suicide gene modified T cells" as an addback after transplant, which can be switched off if they cause GVHD. These may further improve outcomes for patients particularly those with systemic viral infection [5]. We are reaching the situation where there will be a donor for every patient who needs a HSCT, and the technique used can be individualised depending on the patient situation.

Practical Points

- Hematopoietic stem cell transplantation is still the only curative treatment for many primary immunodeficiencies
- The best time to perform HSCT is before the development of potential comorbidities as they could compromise the outcome of the transplant.
- Nowadays, the lack of a matched donor must not be a limitation, thanks to the availability of new techniques to avoid graft versus host disease, while maximising engraftment and immune reconstitution, an example of which is the $CD3^{+}TCR\alpha\beta^{+}/CD19^{+}$ depletion technique used here

References

1. Su HC, Jing H, Zhang Q. DOCK8 deficiency. Ann N Y Acad Sci. 2011;1246:26–33.
2. Biggs CM, Keles S, Chatila TA. DOCK8 deficiency: insights into pathophysiology, clinical features and management. Clin Immunol. 2017;181:75–82.
3. Gennery AR, Slatter MA, Grandin L, Taupin P, Cant AJ, Veys P, Amrolia PJ, Gaspar HB, Davies EG, Friedrich W, Hoenig M, Notarangelo LD, Mazzolari E, Porta F, Bredius RG, Lankester AC, Wulffraat NM, Seger R, Gungor T, Fasth A, Sedlacek P, Neven B, Blanche S, Fischer A, Cavazzana-Calvo M, Landais P. Transplantation of hematopoietic stem cells and long-term survival for primary immunodeficiencies in Europe: entering a new century, do we do better? J Allergy Clin Immunol. 2010;126(3):602–10.e1–11.
4. Pira GL, Montanari SDCM, Moretta L, Manca F. Specific removal of alloreactive T-cells to prevent GvHD in hemopoietic stem cell transplantation: rationale, strategies and perspectives. Blood Rev. 2016;30:297–307.
5. Slatter M, Gennery A. Approaches to the removal of T-lymphocytes to minimize graft-versus-host disease in patients with primary immunodeficiencies who do not have a matched sibling donor. Curr Opin Allergy Clin Immunol. 2017;17:414–20.
6. Slatter MA, Brigham K, Dickinson AM, Harvey HL, Barge D, Jackson A, Bown N, Flood TJ, Cant AJ, Abinun M, Gennery AR. Long-term immune reconstitution after anti-CD52-treated or anti-CD34-treated hematopoietic stem cell transplantation for severe T-lymphocyte immunodeficiency. J Allergy Clin Immunol. 2008;121(2):361–7.
7. Bertaina A, Merli P, Rutella S, Pagliara D, Bernardo ME, Masetti R, Pende D, Falco M, Handgretinger R, Moretta F, Lucarelli B, Brescia LP, Li Pira G, Testi M, Cancrini C, Kabbara N, Carsetti R, Finocchi A, Moretta A, Moretta L, Locatelli F. HLA-haploidentical stem cell

transplantation after removal of alphabeta+ T and B cells in children with nonmalignant disorders. Blood. 2014;124(5):822–6.
8. Balashov D, Shcherbina A, Maschan M, Trakhtman P, Skvortsova Y, Shelikhova L, Laberko A, Livshits A, Novichkova G, Maschan A. Single-center experience of unrelated and haploidentical stem cell transplantation with TCRalphabeta and CD19 depletion in children with primary immunodeficiency syndromes. Biol Blood Marrow Transplant. 2015;21(11):1955–62.
9. Shah RM, Elfeky R, Nademi Z, Qasim W, Amrolia P, Chiesa R, Rao K, Lucchini G, Silva JMF, Worth A, Barge D, Ryan D, Conn J, Cant AJ, Skinner R, Abd Hamid IJ, Flood T, Abinun M, Hambleton S, Gennery AR, Veys P, Slatter M. T-cell receptor alphabeta(+) and CD19(+) cell-depleted haploidentical and mismatched hematopoietic stem cell transplantation in primary immune deficiency. J Allergy Clin Immunol. 2018;141(4):1417–26.e1.
10. Shah NN, Freeman AF, Su H, Cole K, Parta M, Moutsopoulos NM, Baris S, Karakoc-Aydiner E, Hughes TE, Kong HH, Holland SM, Hickstein DD. Haploidentical related donor hematopoietic stem cell transplantation for dedicator-of-cytokinesis 8 deficiency using post-transplantation cyclophosphamide. Biol Blood Marrow Transplant. 2017;23(6):980–90.
11. Teschner D, Distler E, Wehler D, Frey M, Marandiuc D, Langeveld K, Theobald M, Thomas S, Herr W. Depletion of naive T cells using clinical grade magnetic CD45RA beads: a new approach for GVHD prophylaxis. Bone Marrow Transplant. 2014;49(1):138–44.

Chapter 43
Diarrhea Post-HSCT

Beatriz Morillo-Gutierrez and Mary Slatter

A 13-year-old boy presented in the follow-up clinic post hematopoietic stem cell transplantation (HSCT). He was day +90 post-transplant and his chief complaint was daily abdominal pain with watery diarrhea since 2 weeks ago. He had 4–5 daily episodes of loose stools and some isolated vomiting and nausea. He had lost 4 Kg of weight during this period.

The boy had been diagnosed with *CTLA4* haploinsufficiency during investigations for an autoimmune hemolytic anaemia since the age of 8 years and autoimmune enteropathy since the age of 11 years. Due to the lack of control of intestinal symptoms in spite of several courses of immunosuppressive agents, a HSCT was agreed on and performed 3 months prior to this current visit. He had received a HCST from a 10/10 HLA matched unrelated donor, using peripheral blood stem cells. He underwent conditioning with treosulfan, fludarabine and Alemtuzumab. Neutrophil engraftment occurred on day +15 and donor chimerism was proved to be 93% on day +18 post-transplant.

He is currently under anti-infectious prophylaxis with twice daily penicillin V 250 mg, co-trimoxazole 480 mg daily, IVIG 14 g every 3 weeks and posaconazole. For graft-versus-host disease (GVHD) prophylaxis he was on cyclosporine on a weaning dose (target levels 30–60 μ/L). Finally, according to his pre-transplant intestinal symptoms he was on prednisone on a weaning dose.

B. Morillo-Gutierrez
Translational Paediatrics and Infectious Diseases Unit, Santiago de Compostela University Hospital, Santiago de Compostela, Spain

M. Slatter (✉)
Department of Paediatric Immunology, Great North Children's Hospital, Royal Victoria Infirmary, Newcastle upon Tyne, UK

Institute of Cellular Medicine, Newcastle University, Newcastle upon Tyne, UK
e-mail: mary.slatter@nuth.nhs.uk

© Springer Nature Switzerland AG 2020

F. Rahmani, N. Rezaei (eds.), *Pediatric Autoimmunity and Transplantation*,
https://doi.org/10.1007/978-3-030-26280-8_43

Q1. What is the best initial diagnosis?

A. Infectious enterocolitis
B. Reactivation of autoimmune enteropathy
C. Adverse drug reactions and drug toxicity
D. Intestinal GVHD
E. All of the above

Answer: *The correct answer is **E**.*

Infections are a well-known cause of diarrhea in patients with HSCT [1], especially if full immune reconstitution has not yet been achieved. Reactivation of previous viral infections as well as de novo Cytomegalovirus (CMV) or adenovirus infections are both potentially fatal. Community-acquired infection with parasites, such as *Giardia lamblia* should also be considered.

Acute GVHD (aGVHD), described around 50 years ago [2], is still one of the most frequent and life threatening complications post-HSCT, and should always be suspected with post-transplantation diarrhea, particularly during episodes of immunosuppressant weaning, as in our patient. The skin, liver and gastrointestinal tract are most frequently affected, and the pathophysiology of HSCT is known to be basically due to allo-immune humoral and cellular dysregulation. HLA mismatching is a major risk factor, followed by other donor characteristics, such as age or gender, the pre-transplant state of inflammation and other comorbidities [3]. Prophylaxis with anti-GVHD medications (here Alemtuzumab and cyclosporine) is not enough to prevent GVHD from occurring.

Mucositis or necrotizing enterocolitis are suspected with diarrhea in early days post-transplantation, but are not likely in our patient. Transplant-associated thrombotic microangiopathy (TA-TMA), a widespread vasculitis including mesenteric vessels, is also associated with the use of calcineurin-inhibitors (e.g. cyclosporine).

Our first clinical suspicion was of a recrudescence of his CTLA4 associated autoimmune enteropathy. His new graft was still not fully established 3 months after transplant and some residual intestinal symptoms might be possible [4]. He was therefore given a short course of steroids with no response and was admitted to the hospital for assessment and management.

Q2. Which of the following is not among suitable diagnostic options in this condition?

A. Measure his biochemistry including liver enzymes, complete blood count with peripheral film and lymphocyte subsets
B. Comprehensive viral, bacterial and parasitic investigations particularly in stools
C. Perform invasive investigations, such as endoscopies, with biopsies taken
D. Perform a skin, small and large intestine and liver biopsy and begin conservative management before the results are ready

Answer: *The correct answer is **D**.*

Our management would differ completely from one diagnosis to another i.e. increasing immunosuppression would exacerbate an infection.The diagnosis of aGVHD is based on clinical suspicion, and there are clinical scales which classify the grade and stage (Table 43.1) [3]. A gold standard for diagnosis of intestinal GVHD would require a combination of endoscopies with biopsies [5], and further grading depends on pathological findings.

Our patient did not have rash, jaundice or a palpable liver and his CBC and LFT were normal. His stool output was 2 L/day. He had an endoscopy that showed grade 2/3 aGVHD and positive HHV-6 PCR, although negative in blood. No other infectious agents were found in his stool, blood or biopsies. Skin biopsies are not advisable in this case as there is no rash present.

Other useful investigations are the immunereconstitution parameters, including grade of activation (DR expression) of lymphocytes and lymphocyte steroid sensitivity (LSS) numbers.

Q3. All of the following are among the current treatment options, except:

A. Systemic corticosteroids
B. Extracorporeal photopheresis
C. Mycophenolate mofetil
D. Infliximab
E. Resection surgery

***Answer**: The correct answer is **E**.*

Table 43.1 Staging and grading of acute graft versus host disease

Grading of acute graft versus host disease				
Clinical stage	**Lower GI**	**Upper GI**	**Liver (bilirubin, mg/dL)**	**Skin (% rash of BSA)**
1	Diarrhoea <500 mL/d	Nausea/ vomiting	2–3	<25%
2	Diarrhoea 500–1000 mL/d	–	3–6	25–50%
3	Diarrhoea 1000–1500 mL/d	–	6–15	Generalized erythroderma
4	Diarrhoea >1500 mL/d	–	>15	Bullae/ desquamation
Grading of acute graft versus host disease				
Overall clinical grade	**Lower GI**	**Upper GI**	**Liver**	**Skin**
I	0	0	0	1–2
II	1	1	1	3
III	2–3		2–4	–
IV	4		–	4

BSA body surface area, *d* day, *GI* gastrointestinal tract

Generally, the immunosuppression is given in steps, starting with a combination of steroids and another agent and subsequent re-evaluations with increasing dose or changing agents in case of no improvement. There is no preference of one agent over another as there is a lack of adequate randomised studies comparing them [3, 6]. A course of gancyclovir would also be given to treat his HHV6.

In our patient, with grade III aGVHD, systemic steroids were given at 2 mg/kg/day and infliximab 10 mg/kg weekly. A few weeks later, he had not responded and his stool output even deteriorated. Cyclosporine was switched to tacrolimus, mycophenolate mofetil was added and extracorporeal photopheresis (ECP) was started as he was steroid-refractory which can happen in up to 30% of patients.

Other agents that could have been used are: anti-thymocyte globulin (i.e. ATG), anti-IL-2 receptor, anti-cD5-specific immunotoxin, pan T-cell ricin A-chain immunotoxin, ABXcBL –an anti-CD147 monoclonal antibody-, etarnercept, daclizumab, vilizumab and pentostatin [5].

ECP is a leukoapheresis-based therapy with fewer side effects compared to immunosuppressive agents. It is effective for both aGVHD and chronic GVHD. Cells are activated with ultraviolet A radiation after administration of a photosensitiser and a subsequent increase in anti-inflammatory toxins and donor-specific T regs that suppress the effector T cells responsible for GVHD [7]. Side effects mostly relate to catheter infection and haemodynamic instability during and after the procedure, but no toxicity.

Use of HLA-matched mesenchymal stem cells (MSCs), that have immunoregulatory properties and are hypoimmunogenic, is another option. Commercial MSCs preparations can be given, once the diagnosis of GVHD is established, or as prophylaxis along with the infusion of HSC [6].

Current investigations are focused on the identification of biomarkers (e.g. TNF receptor-1, IL-2 receptor, IL-8 and hepatocyte growth factor, elafine) or genetic polymorphisms that could anticipate increased severity of GVHD and response to specific agents [6]. Finally, it is worth mentioning the expanding field in graft manipulation, which allows removal of cells responsible for GVHD, such as CD3 + TCRαβ+/CD19+ lymphocytes, especially when a full HLA -matched donor is unavailable [8].

Practical Points

- Acute graft-versus host disease (GVHD) is one of most frequent complications after a hematopoietic stem cell transplantation
- Acute GVHD is still a cause of significant morbidity and mortality and effort needs to be made in achieving an accurate diagnosis to guide effective management
- The diagnosis of acute GVHD is mostly clinical
- The backbone of treatment is duction of immunosuppression depending on the staging of GVHD
- Prevention of GVHD is of prime importance with the use of good donor matching or specific graft manipulations and adequate pretransplant conditioning

References

1. Robak K, Zambonelli J, Bilinski J, Basak G. Diarrhea after allogeneic stem cell transplantation: beyond graft-versus-host disease. Eur J Gastroenterol Hepatol. 2017;29:495–502.
2. RE B. The biology of graft-versus-host reactions. Harvey Lect. 1996;62:21–78.
3. Nassereddine S, Rafei H, Elbahesh E, Tabbara I. Acute graft versus host disease: a comprehensive review. Anticancer Res. 2017;37:1547–55.
4. Slatter MA, Engelhardt KR, Burroughs LM, Arkwright PD, Nademi Z, Skoda-Smith S, Hagin D, Kennedy A, Barge D, Flood T, Abinun M, Wynn RF, Gennery AR, Cant AJ, Sansom D, Hambleton S, Torgerson TR. Hematopoietic stem cell transplantation for CTLA4 deficiency. J Allergy Clin Immunol. 2016;138(2):615–619.e611.
5. Cruz-Correa M, Poonawala A, Abraham SC, Wu TT, Zahurak M, Vogelsang G, Kalloo AN, Lee LA. Endoscopic findings predict the histologic diagnosis in gastrointestinal graft-versus-host disease. Endoscopy. 2002;34(10):808–13.
6. Dhir S, Slatter M, Skinner R. Recent advances in the management of graft-versus-host disease. Arch Dis Child. 2014;99:1150–7.
7. Das-Gupta E, Dignan F, Shaw B, Raj K, Malladi R, Gennery A, Bonney D, Taylor P, Scarisbrick J. Extracorporeal photopheresis for treatment of adults and children with acute GVHD: UK consensus statement and review of published literature. Bone Marrow Transplant. 2014;49(10):1251–8.
8. Airoldi I, Bertaina A, Prigione I, Zorzoli A, Pagliara D, Cocco C, Meazza R, Loiacono F, Lucarelli B, Bernardo ME, Barbarito G, Pende D, Moretta A, Pistoia V, Moretta L, Locatelli F. gammadelta T-cell reconstitution after HLA-haploidentical hematopoietic transplantation depleted of TCR-alphabeta+/CD19+ lymphocytes. Blood. 2015;125(15):2349–58.

Chapter 44
Follow-Up of a Severe Combined Immunodeficiency, Who Received Bone-Marrow Transplantation Four Decades Ago

Romina Dieli-Crimi and Teresa Español

A 4-month-old boy was born in 1978 to unrelated Spanish parents [1]. His clinical symptoms began with respiratory tract infections and refractory oral candidiasis with persistent thrush, impetigo, recurrent fever, diarrhea and failure to thrive. Absence of tonsils and no prominent lymph nodes were noted on physical exam. The laboratory tests indicated low counts of both T and B lymphocytes and hypogammaglobulinemia (IgG: 121 mg/dL, IgA: 2.4 mg/dL, IgM: 8 mg/dL). In lymphocyte mitogen stimulation test, lymphocytes failed to respond to mitogens, nominal antigens, or allogenic cells. The patient was diagnosed with severe combined immunodeficiency (SCID) in May 1979 and was referred to the Memorial Sloan Kettering Cancer Center in New York, for treatment.

In December 1980 the patient received a first bone marrow transplantation (BMT) from his haploidentical father. Following the procedure, he developed marked hepatosplenomegaly with mild leukopenia and thrombocytopenia. He had developed systemic *Mycobacterium avium* disease, confirmed on the basis of positive sputum culture and presence of abundant acid fast bacilli in a bone marrow sample. Intensive anti-tuberculous therapy was administered until infection was cleared. Because of the failure of this first graft, in March 1981 the patient received a second BMT again from his father. By May 1981, he became afebrile, with gradual resolution of splenomegaly, while leukocyte and platelet counts normalized and smears and cultures of sputum and bone marrow were negative. The HLA analysis revealed total chimerism indicating successful grafting this time. Unfortunately, ototoxicity from ethambutol hydrochloride led to a partial irreversible hearing impairment. From then on, the patient has developed normally and requires nothing but a hearing aid.

At 35 years of age he was living in Barcelona and sought medical consultation because of recurrent respiratory tract infections. The patient complained also of

R. Dieli-Crimi · T. Español (✉)
Clinical Immunologist, Immunology Unit, Hospital Universitario Vall d'Hebron, Barcelona, Spain

© Springer Nature Switzerland AG 2020

F. Rahmani, N. Rezaei (eds.), *Pediatric Autoimmunity and Transplantation*,
https://doi.org/10.1007/978-3-030-26280-8_44

occasional episodes of diarrhea, in one occasion positive for *Giardia lamblia*, and multiple warts in both hands. A CT scan showed diffuse bronchiectasis and slight splenomegaly with several lymphadenopathies.

Because of the SCID, history of BMT and frequent infections, a complete immunological workup and antibody response to vaccines was requested. IgG levels were 477 mg/dL, mostly corresponding to low IgG2. No response to vaccines (*Haemophilus influenza* and *Streptococcus pneumoniae*) was elicited. A marked reduction in B lymphocytes (2% of total lymphocytes) with a decrease in pre-switch and switched memory B cells (1.4% and 0.5%, respectively), low NK cells and normal T cell numbers were found. HLA genotyping showed a mixed chimerism.

Since the original SCID diagnosis was made when molecular biology tests were not readily available a genetic test was requested and a heterozygous mutation in *IL2RG* gene was detected.

Q1. The current clinical picture of the patient is reminiscent of which clinical entity:

A. Common variable immunodeficiency
B. Isolated B lymphocyte deficiency
C. An isolated T lymphocyte deficiency
D. No actual immunodeficiency

Answer: *The correct answer is* ***A.***

The B cells and antibody response were very low and T cell collaboration defect could not be excluded. From the clinical point of view, the clinical picture resembled a common variable immunodeficiency [2–4].

Q2. The patient would benefit from all of the following strategies, <u>expect</u>:

A. Careful workup for chronic rejection
B. Intravenous immunoglobulin infusion
C. Antibiotic prophylaxis
D. HLA-matching with the next best available donor
E. Suppression of bone marrow reactivation through corticosteroids

Answer: *The correct answer is* ***E.***

As the clinical status of the patient was a humoral immunodeficiency. Intravenous immunoglobulin (IVIG), anti-inflammatories and antibiotic prophylaxis was started. Currently the patient has 1.8% pre-switch memory B cells and 0.5% switch memory B cells, he remains asymptomatic with no infections and with a good quality of life. A new CT-scan showed improvement of his bronchiectasis and a reduction of the lymphadenopathies. This case demonstrates that long-term follow up is required even when grafting is correct because the complete recovery of cellular immunity and humoral function occurs only in 50–60% of patients. Although partial immunity function is sufficient to prevent complications for some time, partial immunodeficiency may develop later in life, perhaps due to the immunosenescence of the raft [5].

Practical Points

- Before the availability of gene therapy, bone marrow transplantation was the only available option for primary immunodeficiency diseases
- This case demonstrates that long-term follow up is required even when grafting is correct because the complete recovery of cellular immunity and humoral function occurs only in 50–60% of patients
- Although partial immunity function is sufficient to prevent complications for some time, partial immunodeficiency may develop later in life, perhaps due to the immunosenescence of the graft

References

1. Reisner Y, Kapoor N, Kirkpatrick D, Pollack MS, Cunningham-Rundles S, Dupont B, Hodes MZ, Good RA, O'Reilly RJ. Transplantation for severe combined immunodeficiency with HLA-A,B,D,DR incompatible parental marrow cells fractionated by soybean agglutinin and sheep red blood cells. Blood. 1983;61(2):341–8.
2. Orange JS, Ballow M, Stiehm ER, Ballas ZK, Chinen J, De La Morena M, Kumararatne D, Harville TO, Hesterberg P, Koleilat M, McGhee S, Perez EE, Raasch J, Scherzer R, Schroeder H, Seroogy C, Huissoon A, Sorensen RU, Katial R. Use and interpretation of diagnostic vaccination in primary immunodeficiency: a working group report of the basic and clinical immunology interest section of the American Academy of Allergy, Asthma & Immunology. J Allergy Clin Immunol. 2012;130(3 Suppl):S1–24.
3. Bonilla FA, Barlan I, Chapel H, Costa-Carvalho BT, Cunningham-Rundles C, de la Morena MT, Espinosa-Rosales FJ, Hammarstrom L, Nonoyama S, Quinti I, Routes JM, Tang ML, Warnatz K. International consensus document (ICON): common variable immunodeficiency disorders. J Allergy Clin Immunol Pract. 2016;4(1):38–59.
4. Ting SS, Tangye SG, Wood J, Ffrench RA, Ziegler JB. Reduced memory B-cell populations in boys with B-cell dysfunction after bone marrow transplantation for X-linked severe combined immunodeficiency. Br J Haematol. 2001;112(4):1004–11.
5. Agarwal S, Busse PJ. Innate and adaptive immunosenescence. Ann Allergy Asthma Immunol. 2010;104(3):183–90. quiz 90–2, 210

Chapter 45
Nonalcoholic Steatohepatitis Referred for Liver Transplantation

Laura Cooling

A 14-year-old white female was seen for consultation of possible liver transplantation. She was diagnosed with end-stage liver disease secondary to non-alcoholic steatohepatitis (NASH) approximately 1 year ago. Other significant recent medical history included a "presumed" diagnosis of refractory idiopathic thrombocytopenia that was treated with prednisone for 2 years with no improvement in platelet counts (platelets ranging 60,000–80,000/μL), hypothyroidism, steroid-associated obesity (BMI: 36.3 kg/m^2), and atopy. Her past surgical history was limited to a laparoscopic cholecystectomy 1 year ago. She has no history of transfusion. Over the last year, she has had significant hepatic decompensation and physical decline with worsening ascites requiring several paracenteses, pruritus, fatigue, and deteriorating renal function. Pre-transplant screening laboratories showed mildly elevated bilirubin (4.1 mg/dL), prolonged PT (15 s, INR: 1.8), hemoglobin of 12 g/dL and moderate thrombocytopenia (platelet count 64,000/μL). Screening was negative for red cell alloantibodies and a direct Coombs test was negative. Serology was negative for anti-platelet antibodies. Serum immunoglobulin studies were abnormal with markedly elevated IgG: 2560 mg/dL, and IgM: 205 mg/dL (reference range: 50–70), but low IgA < 6 mg/dL (reference range: 40–350). Serum protein electrophoresis showed decreases in albumin, α1, α2, and β globulins and a polyclonal increase in γ globulins without β-γ bridging.

Q1. Which pre-transplant laboratory test result suggests a potential risk with blood transfusion during transplant surgery?

A. Hemoglobin
B. Platelet count

L. Cooling (✉)
Department of Pathology, University of Michigan, Ann Arbor, MI, USA
e-mail: lcooling@med.umich.edu

© Springer Nature Switzerland AG 2020

F. Rahmani, N. Rezaei (eds.), *Pediatric Autoimmunity and Transplantation*,
https://doi.org/10.1007/978-3-030-26280-8_45

C. Serum immunoglobulins
D. Type and screen

Answer: *The correct answer is* ***C***.

Serum immunoglobulin showed markedly low IgA levels, suggestive of selective IgA deficiency. Individuals with severe IgA deficiency are at a potential risk for transfusion reactions. The low IgA observed cannot be attributed to chronic liver disease, which is typically characterized by hypergammaglobulinemia with elevations in IgG, IgM and IgA [1]. The low IgA in this cirrhotic patient may also explain the absence of β-γ bridging on serum protein electrophoresis: i.e. IgA is more negatively charged than IgG and IgM and migrates ahead of the γ globulin peak, leading to the β-γ bridging, a pattern classically observed in cirrhosis [2]. Her other laboratories are rather typical and mild for patients with chronic liver disease. Although her low platelets and 2-year history of "presumed" idiopathic thrombocytopenic purpura could present a challenge for platelet support during surgery, it is highly unlikely that the patient actually had ITP. Her moderate, steroid-resistant thrombocytopenia is consistent with cirrhosis due to splenomegaly and low hepatic production of thrombopoietin.

Q2. Which adverse reaction is most likely to occur with blood transfusion in this patient?

A. Acute pulmonary edema
B. Severe allergic reaction
C. Acute hemolysis
D. Acute lung injury

Answer: *The correct answer is* ***B***.

Individuals with severe IgA deficiency (IgA < 0.05 mg/dL) may be at risk for severe allergic reactions, including anaphylaxis, due to the presence of pre-formed circulating IgE anti-IgA antibodies [3]. It is reported that 5–20% of all anaphylactic transfusion reactions are due to severe IgA deficiency [4]. Anti-IgA antibodies are present in approximately one-third of severely IgA deficient patients and might be naturally-occurring or immune-stimulated. Although most IgA antibodies are relatively low titer and clinically benign, high-titer antibodies, IgE antibodies and/or antibodies against specific IgA subclasses (IgA1, IgA2) may increase the risk of allergic reactions [3]. IgA deficiency should always be considered in any patient who has had an anaphylactic reaction following transfusion. Interestingly, in Asians, the most common cause of transfusion-associated anaphylaxis is haptoglobin deficiency (1/500–1/4000 Japanese) [5].

Q3. What is the most appropriate method to confirm the diagnosis and assess the risk for future transfusions?

A. Repeat immunoglobulin test using a nephelometry-based assay
B. Challenge the patient with a platelet transfusion

C. Repeat immunoglobulin testing by a more sensitive ELISA-based method
D. Immunofixation electrophoresis

Answer*: The correct answer is* ***C****.*

Most clinical laboratories measure serum IgA levels by nephelometry, which has a lower limit of 5–7 mg/dL. This method is sufficiently sensitive to screen patients for possible IgA deficiency. When the evaluation is performed in the setting of a prior transfusion-related reaction, the diagnosis of severe IgA deficiency (<0.05 mg/dL) requires testing by more sensitive techniques. In this setting, confirmatory testing should be performed at a laboratory approved by the local blood supplier. Methods used for quantitative IgA and anti-IgA measurement include ELISA, as well as agglutination-based assays using IgA-coated red cells (old method) or IgA-coated particles. Of note, these anti-IgA testing methods do not discern the immunoglobulin isotype (such as agglutination-based methods) or often screen for IgG anti-IgA only (such as ELISA), but not IgE anti-IgA.

Q4. All of the following options are correct regarding blood product support for surgery in this patient, <u>except</u>:

A. Autologous blood donation
B. Washed RBC
C. Washed platelets
D. IgA-deficient plasma

Answer*: The correct answer is* ***A****.*

Autologous blood donation might be an option for a minor, non-urgent, scheduled procedure, however, it is not an option for liver transplant in our patient, due to the volume of blood required and short notice (approximately 12 h prior to surgery) [6]. For this patient, 20 units of IgA-deficient FFP was ordered and held on-site. Because washing shortens the shelf-life for RBC to 24 h, and platelets to 4 h, these were only prepared once the surgery time was confirmed (approximately 8 h notice) [7]. In total, 20 units of washed RBC and 3 units of washed platelets were prepared at time of surgery. If the patient had blood needs exceeding these volumes, she was to receive regular, unmodified blood components since any anti-IgA would be "washed out" by the time [8]. This patient did receive 6 units of standard FFP, 4 units platelets and 6 units RBC in the immediate post-operative period without any recorded reactions.

Practical Points

- Individuals with severe IgA deficiency (IgA < 0.05 mg/dL) are at risk for severe allergic reactions, and anaphylaxis, due to the presence of preformed circulating IgE anti-IgA antibodies
- Up to one fifth of all anaphylactic transfusion reactions are due to severe IgA deficiency

- Testing for severe IgA deficiency and anti-IgA antibodies can be done by ELISA and agglutination-based assays
- Autologous blood donation might be an option for a minor, non-urgent, scheduled procedures in patients with selective IgA deficiency in need of blood products

References

1. Mansberg R, Kronenberg H, Pink JM, Ribiero A, Wylie BR, McCaughan G. Transfusion management of a patient with IGA deficiency and anti-IGA during liver transplantation. Aust NZ J Med. 1994;24(6):728.
2. Orange JS, Ballow M, Stiehm ER, Ballas ZK, Chinen J, De La Morena M, Kumararatne D, Harville TO, Hesterberg P, Koleilat M, McGhee S, Perez EE, Raasch J, Scherzer R, Schroeder H, Seroogy C, Huissoon A, Sorensen RU, Katial R. Use and interpretation of diagnostic vaccination in primary immunodeficiency: a working group report of the basic and clinical immunology interest section of the American Academy of Allergy, Asthma & Immunology. J Allergy Clin Immunol. 2012;130(3. Suppl):S1–24.
3. Vamvakas E. Allergic and anaphylactic reactions. Tranfusion reactions. 4th ed. Bethseda: AABB Press; 2012.
4. Vassallo R. Review: IgA anaphylactic transfusion reactions. Part I. Laboratory diagnosis, incidence and supply of IgA-deficient products. Immunohematology. 2004;20(4):226–33.
5. Shimada E, Tadokoro K, Watanabe Y, Ikeda K, Niihara H, Maeda I, Isa K, Moriya S, Ashida T, Mitsunaga S, Nakajima K, Juji T. Anaphylactic transfusion reactions in haptoglobin-deficient patients with IgE and IgG haptoglobin antibodies. Transfusion. 2002;42(6):766–73.
6. Alkhouri N, Hanouneh IA, Zein NN, Lopez R, Kelly D, Eghtesad B, Fung JJ. Liver transplantation for nonalcoholic steatohepatitis in young patients. Transpl Int. 2016;29(4):418–24.
7. Davenport R, Burnie K, Barr R. Transfusion management of patients with IgA deficiency and anti-IgA during liver transplantation. Vox Sang. 1992;63:247–50.
8. Sandler S. How I manage patients suspected of having an IgA anaphylactic transfusion reaction. Transfusion. 2006;46:10–3.

Chapter 46
Acute Respiratory Distress During Stem Cell Infusion

Laura Cooling

A 16-year-old boy, undergoing a related donor, allogeneic stem cell transplant, developed acute respiratory distress during infusion of umbilical cord stem cells. The patient had been premedicated with 100 mg hydrocortisone and 25 mg diphenhydramine. Prior to infusion, he was afebrile with mildly elevated heart rate (102 bpm) but normal blood pressure and respiratory rate. Within 5 min of starting the infusion, the patient developed facial flushing, coughing, anxiety, and chest tightness. His vital signs at the time of the reaction were: T: 36.7 °C, heart rate: 138 bpm, blood pressure: 158/70 mmHg, and respiratory rate of 24/min with 95% O_2 saturation on 4 L flow nasal cannula. On physical exam, the patient had labored breathing with decreased air movement and wheezing bilaterally. A chest X-ray showed no acute disease. Because of the severity of the reaction, the infusion of the remaining stem cell units was postponed to the following day.

The patient's past medical history was significant for Kostmann's congenital neutropenia, chronic sinusitis, asthma, eczema, seasonal allergies and severe allergic reactions to contrast dye, tape, latex and multiple antibiotics. The patient had no history of blood transfusion prior to transplant. His stem cell donor was his 3-year-old healthy, HLA-matched (10/10 match) brother. The donation consisted of both umbilical cord stem cells and cryopreserved bone marrow harvested 1 month earlier. A blood bank evaluation found no clerical errors, no laboratory evidence of hemolysis and a negative direct antiglobulin test. A review of all donor stem cell products showed that both cord and bone marrow were red-cell-depleted and plasma-depleted prior to cryopreservation. The umbilical cord unit was cryopreserved in 10% DMSO and 10% dextran-40 in a final volume of 30 mL, which was then diluted 1:3 in a solution of 8% dextran-40 and 5% human serum albumin in

L. Cooling (✉)
Department of Pathology, University of Michigan, Ann Arbor, MI, USA
e-mail: lcooling@med.umich.edu

© Springer Nature Switzerland AG 2020

F. Rahmani, N. Rezaei (eds.), *Pediatric Autoimmunity and Transplantation*,
https://doi.org/10.1007/978-3-030-26280-8_46

plasmalyte. Bone marrow was cryopreserved in 10% DMSO and 10% plasma in plasmalyte and frozen in 3 units (100 mL each). The patient was successfully infused with all 3 units of cryopreserved bone marrow without incident the next day.

Q1. Which of the following conditions is least likely to explain the patient's symptoms?

A. DMSO toxicity
B. Severe allergic reaction
C. Transfusion-related acute lung injury
D. Cord cell reaction

Answer*: The correct answer is* ***C****.*

DMSO toxicity, a severe allergic/anaphylactoid reaction and a cord cell reaction are all strong considerations in this patient. Allergic reactions occur in 4–5% of allogeneic stem cell transplants [1]. The clinical presentation and vital signs are consistent with a severe allergic/anaphylactoid reaction, particularly in this patient with a history of asthma and atopy [2, 3]. Classic features of severe allergic transfusion reactions are the absence of fever, presence of tachycardia and flushing and hives predominantly along face and truncal areas. In contrast, TRALI is characterized by acute non-cardiogenic pulmonary edema with bilateral pulmonary infiltrates, hypotension, flushing, and fever/chills [1].

An infusion reaction due to DMSO, inflammatory cytokines, and cellular debris from apoptotic, lyzed granulocytes and red cells -which do not survive cryopreservation- must also be considered. Common toxicities associated with cryopreservation and DMSO include hypertension (22–77% patients), headache and bradycardia due to hyperosmolality of the product, cough (25–39%), chest tightness (3–10%) with decreases in forced vital capacity, fever, nausea and vomiting. Although all cryopreserved cell products are associated with some infusion toxicity, umbilical cord stem cells have a particularly high rate of infusion reactions reaching up to 65%. Hypertension and bradycardia are the most common among infusion reactions, followed by nausea, vomiting, chest tightness, and hypoxia. On occasion, cord cell reactions can be life-threatening, with severe cardiopulmonary toxicity suggestive of takotsubo cardiomyopathy [4]. A review by the National Marrow Donor Program (NDMP) found that many of these severe reactions occurred with older, "red cell-replete" cords i.e. unmanipulated cords that contained large quantities of red cells at the time of freezing.

Q2. What is the next best step in the evaluation of this patient?

A. Evaluate level of quantitative IgA
B. Evaluate level of brain-derived natriuretic peptide
C. Perform HLA antibody screening
D. Perform WBC differential count

Answer*: The correct answer is* ***A****.*

Severe IgA deficiency should be considered in any patient who experiences a severe anaphylactic reaction with blood products, especially in naïve patients with no prior history of transfusion. It is reported that 5–20% of all anaphylactic transfusion reactions are due to severe IgA deficiency (IgA < 0.05 mg/dL). The IgA level in this patient was normal (203 mg/dL).

Q3. What is the most likely culprit agent in the anaphylactic reaction?

A. DMSO
B. Dextran
C. Plasmalyte
D. Plasma

***Answer**: The correct answer is **B**.*

Onset of symptoms with cryopreserved umbilical cord cells, but not cryopreserved bone marrow, strongly suggests dextran, as the culprit agent. Dextran is a standard and unique constituent used in cryopreservation of umbilical cord stem cells. Dextran is not used in cryopreservation of marrow, peripheral blood stem cells or other cellular therapy products [5]. In addition, a dextran solution is recommended when diluting umbilical cord cells at the time of thawing and infusion, the so-called dilutional wash-out method. The estimated rate of dextran sensitivity is 1:2000, with 0.01–0.6% of the population at risk for severe grade III-V anaphylactic reactions to dextran, including coronary vasospasm and takotsubo-type cardiotoxicity. Recently, three episodes of severe cardiopulmonary reactions have been reported with red cell-depleted umbilical cord stem cells, raising concerns that dextran may be the actual culprit underlying severe cord-cell reactions [5].

Q4. All of the following options are appropriate in the immediate management of this patient, except:

A. Hydrocortisone
B. Furosemide
C. Albuterol
D. Diphenydramine
E. Famotidine

***Answer**: The correct answer is **B**.*

The patient has hypoxia and clinical findings consistent with bronchoconstriction. He was treated with an additional 100 mg hydrocortisone, 50 mg diphenhydramine, 20 mg famotidine and albuterol. He had complete resolution of his symptoms and discontinuation of supplemental O_2 within 1 h of the reaction. Because of the small volume infused (~100 mL), umbilical cord stem cell transplants are not at risk for volume overload and diuretics are thus not indicated. In contrast, patients undergoing transplant with fresh bone marrow frequently require diuretics due to large infusion volumes (1–2 L) [6].

Practical Points

- Dextran is a standard and unique constituent used in cryopreservation of umbilical cord stem cells
- About 0.01–0.6% of the population are at risk for severe grade III-V anaphylactic reactions, including coronary vasospasm and takotsubo-type cardiotoxicity

References

1. Cooling L, Gorlin J. Transfusion reactions associated with hematopoietic progenitor cell infusion. Transfusion reactions. Bethseda: AABB Press; 2012.
2. Zinderman CE, Landow L, Wise RP. Anaphylactoid reactions to dextran 40 and 70: reports to the United States Food and Drug Administration, 1969 to 2004. J Vasc Surg. 2006;43(5):1004–9.
3. Cooling L, Sankar A, Mody R, Yanik G, Bonifant C, Choi SW. A severe umbilical cord stem cell infusion reaction due to dextran in an atopic pediatric patient. Bone Marrow Transplant. 2017;52(7):1051–3.
4. Konuma T, Ooi J, Takahashi S, Tomonari A, Tsukada N, Kobayashi T, Sato A, Kato S, Kasahara S, Ebihara Y, Nagamura-Inoue T, Tsuji K, Tojo A, Asano S. Cardiovascular toxicity of cryopreserved cord blood cell infusion. Bone Marrow Transplant. 2008;41(10):861–5.
5. Ma R, Kwan J, Ma D, Fay K. Acute life-threatening cardiovascular toxicity with umbilical cord blood infusion: the role of dextran. Am J Hematol. 2010;85:722–4.
6. Choi S, Hoffmann S, Cooling L. Another case of acute cardiopulmonary toxicity with cord blood infusion: is dextran the culprit? Transfusion. 2012;52:207–8.

Chapter 47
Acute Dyspnea After Platelet Transfusion

Laura Cooling

A 16-year-old black boy developed acute dyspnea, rigors and vomiting 20 min after receiving platelet transfusion. His vital signs showed mild fever (T: 37.5 °C), tachycardia (97–120 bpm), tachypnea (RR: 16–28), hypoxia (O_2 saturation: 82% at room air) and a mild drop in blood pressure (138/70–116/60 mmHg). The patient had no prior history of transfusion and was not premedicated prior to transfusion. He was initially treated with demerol and diphenhydramine with resolution of rigors but worsening of hypoxia.

His recent medical history was significant for acute mononucleosis diagnosed 1 week ago, complicated by idiopathic thrombocytopenia purpura (platelet count 2000/μL) requiring hospital admission for high dose parenteral steroid pulse therapy. On the day of admission, he was transfused with platelets following an episode of blood-tinged emesis. His physical examination showed bilateral cervical lymphadenopathy, bloody nasal and oral mucosa including several bleeding ulcers in the oral and pharyngeal cavities, scattered bruises, and labored breathing with fine bibasilar crackles.

Blood bank evaluation confirmed the patients' blood type (group O, Rh+): there were no clerical errors. Transfused platelets were group O. A direct antiglobulin test (DAT) was negative and serum haptoglobin was within normal range. Urinalysis was positive for blood with 3–5 RBC/hpf. A serum total IgA and brain-natriuretic protein levels were normal. Pre- and post-transfusion CBC showed no change in hemoglobin (14.6 g/dL), or platelet count, but a mild drop in WBC (15,200–10,000/μL). An ABG showed pH: 7.36, PaO_2: 97 mm Hg (100% FiO_2), $PaCO_2$: 43 mm Hg, lactate: 0.9 mmol/L (reference range: 0.5–2 mmol/L). A post-transfusion chest X-ray showed bilateral patchy and nodular opacities, more confluent and widespread in the left lung (Fig. 47.1a). A repeat chest X-ray 3 days later is shown in Fig. 47.1b.

L. Cooling (✉)
Department of Pathology, University of Michigan, Ann Arbor, MI, USA
e-mail: lcooling@med.umich.edu

© Springer Nature Switzerland AG 2020

F. Rahmani, N. Rezaei (eds.), *Pediatric Autoimmunity and Transplantation*,
https://doi.org/10.1007/978-3-030-26280-8_47

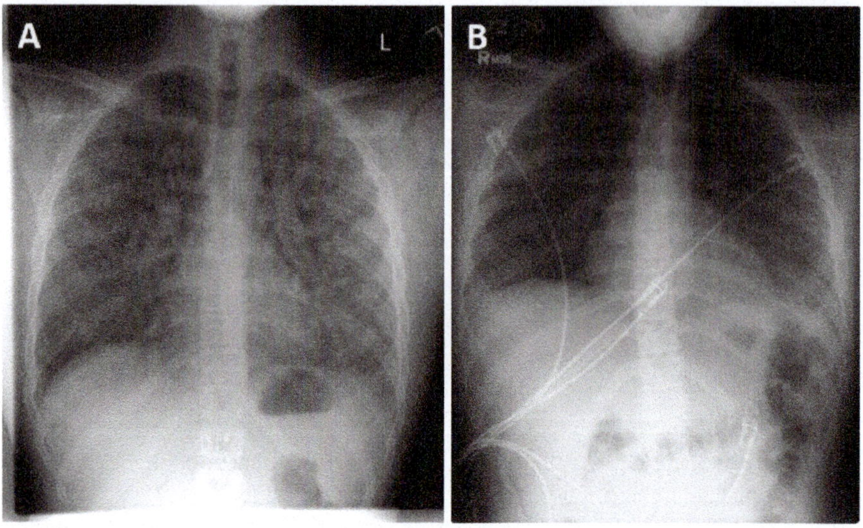

Fig. 47.1 (**a**) Chest x-ray at the time of transfusion reaction, (**b**) and 72 h after transfusion

Q1. What is the most probable diagnosis?

A. Transfusion associated volume overload
B. Transfusion-associated lung injury
C. Septic transfusion reaction
D. Acute hemolytic transfusion reaction
E. Allergic reaction
F. Diffuse alveolar hemorrhage (DAH)

Answer*: The correct answer is* ***B****.*

Although all of the choices listed must be considered in the differential diagnosis for this patient, the presentation, vital signs and immediate post-transfusion laboratories are most consistent with transfusion-associated lung injury (TRALI) [1]. TRALI is defined by the onset of acute, non-cardiogenic pulmonary edema within 6 h of transfusion and the *absence* of pre-existing acute lung injury [2]. Usually, TRALI occurs during or within 1–2 h of transfusion and is typically accompanied by fever, chills/rigors, and decreases in blood pressure or frank hypotension. In some cases, there may be nausea and vomiting. Diagnostic findings are hypoxia (O_2 saturation < 90% in room air), a PaO_2/FiO_2 ratio < 300 mmHg and new bilateral pulmonary infiltrates. A transient post-transfusion decrease in WBC can also be observed in many patients.

Presence of fever, decreased blood pressure and low BNP are against transfusion associated circulatory overload (TACO). Likewise, fever, lack of response to IV antihistamines and normal IgA exclude an anaphylactoid reaction due to IgA deficiency or other allergens. An acute hemolytic transfusion is excluded since: (1) transfused platelets were the same ABO type (group O) as the patient, (2) normal haptoglobin levels, (3) absence of hemoglobinuria (as opposed to hematuria with intact RBC) and (4) stable hemoglobin levels [2]. The latter also argues against significant pulmonary hemorrhage. A septic transfusion reaction must always be considered with platelet transfusions since platelets are stored at room temperature. Septic reactions, however, typically present with fever and chills, accompanied by elevated WBC with left shift.

Q2. All of the following can precipitate this pulmonary reaction in TRALI, except:

A. Anti-HLA class 1 antibodies
B. Anti-HLA class 2 antibodies
C. Anti-granulocyte antibodies
D. Anti-IgA antibodies
E. Bioactive phospholipids

Answer: *The correct answer is* ***D***.

The pathophysiology of TRALI requires an initial priming step, with increased neutrophil adhesion, rigidity and sequestration in the pulmonary microvascular [3]. This priming step is highly dependent on underlying host factors and involves endothelial activation. Blood transfusion elicits a second "hit" with frank neutrophil activation, endothelial damage and interstitial and intra-alveolar edema. Agents in blood that can induce neutrophil and endothelial activation include anti-granulocyte and HLA antibodies [3]. Anti-HLA class 1 antibodies can recognize granulocytes and endothelial cells, leading to cell activation and endothelial damage. Anti-HLA class II antibodies can bind and activate recipient monocytes that yields to the release of proinflammatory cytokines that induce endothelial and neutrophil activation. TRALI can also be precipitated by platelet-activating factor (PAF)-like, lyso-phospholipids generated by oxidation of platelet and red cell membrane phospholipids during storage [4]. These lyso-phospholipids can bind the PAF receptor on neutrophils and activate them. The activation and pulmonary sequestration of neutrophils can lead to a transient (<6 h) decrease in WBC, as was observed in this patient.

Q3. All of additional studies are useful in further evaluation of this patient, except:

A. HLA typing of the platelet donor
B. HLA typing of the patient
C. HLA and granulocyte antibody screen of the platelet donor
D. Crossmatch of patient granulocytes and donor plasma

Answer: *The correct answer is* ***A***.

HLA typing of the donor is not performed, since the primary concern is donor derived, anti-WBC antibodies that are capable of recognizing the patient. Upon notification of a possible TRALI, the blood center will immediately quarantine any products from the donor that are still in inventory and initiate an investigation of the donor, including screening donor plasma for anti-HLA and anti-granulocyte antibodies [5]. If possible, an HLA type of the patient and a crossmatch between patient granulocytes and donor serum may be requested. As part of TRALI risk-reduction strategies, all potential platelet donors with a history of pregnancy or transfusion are now prospectively screened for HLA antibodies. Several countries have also instituted "all male" plasma policies, to further eliminate the risk of TRALI from female donors [4]. As a consequence, the risk for TRALI has decreased from 1:5000 transfusions to 1.8–2 per million RBC and plasma units and 7.3 per million apheresis platelets transfusions.

In this older TRALI case, the donor was a multiparous woman (Gravid 2, Para 2) with high titer, broadly reactive HLA class I (PRA 91%) and class II (PRA 89%) antibodies. No granulocyte-specific antibodies were identified. The granulocyte crossmatch was positive by immunofluorescence and by the granulocyte agglutination assay. Of note, a retrospective review of all donations from this donor identified a prior unreported TRALI in an older female patient, who died within 1 h after being transfused with donor plasma. The donor was permanently deferred from donating any further blood products.

Q4. Which one of the following is indicated in management of this patient's condition?

A. Antihistamine
B. Furosemide
C. High dose steroids
D. Oxygen support

Answer*: The correct answer is* ***D****.*

Patients with TRALI require O_2 supplementation, with up to 72% requiring short-term mechanical ventilation. Symptoms usually resolve within 48–96 h, though pulmonary infiltrates may persist for a week. Surprisingly, high dose steroids have no benefit in TRALI. Because TRALI is a capillary leak syndrome, furosemide or other diuretics should be avoided since they could exacerbate hypotension, which can be unresponsive to fluid resuscitation. Antihistamines are ineffective for TRALI.

Practical Points

- TRALI is defined by the onset of acute, non-cardiogenic pulmonary edema within 6 h, usually the first 1–2 h, of transfusion and the *absence* of pre-existing acute lung injury
- Diagnostic findings are hypoxia (O_2 saturation < 90% in room air), a PaO_2/FiO_2 ratio < 300 mmHg and new bilateral pulmonary infiltrates. A transient post-transfusion decrease in WBC can also be observed in many patients
- With O_2 supplementation, up to 72% of cases of TRALI resolve within 48–96 h
- High dose steroids have no benefit in TRALI

References

1. Kleinman S, Povosky M. TRALI: mechanisms, management and prevention. Bethseda: AABB Press; 2008.
2. Eder A, Dy B, Perez J, Rambaud M, Benjamin R. The residual risk of transfusion-related acute lung injury at the American Red Cross (2008–2011): limitations of a predominantly male-donor plasma mitigation strategy. Transfusion. 2013;53:1442–9.
3. Nagawa M, Toy P. Acute and transient decrease in neutrophil count in transfusion-related acute lung injury: cases at one hospital. Transfusion. 2004;44:1689–94.
4. Stein APDV, Alexander P. Antibody-mediated transfusion-related acute lung injury; from discovery to prevention. Br J Haematol. 2015;170:597–614.
5. Reil A, Keller-Stanislaski B, S SG, Bux JE. Specificities of leucocyte alloantibodies in transfusion-related acute lung injury and results of leucocyte antibody screening of blood donors. Vox Sang. 2008;95:313–7.

Chapter 48
Requiring Immunization After Rescue Autologous HSCT

Darko Richter

Parents of a 6-year-4-months old boy are seeking advice on immunization after rescue hematopoietic stem cell therapy (HSCT) following surgical, radiotherapeutic, chemotherapeutic and myeloablative treatment for his renal clear-cell sarcoma. The boy was well until 3-years and 11-months when he was found to have clear-cell sarcoma of the left kidney with a bone metastasis. Until that age the child had been fully vaccinated in accordance with the local immunization schedule[1]: BCG at birth, a 3-dose primary series of DTaP-IPV-HBV + Hib in infancy, MMR and the first DTaP-IPV-HBV + Hib booster in the second year of life. He also had 3 doses of PCV13. Since he was diagnosed with metastatic left kidney clear-cell sarcoma no further immunizations had been performed since.

At the age of 4-years and 5-months, he underwent leukapheresis with a satisfactory harvest of nucleated peripheral stem cells which were frozen for later autologous transplantation. Eleven months later (age 5-year and 4 months) following an 8-day myeloablative megatherapy he received the rescue autologous peripheral

[1] BCG: Bacillus Calmette Guérin vaccine; DTaP-IPV-HBV + Hib: hexavalent diphteria-tetanus-acellular pertussis-inactivated polio-hepatitis B virus vaccine; DTaP: diphtheria-tetanus acellular pertussis vaccine; DT: diphteria and tetanus toxoids full strength; dT: diphtheria-tetanus toxoids with reduced content of diphtheria; Inf: influenza vaccine; HAV: hepatitis A vaccine; HBV: hepatitis B virus vaccine; Hib: *Haemophilus influenzae* type b vaccine; HPV: human papillomavirus; IPV: inactivated polio vaccine; LAIV: live attenuated influenza vaccine; Men: meningococcal vaccine; MenCV4: 4-valent (A,C,W-135,Y) conjugate meningococcal vaccine; 4CMenB: 4-component meningococcal serogroup B vaccine; MMR: measles-mumps-rubella; OPV: live oral polio vaccine; PCV: pneumococcal conjugate vaccine; RV: rotavirus vaccine; T: tetanus toxoid; Tdpa: tetanus-diphtheria: acellular pertussis with reduced content of diphteria an pertussis antigens; Var: varicella vaccine.

D. Richter (✉)
Pediatric Allergy and Clinical Immunology, University Hospital Center Zagreb, Zagreb, Croatia

Outpatient and Emergency Service, Department of Pediatrics, University Hospital Center Zagreb, Zagreb, Croatia
e-mail: darko.richter@kbc-zagreb.hr

© Springer Nature Switzerland AG 2020

F. Rahmani, N. Rezaei (eds.), *Pediatric Autoimmunity and Transplantation*,
https://doi.org/10.1007/978-3-030-26280-8_48

blood stem cell transplantation (PBSCT). Currently, he is 6 years and 2 months old, 10 months into an uneventful post-HSCT reconstitution and has reached complete remission of his malignant disease. He has been off chemotherapy for the entire course of this period.

The oncologist has suggested that the child now receives a full course of all childhood mandatory vaccines plus pneumococcus, meningococcus and influenza.

Q1. What is your opinion regarding vaccination in this boy?

A. Continue with the second DTaP and IPV booster; add meningococcus and influenza
B. Administer booster D and T vaccines and add meningogoccus and influenza
C. Start all immunizations anew, omitting pertussis; add meningococcus and influenza
D. Boost all previous immunizations, add meningococcus and influenza

Answer: *The correct answer is* ***D.***

The oncologic patient with HSCT should be boosted with the previously received vaccines, adding any potentially missed ones, regardless of the type of transplant, allogeneic or autologous [1]. Although the autologous transplant may, in theory, be considered as being primed by immunizations in the period preceding the illness, this does not appear to be the case and there is insufficient evidence to establish different guidelines for autologous *vs.* allogeneic HSCT [2]. In fact HSCT recipients have a variable, generally significant reduction in protective antibody titers. Up to 95% of HSCT recipients may have protective titers against tetanus, 63% for *Haemophilus influenzae* type b, 60% for measles, 29% for all three types of polioviruses, 11% for meningococcus, and nearly none of the patients receiving HSCT have protective titers for the nine pneumococcal serotypes [3]. It is strongly encouraged that HSCT transplant patients with good engraftment receive the booster for the previously received inactivated childhood vaccines plus seasonal influenza, pneumococcal, meningococcal, and hepatitis A vaccines. Immunization against human papillomavirus is usually recommended.

Inactivated vaccines can generally be given 6 months after HSCT, some even recommend PCV and IPV as soon as 3 months, provided the transplant is engrafted (i.e. no need for red blood cell transfusions, platelets >100,000/μL, total peripheral lymphocyte count >1200/μL), the patient is in remission and off all chemotherapy and immunosuppressants (i.e. for at least 1 month for systemic corticosteroids and up to 6 months after her myeloablative therapy), the last dose of IVIG being infused no sooner than 3 months before, and no intended IVIG infusion for at least the next 1 month following immunization [4, 5].

Our patient has the following laboratory findings: total peripheral lymphocyte count: 1850/μL, $CD4^+$ cell count: 413/μL, IgG level: 4.93 g/L and platelet count: 293,000/μL.

Q2. What immunizations is he qualified to receive at this stage?

A. Inactivated vaccines plus live vaccines
B. Inactivated vaccines only
C. Inactivated vaccines plus MMR
D. Inactivated vaccines plus Var

Answer: *The correct answer is* ***B.***

The child is off anti-cancer therapy for 10 months now (required >6 months), has a satisfactory peripheral lymphocyte count of 1850/μL (required >1200/μL) and marginally sufficient endogenous IgG production of 4.93 g/L (required IgG >5.0 g/L without IVIG).

The immunologic data indicate the capacity to mount an acceptable immune response to inactivated vaccines. With inactivated vaccines, there is no risk of serious or potentially lethal disease due to live vaccine strain. The response, however, may not be optimal [6]. It is suggested to check the specific immune response 1 month following the completion of the full course of immunization [6]. Anti-HBs serology is universally available and a quantitative titer should be obtained. Protective titer should be >10 IU/mL, which often reaches into hundreds. Anti-diphtheria, anti-tetanus and anti-pneumococcal titers can be done in specialized laboratories. Table 48.1 shows the proposed post-transplant schedule of immunizations.

Q3. Which statement is true regarding the possibility for him to receive live-attenuated immunizations?

A. They should not be administered at this stage
B. MMR and Var can be given as soon as there is proof of adequate immune response to inactivated vaccines
C. MMR and Var should be postponed until age 12 years of age
D. MMR only is indicated

Answer: *The correct answer is* ***A.***

HSCT recipients should also be considered for MMR and Var immunizations [8]. Chickenpox will affect an estimated 25% of HSCT recipients and may run a complicated course with visceral involvement. Measles can run a severe course in HSCT recipients as well.

However, immunizing well engrafted HSCT recipients with live vaccines is warranted only when all the requirements minimizing the risk of disseminated disease with the viral strain are met [1–7]:

(a) The time-lag from HSCT should be >24 months,
(b) No GVHD (not applicable in autologous HSCT), and no relapse of cancer,
(c) No immunosuppression for at least 3 months,
(d) Laboratory evidence of sufficient own IgG production (IgG > 5.0 g/L) and T helper count (CD4 > 700/μL),

Table 48.1 Timing and scheduling of post-HSCT immunizations [1, 2, 4, 7]

Level of recommendation	Immunization	Minimum time after HSCT (months)	Schedule (months)[a]	Remark
Strong	DTaP	6	<7 years three-dose series: 0, 2, 4 ≥7 years three-dose series: 0, 2, 4	DTaP not licensed for ≥36 months; however, it is still recommended because low antigen content vaccines may not perform optimally
	Tdpa, DT, dT	6	≥7 years: Tdpa 0 + DT 2 + DT 4/or: Tdpa 0 + dT 2 + dT 4	Low antigen content (except DT). Response may be suboptimal. In line with age specific licensure limitations
	Hib	6	0, 2, 4	
	IPV	3	0, 2, 4	
	HBV	6	0, 2, 4 or 0, 1, 4 or 0, 1, 6, or	
	HAV	6	0, 6	
	Inf	4	<9 years: 2 doses 1 month apart ≥9 years: 1 dose	
	PCV	3	0, 2, 4	PCV13 should be given; PCV10 not licensed ≤5 years
	MenCV4	6	0, 2 or 0, 3	Choice of vaccine depends on regional incidence of meningococcus groups and on age prevalence; both can be given where indicated
	4CMenB		0, 2 or 0, 3	
Medium	HPV	6	9–14 years two-dose series: 0, 6–12; or three-dose series: 0, 2, 6; 15–26 years three-dose series 0, 2, 6	

[a]Temporal spacing of immunization can follow more general rules where not indicated otherwise: not less than 1 month and up to 3 months between 2 same immunizations (e.g. a schedule 0, 2, 4, may in practice be implemented as 0, 3, 6, or 0, 1, 4 etc.); for better immunogenicity longer periods are preferable

(e) Proof of adequate specific immunity following inactivated vaccines should be obtained (see above). Prior to immunization with live vaccines specific serology is warranted, as it may be positive in a number of patients.

(f) In the case of live vaccines, the time since last IVIG should be 8–11 months, or the immunization may fail to induce a good serological response.

The boy does not fulfill criteria (a) and (d), and is not yet initiated on booster inactivated vaccines in order to gain insight into his specific immune response capacity (e).

Other live vaccines are absolutely contraindicated: BCG, LAIV, OPV, RV, oral typhoid vaccine, cholera vaccine, yellow fever and zoster vaccine. LAIV and OPV have inactivated alternatives, RV is contraindicated beyond the age of 24 weeks and is known to be able to cause severe and prolonged intestinal disease in infants with combined immunodeficiency [9], and live zoster vaccine contains several times higher viral titers than Var. Bacterial live vaccines should be equally strictly avoided due to the risk of serious vaccine-induced disease (Table 48.2).

Q4. What can you do if this patient has not yet received MMR and has come in contact with another person with measles?

A. Take urgent blood workup, vaccinate MMR if immunological criteria are met
B. Give measles immunoglobulin
C. Give polyvalent human intravenous immunoglobulin
D. Start MMR vaccination at once

Answer: *The correct answer is* ***C.***

In the case of measles exposure, the patient with HSCT should receive IVIG 0.4 g/kg within the first 48–96 h and no later than the first 6 days. IVIG is in this situation recommended to all HSCT recipients regardless of vaccination status if the time elapsed since HSCT is <12 months, or, if there is any risk of ongoing immunosuppression regardless of time elapsed since HSCT [10]. Measles, and to a certain extent hepatitis A and chickenpox, may be prevented by human normal immunoglobulin (HNIG, a 16% concentrate of polyvalent human immuno-

Table 48.2 Timing and scheduling of post-HSCT live immunizations [1, 2, 4, 7]

Level of recommendation	Immunization	Minimum time after HSCT (months)	Schedule (months)	Remark
Live vaccines generally contraindicated: MMR and Var may conditionally be given	MMR	>24	0, 3	If measles seronegative, no immunosuppression, no GVHD, no cancer relapse; see text for immunological requirements
	Var	>24	0, 3	If varicella seronegative, no immunosuppression, no GVHD, no cancer relapse; see text for immunological requirements

Live post-HSCT immunizations—MMR and Var—should only be done under close surveillance by a competent pediatric immunologist who must carefully evaluate the patient prior to such immunizations

globulin) which is given by IM or SC route. The dose for immunocompromised patients is 0.6 mL/Kg making it a large volume to administer, and therefore preparations that can be given by subcutaneous infusion are preferable [11]. There is no specific anti-measles immunoglobulin, such as the one that exists for varicella.

Patients exposed to chickenpox should receive intramuscular varicella-zoster immunoglobulin (VZIG) ideally within 48–96 h, and at the latest within 10 days of exposure [12]. Dosage varies with weight: 125 units/10 Kg of body weight (maximum dosage 625 units in adult). If VZIG is not available, oral acyclovir or valacyclovir within 48–96 h of exposure should be started (valacyclovir: 20 mg/kg—maximum 1 g 3 times daily for 22 days [12].

HNIG may also have some effect on the prevention of varicella and hepatitis A in case of exposure. Extent of this protection depends on the prevalence of anti-varicella and anti-hepatitis A antibodies in the donor population.

Practical Points

- Patients with successful autologous or allogeneic hematopoietic stem-cell therapy should get booster courses of previous vaccinations
- Additionally, the patient should get inactivated Inf, PCV and Men vaccine
- Inactivated vaccines can generally be started at 6 months post HSCT, provided the child has no immunosuppression for the past 3 months, a lymphocyte count >1200/μL, and endogenous IgG > 500 mg/dL
- Live vaccines are strictly contraindicated. Only MMR and Var can be considered in select well engrafted cases, no sooner than 24 months after HSCT. Requirement is $CD4^+$ count >700/mL, endogenous IgG >500 mg/dL, and adequate serological response to inactivated vaccines, no immunosuppression and no GVHD
- Passive immunoglobulin prophylaxis is established for measles by IVIG and for chickenpox by VZIG
- Chemoprophylaxis with valacyclovir is available for chickenpox, in intramuscular and subcutaneous forms
- The 16% HNIG concentrate can provide passive protection for measles, and to some extent hepatitis A and chickenpox

References

1. Tomblyn M, Chiller T, Einsele H et al. Guidelines for preventing infectious complications among hematopoietic stem cell transplantation recipients: a global perspective. Biol Blood Marrow Transplant. 2009;15(10):1143.
2. Rubin LG, Levin MJ, Ljungman P, Davies EG, Avery R, Tomblyn M, Bousvaros A, Dhanireddy S, Sung L, Keyserling H, Kang I. 2013 IDSA clinical practice guideline for vaccination of the immunocompromised host. Clin Infect Dis. 2014;58(3):309–18.

3. Patel SR, Ortin M, Cohen BJ, Borrow R, Irving D, Sheldon J, Heath PT. Revaccination with measles, tetanus, poliovirus, Haemophilus influenzae type B, meningococcus C, and pneumococcus vaccines in children after hematopoietic stem cell transplantation. Clin Infect Dis. 2007;44(5):625–34.
4. Ljungman P, Engelhard D, de la Camara R, Einsele H, Locasciulli A, Martino R, Ribaud P, Ward K, Cordonnier C. Vaccination of stem cell transplant recipients: recommendations of the infectious diseases working party of the EBMT. Bone Marrow Transplant. 2005;35(8):737–46.
5. Shetty AK, Winter MA. Immunization of children receiving immunosuppressive therapy for cancer or hematopoietic stem cell transplantation. Ochsner J. 2012;12(3):228–43.
6. Richter D, Anca I, Andre FE, Bakir M, Chlibek R, Cizman M, Mangarov A, Meszner Z, Pokorn M, Prymula R, Salman N, Simurka P, Tamm E, Tesovic G, Urbancikova I, Usonis V, Wysocki J, Zavadska D, Central European Vaccination Awareness G. Immunization of high-risk paediatric populations: Central European Vaccination Awareness Group recommendations. Expert Rev Vaccines. 2014;13(6):801–15.
7. Sung L, Heurter H, Zokvic KM, Ford-Jones EL, Weitzman SS, Freeman R, Dupuis LL, Scheifele DW. Practical vaccination guidelines for children with cancer. Paediatr Child Health. 2001;6(6):379–83.
8. Cesaro S, Giacchino M, Fioredda F, Barone A, Battisti L, Bezzio S, Frenos S, De Santis R, Livadiotti S, Marinello S, Zanazzo AG, Caselli D. Guidelines on vaccinations in paediatric haematology and oncology patients. Biomed Res Int. 2014;2014:707691.
9. Patel NC, Hertel MP, Estes MK et al. Vaccine-Acquired Rotavirus in Infants with Severe Combined Immunodeficiency. N Engl J Med 2010; 362:314–9.
10. McLean HQ, Fiebelkorn AP, Temte JL, Wallace GS. Prevention of measles, rubella, congenital rubella syndrome, and mumps, 2013: summary recommendations of the Advisory Committee on Immunization Practices (ACIP). MMWR Recomm Rep. 2013;62(Rr-04):1–34.
11. Centers for Disease Control and Prevention (CDC). FDA approval of an extended period for administering VariZIG for postexposure prophylaxis of varicella. MMWR Morb Mortal Wkly Rep. 2012;61(12):212.
12. Marin M, Guris D, Chaves SS et al. Prevention of varicella: recommendations of the Advisory Committee on Immunization Practices (ACIP). MMWR Recomm Rep. 2007;56:1.

Chapter 49
Fever and Abdominal Pain

Esraa M. Eloseily and Randy Q. Cron

A previously healthy 18-year-old white American female was admitted to the gastroenterology service due to a history of fever for 2 weeks and progressively worsening epigastric pain for 3 days. On examination, she had altered mental status and hepatosplenomegaly. One week after admission, her clinical condition deteriorated and she was transferred to the pediatric intensive care unit. Laboratory findings showed pancytopenia, coagulopathy with elevated D-dimers, liver failure, and inflammation. Lab results are shown in details in the Table 49.1. Work-up for an underlying infectious etiology was negative, including hepatitis A, B and C, HIV-1, Epstein-Barr virus (EBV), cytomegalovirus (CMV), enterovirus, and *Ehrlichia chaffeensis*. She also had undetectable acetaminophen levels.

Q1. Which is the most likely diagnosis?

A. Sepsis
B. Thrombotic thrombocytopenic purpura
C. Malignancy
D. Macrophage activation syndrome
E. Acetaminophen toxicity

Answer: *The correct answer is* ***D.***

E. M. Eloseily
Division of Rheumatology, Department of Pediatrics, University of Alabama at Birmingham, Birmingham, AL, USA

Division of Rheumatology, Department of Pediatrics, Assiut University Children's Hospital, Assiut, Egypt

R. Q. Cron (✉)
Division of Rheumatology, Department of Pediatrics, University of Alabama at Birmingham, Birmingham, AL, USA
e-mail: rcron@peds.uab.edu

© Springer Nature Switzerland AG 2020
F. Rahmani, N. Rezaei (eds.), *Pediatric Autoimmunity and Transplantation*,
https://doi.org/10.1007/978-3-030-26280-8_49

Table 49.1 Laboratory results of an 18-year-old girl with gastric pain

Test	Value	Normal range
White blood cells (WBC)	1720 cells/μL	4500–13,000
Hemoglobin	10.9 mg/dL	12.1–15.3
Platelets	44,000/μL	150–430
Prothrombin time	20.7 s	≤15.2
Partial thromboplastin time	59.2 s	≤36.0
D-dimers	7639 ng/mL	≤240
Fibrinogen	139 mg/dL	164–458
Albumin	2.7 mg/dL	≥3.7
Aspartate aminotransferase (AST)	3487 IU/L	≥30
Alanine aminotransferase (ALT)	523 IU/L	≥35
Aldolase	61.8 U/L	<8.1
Triglycerides	201 mg/dL	≤140
C-reactive protein (CRP)	5.96 mg/dL	≤1.00
Serum ferritin	8446 ng/mL	≤115
ESR	15 mm/h	0–10

Macrophage activation syndrome (MAS), or secondary hemophagocytic lymphohistiocytosis (HLH), has been more commonly diagnosed over the past 30 years, and awareness among physicians is increasing though not yet to the appropriate level. MAS is a life threatening cytokine storm syndrome that is usually diagnosed among febrile hospitalized patients. It presents commonly with unremitting fever and a shock-like multi-organ dysfunction syndrome. Laboratory studies show pancytopenia, elevated liver enzymes, elevated ferritin, and triglycerides, among others [1]. The presented patient had the following laboratory results: soluble CD25: 4171 IU/mL (reference range (<1105), and soluble CD163: 1718 IU/mL (reference range < 1378). She had normal NK cell numbers but absent NK cell function (2% lysis at the 50:1 effector to target cell ratio).

Q2. What is the most common pediatric rheumatologic disease accompanied by MAS?

A. Systemic lupus erythematosus
B. Systemic juvenile idiopathic arthritis
C. Sjogren syndrome
D. Juvenile dermatomyositis
E. Juvenile scleroderma

Answer: *The correct answer is* ***B.***

Secondary HLH is known to be associated with various rheumatologic diseases, where it is often referred to as macrophage activation syndrome or MAS. MAS can be the initial presentation of the disease, or it may be triggered by an infection or a flare of the underlying disease process [2, 3]. Systemic juvenile idiopathic arthritis (SJIA) is the most common of the pediatric rheumatologic diseases that is complicated by MAS (50.2%), followed by systemic lupus erythematosus (22.3%), and Kawasaki disease (5.9%) [2]. MAS develops in about 10% of patients with SJIA [4], though subclinical MAS has been suggested to be far more common (~30–40%) [5]. Mortality of MAS-SJIA reaches 8–22% [5–7].

Q3. According to the HLH-2004 criteria, which of the following criteria is considered enough to make a diagnosis of HLH alone?

A. Serum ferritin >500 ng/ml
B. Two lineage cytopenia
C. Soluble CD25 ≥ 2400 IU/mL
D. Hemophgocytosis in bone marrow, spleen, or lymph nodes
E. Molecular diagnosis

Answer: *The correct answer is* ***E.***

HLH is a clinical diagnosis, and several criteria have been proposed over the years. According to HLH-2004 diagnostic guidelines [8], the diagnosis of HLH can be established in the presence of a molecular diagnosis consistent with HLH, or by fulfilment of five out of eight of the following criteria:

- Fever
- Splenomegaly
- Cytopenia in at least 2 of 3 lineages i.e. hemoglobin below 9 g/dl, platelets below 100,000 per microliter and neutrophils below 1000 per microliter
- Elevated plasma triglyceride and/or low serum fibrinogen levels (triglyceride should be equal or above 265 mg/dl and fibrinogen equal or below ≤1.5 mg/L to fulfil this option
- Hemophagocytosis detected by bone marrow biopsy/aspiration, lymph node or spleen with no evidence suggesting malignancy
- Low to absent natural killer cell activity
- Serum ferritin equal or above 500 ng/mL
- Soluble IL-2 receptor (CD25) equal or above 2400 IU/mL

The presented patient satisfied criteria for HLH with seven of eight features. HLH gene testing was negative for coding mutations in *UNC13D, PRF1, STX11*, and *STXBP2*, but she was found to have a single copy missense mutation in *RAB27A,* which is a known cause of Griscelli type 2, an established cause of familial HLH when present as a homozygous or compound heterozygous mutation [9].

Of note, bone marrow hemophagocytosis is not essential for the diagnosis of HLH since it might be absent, especially early on in the disease course [6, 7, 10]. Moreover, HLH patients are usually critically ill and might not be fit for bone marrow biopsy. Waiting for evidence of hemophagocytosis to make the diagnosis of HLH might lead to a delay in diagnosis and institution of appropriate therapy, which can have dire consequences.

Q4. Mutations associated with familial HLH are thought to cause a defect in which of the following functions of the immune system?

A. Phagocytosis by macrophages and neutrophils
B. Antibody production by B lymphocytes
C. Cytolytic abilities of natural killer cells and CD8+ T lymphocytes
D. MHC II presentation on antigen presenting cells in the bone-marrow

Answer: *The correct answer is* ***C.***

Familial HLH is associated with biallelic defects in gene products involved in the perforin-mediated cytolytic pathway used by NK cells and CD8+ T lymphocytes [11, 12]. Inability to clear the antigenic stimulus and thus turn off the inflammatory response results in hypercytokinemia [13]. Single-copy mutations in these "perforin pathway genes"are been shown to have hypomorphic or dominant negative phenotypes in familial forms of HLH [14–16], and even contribute to sporadic HLH/MAS in older children and adults [16, 17]. On the other hand, a state of inflammation with elevated IL-6 may also reduce the lytic capacity of NK cells and CD8+ T cells [18–20]. MAS and secondary HLH often result from a combination of genetic predisposition, a hyperinflammatory state reducing cytolytic function (e.g., cancer, autoimmunity, and autoinflammation), and an infectious trigger [21–23].

Q5. What is the most common infectious agent associated with HLH?

A. HIV
B. EBV
C. Tuberculosis
D. Ehrlichia
E. Hepatitis A

Answer: *The correct answer is* ***B.***

Epstein-Barr virus is the most commonly reported infectious trigger of HLH [24], with the highest incidence in East Asia [25]. In addition to the traditional treatments for HLH, such as immunosuppressive chemotherapy and hematopoietic stem-cell transplantation, Balamuth et al. [26], reported that adding rituximab to the HLH-2004 treatment protocol improves its efficacy in patients with EBV-HLH. Rituximab is a monoclonal antibody against CD20 on the surface of B cells. As EBV targets B cells in the initial phase of the disease, rituximab's depletion of B cells is thought to inhibit the extent of the infection. In addition, B cells may be a target in EBV-HLH, and rituximab may reduce morbidity and mortality by reducing the circulating B cell population and EBV load [27].

Q6. What is the best initial treatment in this patient?

A. Vancomycin + ceftriaxone + IL-6 inhibitors
B. Emergency Hematopoetic stem-cell transplantation
C. Corticosteroids + cyclosporin A + IL-1 inhibition

D. Etoposide monotherapy
E. Rituximab followed corticosteriods and stem cell transplantation

Answer: *The correct answer is* ***C.***

Different treatment options are now available for HLH/MAS, including etoposide-based regimens such as HLH-94 and HLH-2004 [8]. However, etoposide-based regimens have significant mortality rates during pre- and post-BMT periods [28], and are more commonly reserved for familial forms of HLH. Cytokine targeted biologic therapies have provided a less toxic but effective option for the non-familial or secondary forms of HLH or MAS. Anakinra, a recombinant IL-1 receptor antagonist, has been reported to be efficacious and safe, and is often combined with high dose corticosteroids +/− cyclosporine A [29–32].

The patient presented above was started on high dose intravenous methylprednisolone, cyclosporine A, and the recombinant human interleukin-1 receptor antagonist, anakinra. Her clinical condition and laboratory features dramatically improved, and she was discharged home after 6 days in the hospital. Within 2 weeks of leaving the hospital, she developed bilateral symptomatic chronic anterior uveitis. She later developed HLA-B27–negative spondyloarthritis, and is one of 2 secondary HLH cases reported to run a similar disease course [33].

Practical Points

- Macrophage activation syndrome (MAS), or secondary hemophagocytic lymphohistiocytosis (HLH), is a life-threatening condition
- MAS is usually diagnosed in febrile intensive care unit patients
- MAS can mimic septic shock, systemic inflammatory response syndrome (SIRS), or multi-organ dysfunction syndrome (MODS)
- Timely diagnosis and early treatment are crucial to improve survival
- Serum ferritin is usually highly elevated and will assist in recognizing secondary HLH/MAS in critically ill febrile patients
- Bone marrow hemophagocytosis, while common, is not an essential feature for diagnosis, and its frequently presumed requirement should not cause delay in starting appropriate treatment
- IL-1 inhibition with anakinra has been reported to be safe and efficacious in non-malignancy forms of secondary HLH and MAS

References

1. Grom AA, Mellins ED. Macrophage activation syndrome: advances towards understanding pathogenesis. Curr Opin Rheumatol. 2010;22(5):561–6.
2. Atteritano M, David A, Bagnato G, Beninati C, Frisina A, Iaria C, Cascio A. Haemophagocytic syndrome in rheumatic patients. A systematic review. Eur Rev Med Pharmacol Sci. 2012;16(10):1414–24.

3. Wong K-F, Hui P-K, Chan JK, Chan Y-W, Ha S-Y. The acute lupus hemophagocytic syndrome. Ann Intern Med. 1991;114(5):387–90.
4. Voskoboinik I, Sutton VR, Ciccone A, House CM, Chia J, Darcy PK, Yagita H, Trapani JA. Perforin activity and immune homeostasis: the common A91V polymorphism in perforin results in both presynaptic and postsynaptic defects in function. Blood. 2007;110(4):1184–90.
5. Behrens EM, Beukelman T, Paessler M, Cron RQ. Occult macrophage activation syndrome in patients with systemic juvenile idiopathic arthritis. J Rheumatol. 2007;34(5):1133–8.
6. Sawhney S, Woo P, Murray K. Macrophage activation syndrome: a potentially fatal complication of rheumatic disorders. Arch Dis Child. 2001;85(5):421–6.
7. Stephan J, Koné-Paut I, Galambrun C, Mouy R, Bader-Meunier B, Prieur AM. Reactive haemophagocytic syndrome in children with inflammatory disorders. A retrospective study of 24 patients. Rheumatology. 2001;40(11):1285–92.
8. Henter JI, Horne A, Arico M, Egeler RM, Filipovich AH, Imashuku S, Ladisch S, McClain K, Webb D, Winiarski J, Janka G. HLH-2004: diagnostic and therapeutic guidelines for hemophagocytic lymphohistiocytosis. Pediatr Blood Cancer. 2007;48(2):124–31.
9. Zur Stadt U, Beutel K, Kolberg S, Schneppenheim R, Kabisch H, Janka G, Hennies HC. Mutation spectrum in children with primary hemophagocytic lymphohistiocytosis: molecular and functional analyses of PRF1, UNC13D, STX11, and RAB27A. Hum Mutat. 2006;27(1):62–8.
10. Ravelli A. Macrophage activation syndrome. Curr Opin Rheumatol. 2002;14(5):548–52.
11. Jenkins MR, Rudd-Schmidt JA, Lopez JA, Ramsbottom KM, Mannering SI, Andrews DM, Voskoboinik I, Trapani JA. Failed CTL/NK cell killing and cytokine hypersecretion are directly linked through prolonged synapse time. J Exp Med. 2015;212(3):307–17.
12. Janka G. Hemophagocytic lymphohistiocytosis: when the immune system runs amok. Klin Padiatr. 2009;221(05):278–85.
13. Grom AA. Natural killer cell dysfunction: a common pathway in systemic-onset juvenile rheumatoid arthritis, macrophage activation syndrome, and hemophagocytic lymphohistiocytosis? Arthritis Rheum. 2004;50(3):689–98.
14. Saltzman RW, Monaco-Shawver L, Zhang K, Sullivan KE, Filipovich AH, Orange JS. Novel mutation in syntaxin-binding protein 2 (STXBP2) prevents IL-2-induced natural killer cell cytotoxicity. J Allergy Clin Immunol. 2012;129(6):1666.
15. Spessott WA, Sanmillan ML, McCormick ME, Patel N, Villanueva J, Zhang K, Nichols KE, Giraudo CG. Hemophagocytic lymphohistiocytosis caused by dominant-negative mutations in STXBP2 that inhibit SNARE-mediated membrane fusion. Blood. 2015;125(10):1566–77.
16. Zhang M, Bracaglia C, Prencipe G, Bemrich-Stolz CJ, Beukelman T, Dimmitt RA, Chatham WW, Zhang K, Li H, Walter MR, De Benedetti F, Grom AA, Cron RQ. A Heterozygous RAB27A mutation associated with delayed cytolytic granule polarization and hemophagocytic lymphohistiocytosis. J Immunol. 2016;196:2492–503.
17. Zhang X-Y, Ye X-W, Feng D-X, Han J, Li D, Zhang C. Hemophagocytic lymphohistiocytosis induced by severe pandemic influenza A (H1N1) 2009 virus infection: a case report. Case Rep Med. 2011;2011:951910.
18. Sullivan KE, Delaat CA, Douglas SD, Filipovich AH. Defective natural killer cell function in patients with hemophagocytic lymphohistiocytosis and in first degree relatives. Pediatr Res. 1998;44(4):465–8.
19. Villanueva J, Lee S, Giannini EH, Graham TB, Passo MH, Filipovich A, Grom AA. Natural killer cell dysfunction is a distinguishing feature of systemic onset juvenile rheumatoid arthritis and macrophage activation syndrome. Arthritis Res Ther. 2004;7(1):1.
20. Caiello I, Minnone G, Holzinger D, Vogl T, Prencipe G, Manzo A, De Benedetti F, Strippoli R. IL-6 amplifies TLR mediated cytokine and chemokine production: implications for the pathogenesis of rheumatic inflammatory diseases. PLoS One. 2014;9(10):e107886.
21. Zhang M, Behrens EM, Atkinson TP, Shakoory B, Grom AA, Cron RQ. Genetic defects in cytolysis in macrophage activation syndrome. Curr Rheumatol Rep. 2014;16(9):439.

22. Schulert GS, Grom AA. Macrophage activation syndrome and cytokine-directed therapies. Best Pract Res Clin Rheumatol. 2014;28(2):277–92.
23. Weaver LK, Behrens EM. Hyperinflammation, rather than hemophagocytosis, is the common link between macrophage activation syndrome and hemophagocytic lymphohistiocytosis. Curr Opin Rheumatol. 2014;26(5):562.
24. Chen C, Huang Y, Jaing T, Hung I, Yang C, Chang L, Lin T. Hemophagocytic syndrome: a review of 18 pediatric cases. J Microbiol Immunol Infect. 2004;37(3):157.
25. Elazary AS, Wolf DG, Amir G, Avni B, Rund D, Yehuda DB, Sviri S. Severe Epstein–Barr virus-associated hemophagocytic syndrome in six adult patients. J Clin Virol. 2007;40(2):156–9.
26. Balamuth NJ, Nichols KE, Paessler M, Teachey DT. Use of rituximab in conjunction with immunosuppressive chemotherapy as a novel therapy for Epstein Barr virus-associated hemophagocytic lymphohistiocytosis. J Pediatr Hematol Oncol. 2007;29(8):569–73.
27. Milone MC, Tsai DE, Hodinka RL, Silverman LB, Malbran A, Wasik MA, Nichols KE. Treatment of primary Epstein-Barr virus infection in patients with X-linked lymphoproliferative disease using B-cell–directed therapy. Blood. 2005;105(3):994–6.
28. Henter J-I, Samuelsson-Horne A, Arico M, Egeler RM, Elinder G, Filipovich AH, Gadner H, Imashuku S, Komp D, Ladisch S. Treatment of hemophagocytic lymphohistiocytosis with HLH-94 immunochemotherapy and bone marrow transplantation. Blood. 2002;100(7):2367–73.
29. Bruck N, Suttorp M, Kabus M, Heubner G, Gahr M, Pessler F. Rapid and sustained remission of systemic juvenile idiopathic arthritis-associated macrophage activation syndrome through treatment with anakinra and corticosteroids. J Clin Rheumatol. 2011;17(1):23–7.
30. Kelly A, Ramanan AV. A case of macrophage activation syndrome successfully treated with anakinra. Nat Clin Pract Rheumatol. 2008;4(11):615–20.
31. Nigrovic PA, Mannion M, Prince FH, Zeft A, Rabinovich CE, Van Rossum MA, Cortis E, Pardeo M, Miettunen PM, Janow G. Anakinra as first-line disease-modifying therapy in systemic juvenile idiopathic arthritis: report of forty-six patients from an international multicenter series. Arthritis Rheum. 2011;63(2):545–55.
32. Record JL, Beukelman T, Cron RQ. Combination therapy of abatacept and anakinra in children with refractory systemic juvenile idiopathic arthritis: a retrospective case series. J Rheumatol. 2011;38(1):180–1.
33. Cron RQ, Chatham WW. Development of spondyloarthropathy following episodes of macrophage activation syndrome in children with heterozygous mutations in haemophagocytic lymphohistiocytosis-associated genes. Clin Exp Rheumatol. 2016;34(5):953.

Chapter 50
Prolonged Fever, Rash and Mucosal Bleeding

Beata Derfalvi

A 2-year-old, previously healthy girl was admitted to ICU from the pediatric inpatient ward with a 17-day history of high, non-remitting fever (>39 °C), mucosal bleeding and neurological disturbances including lethargy and irritability. There was no history of prior infections, but her parents noticed that she refused to stand on weight-bearing joints.

On physical exam she had hepatosplenomegaly, lymphadenopathy, petechiae and macular erythematous rash. Laboratory investigations revealed hyperinflammation, three lineage cytopenia, hepatic dysfunction and consumption coagulopathy (Table 50.1). Bacterial and viral throat swabs were negative. Extended investigations for fever of unknown origin (blood, CSF and urine cultures) were negative for bacteria and fungi, as were Epstein-Barr virus (EBV), herpes, cytomegalovirus, and adenovirus PCR in blood. Echocardiography did not show pericarditis or coronary artery dilatation. An initial unremarkable joint exam progressed into arthritis with palpable synovial effusion in knees, ankles and wrists on day 31 since the fever began.

Q1. What is the least likely cause of her symptoms?

A. Lymphoma
B. Systemic juvenile idiopathic arthritis
C. Sepsis
D. Hemophagocytic lymphohistiocytosis

Answer: *The correct answer is* ***C.***

All culture results came back as negative, making sepsis unlikely. Lymphoma is an important differential diagnosis, especially if excessive cytopenia is present.

B. Derfalvi (✉)
Department of Pediatrics, Dalhousie University/IWK Health Centre, Halifax, NS, Canada
e-mail: Beata.Derfalvi@iwk.nshealth.ca

© Springer Nature Switzerland AG 2020

F. Rahmani, N. Rezaei (eds.), *Pediatric Autoimmunity and Transplantation*,
https://doi.org/10.1007/978-3-030-26280-8_50

Table 50.1 Abnormal laboratory results in a 2-year-old girl with prolonged fever

	Patient results	Normal range
Inflammatory parameters	ESR 45 mm/h	1–9 mm/h
	CRP 356 mg/L	0–5.0 mg/L
	ferritin 6,100 ng/mL	12–140 ng/mL
CBC	Hb 9.2 g/dL	102–127 g/dL
	WBC 2,200/μL	4,860–13,180/μL
	ANC 1,200 μ/L	1,600–8,290/μL
	Platelets 14,000 μ/L	189,000–394,000/μL
Liver function tests	AST 248 IU/L	20–60 U/L
	ALT 70 IU/L	5–45 U/L
	γGT 645 IU/L	0–40 U/L
	Total bilirubin 28 μmol/L	0–17 μmol/L
Coagulation parameters	Fibrinogen 76 mg/dL	82–383 mg/dL
	D-dimer >4000 μg/L	<500 μg/L
	INR 1.47	0.88–1.12
Others	Sodium 130 mmol/L	133–148 mmol/L
	Albumin 31 g/L	36–49 g/L
	LDH 3598 IU/L	470–920 IU/L
	TG 4.4 mmol/L	0.24–1.7 mmol/L

γGT gamma glutamyl transferase, *LDH* lactate dehydrogenase, *TG* triglyceride, *ANC* absolute neutrophil count

Bone marrow biopsy is a helpful tool to rule out this diagnosis and there was no evidence of malignancy in our case.

The International League of Associations for Rheumatology (ILAR) classification criteria for systemic juvenile rheumatoid arthritis (SJIA) include fever of at least 2 weeks duration, daily for at least 3 days, and arthritis in at least 1 joint, and at least one of the following: evanescent, i.e. non-fixed, erythematous rash, generalized lymph node enlargement, hepatomegaly and/or splenomegaly and serositis, mainly as pericarditis [1]. A subgroup of SJIA patients present with rather unspecific signs and symptoms initially, with the hallmark fever of unknown origin, but without chronic arthritis, which accounts for the challenging diagnosis. In our case, the rash and arthralgia that evolved to polyarthritis confirmed the diagnosis of SJIA, and the non-remitting, rather than spiking, fever, the encephalopathy, as well as the cytopenias and coagulopathy in laboratory results signaled macrophage activation syndrome (MAS). MAS is considered an acquired or secondary hemophagocytic lymphohistiocytosis (HLH) disorder and has been reported to occur in the context of various rheumatological diseases, such as in our case. MAS presents at onset in up to 22% of patients and in up to 50% in subclinical forms of SJIA, and is considered to be a serious complication with 8–20% mortality risk [2]. Other conditions triggering MAS were unlikely in our patient, since bone marrow biopsy ruled out malignancy, she had no clinical symptoms of an infection, and PCR results confirmed the absence of any herpes virus and adenovirus load in blood.

It is very difficult to distinguish SJIA/MAS from primary HLH, especially in a very young child, since there is great phenotypic similarity. HLH and MAS share common pathogenesis, with uncontrolled activation and hyper-responsiveness of the monocyte/macrophage system, including excessive IL-1β production, suggestive of an autoinflammatory disease, rather than an autoimmune disease.

Q2. All of the laboratory investigation would support the ultimate diagnosis of MAS/HLH in this case, except:

A. Highly increased soluble IL-2 receptor alpha (sIL-2Rα) level
B. Extremely increased ferritin level
C. Increased triglyceride level
D. Increasing erythrocyte sedimentation rate

Answer: *The correct answer is* ***D.***

Paradoxically, an initially high ESR that then drops, despite increasing inflammation, especially with rising ferritin and CRP, is characteristic of MAS/HLH and thought to be secondary to decreasing fibrinogen levels. Decreasing serum fibrinogen results from intravascular coagulopathy, fibrinogen consumption and liver dysfunction [3]. MAS/HLH is defined as an acute episode of overwhelming inflammation, and is characterized by activation and expansion of T lymphocytes and hemophagocytic macrophages and thus secretion of large amounts of inflammatory cytokines, leading to a severe hyperinflammatory state and multiorgan damage [2]. In our case a high sIL-2Rα (or sCD25) level of 5,600 reflects excessive T cell activation. Elevated triglyceride level, due to lipoprotein lipase inhibition by cytokines, and highly elevated serum ferritin level fit well the HLH-2004 diagnostic guideline [4] and also meet validated criteria for MAS in SJIA [5] (Table 50.2).

Q3. Which investigation is most helpful to distinguish between secondary MAS or primary HLH?

A. Detecting hemophagocytosis on bone marrow aspirates, lymph node biopsy, CSF spin or liver biopsy
B. Measurement of soluble CD163 levels in serum

Table 50.2 Diagnosis of macrophage activation syndrome in systemic juvenile idiopathic arthritis (SJA)[a]

A febrile patient with known SJIA and serum ferritin >684 ng/mL	+ any 2 of:	PLT ≤181,000 μ/L
		AST >48 IU/L
		TG >156 mg/dL (1.76 mmol/L)
		Fibrinogen ≤360 mg/dL

PLT platelet, *AST* aspartate aminotransferase, *TG* triglyceride
[a]Based on 2016 EULAR/ACR/PRINTO criteria [5]

C. Next generation sequencing of primary HLH genes (*PRF1*, *UNC13D*, *STXBP2*, *RAB27A*, *STX11*, *SH2D1A*, or *XIAP*)
D. Measurement of NK cell killing potential of FK562 erythroleukemia target cells

Answer: *The correct answer is* ***C.***

Hemophagocytosis is characteristic in both conditions, but is not always present (Fig. 50.1).

Soluble CD163, a scavenger receptor and a marker for alternatively activated macrophages and hemophagocytosis, is markedly elevated both in MAS as well as in HLH. Presence of biallelic pathogenic variants of the above mentioned genes is the most reliable indicator of primary HLH.

Primary or familiar HLH (FHLH) is a genetic disease resulting from recessively inherited defects in the cytolytic pathway, affecting perforin synthesis as well as intracellular vesicular trafficking, and resulting in failure of killing function of NK and cytotoxic T cells. Additionally, primary defects of immune dysregulation, such as oculocutaneous albinisms (Griscelli syndrome type2, Chediak-Higashi syndrome, Hermansky-Pudlak syndrome 2) and EBV-associated lymphoproliferation (X-linked lymphoproliferation), present also with hyperinflammation due to reduced cytotoxic T cell/NK cell degranulation and activity (Table 50.3) [6–8].

The diagnostic immune tests for primary HLH include: detection of perforin in NK, $CD8^+$ cytotoxic T and NK T cells by flow cytometry, assessment of NK cell function by a chromium-release assay measuring target cell killing, and measurement of intracellular vesicular trafficking by the CD107a mobilization assay by flow cytometry.

Interestingly, hypomorphic or heterozygous protein-altering variants of HLH-associated genes (*PRF1*, *UNC13D*, *LYST*, *RAB27* and *STXBP2*), as well as reduced NK cell cytotoxic function have been reported in up to one third of the SJIA patients presenting with MAS, prompting the question whether HLH and MAS are two distinct conditions or a single disease continuum [9–11].

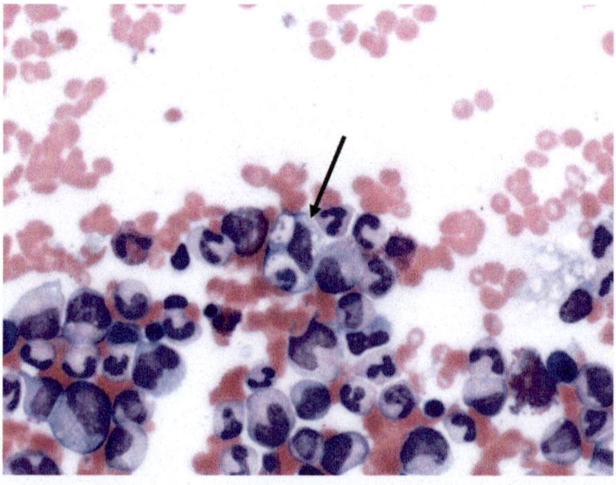

Fig. 50.1 H&E staining of bone marrow biopsy of the patient. The arrow shows hemophagocytosis

Table 50.3 Hereditary causes of HLH

Primary immunodeficiency category	Disease	Involved *Gene*/protein	Cytolytic pathway defect, findings on flow cytometry, distinctive clinical features	
Primary or familiar HLH (FHLH)	FHL2	*PRF1*/Perforin	Pore-forming perforin protein expression low or absent, normal NK degranulation.	
	FHL3	*UNC13D*/MUNC13–4	Defective vesicle priming, NK degranulation	
	FHL4	*STX11*/Syntaxin11	Defective vesicle transport and fusion, NK degranulation	
	FHL5	*STXBP2*/MUNC18–2	Defective vesicle transport and fusion, NK degranulation	
Diseases of immune dysregulation	Griscelli syndrome 2	*RAB27A*	Defective vesicle docking, NK degranulation	Hypopigmentation
	Chediak–Higashi syndrome	*LYST*	Defective vesicle transport, NK degranulation	
	Hermansky–Pudlak syndrome 2	*AP3B1*	Defective NK degranulation	
	XLP1	*SH2D1A*/SAP	SAP expression low or absent. Reduced number of NKT cells. Defective signal transduction and activation of lymphocytes.	EBV associated lymphoproliferation
	XIAP	*BIRC4*/XIAP	XIAP expression low or absent. Reduced number of NKT cells. Defective signal transduction and activation of lymphocytes.	
Immunodeficiencies affecting cellular and humoral immunity	ITK	*ITK*	Reduced number of NKT cells	EBV associated lymphoproliferation
	CD27	*CD27*	Low CD27 expression, hypogammaglobulinaemia	
Autoinflammatory disorder	NLCR4	*NLCR4*	Periodic fever, neonatal enterocolitis, severe MAS	

Modified from Ref. [8], with permission

Q4. Next-generation sequencing detected no pathogenic variant in the known HLH-causing genes in our patient. All of the following options are usually recommended in management of MAS in SJIA, except:

A. Emergency allogeneic hematopoietic stem cell transplant
B. High-dose IVIG infusion + IL-1 blocking biological agents such as anakinra
C. High-dose intravenous corticosteroid monotherapy
D. Monotherapy with calcineurin inhibitor such as cyclosporine

Answer: *The correct answer is* ***A.***

Currently there are no validated evidence-based treatment guidelines on MAS in SJIA. A short-term, high-dose intravenous methylprednisolone therapy is frequently reported as an effective first-line treatment. Alternative therapeutic options for MAS in SJIA include T cell blocking agents such as cyclosporine in conjunction with IL-1 receptor antagonist anakinra, depending on the severity of presentation [12, 13].

Replacement of the defective immune system via HSCT is a lifesaving therapy in primary HLH, but is used only rarely in severe, refractory secondary HLH/MAS cases.

Practical Points

- Macrophage activation syndrome (MAS) presents at onset in up to 22% of patients and in up to 50% in subclinical forms of systemic juvenile idiopathic arthritis (SJIA), and is overt in about 10–15% of children with SJIA during their disease
- It is very difficult to distinguish SJIA/MAS from primary HLH, especially in a very young child
- An initially high ESR that then drops, despite increasing inflammation, is characteristic of MAS/HLH and thought to be secondary to decreasing fibrinogen level
- Elevated triglyceride level, due to lipoprotein lipase inhibition by cytokines
- Currently there are no validated evidence-based treatment guidelines on MAS in SJIA
- A short-term, high-dose intravenous methylprednisolone therapy is frequently reported as an effective first-line treatment

References

1. Petty RE, Southwood TR, Manners P, Baum J, Glass DN, Goldenberg J, He X, Maldonado-Cocco J, Orozco-Alcala J, Prieur AM, Suarez-Almazor ME, Woo P. International League of Associations for Rheumatology classification of juvenile idiopathic arthritis: second revision, Edmonton, 2001. J Rheumatol. 2004;31(2):390–2.
2. Minoia F, Davi S, Horne A, Demirkaya E, Bovis F, Li C, Lehmberg K, Weitzman S, Insalaco A, Wouters C, Shenoi S, Espada G, Ozen S, Anton J, Khubchandani R, Russo R, Pal P, Kasapcopur

O, Miettunen P, Maritsi D, Merino R, Shakoory B, Alessio M, Chasnyk V, Sanner H, Gao YJ, Huasong Z, Kitoh T, Avcin T, Fischbach M, Frosch M, Grom A, Huber A, Jelusic M, Sawhney S, Uziel Y, Ruperto N, Martini A, Cron RQ, Ravelli A. Clinical features, treatment, and outcome of macrophage activation syndrome complicating systemic juvenile idiopathic arthritis: a multinational, multicenter study of 362 patients. Arthritis Rheumatol. 2014;66(11):3160–9.
3. Sen ES, Steward CG, Ramanan AV. Diagnosing haemophagocytic syndrome. Arch Dis Child. 2017;102(3):279–84.
4. Henter JI, Horne A, Arico M, Egeler RM, Filipovich AH, Imashuku S, Ladisch S, McClain K, Webb D, Winiarski J, Janka G. HLH-2004: diagnostic and therapeutic guidelines for hemophagocytic lymphohistiocytosis. Pediatr Blood Cancer. 2007;48(2):124–31.
5. Ravelli A, Minoia F, Davi S, Horne A, Bovis F, Pistorio A, Arico M, Avcin T, Behrens EM, De Benedetti F, Filipovic L, Grom AA, Henter JI, Ilowite NT, Jordan MB, Khubchandani R, Kitoh T, Lehmberg K, Lovell DJ, Miettunen P, Nichols KE, Ozen S, Pachlopnik Schmid J, Ramanan AV, Russo R, Schneider R, Sterba G, Uziel Y, Wallace C, Wouters C, Wulffraat N, Demirkaya E, Brunner HI, Martini A, Ruperto N, Cron RQ. 2016 Classification Criteria for Macrophage Activation Syndrome Complicating Systemic Juvenile Idiopathic Arthritis: A European League Against Rheumatism/American College of Rheumatology/Paediatric Rheumatology International Trials Organisation Collaborative Initiative. Ann Rheum Dis. 2016;75(3):481–9.
6. Bousfiha A, Jeddane L, Al-Herz W, Ailal F, Casanova JL, Chatila T, Conley ME, Cunningham-Rundles C, Etzioni A, Franco JL, Gaspar HB, Holland SM, Klein C, Nonoyama S, Ochs HD, Oksenhendler E, Picard C, Puck JM, Sullivan KE, Tang ML. The 2015 IUIS Phenotypic classification for primary immunodeficiencies. J Clin Immunol. 2015;35(8):727–38.
7. Sepulveda FE, de Saint Basile G. Hemophagocytic syndrome: primary forms and predisposing conditions. Curr Opin Immunol. 2017;49:20–6.
8. Janka GE, Lehmberg K. Hemophagocytic syndromes--an update. Blood Rev. 2014;28(4):135–42.
9. Bracaglia C, Prencipe G, De Benedetti F. Macrophage activation syndrome: different mechanisms leading to a one clinical syndrome. Pediatr Rheumatol Online J. 2017;15(1):5.
10. Kaufman KM, Linghu B, Szustakowski JD, Husami A, Yang F, Zhang K, Filipovich AH, Fall N, Harley JB, Nirmala NR, Grom AA. Whole-exome sequencing reveals overlap between macrophage activation syndrome in systemic juvenile idiopathic arthritis and familial hemophagocytic lymphohistiocytosis. Arthritis Rheumatol. 2014;66(12):3486–95.
11. Zhang M, Behrens EM, Atkinson TP, Shakoory B, Grom AA, Cron RQ. Genetic defects in cytolysis in macrophage activation syndrome. Curr Rheumatol Rep. 2014;16(9):439.
12. Morimoto A, Nakazawa Y, Ishii E. Hemophagocytic lymphohistiocytosis: pathogenesis, diagnosis, and management. Pediatr Int. 2016;58(9):817–25.
13. Brisse E, Matthys P, Wouters CH. Understanding the spectrum of haemophagocytic lymphohistiocytosis: update on diagnostic challenges and therapeutic options. Br J Haematol. 2016;174(2):175–87.

Chapter 51
Recurrent Infections, Diarrhea and Hypereosinophilia

Haskologlu Sule, Islamoglu Candan, and Ikinciogullari Aydan

An 8-month-old boy was admitted to our clinic with a history of recurrent hospitalizations due to fever and diarrhea. He was once diagnosed with septicemia which required intravenous antibiotic treatment. He was the fifth child of consanguineous parents with no history of similar conditions in their families.

In his physical examination a mild dermatitis with skin dryness, failure to thrive, hepatomegaly and splenomegaly were detected. There was no sign of syndromic appearance. Laboratory analysis revealed leukocytosis with eosinophilia (absolute eosinophil count: 6830/μL) and panhypogammaglobulinemia (serum IgA: <6 mg/dL (reference: 7–123), IgG: 494 mg/dL (under IVIG treatment) (reference: 304–1231), IgM: <6 mg/dL (reference: 32–203), and total IgE: <1 (IU/mL). The patient was referred to our clinic with a suspicion of primary immunodeficiency. Results of the lymphocyte subset enumeration are presented in Table 51.1.

Q1. What is the best initial diagnosis?

A. Omenn's syndrome
B. X-linked agammaglobulinemia
C. Severe combined immune deficiency with maternal engrafment
D. Intestinal lymphangiectasia

Answer: *The correct answer is* ***C.***

Severe combined immune deficiency (SCID) is a genetically heterogeneous group of disorders affecting the development and function of T cells. B and NK cells are affected in some cases as well. SCID typically presents early in life with

H. Sule · I. Candan · I. Aydan (✉)
Department of Pediatric Allergy and Immunology, Ankara University School of Medicine, Ankara, Turkey
e-mail: aydani@medicine.ankara.edu.tr

© Springer Nature Switzerland AG 2020

F. Rahmani, N. Rezaei (eds.), *Pediatric Autoimmunity and Transplantation*,
https://doi.org/10.1007/978-3-030-26280-8_51

Table 51.1 Peripheral lymphocyte subsets enumeration of the patient

	% (/μL)	Age references [% (/μL)] [1]
$CD3^+CD16^-CD56^-$	47 (164)	51–79 (1400–11,500)
$CD3^-CD16^+CD56^+$	51 (178)	5–23 (68–3900)
$CD3^+CD4^+$	47 (164)	31–54 (1000–7200)
$CD3^+CD8^+$	0 (0)	10–31 (400–5400)
$CD19^+$	0.3 (1)	14–44 (300–6300)
$CD20^+$	0.1 (0.3)	13–40 (300–6300)
$CD4^+CD45RO^+$	45 (157)	6–21 (800–7200)
$CD4^+CD45RA^+$	0 (0)	25–45 (83–1300)
$HLA\text{-}DR^+$	76	15–48
$CD4^+CD45RA^+CD31^+$ (Trec)	0	(63–81)

Age Ref. [1]

moniliasis, failure to thrive, diarrhea, recurrent infections due to respiratory viruses, herpes viruses, and *Pneumocystis jiroveci* [1]. Lymphopenia is the most common finding in many forms of SCID, while T cells may even be found in normal numbers in some SCID patients. Numerous recently identified defects allow T cell development on one hand, but compromise T cell function on the other, affecting proximal or distal steps of intracellular signaling. These functional T cell immunodeficiencies are characterized by immune dysregulation, autoimmunity, increased risk of malignancies, and infections [2]. Some of these "leaky" phenotypes are due to hypomorphic mutations in SCID-associated genes and some can be attributed to SCID mutations that allow development of a number of residual non-functioning cells [3]. Omenn's syndrome (OS) is a typical example of a unique SCID phenotype that is characterized by impaired T cell differentiation in the presence of abnormal self-reactive cells [4]. These T cells are autoreactive and exhibit uncontrolled proliferation, leading to the infiltration of various organs such as the skin, spleen, liver, and lymph nodes. OS usually present in infancy with recurrent infections, erythroderma, lymphadenopathy and hepatosplenomegaly. In OS absolute lymphocyte count is normal or high due to the presence of oligoclonally expanded T cells. Eosinophilia, elevated IgE, low IgG, IgA, IgM and specific antibody response, normal $CD3^+$ T cell numbers but low T cell receptor excision circles (Trec) level are the major laboratory findings in OS. These activated T cells have a memory (CD45RO) phenotype and are HLA-DR positive. B cell and NK cell counts are variable depending on the type of mutation [4].

SCID newborns fail to eliminate maternal cells and T cell engraftment has been reported in as many as 40% of newborns [5]. Hypofunctioning T cells may facilitate persistent engraftment of maternal T lymphocytes, leading to alloreactive immune response referred as GVHD. Maternal engraftment syndrome thus typically present in a neonate/infant as rash and/or diarrhea. An infant with any of the features suggestive of an immunodeficiency yet with normal lymphocyte count, should be evaluated for maternal T cell engraftment. One indicator that maternal T cell engraftment is present, is predominance of either $CD4^+$ or $CD8^+$ T cells since maternally engrafted cells are oligoclonal. However, this phenotype is not always evident. A majority of the maternally engrafted T cells have an activated or memory phenotype (they express CD45RO). These cell surface markers can be measured by flow cytometry.

OS and maternal T lymphocyte engraftment have many clinical and laboratory features in common, although maternally engrafted T lymphocytes most often result in a milder clinical presentation. These phenotypes can be distinguished by different patterns of cell activity, enumeration and function of regulatory T cells and diversity of the TCR repertoire [5].

Infants with intestinal lymphangiectasia often present with profound lymphopenia and hypogammaglobulinemia and have been mistakenly diagnosed as having SCID. In these patients, there is usually evidence of intestinal protein loss, hypoalbuminemia, and elevated stool alpha-1-antitrypsin [6].

Here in this case, generalized cutaneous eruption, hepatosplenomegaly, recurrent intravenous antibiotic treatment history, diarrhea, failure to thrive, normal levels of circulating lymphocytes (4050/μL) with extreme eosinophilia (6830/μL), and undetectable Trec level, led to a diagnosis of SCID with maternal engrafment. Absence of recent thymic emigrants is also consistent with predominance of memory T cells detected in the patient. These results further support the diagnosis of SCID with maternal T cell engraftment.

Q2. What is the next diagnostic method to confirm SCID with maternal engrafment?

A. Human leucocyte antigen typing
B. The PCR-based short tandem repeat (STR) analysis
C. Fluorescence in-situ hybridization (FISH) analysis
D. All of the above

Answer: *The correct answer is* ***D.***

The peripheral blood of the infant and his mother were tested for HLA-A, HLA-B and HLA-DR using standard serological methods or DNA hybridization with sequence specific oligonucleotide probes in order to define tissue typing. Presence of maternal T cells allows maternal HLA haplotypes to be detected in addition to the inherited paternal haplotype. PCR based STR is another method available that can be performed on peripheral blood or any other DNA-containing material. Since PCR amplification of a sample is routinely performed with less than 2 ng of genomic DNA (equivalent to approximately 300 cells), chimerism testing by this method can be successfully performed. Additionally, maternal engraftment can be detected by analyzing patients' PBMCs by using a combination of noninherited HLAs and FISH [7]. In our patient maternal engraftment was found 25% by PCR-based STR analysis.

Q3. What is the most appropriate treatment modality?

A. Avoid all live vaccines, initiate antiviral, antifungal and antibacterial prophylaxis
B. Start prophylactic intravenous immunoglobulin infusion

C. Consider hematopoietic stem cell transplantation from mother
D. All of the above

Answer: *The correct answer is **D.***

SCID is a pediatric emergency. Early hematopoietic stem cell transplantation (HSCT) is a lifesaving, curative treatment. Evaluation for BMT should be started. Maternal T cell engraftment has been reported in 40% of SCID patients, thus it is a common phenomenon in this patient population and should be prioritized when resolving aberrant HLA typing results. Since the presence of transplacental maternal engrafment is associated with a decreased risk of rejecting a maternal graft, haploidentical HSCT from mother could be a fast and reliable treatment modality in these patients.

Practical Points

- Severe combined immunodeficiency (SCID) newborns fail to eliminate maternal cells and T cell engraftment has been reported in as many as 40% of newborns
- Hypofunctioning T cells may facilitate persistent engraftment of maternal T lymphocytes, leading to alloreactive immune response referred as graft versus host disease (GVHD). Maternal engraftment syndrome thus typically present in a neonate/infant as rash and/or diarrhea
- One indicator that maternal T cell engraftment is present, is predominance of either $CD4^+$ or $CD8^+$ T cells since maternally engrafted cells are oligoclonal. However, this phenotype is not always evident. A majority of the maternally engrafted T cells have an activated or memory phenotype and express CD45RO
- HLA typing, PCR-based short tandem repeat (STR) analysis or fluorescence in-situ hybridization (FISH) analysis, can help detect maternal engrafment syndrome

References

1. Fischer A, Cavazzana-Calvo M, De Saint Basile G, DeVillartay JP, Di Santo JP, Hivroz C, Rieux-Laucat F, Le Deist F. Naturally occurring primary deficiencies of the immune system. Annu Rev Immunol. 1997;15:93–124.
2. Notarangelo LD. Combined immunodeficiencies with nonfunctional T lymphocytes. Adv Immunol. 2014;121:121–90.
3. Notarangelo LD. Partial defects of T-cell development associated with poor T-cell function. J Allergy Clin Immunol. 2013;131(5):1297–305.
4. Villa A, Notarangelo LD, Roifman CM. Omenn syndrome: inflammation in leaky severe combined immunodeficiency. J Allergy Clin Immunol. 2008;122(6):1082–6.
5. Dvorak CC, Cowan MJ, Logan BR, Notarangelo LD, Griffith LM, Puck JM, Kohn DB, Shearer WT, O'Reilly RJ, Fleisher TA, Pai SY, Hanson IC, Pulsipher MA, Fuleihan R,

Filipovich A, Goldman F, Kapoor N, Small T, Smith A, Chan KW, Cuvelier G, Heimall J, Knutsen A, Loechelt B, Moore T, Buckley RH. The natural history of children with severe combined immunodeficiency: baseline features of the first fifty patients of the primary immune deficiency treatment consortium prospective study 6901. J Clin Immunol. 2013;33(7):1156–64.
6. Ingle SB, Hinge Ingle CR. Primary intestinal lymphangiectasia: minireview. World J Clin Cases. 2014;2(10):528–33.
7. Liu C, Duffy B, Bednarski JJ, Calhoun C, Lay L, Rundblad B, Payton JE, Mohanakumar T. Maternal T-cell engraftment interferes with human leukocyte antigen typing in severe combined immunodeficiency. Am J Clin Pathol. 2016;145(2):251–7.

Chapter 52
Liver Transplantation Who Developed Pancytopenia Post-transplantation

Soumya Pandey and Terry Harville

A 12-year-old Caucasian male with end-stage liver disease due to hepatitis C, received orthotopic liver transplantation (OLT) from an 18 year-old male deceased-donor. The patient and donor were both positive for cytomegalovirus and Epstein-Barr virus. Donor HLA typing and fluorescence cytometric crossmatch (FCXM) were performed retrospectively (i.e. post-transplantation). Patient's HLA antibody results showed no evidence of potentially elevated donor-specific antibodies (DSA), and FCXM studies were negative.

Q1. True or False: Studies performed on liver transplant donors at the recipient transplantation medical center are typically performed retrospectively due to the narrow time window between harvesting of the liver and transplantation. This is to prevent cold-ischemic damage to the donor liver

A. True
B. False

Answer: *The correct answer is* ***A.***

Typically, the cold-ischemic time allowed for a donor liver is up to 12 h. Generally, HLA typing and FCXM can be performed and analyzed within 4–5 h. Once the donor becomes deceased, the countdown sets off for the organ to be carefully harvested, packaged, delivered to a transport facility, which is generally an

S. Pandey
Department of Pathology and Laboratory Services, University of Arkansas for Medical Sciences, Little Rock, AR, USA

T. Harville (✉)
Departments of Pathology and Laboratory Services, Pediatrics, and Internal Medicine, University of Arkansas for Medical Sciences, Little Rock, AR, USA
e-mail: harvilleterryo@uams.edu

© Springer Nature Switzerland AG 2020

F. Rahmani, N. Rezaei (eds.), *Pediatric Autoimmunity and Transplantation*,
https://doi.org/10.1007/978-3-030-26280-8_52

airport, transported to the transplant facility and finally surgically placed. The process of harvesting to transportation can take several hours, so that by the time of arrival to the transplant facility, there is insufficient time for HLA matching or laboratory tests within the golden time of cold-ischemic damage [1].

Patient's initial post-OLT course was unremarkable. He received immunosuppressive therapy with basiliximab, mycophenolate mofetil, and tacrolimus. He was discharged on post-operative day 4 (POD 4), seeming to be doing well. On POD 10, the patient was readmitted for complaints of hallucinations and delusions, which were attributed to tacrolimus. Hence, tacrolimus was transitioned to cyclosporine, without further apparent sequelae.

Q2. Basiliximab is a chimeric mouse-human monoclonal antibody to the alpha-chain of the IL-2 receptor. Which of the following statements are true?

1. Anti-chimeric antibodies could reduce the effectiveness of basiliximab
2. Anti-chimeric antibodies could actually enhance the effectiveness of basiliximab by increasing the cross-linking capacity and thereby making it more effective at inhibiting T lymphocytes
3. An inadvertent effect of basiliximab is the inhibition of regulatory T cells (Tregs)
4. The main effect of basiliximab is to over-stimulate effector T lymphocytes, which in turn induces them to undergo apoptosis
5. Basiliximab works by blocking the activation of T lymphocytes via blocking IL-2 signaling

A. All of the above
B. 1, 3, and 5
C. 2, 3, and 5
D. 2 and 4
E. None of the above

Answer: *The correct answer is* ***B.***

Q3. Which statement is most correct about tacrolimus?

A. It has broad immunosuppressive activities, which may include T-lymphocytes, B-lymphocytes, and monocytes
B. It is a very good immunosuppressive agent, since it has minimal renal toxicity
C. It is a calcineurin inhibitor, which blocks the activation of T lymphocytes from the IL-2 receptor
D. It only extremely rarely has systemic side effects
E. Unfortunately, hair loss is a side effect of tacrolimus

Answer: *The correct answer is* ***C.***

Q4. Which medication allowed for successful solid organ transplantation, without the need for careful HLA-matching of patient and donor?

A. Corticosteroids
B. Azathioprine

C. Cyclosporine A
D. Mycophenolate
E. Anti-IL-2 Receptor monoclonal antibodies

Answer: *The correct answer is* ***C.***

As a chimeric monoclonal antibody, basiliximab may be subject to anti-mouse-chimeric antibodies, which block its function. Basiliximab primarily works by blocking the IL-2 receptor and thereby prevent activation of T lymphocytes via IL-2. There are concerns about reduced tolerance induced by Tregs with use of basiliximab, since IL-2 is also critical for the activity and survival of Tregs as well.

Tacrolimus is a calcineurin inhibitor, which blocks the activation of T lymphocytes by blocking signal transduction from the IL-2 receptor, primarily inhibiting T-lymphocytes. Unfortunately, there is a potential for severe renal side effects, which may not reverse upon cessation of the medication. At high plasma levels, tacrolimus can yield to neurologic side effects including seizures. Rapid infusion is one known risk factor for neurologic complications while, oral dosing can also create neurologic issues in some patients, as in ours. Increased hair growth and coarseness of the facial features can be troublesome side-effects in others.

Fortunately, introduction of cyclosporine in early 1970s led to the same success in transplantation of poorly HLA-matched donor and recipients, compared to well HLA-match pairs [2].

The patient was again readmitted on day 26 with a 5-day history of progressive mouth and throat pain, fevers, productive cough, and new-onset diffuse skin rash. Due to the initial suspicion for acute infection, immunosuppressive therapies were discontinued and broad-spectrum antibiotics, micafungin, vancomycin, and cefepime, were begun empirically. Physical examination was notable for erythematous papules coalescing into diffuse erythema on the back, chest, arms, face, and neck, and erythematous papules scattered on thighs, sparing the conjunctiva and scrotum.

Q5. Which of the following conditions should be included in the differential diagnosis list? (select the best answer)

1. Viral eruption
2. Medication hypersensitivity
3. Fungal rash
4. Graft rejection
5. Graft versus host disease

A. All of the above
B. 1, 2, and 3
C. 1, 2, 3, and 4
D. 1, 2, 3, and 5
E. None of the above

Answer: *The correct answer is* ***D.***

Mouth and throat involvement along with fevers and rash, in an immunosuppressed patient would be suggestive of viral infection. In immunosuppressed individuals, multiple infections, including bacterial and fungal, as well as opportunistic infections may also be present. Yet, these are also symptoms consistent with medication hypersensitivity. These are also features of graft versus host disease (GVHD), given the fact that as many as 2% of patients receiving donor livers might develop GVHD. The liver is a large repository of donor lymphocytes. Depending on circumstances, including HLA similarities between the patient and donor and extent of immunosuppression in the patient, the donor lymphocytes may be activated sufficiently to "over-power" the host lymphocytes and result in GVHD.

Viral studies were negative. Liver function tests were within normal limits and stayed within normal limits throughout his course. CBC demonstrated severe pancytopenia. A bone marrow biopsy to revealed diffuse necrosis with absent viable cells of any hematopoietic lineage. Skin biopsy of the right arm lesion revealed interface dermatitis with vacuolar alterations. While medication hypersensitivity could not be fully excluded, the findings were considered most consistent with acute GVHD. Treatment with intravenous methylprednisolone and tacrolimus were initiated for acute grade IV GVHD.

The patient and donor HLA typing results were reviewed for potential disclosure of the risks for GVHD due to specific locus matching and homozygosity. Low-resolution, serologic-equivalent HLA typing revealed apparent homozygosity in favor of graft rejection, however, high-resolution HLA typing results did not demonstrate homozygosity or specific risks for GVHD (Table 52.1).

High-resolution HLA typing was performed on the lymphocytes from the bone marrow specimen. The results demonstrated a mixed chimerism with a strong presence of the donor HLA type, consistent with donor lymphocyte infiltration of the bone marrow and GVHD (Table 52.2). An emergent bone marrow donor search was initiated, however, despite therapeutic interventions the patient died before a donor could be identified.

As seen in Table 52.2, HLA typing was performed using Luminex® technology by the rSSO technique. Essentially 100 beads with probes attached were used to resolve the HLA type of each locus. The specific beads, which are positive at each locus are listed according to the positive bead number, for the patient, the donor, and the patient's bone marrow following emergence of symptoms. Positive beads found only in the patient are shown in "green", whereas beads only positive in the donor are shown in "red". Both beads/HLA loci, from the patient (expected) and donor (not-expected) are found in the patient's bone marrow. This indicates chimerism and confirms the diagnosis of GVHD in this patient. The probable source of the donor lymphocytes is the transplanted liver [3].

Acute GVHD is a frequent complication after hematopoietic cell transplantation (HCT), but occurs less commonly after solid organ transplantation. GVHD after OLT occurs in as many as 2% of cases, and is due to passenger lymphocytes passing from the donor liver into the recipient. It is generally thought that sharing of

Table 52.1 Patient and donor HLA typing results in this case of liver transplantation (apparent serologic homozygosity) (high-resolution homozygosity)

Class I	A		B		C							
Patient	2	3	7	44	5	7						
	02:01	03:01	07:02	44:02	05:01	07:01						
Donor	23	3	65	44	4	8						
	23:01	03:01	14:02	44:03	04:01	08:02						
Class II	DRB1		DRB3/4/5		DQA1		DQB1		DPA1		DPB1	
Patient	15	13	51	52	-	-	6	6	-	-	4	4
	15:01	13:01	5*01	3*01	01:03	01:02	06:03	06:19	01:03	01:03	04:01	04:01
Donor	7	13	53	52	-	-	2	6	-	-	4	5
	07:01	13:02	4*01	3*03	02:01	01:02	02:02	06:09	02:01	01:03	04:02	05:01

Patient donor HLA typing results are compared at the serologic equivalence level and at high-resolution. There is apparent serologic homozygosity between the patient and donor, but this resolves at high-resolution. The presence of apparent serologic Class II homozygosity at DQB1 and DPB1 in the recipient may be predictive for host versus graft direction (predictive of graft rejection), due to disparity with the second donor allele. These differences also disappeared at high-resolution, while HLA typing differences were not predictive of GVHD. in this setting

some HLA alleles between patient and donor, with homozygosity of loci in the donor may result in the inability of the patient to recognize the donor as foreign. Meanwhile, the heterozygosity of a specific locus in the patient (two different alleles present in a locus, one of which is shared with the donor, who is homozygous at the locus) allows the donor lymphocytes to recognize the patient as non-self, with activation and subsequent features of GVHD. Multiple tissues may be affected, with skin, GI tract, and the hematopoietic system being common. Importantly, since the lymphocytes causing GVHD are from the donor, the donor-liver is spared from GVHD, in contrast to allogeneic HCT, where the liver is typically greatly involved. Severe bone marrow aplasia may occur, which can precipitate the extent of morbidity and risk for mortality, as in this patient. Additionally, graft rejection does not occur [4].

Diagnosis can often be challenging as the clinical findings and laboratory results are non-specific and can mimic drug reaction or infections. Given the dismal outcomes of GVHD post-OLT, early recognition and treatment is necessary.

Most therapeutic interventions are not successful and emergent HLA-matched HCT is deemed the most likely successful intervention. The patient must be aggressively supported while waiting for a compatible HCT donor.

Table 52.2 High-resolution HLA typing of patient's bone marrow cells, revealing donor chimerism for solid organ transplantation

Source	Molecular Typing	Bead Number
Patient	A*02:01, *03:01	1, 11, 13, 20, 23, 31, 32, 38, 39, 43, 46, 47, 52, 54, 56, 57, 64, 65, 66, 68, 72, 75, 87
Donor	A*03:01, *23:01	1, 11, 12, 13, 17, 20, 27, 31, 32, 33, 39, 40, 43, 46, 47, 52, 54, 56, 57, 58, 64, 72, 75, 87
Bone Marrow		1, 11, 12, 13, 17, 20, 23, 27, 31, 32, 33, 38, 39, 40, 43, 46, 47, 52, 54, 56, 57, 58, 64, 65, 66, 68, 72, 75, 87
Patient	B*07:02, *44:02	1, 4, 8, 13, 18, 20, 23, 24, 26, 27, 30, 32, 39, 41, 44, 46, 50, 51, 55, 66, 67, 69, 70, 71, 73, 75, 86, 89, 95
Donor	B*14:02 , *44:03	4, 11, 13, 18, 20, 24, 26, 27, 30, 32, 42, 44, 45, 50, 55, 64, 66, 67, 68, 71, 73, 74, 85, 86, 88, 89, 95
Bone Marrow		1, 4, 8, 11, 13, 18, 20, 23, 24, 26, 27, 30, 32, 39, 41, 42, 44, 46, 50, 51, 55, 66, 67, 68, 69, 70, 71, 73, 74, 75, 85, 86, 89, 95
Patient	C*05:01, *07:01	1, 3, 4, 5, 11, 13, 14, 19, 20, 23, 26, 28, 32, 37, 39, 47, 49, 50, 51, 53, 56, 60, 61, 63, 65, 74
Donor	C*04:01, *08:02	1, 2, 3, 4, 11, 13, 19, 20, 23, 28, 32, 39, 45, 47, 49, 50, 51, 56, 60, 61, 62, 74
Bone Marrow		1, 3, 4, 5, 11, 13, 14, 19, 20, 23, 26, 28, 32, 37, 39, 45, 47, 49, 50, 51, 53, 56, 60, 61, 62, 65, 74
Patient	DRB1*13:01, *15:01	2, 7, 10, 15, 16, 33, 34, 39, 42, 43, 60, 82
Donor	DRB1*07:01, *13:02	1, 2, 10, 12, 16, 34, 39, 42, 43, 44, 63, 66, 71, 75, 82
Bone Marrow		1, 2, 7, 10, 12, 15, 16, 33, 34, 39, 42, 43, 44, 60, 63, 66, 71, 75, 82
Patient	DRB3*01, DRB5*01	2, 28, 34, 36, 38, 49, 50, 51, 63, 81
Donor	DRB3*03:01, DRB4*01	1, 20, 25, 34, 42, 49, 61, 64
Bone Marrow		2, 25, 28, 34, 36, 42, 49, 50, 51, 61, 64, 81

Table 52.2 (continued)

Patient	DQA1*01:02, *01:03; DQB1*06:03, *06:19	1	2	4	7		9				18	22	28			34	36		43	45	46		50	51	54	55	59	60	64	65	69		93	94	95			
Donor	DQA1*01:02, *02:01; DQB1*02:02, *06:09		2	4				11	16	17				29	30	34	36	38		45	46	47	50	51	55	59		60	64	65	69	85	93	94	95			
Bone Marrow			2	4	7	8			16			22	28	29		34	36	38	43	45	46		50	51	54	55	59	60	64	65	69			94	95			
Patient	DPA1*01:03, *01:03; DPB1*04:01, *04:01	3		8	9			19	22			32		34	36		42		45	51	52	54			60		62	67	68		73	75		93				
Donor	DPA1*01:03, *02:01; DPB1*04:02, *05:01	3	5			10	17	19	22	23	31	32	33	34	36	41	42	43	45	51		54	55	58	60	61	62	67	68	70		75	76	93	95			
Bone Marrow		3	5	8	9	10	17	19	22	23	31	32	33	34	36		42	43	45	51	52	54	55	58	60	61	62	67	68	70		75	76	93	95			

High-resolution HLA typing of patient bone marrow cells, revealing donor chimerism in a patient with liver transplantation

Q6. Which of the following statements is most correct?

A. HLA Class II are primarily expressed on specific antigen-presenting cells and are therefore the most likely cause of cellular organ rejection or GVHD

B. HLA Class I are found expressed on essentially all nucleated cells in the body and are therefore the most likely target involved with cellular organ rejection, but not GVHD

C. HLA Class I are found expressed on essentially all nucleated cells in the body and are therefore the most likely target involved with cellular organ rejection and GVHD

D. HLA Class I are found expressed on essentially all nucleated cells in the body and are therefore the most likely target involved with GVHD, but not cellular organ rejection
E. Anti-HLA antibodies play a major role in cellular rejection and GVHD

Answer: *The correct answer is* ***C.***

Q7. Which of the following statements is most correct?

A. HLA Class II present endogenous antigens to $CD8^{+}$ T-lymphocytes as the initial step in activation towards organ rejection or GVHD
B. HLA Class I present endogenous antigens to $CD8^{+}$ T lymphocytes as surveillance for foreign antigens, which can be involved with organ rejection or GVHD
C. HLA Class II present exogenous antigens to $CD8^{+}$ T-lymphocytes precipitating organ rejection or GVHD
D. HLA Class I present exogenous antigens to $CD4^{+}$ T-lymphocytes precipitating organ rejection of GVHD
E. HLA Class I and Class II presentation of antigens to $CD8^{+}$ T-lymphocytes have equal roles in causing organ rejection or GVHD

Answer: *The correct answer is* ***B.***

Class I HLA molecules are comprised of the HLA-A, -B, and -C loci, and are found expressed on essentially all nucleated cells in the body. HLA class I primarily present endogenous antigens (i.e., peptides from inside the cell) to $CD8^{+}$ T lymphocytes, responsible for defense against viral infections and cancer immunosurveillance. HLA class II is comprised of the HLA-DR, -DQ, and -DP loci, and primarily present exogenously derived antigens to $CD4^{+}$ T lymphocytes. HLA class II are expressed primarily on specific, "professional" antigen-presenting cells (APC), such as macrophages and dendritic cells, and on B-lymphocytes. The primary source of incompatibility in solid-organ transplantation will therefore be most noticeable with the HLA class I molecules, since these are uniformly expressed on the cells from the donor organ. Further, donor T lymphocytes with different HLA class I expression introduced into the patient will be seeing everything around them as foreign in the setting of GVHD. Event in a fully HLA-matched HCT setting, self-antigens presented by the self HLA-class I form a complex that may elicit a response with the donor T lymphocytes.

Practical Points

- Once the donor becomes deceased, the countdown sets off for the organ to be carefully harvested, packaged, delivered to a transport facility, transported to the transplant facility and finally surgically placed.
- The cold-ischemic time allowed for a donor liver is up to 12 h
- The liver is a large repository of donor lymphocytes and as many as 2% of patients receiving donor livers might develop graft versus host disease

References

1. Brent L. A history of transplantation immunology. San Diego: Academic Press Inc.; 1996.
2. Cruse J, Lewis R. Historical atlas of immunology. London: Taylor and Francis Group; 2005.
3. Amico P, Hönger G, Mayr M, Steiger J, Hopfer H, Schaub S. Clinical relevance of pretransplant donor-specific HLA antibodies detected by single-antigen flow-beads. Transplantation. 2009;87(11):1681–8.
4. Pandey S, Rhodes-Clark B, Borja-Cacho D, Jethava Y, Harville T. P159 High-resolution HLA-typing can confirm diagnosis of graft versus host disease after orthotopic liver-transplantation. Hum Immunol. 2016;77:153.

Chapter 53
Kidney Transplant Candidate Showing Presence of Pre-formed Donor-Specific Antibodies Against a Prospective Living Donor

Soumya Pandey and Terry Harville

A 16-year-old Caucasian male with end-stage renal disease secondary to IgA nephropathy underwent evaluation for kidney transplantation.

Q1. Which of the following tests is indicated as initial pre-transplant workup for kidney transplant candidates?

A. HLA typing
B. Anti-HLA antibody studies
C. HLA typing and anti-HLA antibody studies
D. Evaluation of potential donors for anti-HLA antibodies
E. None of the above

Answer: *The correct answer is* ***C.***

Routine pre-transplantation HLA workup on a transplant candidate include at least an initial HLA typing and anti-HLA-antibody screening. In case a sensitization event occurs, e.g. blood product transfusion, serum for anti-HLA antibody studies are collected from the patient each month and analyzed on at least a quarterly basis, to determine any change in anti-HLA antibody pattern. Presence of elevated donor-specific antibodies (DSA) or antibodies directed against the donor HLA type can only be ascertained once a potential donor is identified. Main concern

S. Pandey
Department of Pathology and Laboratory Services, University of Arkansas for Medical Sciences, Little Rock, AR, USA

T. Harville (✉)
Departments of Pathology and Laboratory Services, Pediatrics, and Internal Medicine, University of Arkansas for Medical Sciences, Little Rock, AR, USA
e-mail: harvilleterryo@uams.edu

© Springer Nature Switzerland AG 2020
F. Rahmani, N. Rezaei (eds.), *Pediatric Autoimmunity and Transplantation*,
https://doi.org/10.1007/978-3-030-26280-8_53

is that the presence of DSA can result in poor outcomes including poor graft function and antibody-mediated rejection (AMR) [1].

Anti-HLA antibody studies revealed presence of multiple antibodies including elevated class I anti-HLA-B44 (anti-HLA-B*44:02 and anti-B*44:03 with mean fluorescent intensity (MFI) >5000). In case of our patient, these antibodies persisted on routine quarterly testing while other class I anti-HLA antibodies with lower MFI values were also present. No significant Class II anti-HLA antibody was noted. Importantly, the MFI values greater than 1000 correlate with positive fluorescence cytometric crossmatches (FCXM) [2].

Nineteen months after the patient's initial work-up, he received a potential offer from an altruistic, unrelated living-donor. As listed in Table 53.1, patient and donor were a 1 of 6 HLA match at the serologic equivalent level (HLA-DR4 match, of HLA-A, -B, and -DR). Unfortunately, this potential donor expressed HLA-B*44:02, to which the patient has apparent antibodies present.

Q2. True or False: Renal transplantation should only be performed when the transplant candidate and the donor match at 6 HLA loci (HLA-A, -B, and -DR) at the serologic equivalent level

A. True
B. False

Answer: *The correct answer is* ***B.***

Q3. True or False: "Virtual Crossmatch" can be performed by comparing the HLA type of the potential donor with the recipient's anti-HLA antibody profile. In this case, the patient donor pairing would appear unsuitable by "Virtual Cross-matching", due to a risk for a positive crossmatch

A. True
B. False

Answer: *The correct answer is* ***A.***

Table 53.1 HLA Typing results for solid organ transplantation of the 16-year-old boy candidate for kidney transplantation

	A	B	C	DRB1	DRB3/4/5	DQB1	DQA1
Patient	*01:01	*08:01	*07:02	*04:01	4*01:01	*03:01	*03:02
	*34:02	*08:01	*07:02	*13:02	3*03:01	*06:04	*01:02
Serologic	1, 34	8, x	7, x	4, 13	53, 52	7, 6	–
Potential donor	*32:01	*44:02	*05:01	*04:03	4*01:01	*03:02	*03:01
	*32:01	*15:09	*07:04	*12:01	3*02:02	*03:01	*05:05
Serologic	32, x	44, 70	5, 7	4, 12	53, 52	8, 7	–

The molecular and serologic equivalent results are listed for each HLA locus for the patient (upper three rows) and potential donor (bottom three rows). Note: When only one serologic allele can be detected at a locus, the naming convention is to list that particular HLA type and use an "x" in the second position. There are no serologic equivalent names for HLA-DQA1 alleles

In contrast to hematopoietic cell transplantation, where HLA matching criteria are very stringent, renal transplantation does not require HLA matching between the recipient and the donor. There are several reasons for this including equitable allocation of deceased-donor kidneys into all ethnic groups in the transplantation list, which would be restricted using HLA matching as a major criteria. Moreover, once cyclosporine A was introduced as an anti-rejection, immunosuppressive agent, the need for close HLA matching between the donor and recipient was reduced, approaching the goal of equal organ allocation. Nonetheless, presence of DSA against the mismatched donor HLA is more relevant in determining donor compatibility. In this case, the donor expressing HLA-B∗44:02 would be incompatible with a patient with anti-B44 antibodies present [3].

Q4. A renal transplant recipient is found to have apparent DSA against a potential donor. Which of the following statements is most correct?

A. The donor should be immediately deemed incompatible and no further workup should be performed.
B. The anti-HLA antibody profile in the patient should be scrutinized for validity of the apparent DSA.
C. The recipient should receive the transplant along with additional immunosuppressive treatment, and additional modalities for reduction of DSA including, plasmapheresis, rituximab, intravenous immunoglobulin, etc.
D. The potential donor should have their HLA typing redone to verify the results.
E. None of the above

Answer: *The correct answer is* ***B.***

In some instances, the concentration and "strength" of the detected anti-HLA antibody may be below the threshold to induce tissue damage, yet is detected above the defined cut-off in the assay. Therefore, not all anti-HLA antibodies are clinically relevant. Additionally, during the manufacturing process of the reagents used for detection of anti-HLA antibodies, some of the HLA molecules attached to reagents beads, may become denatured resulting to the exposure of otherwise "non-exposed epitopes" to which certain antibodies may bind. In the "native" (i.e. non-denatured) state, only exposed surface epitopes of the HLA molecule are expected to have clinical relevance. Therefore, it is imperative to evaluate the antibody profile in each patient to determine whether the pattern is consistent with antibodies directed to "exposed" epitopes only, which indicates clinical relevance. While, it is clearly important to screen the potential donor's HLA type versus the recipient's antibody profile, i.e. a virtual crossmatch, these future confirmation steps are crucial to verify which anti-HLA antibodies have clinical relevance. This should help prevent excluding a donor, who may actually work well for a patient, based on what may be considered as a "false-positive/relevant" anti-HLA antibody detection. Finally, performing a "physical crossmatch" can ultimately answer the question of compatibility. This remains the "gold-standard" in most situations [2].

The anti-HLA antibody profile in organ transplantation *Case 18.2* did not have a pattern consistent with exposed epitopes. Each HLA class I molecule contains ~50 epitopes, with usually ~30 exposed-epitopes, hence there may be nearly 300 total HLA class I epitopes with nearly 180 exposed epitopes per person. Comparison of this patient and potential donor revealed that their class I HLA types shared ~250 epitopes, so that ~50 epitopes are different between these two. Comparison of the "non-shared" epitopes revealed that none of the HLA molecule surface-exposed epitopes were present in the antibody profile. No antibody against shared exposed epitopes were present in the antibodies detected in the assay. Thus, the anti-B44 antibody was in essence, a false positive result, due to antibodies binding to denatured epitopes. While, this patient-donor pairing could have been excluded via virtual crossmatch, whereas, further testing was capable of demonstrating compatibility for this potential donor.

Moreover, the risks of hyperacute antibody-mediated rejection were considered to be minimal.

The patient is currently more than 5 years post-transplantation without signs of rejection. Post-transplant monitoring by routine anti-HLA detection assays, finds the same anti-B∗44:02 antibody (MFI ~1500–2000), with the same overall antibody profile as previously detected. Thus, the antibodies to denatured antigens are remaining present, which means that he has not produced anti-HLA antibodies to exposed epitopes.

Additional assays are available to helping distinguish antibodies, which may be more clinically relevant due to their ability to activate complement. The C1q binding assay is one such test. Binding of C1q to the constant domain of antibodies -typically, IgG1, IgG2, IgG3, and IgM- is the first step towards the activation of complement. IgG1, IgG2, and IgG3, anti-HLA antibodies are thought to be the ones most capable of inflicting antibody-mediated damage or rejection, because of their ability to activate complement, while IgM anti-HLA antibodies are thought not to be as important, but there are reports where they have inflicting the damage. The negative C1q assay results, both prior to and post-transplantation have provided another component of relief regarding risks for antibody-mediated rejection in this patient [2].

This case illustrates important issues in the complexities of solid organ transplantation. The assays are becoming more sensitive, resulting in the detection of anti-HLA antibodies, which have no clinical relevance. First, the antibody profile can be scrutinized for whether exposed or non-exposed epitopes are being shared amongst the detected antibodies. Additional assays for evaluating the relevance of the antibodies, such as the C1q assay can be quite helpful. When possible, performing actual crossmatches with the potential donor or surrogate donors are considered gold standard. Surrogate donors are volunteer cell donors who share the HLA type with prospective donors, or who have HLA types to which the patient appears to have DSA against. Every patient deserves every chance possible to receive a compatible transplant.

Q5. True or False: IgA anti-HLA antibodies are important in pre-transplant monitoring of kidney transplantation as they may precipitate IgA nephropathy

A. True
B. False

Answer: *The correct answer is **B.***

Q6. True or False: Anti-HLA antibodies, which do not have the ability to activate complement, are as detrimental as those able to activate the complement

A. True
B. False

Answer: *The correct answer is **B.***

IgA anti-HLA antibodies have not been shown to be relevant towards renal disease or transplantation [2]. IgA nephropathy is thought to have a genetic contribution, which may include altered glycosylation patterns of IgA, which therefore allows deposition in glomerular tissue, and results in the damage.

Practical Points

- Routine pre-transplantation HLA workup on a transplant candidate include at least an initial HLA typing and anti-HLA-antibody screening
- Presence of donor specific antibodies (DSA) or antibodies directed against the donor HLA type can only be ascertained once a potential donor is identified
- Main concern is that the presence of DSA can result in poor outcomes including poor graft function and acute antibody-mediated rejection
- Not all anti-HLA antibodies are clinically relevant. Exposure of otherwise "non-exposed epitopes" in the HLA reagents, or presence of anti-HLA antibodies below threshold of reaction are some instances
- Performing a "physical crossmatch" can ultimately answer the question of compatibility. This remains the "gold-standard" is most situations

References

1. Valenzuela N, Reed E. Antibody-mediated rejection across solid organ transplants: manifestations, mechanisms, and therapies. J Clin Invest. 2017;127(7):2492–504.
2. Liwsk R, Gebel H. Of cells and microparticles: assets and liabilities of HLA antibody detection. Transplantation. 2018;102(1S Suppl 1):S1–6.
3. Lan J, Tinckam K. Clinical utility of complement dependent assays in kidney transplantation. Transplantation. 2018;102(1S Suppl 1):S14–22.

Chapter 54
Heart Transplant Candidate Who Required Extra-Corporal Membrane Oxygenation (ECMO)

Soumya Pandey and Terry Harville

Our patient is a 14-year-old heart transplant candidate with dilated cardiomyopathy. HLA typing and anti-HLA antibody testing were performed as a part of initial pre-transplant work-up (Tables 54.1 and 54.2). The patient became quite ill while awaiting for a donor heart, and was placed on extra-corporal membrane oxygenation (ECMO) for ~9 days before being able to undergoing orthotopic heart transplantation. During this time, he also received multiple blood product transfusions including RBC and platelets. Results of pre-transplantation anti-HLA antibody studies are shown in Table 54.3.

Q1. Regarding the information in Tables 54.1 and 54.3, which statement is most correct?

A. This potential donor is not a suitable candidate, due to multiple HLA locus mismatches and presence of DSA, which could result in hyperacute rejection at the time of transplantation
B. A "virtual crossmatch" indicates this pair to be incompatible
C. The only potential DSA detected is anti-HLA-A∗02:06 with an MFI = 249, indicating this donor-patient pairing is compatible for transplantation
D. No further studies are required prior to transplantation

S. Pandey
Department of Pathology and Laboratory Services, University of Arkansas for Medical Sciences, Little Rock, AR, USA

T. Harville (✉)
Departments of Pathology and Laboratory Services, Pediatrics, and Internal Medicine, University of Arkansas for Medical Sciences, Little Rock, AR, USA
e-mail: harvilleterryo@uams.edu

© Springer Nature Switzerland AG 2020
F. Rahmani, N. Rezaei (eds.), *Pediatric Autoimmunity and Transplantation*,
https://doi.org/10.1007/978-3-030-26280-8_54

Table 54.1 Patient and donor HLA typing results for a heart transplant candidate

	A	B	C	DRB1	DRB3/4/5	DQB1	DQA1
Patient	*03:01	*07:02	*04:01	*01:01	–	*05:01	*01:01
	*03:01	*35:01	*07:01	*15:01	5*01:01	*06:02	*01:02
Serologic	3, 3	07 (Bw6), 35 (Bw6)	4, 7	1, 15	51, –	5, 6	–
Potential donor	*02:06	*35:01	*04:01	*08:02	–	*04:02	*04:01
	*32:01	*44:02	*07:01	*11:01	3*02:02	*03:01	*05:05
Serologic	2, 32	35 (Bw6), 39 (Bw6)	4, 7	8, 11	52, –	7, 4	–

The molecular and serologic equivalent HLA Typing results are presented by each locus for the patient in the upper three rows and potential donor in the bottom three rows. Note: HLA-DR1, –DR8, –DR10, and –DR103 do not typically express HLA-DRB3 (HLA-DR52), –DRB4 (–DR53), or –DRB5 (–DR51). HLA-DQA1 does not have a serologic equivalent. For absent alleles "–" is presented

Table 54.2 Anti-HLA antibody studies for a heart transplantation candidate

Serum date	Class I specificities (MFI)	Class II specificities
Two weeks pre-transplant	A*02:06 (249) A*02:01 (315) A*02:03 (420)	No significant DSA
At the time of transplant	A*02:06 (8092) A*02:01 (9551) A*02:03 (10,463)	No significant DSA
Day 2 post-transplant	A*02:06 (3043) A*02:01 (4662) A*02:03 (6139)	No significant DSA
Day 6 post-transplant	A*02:06 (1198) A*02:01 (1558) A*02:03 (1768)	No significant DSA
Day 9 post-transplant	A*02:06 (10,024) A*02:01 (11,999) A*02:03 (12,426)	No significant DSA
Day 25 post-transplant	A*02:06 (8480) A*02:01 (11780) A*02:03 (13,723)	No significant DSA
Day 60 post-transplant	A*02:06 (4075) A*02:01 (6088) A*02:03 (7601)	No significant DSA

The progressive changes in the anti-HLA antibody levels beginning pre-transplantation and extending to 2 months post-transplantation are listed. The MFI values are listed in the parentheses

Table 54.3 Pre-transplantation anti-HLA antibody studies for a heart transplant candidate

Serum date	Class I specificities	Class II specificities
Pre-transplant	A*02:06 (249 MFI) A*02:01 (315 MFI) A*02:03 (420 MFI)	No significant DSA

The anti-HLA Class I and Class II antibody specificities are listed from serum obtained at the initial evaluation. Donor-specific antibodies (DSA) with MFI > 1000 may result in positive fluorescence cytometric crossmatch (FCXM) [1]. DSA with MFI < 300 are likely clinically insignificant

E. The transfusions during ECMO are unlikely to have prompted antibody formation due to the short time before transplantation

Answer: *The correct answer is* ***C.***

This patient and donor were mismatched at multiple loci, but a careful scrutiny of the anti-HLA antibody results revealed absence of significant anti-class II DSA and no significant anti-class I DSA (A∗02:06 with 249 MFI). Based on the absence of DSA, a virtual crossmatch would be predicted to be negative.

Prospective testing, prior to transplantation, can be challenging for cardiac transplantation. The potential donor will be HLA typed by the originating organ procurement organization (OPO), for the information to be submitted to United Network for Organ Sharing (UNOS), in order for donor organ to be allocated. The patient will have studies performed at the transplant center, typically an initial anti-HLA antibody evaluation. Depending on the relative urgency of the need for transplantation, HLA typing of the patient may be deferred until the time of transplantation. In this case, though, the severity of the illness led to a more complete "up-front" evaluation with completion of HLA typing. When the patient is listed in UNOS as needing organ transplantation, anti-HLA antibodies deemed as relevant are inserted as "avoidance antigens" for the HLA types to which the antibodies are directed. This helps the allocation process by not offering the organ to a recipient who will likely have a positive crossmatch [2]. In this case, there were no avoidance HLA antigens listed, since no significant anti-HLA antibodies were originally detected. Once UNOS assigns a potential donor to a patient in the registry, the transplant center is alerted and is given an hour to determine whether they will accept the donor organ for transplantation. After the donor organs have been allocated and accepted at their respective transplant centers, the donor is removed from life-support and upon recognition of being deceased, the organs are harvested. Sometimes, the harvests are performed by the actual transplantation surgical team, who then fly with the organ back to the transplant center to perform the transplantation. Regardless, once harvested, there are only 4–6 h of time to complete the transplantation of a heart before it will become irreparably damaged due to the cold-ischemic time. The HLA laboratory typically requires 4–5 h to perform HLA typing studies (i.e. confirmatory typing for an imported organ) and the fluorescence cytometric crossmatch (FCXM), which is the current standard approach for determining compatibility for transplantation. Thus, the heart must be transplanted prior to knowing the confirmatory typing results and FCXM results. The FCXM is therefore known as a "retrospective" study, yet remains critically important for further decision making.

Q2. Which of the following actions is mandatory to perform prior to heart transplantation?

A. Matching HLA types of the donor and recipient
B. Proof that total anti-HLA antibodies below a certain cut-off to prevent rejection

C. Testing and confirmation of the ABO type of the donor and recipient on two separate specimens
D. A negative crossmatch must be confirmed negative a second time for validity
E. None of the above

Answer: *The correct answer is* ***C.***

Isohemagglutinins are the first and perhaps greatest impediment to successful solid organ transplantation. Indeed, the initial step in the allocation process is screening of the donor and recipient blood types. Due to instances in which ABO incompatible organs were transplanted a number of years ago, rules were placed to prevent this from being overlooked in the haste to transplant, when HLA studies appeared to demonstrate compatibility. The guidelines explicitly state, blood to "be drawn on two separate occasions, have different collection times, be submitted as separate samples, and have results indicating the same blood type". In addition, two different qualified health care professionals must evaluate the two results and sign-off on them. Just as anti-HLA antibodies can bind to the HLA expressed on endothelial cells, initiate complement activation, and promote vascular damage, the ubiquitous expression of type A and type B antigens on endothelial cells can result in vascular damage if the corresponding isohemagglutinin is present.

The FCXM was retrospectively performed using serum from the day of transplantation and was positive, whereas the initial serum specimen from 14 days earlier was negative. The FCXM is performed by incubating donor lymphocytes with patient/recipient serum, and using an anti-CD3 monoclonal antibody to identify T lymphocytes and an anti-CD19 monoclonal antibody to identify B lymphocytes. Human antibodies from the recipient serum binding to proteins expressed on the donor lymphocytes are detected using an anti-human IgG antibody. If the level of detection is above the defined cutoff, a positive crossmatch is reported. Under most circumstances, the major polymorphic cell-surface proteins to which antibodies can bind are HLA proteins. Thus, a positive FCXM generally indicates that DSA are present.

Q3. Select the most correct statement:

A. A T positive and B positive FCXM would indicate that only anti-class I antibodies are present, since HLA class I is expressed on essentially all nucleated cells
B. A T positive and B positive FCXM would indicate that only anti-class II antibodies are present, since HLA class II is expressed on essentially all nucleated cells
C. A T positive and B negative FCXM would be indicative of the presence of anti-class I antibodies, since B lymphocytes express much lower levels of class I HLA than T lymphocytes
D. A T positive and B positive FCXM would indicate that anti-class I antibodies are present, but cannot exclude the presence of anti-class II antibodies

Answer: *The correct answer is* ***D.***

Q4. Which statement is most correct?

A. The positive crossmatch at the time of transplantation was unlikely due to anti-HLA antibodies, as the 2 week interval from the initial specimen is not the sufficient time for anti-HLA antibodies of enough strength to develop and result in a positive crossmatch
B. The positive crossmatch indicates that anti-HLA antibodies are present
C. A positive crossmatch must always be considered with caution as possibly "false positive" in someone who has recently been anticoagulated on ECMO and has received blood product transfusions
D. Since a positive crossmatch indicates that the recipient has antibodies to both T and B lymphocytes from the donor, it is likely that both anti-class I and anti-class II antibodies are present
E. A retrospective crossmatch has less validity than a prospective crossmatch, considering the fact that the organ is already transplanted and functioning well

Answers: *The correct answer is* ***B.***

HLA proteins are the most polymorphic of all proteins expressed in human being. HLA will most likely be the target of antibody production when someone is exposed to someone else's blood product transfusions, organ transplantation, or during pregnancy. Someone with cardiac disease may be exposed during surgery, especially if undergoing heart-bypass, which requires donor blood to fill the machinery. HLA class I is found expressed on essentially all nucleated cells in the body, including T and B lymphocytes. While some differences in the HLA class I expression level may occur between T and B lymphocytes, depending on states of activation, the differences are typically not sufficient to result in a T positive B negative crossmatch, or vice versa. Thus the presence of anti-HLA class I DSA are expected to result in both T positive and B positive crossmatch. HLA class II is expressed on certain antigen-presenting cells, including B lymphocytes. Thus, a T negative and B positive crossmatch indicates the likely presence of anti-HLA class II DSA. Further, the presence of anti-HLA class I DSA may partially mask the presence of anti-HLA class II DSA, since the former will also result in a positive B lymphocyte crossmatch. Therefore, one cannot typically exclude the presence of anti-HLA class II DSA in the presence of anti-HLA class I DSA.

There were 2 weeks between the initial serum obtained without DSA being present, and the pre-transplant serum which produced a positive crossmatch due to DSA. During the last 9 days of the period, there were blood product exposures. Packed RBC generally have no more than one lymphocyte per microliter of blood. Conversely, platelets may have 500 lymphocytes per microliter. In addition, RBC do not typically have HLA expression (as they are non-nucleated cell), but platelets express class I HLA, which comes along with the budding membranes from their progenitor cells, megakaryocytes. Thus, platelet transfusions can generate a tremendous exposure to other person's HLA class I. During the primary immune response, we expect several days between the initial exposure and first IgM production, and another 10–14 days to have the HLA class I switched to IgG [3]. In this case, IgG anti-HLA production is "ramping up" in under 10 days. As noted, in patients with cardiac disease, prior exposure to other's HLA types is very likely, thus, this patient experienced a secondary antibody recall response, which allowed for the rapid escalation in DSA (Table 54.2).

Q5. Which of the following statements is most correct?

A. There is a continuing increase in DSA MFI during the time of study
B. The DSA MFI values fluctuation over the noted time intervals is occurring in a not-unexpected manner
C. The higher MFI values of the non-DSA antibodies is of concern
D. These results do not help explain the positive FCXM noted after transplantation

Answer: *The correct answer is* ***B.***

Q6. True or False: Exposure to transfused platelets during ECMO explains the positive anti-class I DSA

A. True
B. False

Answers: *The correct answer is* ***A.***

In this case, the DSA corresponds to anti-HLA-A∗02:06. Comparisons of epitopes for HLA-A∗02:06, A∗02:01, and A∗02:03 (http://www.epregistry.com.br/index/databases/database/ABC/), reveals that these do not share any exposed epitopes (although, they do share a non-exposed epitope). Thus, antibodies detected to each will be unique. As a consequence, only anti-A∗02:06, as a DSA, is relevant. In Table 54.2, there are initial low MFI values, which have greatly expanded within 9 days, and have resulted in a positive FCXM. This expansion is likely a secondary, or even tertiary, response to prior exposure to these specific HLA types. Also note the large fall in MFI noted on days 2 and 6 post-transplantation. This effect is thought to occur as antibodies in the circulating blood are binding the HLA expressed on the donor tissue, thereby reducing the serum levels detected. By 9 days post-transplantation, an increase is again noted, which is compatible with the timeframe required for memory B cells activation. Subsequently, the DSA begins to fall, but does not go away. Part of this may be due to some induced tolerance, as well as due to successful immunosuppressive therapy [2, 4, 5].

Endomyocardial biopsy performed on day 2 post-transplantation was interpreted as mild antibody-mediated rejection (i.e. AMR) with slight C4d deposition (positivity) noted. The detection of C4d is used as an indicator of complement deposition in AMR. The patient was treated with bolus corticosteroids, plasmapheresis, and intravenous immunoglobulin. During all this time, the patient was clinically stable. On the 24th day after transplantation, the patient began to experience chest pain. The follow-up endomyocardial biopsy was performed the next day and revealed no evidence for antibody-mediated rejection and C4d was negative, despite the continued presence of DSA. However, moderate acute cellular rejection (ISHLT Grade 2R) was diagnosed from the biopsy, and he subsequently received appropriate treatment.

Potential DSA can only be identified once a potential donor is identified. The presence of DSA results in risks for AMR. Yet, despite DSA remaining detectable there may not be clinically or biopsy apparent AMR in a patient, after successful treatment. Even a resolution of an originally present AMR might occur post transplantation. Further, treatment for AMR does not preclude the subsequent development of cellular-mediated rejection.

Q7. True or False: C1q study would be useful in this patient

A. True
B. False

Answer: *The correct answer is* **A.**

C1q analyses were performed. C1q was negative in the pre-transplantation specimen. Serum from at the time of transplantation through the specimen from the post-transplantation day 9 did have elevated anti-A*02:06 C1q MFI values. These would be consistent with the deposition of C4d and diagnosis of AMR. In contrast, by day 25 and the second month post-transplantation, the C1q assay did not detect any elevated MFI values. Thus, DSA capable of activation of complement appeared to have subsided and what is described as accommodation appears to have occurred. This further helps to explain the lack of evidence of AMR and C4d deposition at the day 25 biopsy.

Practical Points

- The HLA laboratory typically requires 4–5 h to perform HLA typing studies and fluorescence cytometric crossmatch (FCXM), therefore, the heart is typically transplanted prior to knowing the confirmatory typing and FCXM results
- The FCXM is therefore known as a "retrospective" study, yet remains critically important for further decision making
- The FCXM is performed by incubating donor lymphocytes with patient/recipient serum, and using an anti-CD3 monoclonal antibody to identify T lymphocytes and an anti-CD19 monoclonal antibody to identify B lymphocytes. Human antibodies from the recipient serum binding to proteins expressed on the donor lymphocytes are detected using an anti-human IgG antibody
- Detection of C4d deposition in endomyocardial biopsy confirms antibody-mediated rejection

References

1. Sullivan H, Gebel H, Bray R. Understanding solid-phase HLA antibody assays and the value of MFI. Hum Immunol. 2017;78(7–8):471–80.
2. Petersdorf EW, Gooley T, Malkki M, Horowitz M. Clinical significance of donor-recipient HLA matching on survival after myeloablative hematopoietic cell transplantation from unrelated donors. Tissue Antigens. 2007;69(Suppl 1):25–30.
3. Rosenbaum EPS, Harville TO, Drobena GA, Cottler-Fox M. Flow cytometric panel-reactive antibody results and the ability to find transfusion-compatible platelets after antibody-desensitization for allogeneic bone marrow transplant. Ann Clin Lab Sci. 2016;46(6):662–5.
4. Kampmann B, Hemingway C, Stephens A, Davidson R, Goodsall A, Anderson S, Nicol M, Scholvinck E, Relman D, Waddell S, Langford P, Sheehan B, Semple L, Wilkinson KA, Wilkinson RJ, Ress S, Hibberd M, Levin M. Acquired predisposition to mycobacterial disease due to autoantibodies to IFN-gamma. J Clin Invest. 2005;115(9):2480–8.
5. Amico P, Hönger G, Mayr M, Steiger J, Hopfer H, Schaub S. Clinical relevance of pretransplant donor-specific HLA antibodies detected by single-antigen flow-beads. Transplantation. 2009;87(11):1681–8.

Chapter 55
Acute Antibody-Mediated Rejection of Transplantation with Negative Prospective Crossmatch Results

Soumya Pandey and Terry Harville

The patient is a 16-year-old African American female with end-stage renal disease (ESRD) due to unknown cause, and requires renal transplantation. The patient underwent HLA typing and routine quarterly testing for anti-HLA antibodies as part of the pre-transplantation work-up. Pre-transplantation anti-HLA antibody testing showed consistent patterns of positive anti-B57, -B58, -B76, -C15 and -DP1 antibodies, for more than 2 years. Patient received several deceased-donor kidney offers, over the 5 years after being listed, finally being transplanted with the fifth potential donor at age 18 years (Table 55.1).

Q1. Based on the patient and potential donor HLA typing results in Table 55.1, which of the potential donors would you expect to have a positive virtual cross-match?

A. Potential donors 1, 2, and 3
B. Potential donors 4 and 5
C. Potential donor 3
D. All of the above
E. None of the above

Answer: *The correct answer is* ***E.***

S. Pandey
Department of Pathology and Laboratory Services, University of Arkansas for Medical Sciences, Little Rock, AR, USA

T. Harville (✉)
Departments of Pathology and Laboratory Services, Pediatrics, and Internal Medicine, University of Arkansas for Medical Sciences, Little Rock, AR, USA
e-mail: harvilleterryo@uams.edu

© Springer Nature Switzerland AG 2020

F. Rahmani, N. Rezaei (eds.), *Pediatric Autoimmunity and Transplantation*,
https://doi.org/10.1007/978-3-030-26280-8_55

Table 55.1 HLA-typing results for kidney transplant candidate patient

	A	B	C	DRB1	DRB3/4/5	DQB1
Patient	33	53	4	8	–	4
	68	x	x	18	52	5
Potential donor 1	3	51	14	8	–	5
	33	63	16	13	52	7
Potential donor 2	26	71	6	10	–	5
	29	13	10	16	51	5
Potential donor 3	2	7	1	103	–	6
	3	27	7	15	51	7
Potential donor 4	31	39	7	9	53	7
	68	x	12	14	–	9
Potential donor 5	1	7	7	103	–	2
	2	8	x	17	52	5

The serologic equivalent typing results are listed for the patient and potential donors for each HLA locus. When a second, different allele cannot be identified, or homozygosity may be present for an HLA locus, an "x" is listed. When an allele is not present, a dash, "–", is listed

In the absence of any significant elevated donor-specific antibodies (DSA) in the recipient, a crossmatch is expected to be negative. Typically, DSA with mean fluorescence intensity (MFI) >1000 could result in a positive fluorescence cytometric crossmatch (FCXM) with risks for antibody-mediated rejection (AMR) [1]. As noted above, the patient had anti-HLA antibodies against HLA-B57, -B58, -B76, -C15 and -DP1. Evaluation of patient's anti-HLA antibody profile and potential donor HLA typing results indicated that no significant DSA were present. Hence, a predicted virtual crossmatch should be negative with each of these donors [2].

Patient underwent FCXM at each time an offer was made. The first deceased-donor kidney offer revealed both T and B lymphocyte FCXM positive, despite absence of any potentially significant DSA with MFI > 1000. Patient did not receive the transplant. FCXM studies with a second donor were compatible, however, the kidney was transplanted to another recipient that was higher on the allocation list. Patient showed positive T and B lymphocyte FCXM with both third and fourth potential donors, despite the absence of potentially significant DSA with MFI >1000. Patient did not therefore receive the transplant from either potential donors 3 or 4.

When an offer was received from a fifth potential donor, lack of potentially significant DSA with MFI >1000 was again noted. FCXM was negative for both T and B-lymphocytes, and the patient was successfully transplanted, although there was concern about a prolonged cold-ischemic time prior to transplantation. The transplanted kidney began with poor function, consistent with this. It was thought that by 5 days post-transplantation the kidney function should have improved, but it was not. The transplant site was tender on palpation. The patient's heart rate and temperature had increased. Doppler ultrasound study demonstrated that there was reduced blood flow through the transplanted kidney.

Q2. Which statement is most correct?

A. The symptom and findings are consistent with prolonged acute tubular necrosis due to the prolonged cold-ischemic time.
B. The findings are most consistent with acute post-transplantation cellular rejection.
C. The findings are most consistent with reactivation of CMV due to the immunosuppressive therapy.
D. The findings are most consistent with development of BK viral infection of the urinary tract
E. The findings are most consistent with humoral rejection of the transplanted kidney

Answer: *The correct answer is* ***E.***

Increased cold-ischemic time can result in acute tubular necrosis (ATN). The symptoms are initially decreased urine output, with rise in serum creatinine, typically followed in 3–5 days by increased urine output. Hemofiltration or dialysis may be required as the kidney recovers. Our patient had no reported change in urine output. It would be rare for acute cellular rejection to occur so soon after transplantation. Moreover, we do not expect to find the reduction in blood flow acute rejection. CMV may reactivate, and can actually precipitate rejection, but again will not explain the reduction in blood flow, so soon after transplantation. BK viral infections of the urinary tract are recognized as problematic for transplanted patients, but this is not usually an acute post-transplantation issue. Humoral rejection is another term used to represent presence of AMR. Indeed, the word "humoral" may be a more correct term to use, as activation of the complement system, following antigen: antibody binding, is the reason for endothelial damage of the glomerular capillaries [2]. Activation of the complement system and ensuing cell damage, promotes clot formation and occlude the capillaries. Thus, reduction in blood flow through the transplanted kidney is an ominous finding for AMR or humoral rejection. The histopathologic findings include inflammation and damage of the capillaries with a neutrophilic infiltrate, as found in vasculitis, justifying the use of the term "vascular rejection".

A renal biopsy was then performed: the glomerular capillaries were swollen, clots were present, and neutrophils were found in, and surrounding the vessels. IgG, C3, C4, and C4d were detected in the capillaries by immunofluorescence studies, all compatible with a diagnosis of acute AMR (i.e. humoral or vascular rejection). The tissue also appeared to become necrotic. Unfortunately, serum creatinine levels increased back to pre-transplant status and the following day, a nephrectomy was performed. The histopathologic diagnosis from the explant was the same as from the biopsy, severe antibody-mediated rejection.

A quandary was present. The course and histopathologic evidence was compatible with AMR, yet DSA were not present for at least 2 years prior to transplantation, which is a common interval to justify reexamination. Follow-up anti-HLA antibodies studies were performed (Table 55.2).

Table 55.2 Anti-HLA antibody results from the patient undergoing kidney transplantation in different time periods

Serum date	Anti-HLA Class I specificities (MFI)	Anti-HLA Class I specificities (MFI)
Pre-transplantation	B57 (~12 K) B58 (~8 K) B76 and Cw15 (1000–3000)	DP1 (1000–3000 MFI)
6 days post-transplantation	B57, B58, A2* (>10,000) B8* (5000-10,000) B63 (3000–5000) B73, B59, Cw15 (1000–3000)	DR103*, DR51, DR1, DR9 (5000–10,000) DR15, DR16 (3000–5000) DP28, DP4, DP1, DP18, DP2, DP23 (1000–3000)
5 months post-transplantation	B57, B58, A2*, B8* (>10,000) B7*, 67, 81, 2708, 42, 44, 56, 59, 82, A1* (5000–10,000) B54, 60, 27, 61, 48, 76 (3000–5000) B39, 50, 41, 35, 18, 72, 61, 45, 73, 62, 75, 46, 71, 78, 64, 65, Cw10, 9, A36 (1000–3000)	DR103* (3000–5000) DR15, DR16, DR1, DR51, DR9, DQ2* (1000–3000)

Anti-HLA Class I and Class II antibodies are listed by their specificities, with the MFI values in parentheses. "*": DSA: donor-specific antibodies

Please compare the above to results presented in Tables 55.1 and 55.2.

Q3. True or False: Elevated donor-specific antibodies were detected at the time AMR was diagnosed

A. True
B. False

Answer: *The correct answer is* ***A.***

Q4. Which of the statements below is most correct?

A. Development of DSA from primary exposure can be expected within 5 days of transplantation
B. De novo antibody production is a common cause of acute AMR in the first 7–10 days post-transplantation
C. DSA developing within 5 days of transplantation indicates there had been prior exposure to the antigen
D. Pre-formed anti-HLA antibodies could be responsible for the negative cross-match and evidence of rejection on day 5
E. Anti-HLA class II antibodies are more likely responsible for the histopathologic changes observed in this case, than anti-class I antibodies

Answers: *The correct answer is* ***C.***

The data in Tables 55.1 and 55.2 indicate anti-A2, anti-B8, and anti-DR103 DSA were detectable by the time AMR was diagnosed. Yet, these had not been detected for the two-years prior to transplantation. Flash back over of the patients records did indicate that early in her course of disease, she required blood product transfusions, and 5 years prior to transplantation anti-A2 was detected on two occasions at ~1500 MFI and ~2000 MFI, but subsequently was <500 MFI on some 16 additional analyses later performed. Therefore, there is evidence for prior exposure with blood products and prior presence of DSA. In order to facilitate renal transplantation, most specialists review data from at least 2 years prior to transplantation to make decision regarding the particular donor to be used for transplantation. It is thought to be rare for an antibody detected previously, to resurface and increase so rapidly post-transplantation. This case is exceptional, but does demonstrate the rapidity of a secondary or tertiary antibody response to recall antigen. Antibody response to de novo exposure is not expected to result in significant DSA titters, not until at least 14 days post-transplantation. It might take up to a month before DSA levels are sufficiently high to result in AMR. Moreover, cells are armed with surface complement regulatory proteins to help prevent alternative activation of complement pathway. Thus, there is a threshold, beyond which, there is sufficient concentration and antibody affinity to allow antibodies to be able to initiate complement activation, and subsequent AMR. Anti-HLA class I antibodies mediate endothelial damage, due to the ubiquitous presence of expression of HLA class I on nucleated cells in the body.

The C1q assay is very useful for indicating the antibodies most likely to activate complement through the initial binding of C1q. For this purpose, patient's samples of stored serum, dating back 3 years ago, all through the post-transplantation period were reevaluated. All the pre-transplantation specimens DSA had 0 MFI values for the C1q assay. The post-transplantation specimens had MFI values similar to the routine assay results [1]. Thus, the post-transplantation results were suggestive for an ability to mount complement response by the detected DSA, whereas the pre-transplantation specimens did not.

Q5. True or False: Based on the C1q information, the patient: donor pairing should have been deferred, despite the negative FCXM

A. True
B. False

Answer: *The correct answer is **B.***

DSA were not detected for more than 4 years prior to the transplant. C1q results were negative for 3 years prior to the transplant. The FCXM were negative in the current fresh serum from the patient obtained on the day of transplantation, as well as three prior sera spanning the previous 2 years. This accelerated form of antibody-mediated rejection would have been impossible to predict.

Practical Points

- This case illustrates there will always be additional factors present that can interfere with successful transplantation.
- When an unexpected acute/hyper acute rejection occurs, all data are reviewed and results of all donor specific antibodies (DSA) and fluores-

cence cytometric crossmatch (FCXM) are recollected, even if a particular DSA was previously elevated only in the remote past
- If there may be a more suitable recipient available for the donor, then it might be reasonable to defer the donor to those who do not have DSA or positive FCXM, even if positive only in one occasion

References

1. Sullivan H, Gebel H, Bray R. Understanding solid-phase HLA antibody assays and the value of MFI. Hum Immunol. 2017;78(7–8):471–80.
2. Schinstock C, Gandhi M, Stegall M. Interpreting anti-HLA antibody testing data: a practical guide for physicians. Transplantation. 2016;100(8):1619–28.

Chapter 56
Kidney Transplantation in a Patient with End Stage Renal Disease (ESRD) Secondary to Focal Segmental Glomerulosclerosis

Soumya Pandey and Terry Harville

The patient is a 16-year-old Caucasian male with end stage renal disease (ESRD) secondary to focal segmental glomerulosclerosis (FSGS) requiring renal transplant. Patient underwent evaluation for HLA typing and anti-HLA antibody testing as part of the routine pre-transplantation workup. Anti-HLA antibodies were not detected in the patient [1]. A potential living-donor became available (Table 56.1).

Q1. Which statement is most correct?

A. The patient and potential donor share a compatible haplotype including HLA-B44, HLA-Cw7, and HLA-DR52
B. A predicted virtual crossmatch would be positive in this scenario
C. This potential living-donor would appear to be compatible for transplantation

Table 56.1 HLA typing results for the patient and his potential donor undergoing kidney transplantation

	A	B	C	DR	DR(51, 52, 53)	DQ
Patient	11	8	5	17	52	2
	32	44	7	12	52	7
Potential living-donor	2	7	7	13	52	6
	29	44	16	15	51	6

The serologic equivalent HLA type is list by each locus for the patient and potential living-donor

S. Pandey
Department of Pathology and Laboratory Services, University of Arkansas for Medical Sciences, Little Rock, AR, USA

T. Harville (✉)
Departments of Pathology and Laboratory Services, Pediatrics, and Internal Medicine, University of Arkansas for Medical Sciences, Little Rock, AR, USA
e-mail: harvilleterryo@uams.edu

© Springer Nature Switzerland AG 2020

F. Rahmani, N. Rezaei (eds.), *Pediatric Autoimmunity and Transplantation*,
https://doi.org/10.1007/978-3-030-26280-8_56

D. The overall lack of HLA-matching argues against renal transplantation
E. Patients with FSGS generally do very well with renal transplantation, with low risk of graft loss

Answer: *The correct answer is* ***C.***

An HLA haplotype includes all of the HLA loci from one chromosome, therefore this patient: donor pair do not share a haplotype. Based on the HLA typing results, the patient and donor are 1/6 matched: mismatched at both HLA-A loci, one -B locus, and both -DR loci. A virtual crossmatch would be predicted to be negative, since the patient has no anti-HLA antibodies detected. Since the introduction of calcineurin inhibitors HLA matching is not considered an important criterion for donor selection, therefore, this pair would appear to be compatible. An issue to be always considered is FSGS recurrence in transplanted kidney allograft which is reported to be as high as 50% in some cohorts [2, 3]. A physical examination was performed and was negative.

Q2. Which of the following is a primary concern in the initial donor selection?

A. Donor gender match with the patient to minimize disease recurrence risks
B. Donor ethnicity match with the patient to minimize disease recurrence risks
C. Donor ABO status match with the patient to minimize risk of acute rejection
D. Donor risk factors for developing FSGS to minimize disease recurrence risks
E. All of the above

Answer: *The correct answer is* ***C.***

The initial primary consideration for potential donor selection is always the matching of ABO blood type between the patient and the potential donor. There are a few centers, which have protocols for "desensitizing" the patient in order to receive an ABO-mismatched transplant, but most centers transplant via UNOS allocation with ABO-matching as the initial, critical decision step. While it may be difficult to find a suitable donor for a multiparous female patient, with multiple positive elevated donor-specific antibodies (DSA), in comparison with a young male with no history of prior transfusions or transplantation, the patient and donor gender mismatch does not generally have additional consequences. However, there have been concerns about such as female immune reactivity against male Y-antigen (i.e. male donor into female recipient), but for the most, such concerns have not transpired into clinical consequences. Immunologic issues associated with HLA type variability due to ethnic differences, have been overcome through the use of calcineurin inhibitors for immune suppression.

The underlying diagnosis resulting in renal loss may also be an important consideration, particularly when a living donor is being considered, as in this case. Many conditions, which result in renal loss, may recur after transplantation. Systemic lupus erythematosus (SLE) recurrence is as high as 30%, which may result in a 5% loss of transplanted kidneys. Membranoproliferative glomerulonephritis recurrence may be as high as 100% and result in a 60% loss of transplanted kidneys. Atypical HUS recurrence may be as high as 80% and may result in an 80%

loss of transplanted kidneys [4]. Finally, FSGS may return in 50% of the patients with a 60% loss of the transplanted kidneys [4].

Thus, the decision to use a living- or a deceased-donor in such situations may not be easy. There may be loss of the transplanted kidney due to disease recurrence. Moreover, while the risk of renal failure in a donor is somewhat low, there is risk for the donor to need a kidney transplant. UNOS prioritizes previous living-donors if they subsequently need a kidney transplant. Additionally, there are potentials for morbidity and mortality in the donor from the procedures used for harvesting the donor organ. The patient and donor need to understand fully the potential risks.

Q3. Which statement is most correct regarding patients who develop end-stage renal disease due to SLE?

A. The patient should forgo dialysis and be transplanted via a living- or deceased donor, in order to reduce the morbidity associated with dialysis
B. Living-donation should not be considered due to recurrence risks
C. When disease is in full remission, at least 2 years after renal failure and dialysis, disease recurrence in the transplanted kidney is low
D. Late recurrence in the transplanted kidney is common, due to resurgence of remitted disease in SLE
E. SLE rarely goes into remission after renal failure

Answer: *The correct answer is* ***C.***

Fortunately, for patients with SLE, after the onset of renal failure, disease may begin to go into remission. Many physicians prefer to allow the patient with ESRD resulting from SLE to go on dialysis for a couple of years, test and demonstrate laboratory evidence of remission, and then list for transplantation.

Q4. Which of the following statements is most correct, regarding patients with FSGS and ESRD?

A. The patient should be maintained on dialysis and forgo transplantation due to recurrence risks
B. Living-donation should not be considered due to recurrence risks
C. Patient should be eligible for transplantation with ESRD
D. Late recurrence in the transplanted kidney is common, due to resurgence of remitted disease with FSGS
E. FSGS rarely goes into remission after renal failure

Answer: *The correct answer is* ***C.***

The recurrence rate for FSGS may be as high as 50% in the transplanted kidney, with as high as 60% graft loss [5]. Yet, modern therapy, such as plasmapheresis, intravenous immunoglobulin, rituximab, and abatacept, have demonstrated great beneficial effects for disease treatment, as well as, with disease recurrence in renal allografts [2]. This has provided a momentum by some, to transplant patients with FSGS with living-donors, which seem to have better outcomes as reported by some studies. Deceased-donors may also be used and are reported to have better outcomes in some studies.

From the ethical perspective, we must consider the potential morbidity and mortality to the donor and patient, as well as, greatly increased costs for dealing with the consequences, to the patient, family, and society, in case of disease recurrence in the living-donor kidney allograft [2]. Additional consideration is the potential loss of deceased-donor organ, which could have been successfully transplanted into someone else. Nonetheless must also advocate for the patient with FSGS to receive a kidney transplant to help with their quality of life, one half or more will not experience recurrence, and even in those who have, up to 40% maintain their allograft [5]. This can be a difficult situation to make decision and requires good physician: patient communication.

In this particular case, the donor and patient were ABO matched and cross-match compatible. Both donor and patient underwent counselling and decided not to proceed with transplantation. The patient was ultimately transplanted with a compatible deceased-donor kidney, and has continued to do well.

Practical Points

- Successful solid organ transplantation is a result of good communication between the laboratories and physician
- The technology continues to advance, sometimes at a pace that transcends the interpretation and implementation of the results
- We shall continue to educate ourselves, to better understand what is going on and to provide the best care possible for our patients

References

1. Abbott K, Sawyers E, Oliver JD 3rd, Ko C, Kirk A, Welch P, Peters T, Agodoa L. Graft loss due to recurrent focal segmental glomerulosclerosis in renal transplant recipients in the United States. Am J Kidney Dis. 2001;37(2):366–73.
2. Cibrik D, Kaplan B, Campbell D, Meier-Kriesche H. Renal allograft survival in transplant recipients with focal segmental glomerulosclerosis. Am J Transplant. 2003;3(1):64–7.
3. South A, Grimm P. Transplant immuno-diagnostics: crossmatch and antigen detection. Pediatr Nephrol. 2016;6:897–905.
4. Cochat P, Fargue S, Mestrallet G, Jungraithmayr T, Koch-Nogueira P, Ranchin B, Zimmerhackl L. Disease recurrence in paediatric renal transplantation. Pediatr Nephrol. 2009;24:2097–108.
5. Kang HG, Ha I-S, Cheong HI. Recurrence and treatment after renal transplantation in children with FSGS. Biomed Res Int. 2016;2016:1–7.

Chapter 57
Itchy Violaceous Plaques

Yan Ling Kong and Emily Yiping Gan

A 12-year-old girl presented with a 5-year history of photo-aggravated rashes that started on her arms, but gradually progressed to involve her trunk, limbs and then face. The rash was occasionally itchy. Mucosal surfaces were uninvolved and there was no associated hair loss. She had tried application of topical steroids of various potencies, with no improvement. On examination, there were violaceous, hyperpigmented indurated plaques with atrophic scarring and overlying thick adherent scales on her forehead, extending to the frontotemporal scalp and involving the ears, cheeks, nose, arms, elbows and shins (Fig. 57.1). There was no scalp alopecia. She had two elder siblings with no similar complaints, and there was no family history of skin diseases or autoimmune conditions.

Laboratory data revealed: WBC: 3500/μL (neutrophils: 52.5%, lymphocytes: 36%, monocytes: 11%, eosinophils: 0.5%), hematocrit: 35%, Hb: 11.7 g/dL, platelet: 321,000/μL and ESR: 34 mm/h. Anti-nuclear antibody was positive with a titter of 1:100 with speckled pattern, along with anti-double stranded DNA antibody (anti-dsDNA), and anti-ribonucleoprotein. Serum C3 (10.7 mg/L) and C4 (23 mg/L) were normal.

Q1. What is the most likely diagnosis?

A. Acute cutaneous lupus erythematosus
B. Subacute cutaneous lupus erythematosus
C. Discoid lupus erythematosus
D. Lichen planus

Answer: *The correct answer is* ***C.***

Y. L. Kong
National Skin Centre, Singapore, Singapore

E. Y. Gan (✉)
Dermatology Service, KK Women's and Children's Hospital, Singapore, Singapore

© Springer Nature Switzerland AG 2020

F. Rahmani, N. Rezaei (eds.), *Pediatric Autoimmunity and Transplantation*,
https://doi.org/10.1007/978-3-030-26280-8_57

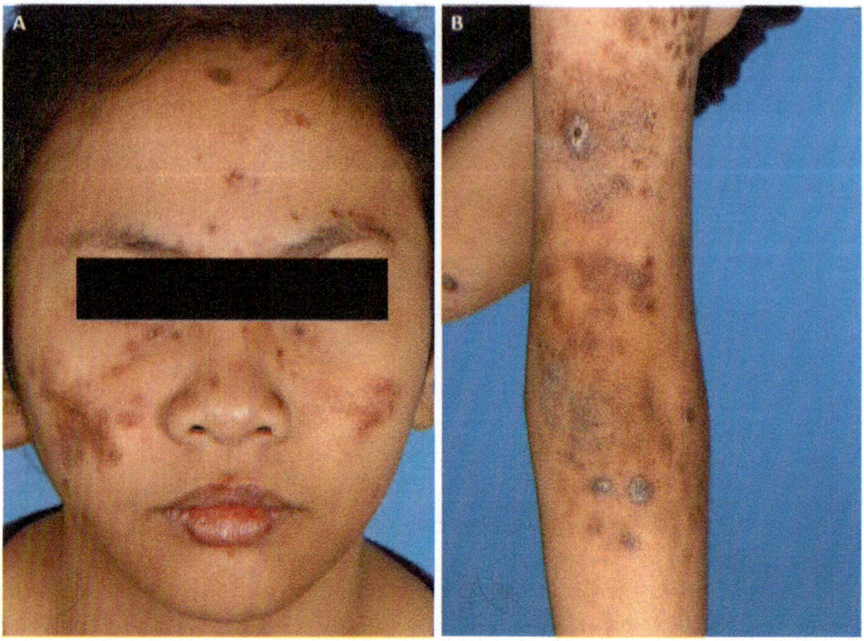

Fig. 57.1 Hyperpigmented plaques and papules with thick adherent scales over the patient's (**a**) face and (**b**) upper limb

Table 57.1 Lupus erythematosus specific skin disease

A. Acute Cutaneous LE (ACLE)	1. Localized ACLE (malar rash) 2. Generalized ACLE (morbiliform) 3. Toxic epidermal necrolysis-like ACLE
B. Subacute Cutaneous LE (SCLE)	1. Annular SCLE 2. Papulosquamous SCLE 3. Toxic epidermal necrolysis-like SCLE
C. Chronic Cutaneous LE (CCLE)	1. Discoid LE (DLE) (a) Classic DLE • Localized DLE • Generalized DLE (b) Hypertrophic DLE (c) Mucosal DLE • Oral DLE • Conjunctival DLE • Nasal DLE • Genital DLE 2. Tumid LE 3. Lupus panniculitis 4. Chilblain LE 5. Lichenoid LE (LE-lichen planus overlap)

LE lupus erythematosus

Cutaneous lupus erythematosus may occur independently, or as a feature of systemic lupus erythematosus (SLE). Cutaneous lupus erythematosus (LE) includes three subtypes as illustrated in Table 57.1: acute cutaneous lupus erythematosus

(ACLE), subacute cutaneous lupus erythematosus (i.e. SCLE), and chronic cutaneous lupus erythematosus (CCLE) [1].

This patient has discoid lupus erythematosus (DLE), which is the most common subtype of CCLE [2]. It is characterized by well demarcated erythematous papules or plaques with an adherent scale, extending down into follicular orifices. With time, skin lesions demonstrate a depressed, depigmented and scarred center with peripheral hyperpigmentation. Progression of follicular involvement eventually results in scarring alopecia. Commonly affected sites include the scalp, face, ears (at the external canal and conchal bowl), V-part of the neck and the extensors arms. Patients may also develop nail changes including dystrophy, pitting, leukonychia striata, onycholysis, clubbing, nail bed erythema and telangiectasia [3]. DLE is in turn subdivided into localized DLE, where lesions are found only above the neck, and the generalized form, where lesions may occur both above and below the neck [2]. Anti-RNP antibodies are present in approximately 20–30% of patients with SLE, but are uncommon in patients with DLE only [4, 5]. The presence of high levels of anti-RNP antibodies in patients presenting with lesions consistent with DLE might be indicative of associated SLE [5].

Q2. A skin biopsy was performed. What are the expected histology and direct immunofluorescence (DIF) findings?

A. Spongiotic dermatitis, basement membrane thickening, increase in dermal mucin; negative DIF
B. Interface dermatitis, basement membrane thickening, increase in dermal mucin; linear IgG and C3 at the dermal-epidermal junction
C. Psoriasiform dermatitis, no basement membrane thickening, increase in dermal mucin; granular band-like C3, IgG, IgM, C1q at the dermal-epidermal junction
D. Interface dermatitis, basement membrane thickening, increase in dermal mucin; granular band-like C3, IgG, IgM, C1q at the dermal-epidermal junction

Answer: *The correct answer is* ***D.***

Histologically, DLE is characterized by the presence of hyperkeratosis, epidermal hyperplasia, follicular plugging and interface dermatitis (Fig. 57.2). The basement membrane is usually thickened and there is an increase in dermal mucin (Fig. 57.3). Mononuclear cell infiltrates are also present in the perivascular, perifollicular areas and at the dermal-epidermal junction [3]. DIF demonstrates granular band-like immune deposits in multiple classes of C3, IgG, IgM and C1q at the dermal-epidermal junction, also known as the "lupus band test"[3, 6]. Positive DIF is found in up to 60% of patients with DLE, especially when the specimen is taken from a longstanding lesion (>2 months) on sun-exposed skin [7]. Positive DIF on non-lesional skin of a patient with DLE may be predictive of conversion to SLE.

Q3. What is the first-line oral agent used to treat this condition?

A. Hydroxychloroquine
B. Azathioprine
C. Methotrexate
D. Acitretin

Answer: *The correct answer is* ***A.***

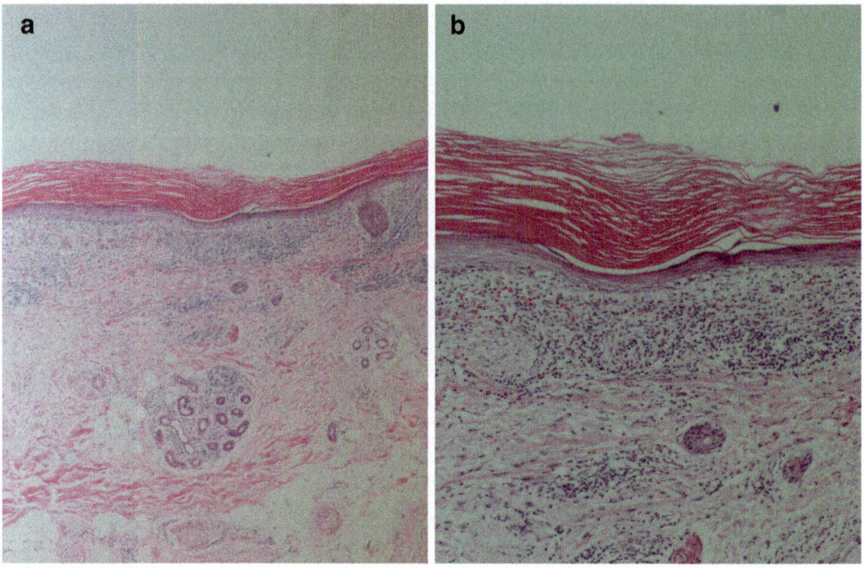

Fig. 57.2 Skin biopsy demonstrating hyperkeratosis, epidermal hyperplasia, follicular plugging and interface dermatitis (**a**) Hematoxylin and eosin, magnification ×40, (**b**) Hematoxylin and eosin, magnification ×100

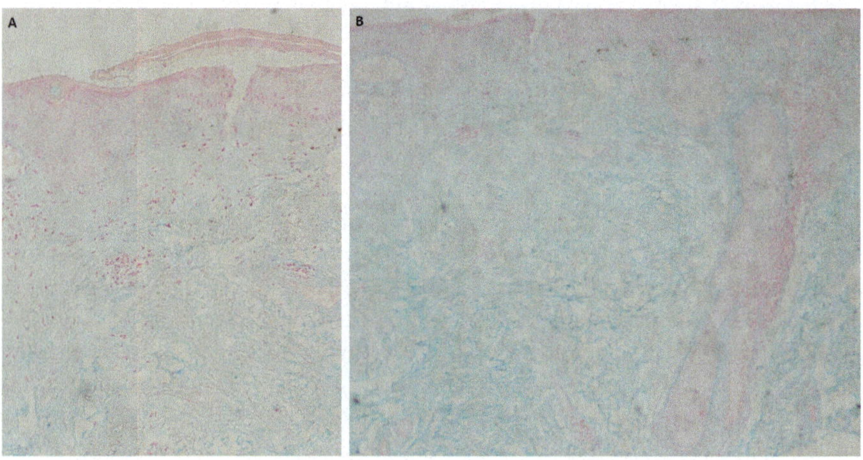

Fig. 57.3 (**a**) and (**b**): Increased mucin in the dermis (Alcian blue, magnification ×40)

Systemic antimalarial agents are the main class of drugs used in the treatment of all subtypes of cutaneous LE. Examples of antimalarial agents include hydroxychloroquine, quinacrine and chloroquine [7]. They provide effective immunomodulation by inhibiting the activation of intracellular toll-like receptors 7 and 9, which in turn downregulates interferon-alpha, a key cytokine in the pathogenesis of lupus [8]. Response to antimalarial drugs is slow and effect is seen only after 1–2 months.

The patient was started on the drug above. Five-years after initiation of treatment, she started complaining of blurred vision and reduced color vision.

Q4. What is the most serious eye complication associated with the use of the above drug?

A. Retinal detachment
B. Bull's eye maculopathy
C. Closed-angle glaucoma
D. Anterior uveitis

Answer: *The correct answer is* ***B.***

The most concerning side effect of antimalarial agents is retinal toxicity. Risk of retinopathy is dependent on daily dose and duration of use. Risk of retinopathy is higher when the daily dose of hydroxychloroquine exceeds 5 mg/Kg of actual body weight, or 2.3 mg/Kg of actual body weight for chloroquine [9]. At recommended doses, the risk of toxicity remains under 2% up to the first 10 years of use, but rises to almost 20% after 20 years [9]. Other risk factors include extremes of weight, impaired renal or liver function, and presence of pre-existing retinal or macular disease [9, 10].

Earliest retinal abnormalities are asymptomatic and can only be detected by ocular examination. Findings include fine pigment stippling and edema of the macula, increased pigmentation, and loss of the foveal reflex. At this stage, the retinopathy is reversible upon discontinuation of the culprit drug. In advanced macular disease, an irregular central pigmentation of the macula is surrounded a zone of depigmentation of the retinal pigment epithelium, termed as "bull's eye maculopathy". This is a true retinopathy that is generally not reversible [10].

As per the recommendations from the American Academy of Ophthalmology, a baseline fundus examination should be performed for all patients prior to initiating antimalarial agents, to rule out pre-existing maculopathy. Annual screening should begin 5 years after starting the therapy for patients on recommended dosages and with no other risk factors. Regular screening may be commenced earlier for patients with risk factors [9].

Q5. How would you estimate her risk for developing systemic lupus erythematosus?

A. 1–2%
B. 5–10%
C. 15–30%
D. 50–60%
E. 80–90%

Answer: *The correct answer is* ***C.***

Data on the risk for progression of DLE to SLE is limited to retrospective and cross-sectional studies. Progression to SLE is more likely with generalized DLE (15–30%) than with localized disease (5–10%) [11, 12]. Other risk factors for progression of DLE to SLE include: presence of arthritis and hematological abnormalities in terms of elevated ESR, high anti-nuclear antibody (ANA) titers, leukopenia, lymphopenia and anemia [11]. Association of SLE is strongest in patients with ACLE (>90%), followed by SCLE (50%) [13, 14]. Patients with lupus panniculitis (5–10%) and tumid LE rarely develop SLE [15].

Practical Points

- Discoid lupus erythematosus is the most common subtype of chronic cutaneous lupus erythematosus and is characterized by well-demarcated scaly erythematous papules or plaques extending down into follicular orifices
- Discoid lupus erythematosus may be localized or generalized. The generalized form has a stronger association with SLE
- Hyperkeratosis, epidermal hyperplasia, follicular plugging, interface dermatitis, thickened basement membrane and an increase in dermal mucin are histological features of discoid lupus erythematosus
- Direct immunofluorescence demonstrates granular band-like deposition of C3, IgG, IgM and C1q at the dermal-epidermal junction
- Systemic anti-malaria drugs, such as hydroxychloroquine, are the mainstay treatment for all subtypes of cutaneous lupus erythematosus
- The most concerning adverse effect of anti-malaria drug is retinal toxicity
- Advanced retinopathy as a result of anti-malaria drugs is generally irreversible

References

1. Grönhagen CM, Nyberg F. Cutaneous lupus erythematosus: an update. Indian Dermatol Online J. 2014;5(1):7–13.
2. Ribero S, Sciascia S, Borradori L, Lipsker D. The cutaneous spectrum of lupus erythematosus. Clin Rev Allergy Immunol. 2017;53(3):291–305.
3. Rothfield N, Sontheimer RD, Bernstein M. Lupus erythematosus: systemic and cutaneous manifestations. Clin Dermatol. 2006;24(5):348–62.
4. Cozzani E, Drosera M, Gasparini G, Parodi A. Serology of lupus erythematosus: correlation between immunopathological features and clinical aspects. Autoimmune Dis. 2014;2014:321359.
5. Vasquez R, Tseng LC, Victor S, Zhang S, Chong BF. Autoantibody and clinical profiles in patients with discoid lupus and borderline systemic lupus. Arch Dermatol. 2012;148(5):651–5.
6. Ohata C, Ohyama B, Nagata H, Furumura M, Nakama T. Comparative study of direct immunofluorescence in discoid lupus erythematosus and bullous pemphigoid. Am J Dermatopathol. 2016;38(2):121–3.
7. Ng PP, Tan SH, Koh ET, Tan T. Epidemiology of cutaneous lupus erythematosus in a tertiary referral Centre in Singapore. Australas J Dermatol. 2000;41:229–33.
8. Costedoat-Chalumeau N, Dunogue B, Morel N, Le Guern V, Guettrot-Imbert G. Hydroxychloroquine: a multifaceted treatment in lupus. Presse Med. 2014;43(6. Pt 2):e167–80.
9. Marmor MF, Kellner U, Lai TY, Melles RB, Mieler WF. Recommendations on screening for chloroquine and hydroxychloroquine retinopathy (2016 revision). Ophthalmology. 2016;123(6):1386–94.

10. Geamanu Panca A, Popa-Cherecheanu A, Marinescu B, Geamanu CD, Voinea LM. Retinal toxicity associated with chronic exposure to hydroxychloroquine and its ocular screening. Review. J Med Life. 2014;7(3):322–6.
11. Chong BF, Song J, Olsen NJ. Determining risk factors for developing systemic lupus erythematosus in patients with discoid lupus erythematosus. Br J Dermatol. 2012;166(1):29–35.
12. Vera-Recabarren MA, Garcia-Carrasco M, Ramos-Casals M, Herrero C. Comparative analysis of subacute cutaneous lupus erythematosus and chronic cutaneous lupus erythematosus: clinical and immunological study of 270 patients. Br J Dermatol. 2010;162(1):91–101.
13. Watanabe T, Tsuchida T. Classification of lupus erythematosus based upon cutaneous manifestations. Dermatological, systemic and laboratory findings in 191 patients. Dermatology. 1995;190(4):277–83.
14. Sontheimer RD. Subacute cutaneous lupus erythematosus: 25-year evolution of a prototypic subset (subphenotype) of lupus erythematosus defined by characteristic cutaneous, pathological, immunological, and genetic findings. Autoimmun Rev. 2005;4(5):253–63.
15. Watanabe T, Tsuchida T. Lupus erythematosus profundus: a cutaneous marker for a distinct clinical subset? Br J Dermatol. 1996;134(1):123–5.

Chapter 58
Photosensitivity and Bullous Lesions

Ashi and Piyush Kumar

An 11-year old girl presented with crusted lesions over face (Fig. 58.1), upper limbs and lower back (Fig. 58.2), since 15 days. She also had oral erosions leading to difficulty in eating for the last 10 days. Lesions started as fluid-filled vesicles over her face, upper limbs, and lower back after prolonged sun-exposure while working in farm, associated with itching and burning sensation and finally rupturing to form crusts. She had on and off fever without chills or rigor, joint pain of both small and large joints, joint swelling, and also photosensitivity for the past 1 month. The rest of her physical examination and past medical history were not significant. There was no history of similar illness in family members.

Laboratory data revealed: WBC: 5500/μL (neutrophils: 72%, lymphocytes: 24%, monocytes: 3%, eosinophils: 1%); hematocrit: 38%, Hb: 8 g/dL, platelet: 120,000/μL, FBS: 72, ESR: 60 mm/h, CRP:4 mg/dL. Liver and renal function tests were within normal range, yet she had albumin in her urinalysis. Her antinuclear antibody was positive with a titre of 1:2560, as well as anti-double-stranded DNA antibody (anti-dsDNA). Her anti-Smith, anti-histone-negative, and anti-ribosomal-P- antibodies were negative. Based on clinical presentation and investigation findings, her condition was diagnosed as systemic lupus erythematosus (SLE). Her skin condition was as bullous SLE.

Systemic lupus erythematosus (SLE) is an autoimmune connective tissue disorder characterized by multisystem organ inflammation, most commonly the skin, joints and vasculature, and associated immunological abnormalities [1]. The first classification criteria were developed by the American College of Rheumatology (ACR) in 1971 and were modified in 1982 [1]. It consists of 11 criteria out of which at least 4 should be fulfilled to diagnose SLE in a patient. Recent systemic lupus

Ashi
Gauhati Medical College, Guwahati, Assam, India

P. Kumar (✉)
Department of Dermatology, Katihar Medical College, Katihar, Bihar, India

© Springer Nature Switzerland AG 2020

F. Rahmani, N. Rezaei (eds.), *Pediatric Autoimmunity and Transplantation*,
https://doi.org/10.1007/978-3-030-26280-8_58

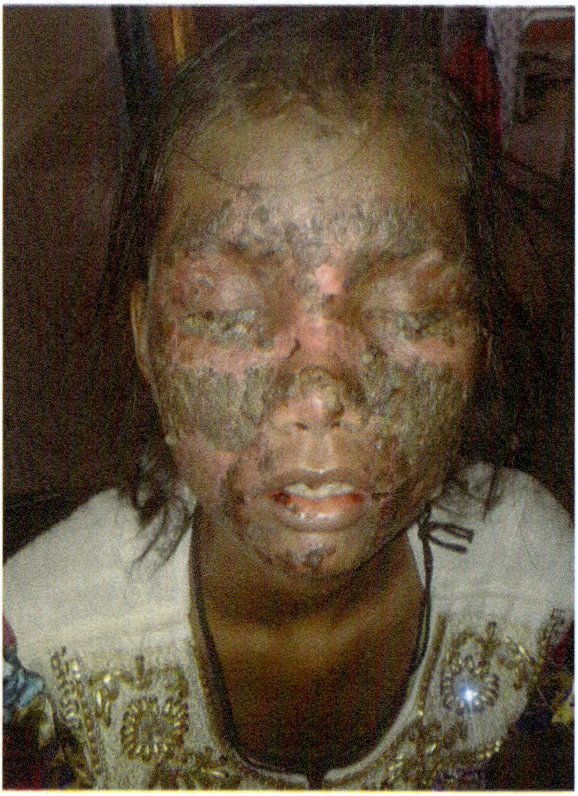

Fig. 58.1 Crusted lesions on the face of an 11-year-old girl

international collaborating clinics (SLICC) criteria has been shown to have greater sensitivity (94% versus 86%) and equal specificity (92% versus 93%) when compared to ACR criteria [2].

Diagnosis of systemic lupus erythematosus cannot be made by serology for antinuclear antibody (ANA) or anti- dsDNA antibody alone. ANA is non-specific and can be found in many autoimmune conditions like dermatomyositis and scleroderma as well. Though anti-dsDNA is specific for lupus, but not all cases of SLE exhibit anti-ds DNA antibody [2].

Q1. All of the following tests are mandatory in this patient, except:

A. Chest X-ray
B. 24-hours urinary protein
C. Ultrasonography of whole abdomen
D. Echocardiography

Answer: *The correct answer is* ***D.***

Since SLE is a disease with systemic involvement, chest X-ray and abdominal ultrasonography should be done to rule out serositis which is also one of the criteria of SLE.

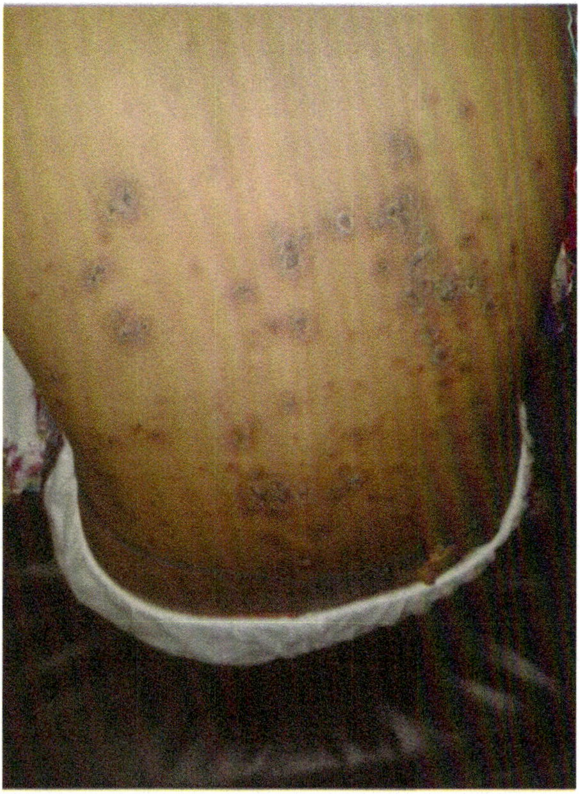

Fig. 58.2 Crusted lesions on the sun-covered areas of the back in an 11-year-old girl

24-hours urinary protein will help to rule out renal involvement as a value greater than 500 mg is suggestive of renal involvement which warrants renal biopsy [2]. Echocardiography is not necessary as pericardial or pleural friction rub can easily be detected via stethoscope. No further cardiac workup is necessary if the patient does not have any complaints.

Q2. What is the significance of ordering histopathology and direct immunofluorescence in this patient?

A. To categorize patient into acute or chronic lupus erythematosus
B. To differentiate between bullous SLE and SLE with lupus-specific bullous lesions
C. To differentiate the condition from epidermolysis bullosa acquisita
D. All of the above

Answer: *The correct answer is* ***D.***

Blistering is uncommon in SLE. Blisters can occur in three different settings in patients with SLE:

1. Bullous lesions arising in the setting of LE-specific skin lesions:

   In cases of LE specific cutaneous lesions such as acute and subacute lupus erythematosus, sub-epidermal bullae formation can sometimes occur due to separation of epidermis and dermis as a result of intense interface dermatitis leading to hydropic degeneration of the basal cell layer and edema of the papillary dermis. This represents severe inflammation in the setting of LE specific cutaneous disease (ALE and SCLE) and resemble erythema multiformis (Rowell syndrome) or toxic epidermal necrolysis (TEN). This type of lesions rarely occur with chronic LE or DLE [2–4]
2. Bullous systemic lupus erythematosus (BSLE); a non-specific LE cutaneous lesion:

   A distinct type of autoantibody mediated cutaneous SLE that results in a sub-epidermal blister and is termed as bullous SLE (BSLE). Injury to the dermoepidermal junction by the interface dermatitis may expose new epitopes and thus lead to the development of newer autoantibodies targeting more antigens of basement membrane zone (BMZ). Thus, immune mediated tissue damage is amplified, leading to severe skin damage and bulla formation. The cartilage matrix protein (CMP) subdomain of the NC1 domain of type VII collagen which are localized to lamina densa have been shown to bind to antibodies from patients with BSLE, suggesting that this subdomain serves as an immunodominant antigenic epitope in these patients [5].

   Salient features of these conditions have been summarized in Table 58.1
3. LE associated autoimmune bullous disorders:

   SLE can sometimes be associated with other autoimmune bullous diseases such as dermatitis herpetiformis, pemphigus vulgaris, pemphigus foliaceus, bullous pemphigoid [5, 6].

   Camisa and Sharma proposed criteria for the diagnosis of bullous SLE [6]:

1. A diagnosis of SLE based on ACR criteria.
2. Vesicles and bullae arising on, but not limited to, sun exposed skin,
3. Histopathology showing subepidermal blister with neutrophilic infiltrate in the dermis
4. Indirect immunofluorescence (IIF) showing antibodies to type VII collagen.
5. Direct IF revealing IgG and/or IgM and often IgA at dermoepidermal junction.

Epidermolysis bullosa (EB) acquisita and BSLE share the same target antigen, causing diagnostic difficulties. A recent study using immunochemical and immune-ultrastructural analysis has demonstrated circulating IgG autoantibodies that are indistinguishable from those found in EB acquisita, in patients with BSLE [1, 2]. However, unlike EB acquisita, BSLE tends to respond dramatically to treatment with dapsone [1].

Q3. How common is pediatric SLE among all SLE patients?

A. 50–70%
B. 80–90%
C. 10–20%
D. Less than 5%

Table 58.1 Bullous lesions in systemic lupus erythematosus (SLE)

Differentiating features	Non-bullous specific cutaneous LE disease	Bullous lesions arising in the setting of specific cutaneous LE disease	Bullous SLE: A non-specific cutaneous LE disease
Pattern and distribution of lesions	Typical lesions of ALE, SCLE and DLE mainly on sun-exposed sites	Blistering lesions mainly on sun-exposed sites typified by TEN-like SLE & Rowell syndrome Nikolsky positive	Blistering lesions on sunexposed as well as non-sunexposed sites (As in our patient). Nikolsky negative
Histopathology	Well-established lesions show prominent vacuolar degeneration of the basal membrane, edema, extravasation of erythrocytes, and a lymphocytic infiltrate in the upper dermis. Fibrinoid material may be present in the dermis around vessels and between collagen strands.	TEN-like LE: Full-thickness epidermal necrosis and a sparse lymphocytic infiltrate in the upper dermis Rowell syndrome: Vacuolar interface dermatitis with lymphocyte exocytosis; prominent necrotic keratinocytes in all layers of the epidermis; a mild, superficial, perivascular lymphocytic infiltrate; and dermal edema.	Dermoepidermal separation beneath an intact epidermis. An oedematous upper dermis with predominantly neutrophilic infiltrate
Associated illness	Lupus nephritis or cerebritis depending on severity of systemic involvement	Patients of TEN-like LE have significant associated systemic disease activity (lupus nephritis or cerebritis).	Parallel exacerbation of lupus nephritis may be present but doesn't necessarily correlate with it.
Severity and prognosis	Prognosis depends on the severity of systemic involvement	Represents more severe cutaneous LE and often more severe systemc involvement	No direct correlation present with systemic involvement, responds well to treatment
Treatment	Corticosteroids & other immunomodulators	Corticosteroid& other immunomodulators	Responds well to dapsone & corticosteroids

TEN toxic epidermal necrolysis, *ALE* acute lupus erythematosus, *ACLE* acute cutaneous lupus erythematosus, *DLE* discoid lupus erythematosus

Answer: *The correct answer is* ***C.***

Childhood SLE accounts between 10 and 20% of all new cases of SLE [1, 2]. Mean age of onset in children is between 11 and 14 years and SLE is rare before 5 years of age. It is more prevalent in black, Hispanic, and Caucasian girls in descending order [7].

Childhood-onset SLE has a worse prognosis compared to adult-onset SLE. The most common presenting features for pediatric SLE include fever, nephropathy, and lymphadenopathy [8]. SLE in children is more active during presentation as well as at follow-up as compared to adults with SLE. Children usually present with more active disease status, and eventually need more intensive drug therapy with steroids and cytotoxic agents compared to adults.

Neuropsychiatric features are more prevalent in juvenile-onset SLE compared to adults and most common manifestations are headache and seizures.

Even though 10 year survival rates for pediatric SLE have improved over the last decade, ranging 80–90%, children end up suffering extensive morbidity because of the longer duration of disease as well as the adverse effects from medication [6]. The earlier age of onset also correlates with a more severe disease [7].

Q4. Premature ovarian failure is a side-effect of which of the following drugs?

A. Hydroxychloroquine
B. Corticosteroids
C. Cyclophosphamide
D. Mycophenolate mofetil

Answer: *The correct answer is* ***C.***

Cyclophosphamide is mainly used for the management of severe SLE, including lupus nephritis, life-threatening organ involvement, and neuropsychiatric manifestations. It can also permanently alter the ovarian reserve in a dose-, duration- and age- dependent manner. This loss of ovarian reserve may manifest as infertility and premature ovarian failure [8].

Early and reversible adverse effects of steroids include endocrine manifestations such as hyperglycemia and weight gain. Long term steroid treatment may result in diabetes mellitus, obesity, hypertension, hyperlipidemia, atherosclerosis, stunted growth, osteoporosis, cataracts and glaucoma [8]. The hallmark adverse effect of hydroxychloroquine is retinopathy, which can present insidiously with subtle color vision changes and paracentral scotoma, making early detection difficult. Cytopenias, and teratogenicity are major adverse effects of mycophenolate mofetil [8].

Practical Points

- Blisters can rise as an lupus erythematosus specific skin lesion, as bullous systemic lupus erythematosus (BSLE) or due to other associated autoimmune bullous disorders
- Systemic lupus erythematosus (SLE) can sometimes be associated with other autoimmune bullous diseases such as dermatitis herpetiformis, pemphigus vulgaris, pemphigus foliaceus, bullous pemphigoid
- Childhood-onset SLE has a worse prognosis compared to adult-onset SLE
- The most common presenting features for pediatric SLE include fever, nephropathy, and lymphadenopathy
- Neuropsychiatric features are more prevalent in juvenile-onset SLE compared to adults
- Cyclophosphamide can permanently alter the ovarian reserve in a dose-, duration- and age- dependent manner
- The hallmark adverse effect of hydroxychloroquine is retinopathy, which can present insidiously with subtle color vision changes and paracentral scotoma

References

1. Rowell NR. Some historical aspects of skin disease in lupus erythematosus. Lupus. 1997;6(2):76–83.
2. Grover C, Khurana A, Sharma S, Singal A. Bullous systemic lupus erythematosus. Indian J Dermatol. 2013;58(6):492.
3. Rappersberger K, Tschachler E, Tani M, Wolff K. Bullous disease in systemic lupus erythematosus. J Am Acad Dermatol. 1989;21(4. Pt 1):745–52.
4. Meislin AG, Rothfield N. Systemic lupus erythematosus in childhood. Analysis of 42 cases, with comparative data on 200 adult cases followed concurrently. Pediatrics. 1968;42(1):37–49.
5. Font J, Cervera R, Espinosa G, Pallares L, Ramos-Casals M, Jimenez S, Garcia-Carrasco M, Seisdedos L, Ingelmo M. Systemic lupus erythematosus (SLE) in childhood: analysis of clinical and immunological findings in 34 patients and comparison with SLE characteristics in adults. Ann Rheum Dis. 1998;57(8):456–9.
6. Spinosa MJ, Bandeira M, Liberalesso PB, Vieira SC, Janz LL Jr, Sa EG, Lohr A Jr. Clinical, laboratory and neuroimage findings in juvenile systemic lupus erythematosus presenting involvement of the nervous system. Arq Neuropsiquiatr. 2007;65(2b):433–9.
7. Thakral A, Klein-Gitelman MS. An update on treatment and management of pediatric systemic lupus erythematosus. Rheumatol Ther. 2016;3(2):209–19.
8. Descloux E, Durieu I, Cochat P, Vital Durand D, Ninet J, Fabien N, Cimaz R. Paediatric systemic lupus erythematosus: prognostic impact of antiphospholipid antibodies. Rheumatology (Oxford). 2008;47(2):183–7.

Chapter 59
Recurrent Bullous Lesions

Santoshdev P. Rathod and Piyush Kumar

A 9-year-old-girl presented to our outpatient clinic with multiple erosions and crusted lesions over face, scalp, trunk and both upper and lower limbs.

The patient was asymptomatic until 2 years ago, when she developed fluid filled skin lesions, initially over the scalp, spreading to involve the face, trunk and both upper and lower limbs within a period of 15 days. The lesions were associated with itching and ruptured spontaneously leaving behind bare areas of the skin which would then go on to heal within a week, forming thin crusts (Fig. 59.1). There was also no mucosal involvement. There was no concomitant medical illness or significant past medical history. The patient took oral and intravenous antibiotics prior to presentation to our outpatient department with no improvement in symptoms. Tzanck smear from bulla showed acantholytic cells. Biopsy of her skin revealed sub-corneal blister formation in epidermis and superficial lymphocytic infiltrate in the dermis. Desmoglein (Dsg) titres was found as follow anti-Dsg-1: 252 IU/mL, anti-Dsg-3: 13.7 IU/mL (reference range: 0–14 IU/mL: negative, 14–20 IU/mL: intermediate and > 20 U/mL: positive).

Q1. What is the most likely diagnosis?

A. Pemphigus vulgaris
B. Pemphigus foliaceus
C. Chronic bullous disease of childhood
D. Epidermolysis bullosa simplex

Answer: *The correct answer is **B**.*

S. P. Rathod
Department of Dermatology, Smt. NHL Municipal Medical College, Ahmedabad, Gujarat, India

P. Kumar (✉)
Department of Dermatology, Katihar Medical College, Katihar, Bihar, India

© Springer Nature Switzerland AG 2020

F. Rahmani, N. Rezaei (eds.), *Pediatric Autoimmunity and Transplantation*, https://doi.org/10.1007/978-3-030-26280-8_59

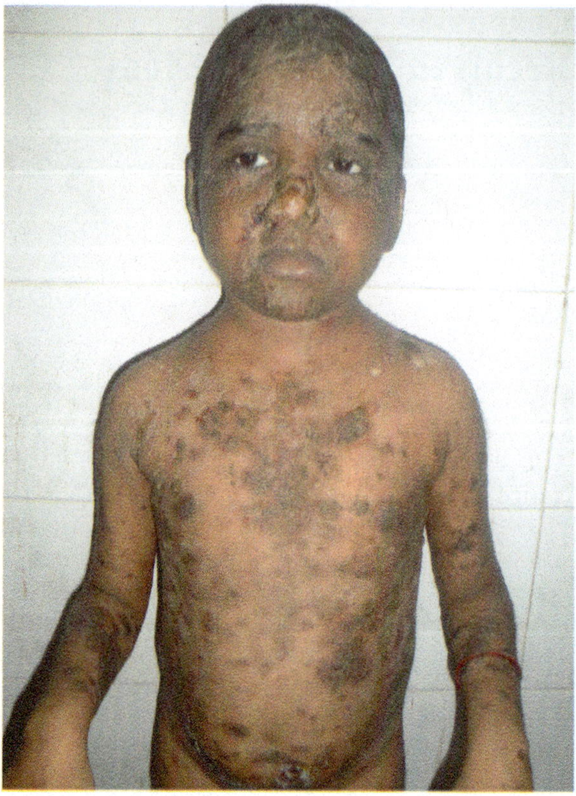

Fig. 59.1 Moist crusted lesions and erosions on face, scalp and trunk in a patients with pemphigus foliaceus (*Courtesy of: Dr. Raju Chaudhary, Professor, Smt. NHL Municipal medical college*)

Table 59.1 Differentiating features of pemphigus vulgaris and pemphigus foliaceus

Features	Pemphigus vulgaris	Pemphigus foliaceus
Site of involvement	Generalized	Preferentially seborrheic areas
Mucosal involvement	Yes	No
Blister on histopathology	Suprabasal	Subcorneal
Other key features on histopathology	Row of tombstones appearance	Dyskeratotic cells
Antibody against	Desmoglein 3 (Dsg-3)	Desmoglein 1 (Dsg-1)

Both pemphigus vulgaris (PV) and pemphigus foliaceus (PF) are autoimmune intraepidermal blistering disorders, clinically characterized by flaccid blisters, erosions and crusts. They are differentiated by the features presented in Table 59.1 [1].

Chronic bullous disease of childhood is an autoimmune subepidermal vesiculobullous disease that presents with clear and/or hemorrhagic bullae on normal, erythematous, or urticarial skin often arranged in herpetiform pattern i.e. described as the cluster of jewels sign. Alternatively, vesicles and bullae may appear at the edge of healing lesions, resulting in annular or polycyclic lesions, described as the string of beads sign. Direct immunofluorescence study typically shows linear deposition of IgA at the basement membrane zone [1].

Epidermolysis bullosa simplex denotes a group of inherited vesicobullous disorders resulting from keratin gene mutations and is characterized by non-inflammatory intraepidermal blistering. It presents within first few months of life. The formation of bulla is often precipitated by mechanical trauma and bulla mostly appears on trauma prone or acral parts. It can be localized or generalized and may have extracutaneous manifestations such as muscular dystrophy or pyloric atresia [1].

Q2. Which of the following is a treatment option in childhood pemphigus foliaceus?

A. Corticosteroids
B. Dapsone
C. Hydroxychloroquine
D. All of the above

Answer: *The correct answer is* ***D.***

Childhood PF is rare and evidence based treatment guidelines have not been established yet. Corticosteroids, both oral and topical have been used as a first line drug in mild cases of this condition. Dapsone appears to be the most popular steroid sparing agent and its safety and efficacy is well documented [2]. Hydroxychloroquine finds efficacy mostly in patients with predominant photodistributed lesions [3]. Apart from mentioned drugs, erythromycin, chloroquine, methotrexate, sulfapyridine, azathioprine [2], and rituximab [4] have been used to treat PF as well.

Q3. Which of the following is associated with an increased risk for pemphigus foliaceus?

A. Sunlight
B. Drugs
C. *Simulium* (black fly) bites
D. All of the above

Answer: *The correct answer is* ***D.***

Both sunlight and drugs (e.g. penicillamine, nifedipine, captopril, and quinolones) are known to be associated with the development of non-endemic forms of PF [4]. Drugs as etiology are implicated in adult PF, and evidence for their role in childhood cases is limited.

Fogo selvagem is an endemic form of PF with major endemic foci are South American countries, such as Brazil, Colombia, Ecuador, Peru, Paraguay, Venezuela and African continent such as Tunisia. In genetically predisposed individuals, bites of hematophagous insects like *Simulium*, *Triatoma*, and *Cimex* precipitate the disease. Clinically, both localized (confined to face) and generalized forms are described [5].

Q4. What is the target antigen in pemphigus foliaceus?

A. Desmoglein 1 & 3
B. Desmoglein 1
C. BP 180 and 230
D. Type VII antigen

Answer: *The correct answer is* ***B.***

Circulating autoantibodies which are targeted against keratinocyte cell surfaces are pillars of pemphigus pathology. Circulating IgG subclass antibodies bind to desmogleins 1 and 3 in PV and desmoglein 1 in PF. BP 180 and BP 230 are target antigens in bullous pemphigoid. Finally, type VII is target antigen in EB acquisita [1].

Practical Points

- Pemphigus foliaceus is an autoimmune intraepidermal blistering disorder, clinically characterized by flaccid blisters, erosions and crusts
- Childhood PF is rare and evidence based treatment guidelines have not been established yet
- Corticosteroids, both oral and topical (in mild cases of PF) have been used as a first line drug
- Dapsone appears to be the most popular steroid sparing agent and its safety and efficacy are well documented
- Sunlight and drugs such as penicillamine, nifedipine, captopril, and quinolones are known aggravating factors

References

1. Lara-Corrales I, Pope E. Autoimmune blistering diseases in children. Semin Cutan Med Surg. 2010;29(2):85–91.
2. De DKA. Childhood pemphigus. Indian J Dermatol Venereol Leprol. 2006;51:89–95.
3. Metry DW, Hebert AA, Jordon RE. Nonendemic pemphigus foliaceus in children. J Am Acad Dermatol. 2002;46(3):419–22.
4. Loh TY, Paravar T. Rituximab in the management of juvenile pemphigus foliaceus. Dermatol Online J. 2017;23(6):13030/qt0415n1r5.
5. Aoki V RE, Diaz LA, Cooperative Group on Fogo Selvagem Research. Update on fogoselvagem, an endemic form of pemphigus foliaceus. J Dermatol. 2015;42(1):18–26.

Chapter 60
Refractory Blisters and Erosions

Ziying Vanessa Lim and Emily Yiping Gan

A 10-year-old boy presented with widespread scalp erosions and extensive flaccid blisters over his face, trunk and limbs involving more than 50% of his body surface area (Figs. 60.1, 60.2 and 60.3). He was diagnosed with pemphigus vulgaris (PV) in 2010 with consistent skin biopsy, immunofluorescence and serology findings. At diagnosis, indirect immunofluorescence (IIF) titre was 1:160, with an intercellular pattern. His condition was difficult to control with several relapses that required various immunosuppressive agents over the subsequent years. Apart from topical tacrolimus and corticosteroids, he was on long-term prednisolone, and had been trialled with azathioprine, methotrexate, and mycophenolate mofetil. He eventually responded to intravenous rituximab, which was given in mid-April 2011. Repeat IIF was negative in April 2015, when his disease was in quiescence.

Q1. What histological findings do you expect to find in skin biopsy of pemphigus vulgaris (Fig. 60.4)?

A. Subcorneal acantholysis in the epidermis with a prominent granular layer
B. Suprabasilar acantholysis in the epidermis with the floor of the blister lined with intact keratinocytes
C. Intraepidermal acantholysis giving rise to a "dilapitated brick wall" appearance
D. Suprabasal clefting with acantholysis and dyskeratosis

Answer: *The correct answer is* ***B.***

The typical histological finding in PV is suprabasilar acantholysis in the epidermis with the floor of the blister lined with intact keratinocytes resulting in a "tombstone

Z. V. Lim
National Skin Centre, Singapore, Singapore

E. Y. Gan (✉)
National Skin Centre, Singapore, Singapore

Dermatology Service, KK Women's and Children's Hospital, Singapore, Singapore

© Springer Nature Switzerland AG 2020

F. Rahmani, N. Rezaei (eds.), *Pediatric Autoimmunity and Transplantation*,
https://doi.org/10.1007/978-3-030-26280-8_60

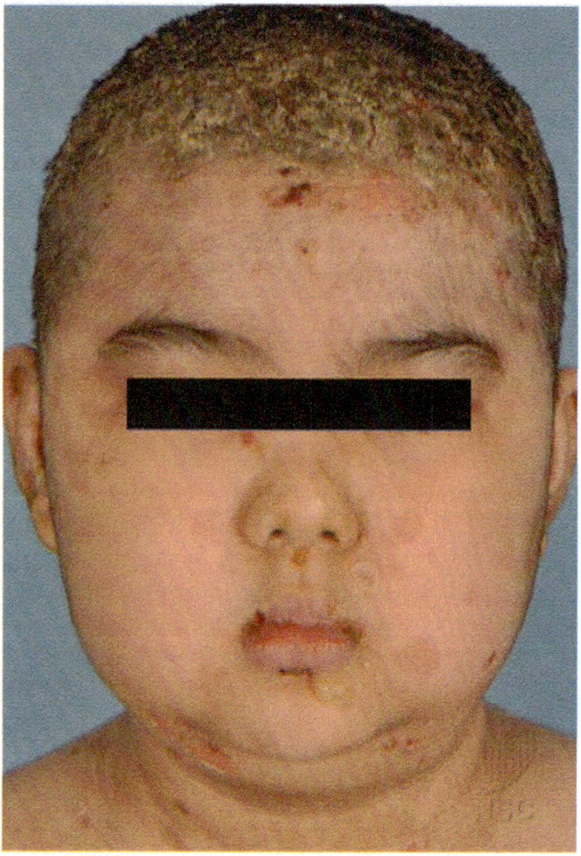

Fig. 60.1 Flaccid blisters and erosions affecting the face, scalp and lips

pattern"[1]. In PF, the epidermal split is more superficial at the subcorneal level, which often leads to the loss of the stratum corneum and a prominent granular layer [1].

In Hailey-Hailey disease, or familial benign chronic pemphigus, the acantholysis affects the whole epidermis, giving rise to the classical "dilapidated brick wall" appearance [1]. In Darier's disease, there is suprabasal clefting with acantholysis and dyskeratosis in the form of corps ronds and grains [1].

Q2. All of the statements are correct regarding anti-desmoglein antibodies in pemphigus, except:

A. Anti-Dsg 1 is associated with mucosal limited pemphigus vulgaris
B. Dsg 1 is found throughout the epidermis and minimally expressed in oral mucosa, and Dsg 3 is expressed in the basal epidermis with higher expression on mucosal surfaces
C. The extended desmoglein compensation theory explains cases of cutaneous pemphigus vulgaris without anti-Dsg 1
D. Anti-Dsg 1 expression is the key driver of disease activity in pemphigus vulgaris

Answer: *The correct answer is* ***A.***

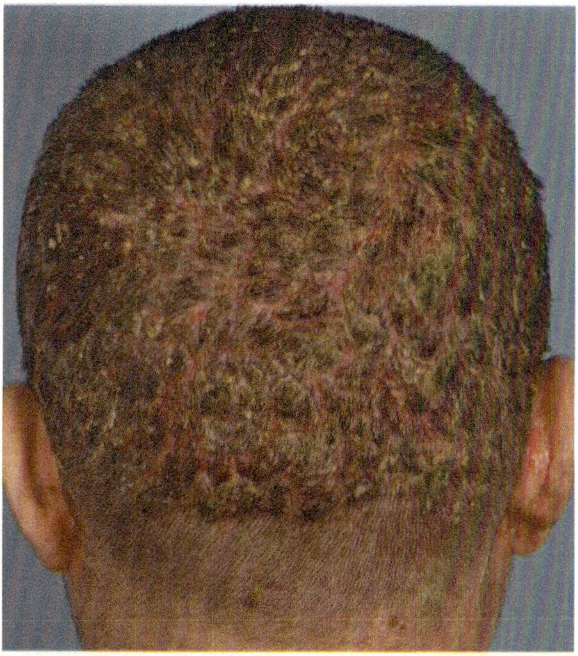

Fig. 60.2 Widespread crusts and erosions affecting the entire scalp

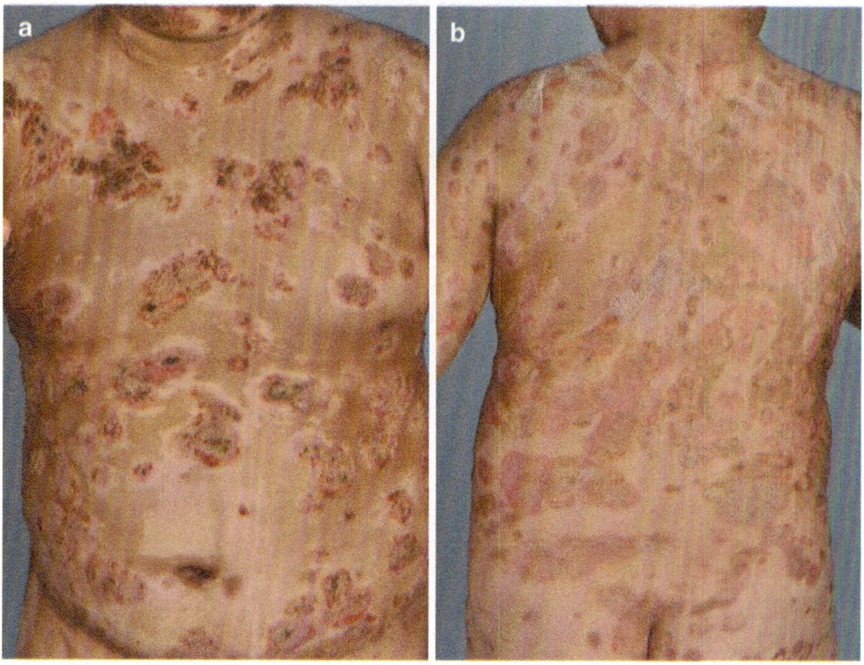

Figs. 60.3 Extensive flaccid blisters and erosions over the anterior (**a**) and posterior (**b**) trunk

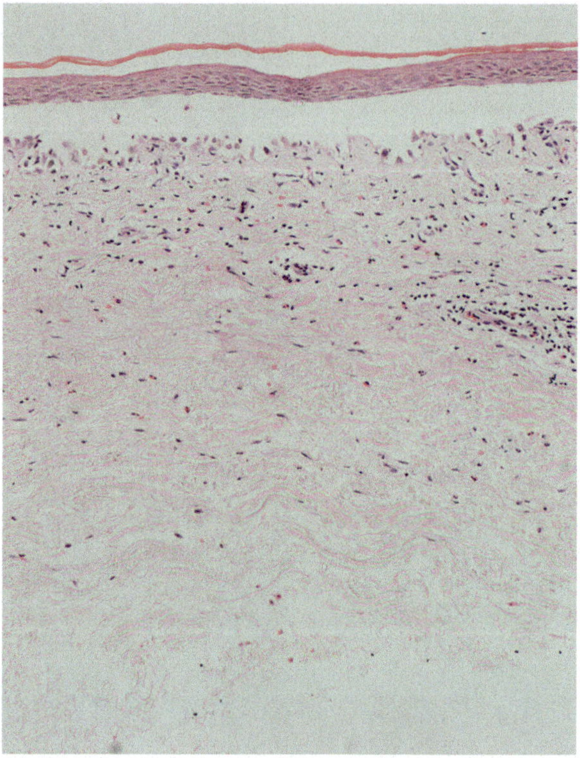

Fig. 60.4 There is suprabasilar acantholysis in the epidermis and the floor of the blister is lined with intact keratinocytes (Hematoxylin & Eosin stain, original magnification ×100)

Desmogleins are transmembrane glycoproteins that play an important role in cell-cell adhesions within the skin. Dsg 1 is located throughout the epidermis and is only minimally expressed in the mucosa, whereas Dsg 3 is expressed only in the basal epidermis with higher expression on the mucosal surfaces [2]. As desmogleins are differentially distributed in the skin and mucosa, the desmoglein compensation theory postulates that Dsg 1 and Dsg 3 compensate for each other when one is disrupted by autoantibodies [2, 3]. The extended desmoglein compensation theory suggests that Dsg autoantibodies have variable pathogenic potential, where weaker or non-pathogenic forms of Dsg 3 antibodies may be only sufficient to block Dsg 3 in the skin but not in the mucosa [2]. This explains patients with cutaneous PV who present with absence of serum anti-Dsg 1 antibodies.

Patients in the active phase of PV, defined by lesions lasting more than a week, have significantly higher levels of anti-Dsg 1 and/or 3 compared to patients in disease remission and healthy controls [4]. Serum from the majority of samples from patients with active PV are positive for anti-Dsg 3 by ELISA (levels >20 IU/mL) (78%), whereas a smaller proportion of patients (39%) are positive for anti-Dsg 1 [4]. In patients who are anti-Dsg 1 positive, the anti-Dsg 1 levels demonstrate a corresponding decline when moving from the active to remission phase. In contrast, anti-Dsg 3 levels remain elevated throughout the course of disease [4]. The persistently elevated anti-Dsg 3 levels may be explained by ongoing transient lesional activity, lasting less than 1 week in the patients [4]. Table 60.1 shows trend of anti-desmoglein 1 and 3 titers over time in our patient.

Q3. Corticosteroids are the mainstay of therapy in pemphigus vulgaris. What is the postulated mechanism of action of corticosteroids?

A. Decreases circulating pathogenic anti-desmoglein antibodies
B. Induces increase in catabolism of anti-desmoglein antibodies
C. Increases the synthesis of desmogleins in keratinocytes
D. Depletes CD20+ peripheral B cells

Answer: *The correct answer is* ***C.***

Corticosteroids are postulated to act very quickly in PV by increasing the synthesis of desmogleins in keratinocytes, which may then overcome the ability of the anti-desmoglein antibodies to internalize the newly synthesized desmogleins. They may also work by increasing synthesis of desmoglein isoforms that are not targeted by pemphigus antibodies, which compensate in function for the loss of the desmogleins targeted by the pemphigus antibodies [5].

Intravenous immunoglobulin decreases the levels of pathogenic anti-Dsg antibodies by increasing the catabolism of anti-desmoglein antibodies [5]. Rituximab is a chimeric monoclonal antibody that binds to the CD20 cell surface receptor of B-cells leading to profound depletion of B-cell repertoire, and has been shown to induce clinical remission in more than 50% of patients with PV [6]. In particular, there have been several reports of successful treatment with rituximab in childhood PV [7].

Table 60.1 Trend of Anti-desmoglein 1 and 3 titers over time in a patient with pemphigus vulgaris

	January 2011 (at diagnosis)	April 2011 (before IV rituximab given on 13–14 April 2011)	March 2012	November 2012	May 2013 (relapse)	March 2014	May 2014
Anti-desmoglein 3 level (U/mL)	143.7	128.3	Negative	20.1	116.9	105.3	61.0
Anti-desmoglein 1 level (U/mL)	198.7	133.8	Negative	2.6	6.7 (negative)	7.5 (negative)	3.1 (negative)

Q4. Use of oral corticosteroids in treatment of pemphigus vulgaris may lead to elevation of blood pressure. Which class of anti-hypertensive medication might exacerbate symptoms of pemphigus vulgaris and is hence contraindicated?

A. Thiazides
B. Calcium channel blockers
C. Beta-blockers
D. Angiotensin converting enzyme inhibitors

Answer: *The correct answer is* ***D.***

Angiotensin converting enzyme inhibitors, which can work immediately by venodilatation to reduce intra-capillary pressure, are the most commonly reported anti-hypertensive class of drugs to be associated with PV. Captopril, enalapril and ramipril are commonly prescribed examples [8]. Thiazides act by inhibiting electrolyte transport and decreasing the glomerular filtration rate in the kidneys. Indapamide, a thiazide-like diuretic, has been reported as a possible cause of PF [9]. Calcium channel blockers promote vasodilatory effects, thus reduce blood pressure. There has been one case report of nifedipine inducing PV [8], and in-vitro studies demonstrating pemphigus and pemphigoid-like effects on cultured normal human skin explants [10]. Beta-blockers, such as propanolol, have also been reported to incite pemphigus [7].

Q5. The prognosis of childhood pemphigus vulgaris is overall better than adults, but is highly variable. All of the following factors can predict remission in childhood PV, <u>except</u>:

A. Disease severity at time of diagnosis
B. Early response to treatment
C. Levels of indirect immunofluorescence
D. Direct immunofluorescence findings

Answer: *The correct answer is* ***D.***

PV was often a severe fatal condition before the widespread use of systemic corticosteroids. With the advent of systemic corticosteroids, mortality rates have markedly reduced from 70 to 30%. Reported remission rates with treatment now stand at approximately 30% [10]. Prognostic factors include disease severity at time of diagnosis, early response to treatment, and levels of IIF and ELISA titers [3]. The direct immunofluorescence findings in PV are not known to bear a prognosis.

Practical Points

- The histological findings in pemphigus vulgaris are suprabasilar acantholysis in the epidermis with the floor of the blister lined with intact keratinocytes. Direct immunofluorescence findings are intercellular IgG and/or C3 in the epidermis

- Anti-Dsg1 levels decline when moving from active to remission phase of the disease, but anti-Dsg3 levels remain elevated throughout
- Corticosteroids are the mainstay of treatment for pemphigus vulgaris and work quickly within days by overcoming the effect of anti-desmoglein antibodies
- Angiotensin converting enzyme inhibitors, such as captorpil, enalapril and ramipril, are the most commonly reported anti-hypertensive drugs to be associated with pemphigus vulgaris
- Prognostic factors of pemphigus vulgaris include disease severity at time of diagnosis, early response to treatment, and levels of indirect immunofluorescence and ELISA titers

References

1. Elston DM, Ferringer T. Dermatopathology. 2nd ed. London: Elsevier; 2014.
2. Carew B, Wagner G. Cutaneous pemphigus vulgaris with absence of desmoglein 1 autoantibodies. An example of the extended desmoglein compensation theory. Australas J Dermatol. 2014;55(4):292–5.
3. Naseer SY, Seiffert-Sinha K, Sinha AA. Detailed profiling of anti-desmoglein autoantibodies identifies anti-Dsg1 reactivity as a key driver of disease activity and clinical expression in pemphigus vulgaris. Autoimmunity. 2015;48(4):231–41.
4. Hammers CM, Stanley JR. Mechanisms of disease: pemphigus and bullous pemphigoid. Annu Rev Pathol. 2016;11:175–97.
5. Heelan K, Al-Mohammedi F, Smith MJ, Knowles S, Lansang P, Walsh S, Shear NH. Durable remission of pemphigus with a fixed-dose rituximab protocol. JAMA Dermatol. 2014;150(7):703–8.
6. Kanwar AJ, Sawatkar GU, Vinay K, Hashimoto T. Childhood pemphigus vulgaris successfully treated with rituximab. Indian J Dermatol Venereol Leprol. 2012;78(5):632–4.
7. Thami GP, Kaur S, Kanwar AJ. Severe childhood pemphigus vulgaris aggravated by enalapril. Dermatology. 2001;202(4):341.
8. Pietkiewicz P, Gornowicz-Porowska J, Bowszyc-Dmochowska M, Dmochowski M. A retrospective study of antihypertensives in pemphigus: a still unchartered odyssey particularly between thiols, amides and phenols. Arch Med Sci. 2015;11(5):1021–7.
9. Brenner S, Ruocco V, Bialy-Golan A, Tur E, Flaminio C, Ruocco E, Lombardi ML. Pemphigus and pemphigoid-like effects of nifedipine on in vitro cultured normal human skin explants. Int J Dermatol. 1999;38(1):36–40.
10. Baratta A, Camarillo D, Papa C, Treat JR, Payne AS, Rozenber SS, Yan AC. Pediatric pemphigus vulgaris: durable treatment responses achieved with prednisone and mycophenolate mofetil (MMF). Pediatr Dermatol. 2013;30(2):240–4.

Chapter 61
Annular Blisters and Erosions

Soner Uzun and Aslı Bilgic-Temel

A 7-year-old girl was referred to our clinic with a 1-month history of widespread annular erythematous lesions with blisters and erosions on her skin. Dermatological examination revealed well-demarcated, erythematous squamous lesions with annular bullous eruption on the scalp, face, trunk and her back (Fig. 61.1).

There were no mucosal lesions. She had reached all the developmental milestones appropriate for her age with no abnormalities on physical examination apart from her skin lesions. Family history was negative for similar signs or symptoms. Parents were not consanguineous.

Q1. What is the most likely diagnosis?

A. Pemphigus foliaceus
B. Pemphigus vulgaris
C. Bullous pemphigoid
D. Necrolytic migratory erythema

Answer: *The correct answer is* **A.**

Pemphigus encompasses a group of life-threatening autoimmune bullous diseases characterized by flaccid blisters and erosions of the mucous membranes and skin. Pemphigus is rare in children and is called as juvenile pemphigus. Pemphigus vulgaris (i.e. PV) and pemphigus foliaceus (i.e. PF) are the most common forms of pemphigus [1–6]. Regarding the pathophysiology, the underlying intraepithelial

S. Uzun (✉)
Department of Dermatology and Venereology, School of Medicine, Akdeniz University, Antalya, Turkey
e-mail: sonuzun@akdeniz.edu.tr

A. Bilgic-Temel
Seydisehir State Hospital, Dermatology Clinic, Konya, Turkey

© Springer Nature Switzerland AG 2020

F. Rahmani, N. Rezaei (eds.), *Pediatric Autoimmunity and Transplantation*,
https://doi.org/10.1007/978-3-030-26280-8_61

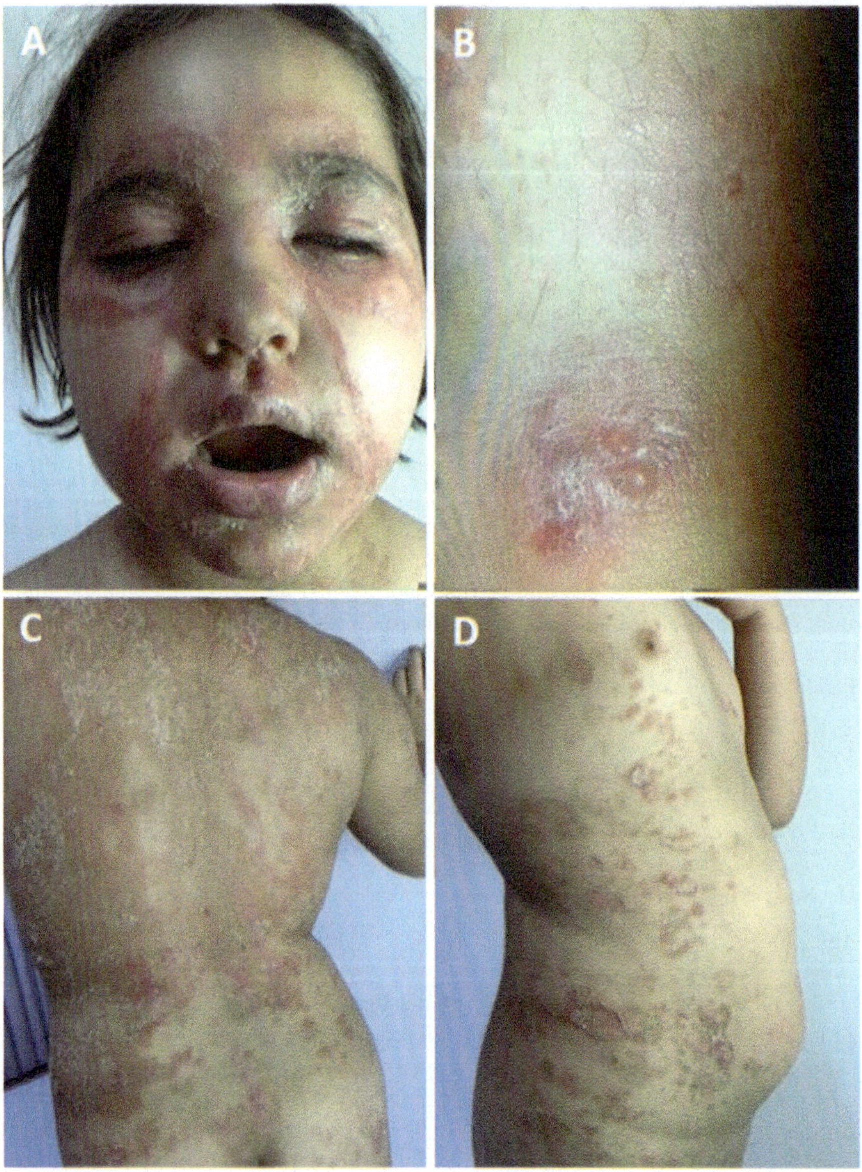

Fig. 61.1 Clinical findings of the patient on her (**a**) face, (**b**) upper arm, (**c**) abdomen and (**d**) back of the girl

blister formation is caused by IgG autoantibodies against the desmosomal adhesion proteins, desmoglein 3 and/or desmoglein 1, on epidermal keratinocytes [7].

PV usually begins by with oral mucosal lesions as buccal and/or gingival painful, persisting erosions. Cutaneous involvement may appear several weeks or months after the first appearance of mucosal lesions with flaccid bullae with clear content on non-erythematous skin, quickly transforming into post-bullous erosions.

PF has sharply demarcated lesions, confined mainly to the seborrheic areas such as face, scalp and upper part of the chest [1, 2]. Sporadic PF, which is very rare in pediatric cases, follows a mild and benign course with most cases reported to resolve with minimal treatment within 1 year [3]. Intact bullous lesions in PF are infrequently observed as the acantholysis is superficial, i.e. within the subcorneal area or stratum granulosum layer, leaving the overlaying skin of the bullae with almost no physical barrier [4].

Q2. What is the most appropriate first step laboratory test in this patient?

A. Indirect immunofluorescence test/IIF
B. Direct immunofluorescence test/DIF
C. ELISA
D. Tzanck smear

Answer: *The correct answer is* ***D.***

Acantholytic cells which indicate pemphigus were seen in the examination of the smear prepared from patient's blisters. Tzanck smear is a cutaneous cytological test may be used as a bedside test in the diagnosis of pemphigus. Samples for this cytological examination are prepared by scraping the youngest vesicle or bullae [7]. While the specimen is being taken, the vesicle's ceiling is removed first. The base of the lesion should be gently scraped with the help of a blunt tipped spatula or brush, avoiding bleeds. The sample should then be spread to form a thin layer on at least two slides to be stained with Giemsa and examined on microscope. Round or oval shaped acantholytic cells that appear single or clustered characterize pemphigus on Tzanck cytology smear [8]. There is a narrow basophilic cytoplasm pallor around the nucleus, the perinuclear halo that gets darker at the periphery (Fig. 61.2).

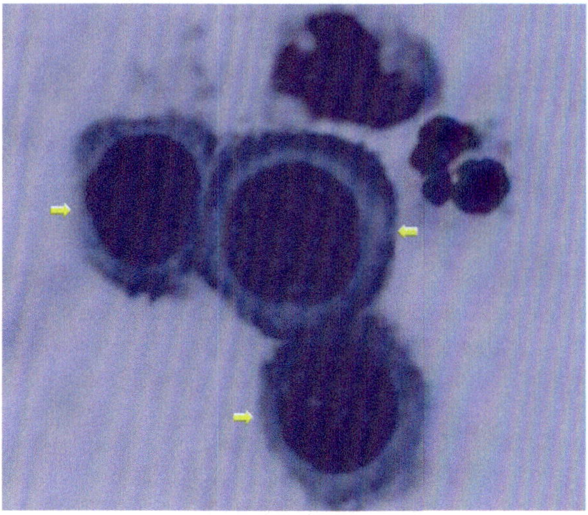

Fig. 61.2 Acatholytic cells (yellow icons) in Tzanck smear of the lesions

Despite emerging new methods to diagnose autoimmune cutaneous disorders, cytology is still a fast, inexpensive and easily applicable diagnostic method that is used to differentiate pemphigus from other autoimmune diseases [6, 9].

Q3. Which of the following tests would reveal the definite diagnosis?

A. Histopathology
B. Indirect immunofluorescence test
C. ELISA
D. Direct immunofluorescence test

Answer: *The correct answer is* ***D.***

The presence of subcorneal splitting, acantholic cells and eosinophilic spongioses, and/or the presence of dyskeratotic keratinocytes are the main histological features, prompting a diagnosis of PF [10, 11]. Biopsy from the bullous lesions of our patient revealed findings compatible with PF. Subcorneal split was seen in histopathological examination.

Enzyme-Linked Immunosorbent Assay (i.e. ELISA) is based on the detection of autoantibodies in skin and/or serum specimens of patients to diagnose autoimmune bullous diseases [12–14]. In addition to its diagnostic value, ELISA is also used to evaluate the response to treatment. There is a positive correlation between clinical activity of pemphigus disorders and ELISA antibody titters [15, 16]. In our patient, positive results for anti-desmoglein-1 antibody (138 U/ml) in ELISA, put further spin on the diagnosis.

DIF is considered the gold standard in diagnosis of pemphigus, and should be performed in all patients if possible [17–19]. A green apple colour epidermal intercellular staining with IgG and/or C3 in a fishnet or chicken wire appearance is pathognomonic finding for pemphigus (Fig. 61.3). In contrast to the Tzanck smear, the most suitable samples for DIF investigation are the biopsy samples taken from "normal-appearing" area close to a fresh lesion. In our patient C3 deposition was seen as "fishnet pattern" in intercellular area in DIF examination of the biopsy.

Q4. What is the first-line treatment option for this patient?

A. Azathioprine
B. Corticosteroids
C. Methotrexate
D. Cyclophosphamide

Answer: *The correct answer is* ***B.***

Prognosis of untreated PF is much better than PV. This is due to lower rate of infection and metabolic disorders and low potential for fluid loss. Although high dose systemic treatment is warranted in treatment of resistant PF cases, patients with PF typically need much lower doses of systemic treatment [20–22].

Systemic corticosteroid therapy is almost always the initial treatment for pemphigus. Generally, moderately effective corticosteroids, such as prednisolone or methylprednisolone, are used as prednisone has a relatively low risk of adverse effects, such as avascular bone necrosis [23]. Superpotent topical corticosteroids such as

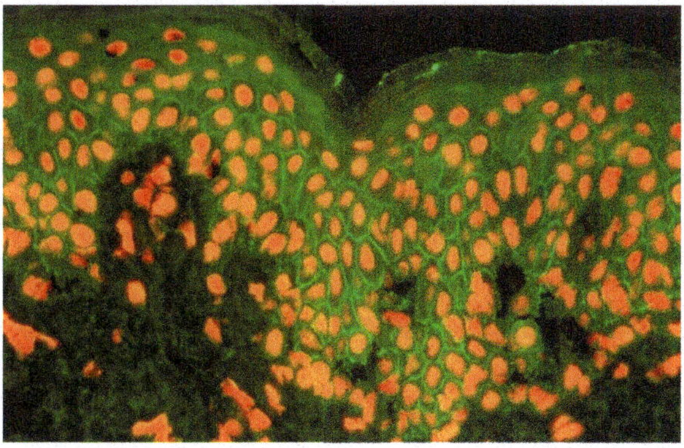

Fig. 61.3 Positive DIF for pemphigus. Green apple colour epidermal intercellular staining with IgG and C3 in a fishnet or chicken wire

clobetasol propionate, and low-dose alternate daily systemic corticosteroids may be the first step in patients with mild to moderate pemphigus. Systemic corticosteroid therapy at a dose of 0.5–1.5 mg/Kg/day prednisolone is warranted in resistant cases.

Dapsone is a well-known, less-used adjuvant in pemphigus, while being a standard treatment in bullous pemphigoid [24, 25]. Dapsone can be considered as an adjuvant in patients with pemphigus. It is also an inexpensive and relatively safe adjuvant. However, glucose-6-phosphate dehydrogenase (G6PD) levels should be checked before the treatment.

Our patient was treated with topical corticosteroids for 1 month without remarkable improvement. Due to lack of response to topical treatment, systemic corticosteroid was initiated with a dose of 1 mg/Kg/day. Dapsone (25 mg per day) was added as an adjuvant a month later, due to side effects of systemic steroids. Systemic steroid therapy was tapered and discontinued. She has maintained her complete remission on dapsone therapy for 3 months.

Practical Points

- Pemphigus is rare in children and is called as juvenile pemphigus
- The intraepithelial blister formation in pemphigus is caused by IgG autoantibodies against the desmosomal adhesion proteins, desmoglein 3 and/or desmoglein 1, on epidermal keratinocytes
- Direct immunofluorescence is considered the gold standard in diagnosis of pemphigus
- Prognosis of untreated PF is much better than PV. This is due to lower rate of infection and metabolic disorders and low potential for fluid loss

References

1. Küçükoglu RB, Babuna G. The clinical diagnosis of autoimmune bullous diseases. Türkderm. 2011;45:16–25.
2. Ioannides D, Lazaridou E, Rigopoulos D. Pemphigus. J Eur Acad Dermatol Venereol. 2008;22(12):1478–96.

3. Marathe K, Lu J, Morel K. Bullous diseases: kids are not just little people. Clin Dermatol. 2015;33(6):644–56.
4. Uzun S, Durdu M, Akman A, Gunasti S, Uslular C, Memisoglu H, Alpsoy E. Pemphigus in the Mediterranean region of Turkey: a study of 148 cases. Int J Dermatol. 2006;45(5):523–8.
5. Haber H. Cytodiagnosis in dermatology. Br J Dermatol. 1954;66:79–94.
6. Yazganoğlu KD, Baykal C, Küçükoğlu R. Childhood pemphigus vulgaris: five cases in 16 years. J Dermatol. 2006;33:846–9.
7. Ruocco V. Cytodiagnosis in dermatology. Naples: Cooperativa Libraria Universitaria; 1980. p. 20–110.
8. Blank H, Burgoon C. Abnormal cytology of epithelial cells in pemphigus vulgaris: a diagnostic aid. J Invest Dermatol. 1952;18:213–23.
9. Durdu M, Baba M, Seçkin D. The value of Tzanck smear test in diagnosis of erosive, vesicular, bullous, and pustular skin lesions. J Am Acad Dermatol. 2008;59(6):958–64.
10. Erkin G. The histopathological diagnosis of autoimmune bullous diseases. Türkderm. 2011;45(Special edition 1):26–30.
11. Elston D, Ferringer T, Ko C, Peckham S, High W, DiCaudo D. Blistering diseases. In: Dermatopathology. 2nd ed. Philadelphia: Elsevier Ltd.; 2009.
12. Probst C, Schlumberger W, Stöcker W, Recke A, Schmidt E, Hashimoto T, Zhu XJ, Zillikens D, Komorowsk L. Development of ELISA for the specific determination of autoantibodies against envoplakin and periplakin in paraneoplastic pemphigus. Clin Chim Acta. 2009;410(1–2):13–8.
13. Remington J, Chen M, Burnett J, Woodley D. Autoimmunity to type VII collagen: epidermolysis bullosa acquisita. Curr Dir Autoimmun. 2008;10:195–205.
14. Bekou V, Thoma-Uszynski S, Wendler O, Uter W, Schwietzke S, Hunziker T, Zouboulis C, Schuler G, Sorokin L, Hertl M. Detection of laminin 5-specific auto-antibodies in mucous membrane and bullous pemphigoid sera by ELISA. J Invest Dermatol. 2005;124(4):732–40.
15. Amagai M, Komai A, Hashimoto T, Shirakata Y, Hashimoto K, Yamada T, Kitajima Y, Ohya K, Iwanami H, Nishikawa T. Usefulness of enzyme-linked immunosorbent assay using recombinant desmogleins 1 and 3 for serodiagnosis of pemphigus. Br J Dermatol. 1999;140(2):351–7.
16. Sitaru C, Dahnrich C, Probst C, Komorowski L, Blocker I, Schmidt E, Schlumberger W, Rose C, Stocker W, Zillikens D. Enzyme-linked immunosorbent assay using multimers of the 16th non-collagenous domain of the BP180 antigen for sensitive and specific detection of pemphigoid autoantibodies. Exp Dermatol. 2007;16(9):770–7.
17. Uzun S. Dermatolojide immünofloresan teknikler. Deri Sorunlarında Adım Adım Tanısal Yaklaşımlar. Istanbul: Mart Matbaacılık; 2006.
18. Mutasim D, Adams B. Immunofluorescence in dermatology. J Am Acad Dermatol. 2001;45(6):803–22.
19. Uzun S. Immunofluoresecence findings in the diagnosis of autoimmune bullous diseases. Türkderm. 2011;45(Special edition 1):31–5.
20. James W, Berger T, Elston D. Andrew's diseases of the skin clinical dermatology. Canada: Saunders Elsevier; 2006.
21. Wien MH. Pemhigus. In: Wien MH, editor. Autoimmune diseases of the skin. Vienna: Springer; 2005.
22. Bystryn J, Rudolph J. Pemphigus. Lancet (London, England). 2005;366:61–73.
23. Uzun S. Current management of pemphigus: review. Turk J Dermatol. 2012;6:91–101.
24. Kasperkiewicz M, Schmidt E, Zillikens D. Current therapy of the pemphigus group. Clin Dermatol. 2012;30(1):84–94.
25. Werth VP, Fivenson D, Pandya AG, Chen D, Rico MJ, Albrecht J, Jacobus D. Multicenter randomized, double-blind, placebo-controlled, clinical trial of dapsone as a glucocorticoid-sparing agent in maintenance-phase pemphigus vulgaris. Arch Dermatol. 2008;144(1):25–32.

Chapter 62
Vesicular Pruriginous Lesions

Dario Didona and Biagio Didona

An 11-year-old boy presented to our department with a 10-months history of pruriginous vesicular and squamous erythematous lesions on the chest and axilla (Fig. 62.1). No erosions were detected in the oral and nasal mucosa. His past medical history was positive for mild vulgar psoriasis, but negative for autoimmune diseases or infections. He denied any new exposures to drugs. His family history was negative for autoimmune or inherited diseases. Routine laboratory tests were all negative. Skin culture was positive for *Staphylococcus aureus*. Initially, the patient

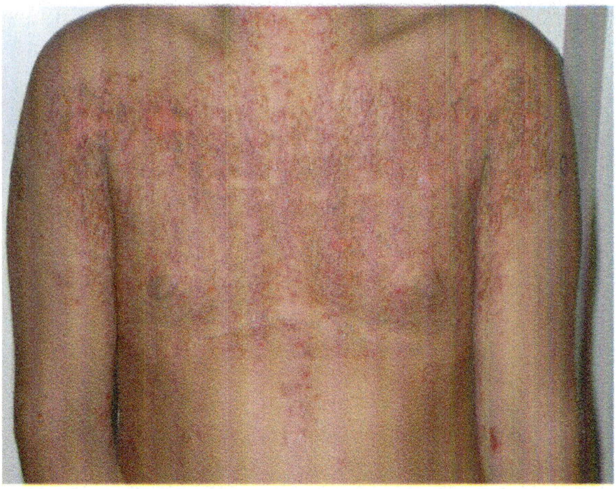

Fig. 62.1 Vesicular, erythematous lesions on the chest of an 11-year-old boy

D. Didona (✉)
Department of Dermatology and Allergology, Philipps University, Marburg, Germany

B. Didona
First Division of Dermatology, Istituto Dermopatico dell'Immacolata-IRCCS, Rome, Italy

© Springer Nature Switzerland AG 2020

F. Rahmani, N. Rezaei (eds.), *Pediatric Autoimmunity and Transplantation*,
https://doi.org/10.1007/978-3-030-26280-8_62

was started on prednisone (1.5 mg/Kg per day) and antihistamines with slight improvement. Six days after, he developed erythematous and exudative lesions on the chest and upper limbs.

Q1. What is the most likely diagnosis?

A. Eczema
B. Impetigo
C. Pemphigus foliaceus
D. Dermatitis herpetiformis

Answer: *The correct answer is* ***C.***

Although skin culture was positive for *Staphylococcus aureus,* the clinical picture led to a diagnosis of pemphigus foliaceus (PF), due to the presence of long-lasting vesicular lesions on an erythematous background in an asymptomatic patient. PF is a rare, acquired, autoimmune blistering disease that belongs to the group of superficial pemphigus. It's target antigen is desmoglein 1, which is present in skin but not in mucous membranes [1]. PF is a chronic disease, characterized by loss of intercellular adhesion of keratinocytes in the superficial epidermal layer of the skin, leading to superficial bullous lesions on the skin, while mucosal surfaces are spared. Clinically, PF can be differentiated from the more severe pemphigus vulgaris (PV), as PV shows a more widespread distribution and usually involves mucous membrane [1]. In addition, in comparison with pediatric PV, pediatric PF appears to follow a benign course, characterized by a relatively short duration [2, 3].

PF's mean age at onset is 7.7 years and the male-to-female ratio is 1.33:1 [2]. PF patients show usually crusted plaques and erosions [2, 3], while flaccid vesicels and bullae are also often observed. Less frequently, intact vesiculobullae are present, which are usually observed on the lower legs, showing a grouped or a linear pattern. The most commonly involved sites are the scalp and the face, followed by the trunk or upper extremities [2, 3]. Although our patient complained about pruritus, it is not a main symptom in PF [2, 3]. Indeed, most patients are often asymptomatic. Pain could be present in case of a secondary infection of the lesions. Several provoking factors have been reported in the literature, including sunlight exposure, drugs, cytomegalovirus, and bacterial infections.

Q2. What is the next best diagnostic test for this patient? (dsg: desmoglein, ANA: anti-nuclear antibody, ENA: extractable nuclear antigen)

A. Skin Punch biopsy
B. Serum ANA and ENA levels
C. Serum Anti-dsg 1 and 3 levels

Answer: *The correct answer is* ***C.***

Presence of serum anti-dsg 1 and 3 autoantibodies are one of the main features of autoimmune blistering diseases that belong to the pemphigus group. Dsgs belong to the cadherins family and are components of cell adhesion complexes, called desmosomes [4]. The antidesmogelin 1 autoantibodies found in the sera of patients with PF are probably responsible for the superficial acantholysis that characterize PF [4]. Serum anti-dsg 3 autoantibodies should be looked for, to rule out the diagnosis of PV. Nevertheless, several cases of isolated mucosal or skin bullous lesions have been reported in patients with only anti-dsg1 or 3 respectively [4]. Although serum IgG anti-dsg 1 antibodies are considered as pathogenic for pemphigus foliaceus, IgE anti-dsg autoantibodies can also be detected in the serum of these patients [4].

Q3. Which of the following pathological findings gives you a major clue for the diagnosis of PF?

A. Cleavage at the substratum corneum
B. Sub-epidermal cleavage
C. Supra-basal blistering
D. Acanthosis and neutrophilic infiltration

Answer: *The correct answer is* ***A.***

Pathologically, PF is characterized by a subcorneal acantholytic blister, usually filled with neutrophils [4]. In addition, a slight inflammatory infiltration of the upper dermis can be detected, such as perivascular infiltrates of lymphocytes and neutrophils in the papillary dermis. H&E staining of biopsy specimen is mandatory to differentiate PF from PV which often have a lot of clinical resemblance [4]. PV is pathologically characterized by intraepidermal and suprabasal acantholysis, loss of keratinocytes adhesion, neutrophilic and eosinophilic infiltrate, and a scant perivascular round-cell infiltrate in the upper dermal vascular plexus [4]. Figure 62.2 shows H&E staining of the sample we obtained from the base of our patients lesions.

Q4. What is the next best step to confirm the diagnosis?

A. Evaluation of ANA autoantibodies
B. Direct and indirect immunofluorescence microscopy

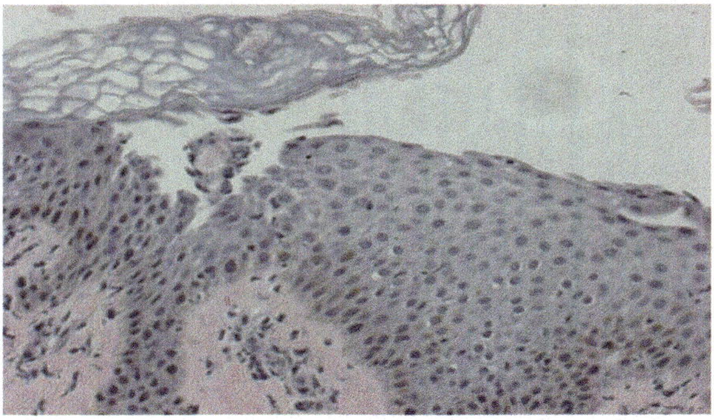

Fig. 62.2 Sub-corneal acantholytic blister (H&E 30x) in an 11-year-old boy with vesicular pruriginous lesions

C. Evaluation of lymphocyte subsets and serum antibody levels
D. Electron microscopy of skin biopsy

Answer: *The correct answer is* ***B.***

Direct and indirect immunofluorescence (DIF and IIF) are extremely useful to confirm the diagnosis of PF [4]. DIF on perilesional skin shows an intercellular, reticular pattern of fluorescence of IgG autoantibodies in the epidermis. C3 could be also detected at the same site by DIF. IIF may be used to identify circulating autoantibodies in patients serum. Both studies are also extremely useful to differentiate diseases of the pemphigus group from other similar bullous diseases, such as bullous lupus erythematosus.

Q5. What is the main underlying mechanism of this disorder?

A. Humoral autoimmunity and type II hypersensitivity reaction
B. Cellular autoimmunity and delayed type hypersensitivity
C. Monogenic mutations
D. Multigenic disorders with infectious trigger

Answer: *The correct answer is* ***A.***

Anti-dsg 1 IgG autoantibodies have been reported as pathogenic. However, other non-dsg autoantibodies could be detected in PF whose role in pathogenesis is now under debate, including anti-thyroglobulin antibodies [1]. Autoreactive $CD4^{+}$ T cells appear to play a pivotal role in autoantibody production [1]. These are mainly T helper 2 cells which regulate autoantibody production, via secretion of interleukins 4, 5, and 13b [1].

Q6. What is the mainstay therapeutic option for pemphigus vulgaris?

A. Glucocorticoids
B. Cyclosporine
C. Methotrexate
D. Azathioperin

Answer: *The correct answer is* ***A.***

Up to this date, less than 40 cases of pediatric PF are reported in the literature [2]. Therefore, the standard therapy is based on the ones used in adult patients. In the majority of cases, systemic corticosteroids represent an adequate and safe therapy, although in mild cases, topical steroids may be effectively used [2]. Dapsone is the most commonly used adjuvant drug [2]. Several other treatments have been proposed in the literature, including chloroquine, methotrexate, and azathioprine [2].

Practical Points

- No more than 40 cases of pemphigus foliaceus are reported in pediatric patients
- Direct immunofluorescence study is mandatory to confirm the diagnosis of pemphigus foliaceus
- Systemic steroids are the first choice therapeutic option in management of pemphigus foliaceus

References

1. Di Zenzo G, Amber KT, Sayar BS, Muller EJ, Borradori L. Immune response in pemphigus and beyond: progresses and emerging concepts. Semin Immunopathol. 2016;38(1):57–74.
2. Metry DW, Hebert AA, Jordon RE. Nonendemic pemphigus foliaceus in children. J Am Acad Dermatol. 2002;46(3):419–22.
3. Marathe K, Lu J, Morel KD. Bullous diseases: kids are not just little people. Clin Dermatol. 2015;33(6):644–56.
4. Kasperkiewicz M, Ellebrecht CT, Takahashi H, Yamagami J, Zillikens D, Payne AS, Amagai M. Pemphigus. Nat Rev Dis Primers. 2017;3:17026.

Chapter 63
Widespread Vesiculobullous Rash

Soner Uzun and Aslı Bilgic-Temel

A 26-month-old boy presented with a widespread vesiculobullous rash. Dermatological examination revealed symmetrically distributed and grouped blisters, erosions and crusts rising over an urticarial ground on face, trunk, limbs and palmoplantar areas (Fig. 63.1). The patient had experienced the same episodes at 3 months of age, similarly accompanied by a severe itch. There were also mucosal erosions and intact blisters. He had no abnormalities on physical examination apart from skin lesions. There was no family history for similar signs or symptoms. Parents were not related.

Q1. What is the most likely diagnosis?

A. Hereditary epidermolysis bullosa
B. Bullous impetigo
C. Bullous pemphigoid
D. Bullous drug eruption

Answer: *The correct answer is* ***C.***

Bacterial or viral skin infections, drug eruptions and genodermatoses, such as hereditary epidermolysis bullosa, should also be included in the differential diagnosis of children presenting with vesiculobullous eruption. Age of presentation, patient's general condition, morphology and distribution of the lesions as well as

S. Uzun (✉)
Department of Dermatology and Venereology, School of Medicine, Akdeniz University, Antalya, Turkey
e-mail: sonuzun@akdeniz.edu.tr

A. Bilgic-Temel
Seydisehir State Hospital, Dermatology Clinic, Konya, Turkey

© Springer Nature Switzerland AG 2020
F. Rahmani, N. Rezaei (eds.), *Pediatric Autoimmunity and Transplantation*,
https://doi.org/10.1007/978-3-030-26280-8_63

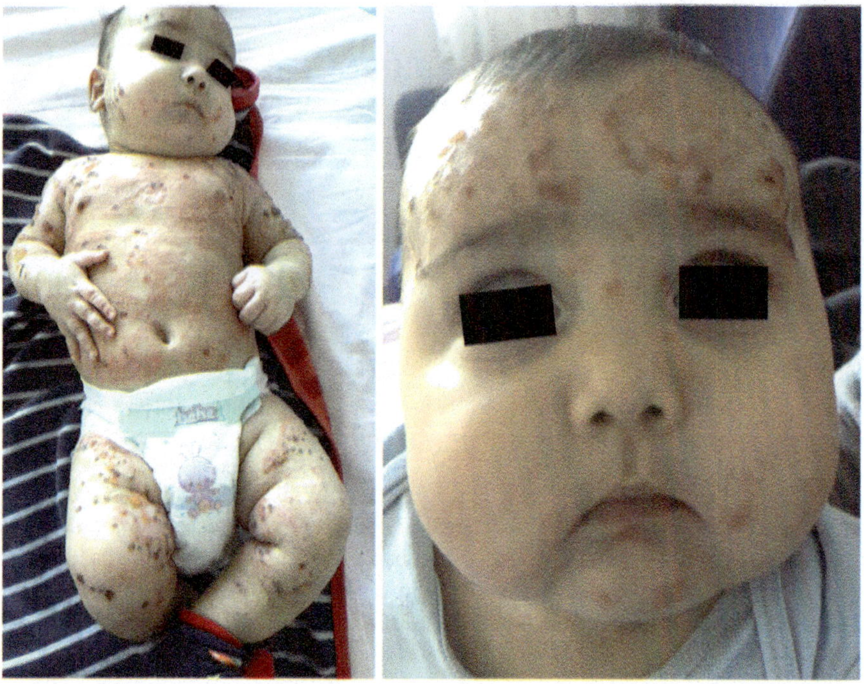

Fig. 63.1 Widespread vesiculobullous rash of a 26-month-old boy

family history are important elements of history that would help differentiate between these conditions [1].

For instance, bullous impetigo is the most common bacterial skin infection in children. It is a highly contagious infection of the superficial epidermis and frequently affects children between 2 and 5 years of age. Bullous impetigo often heals without scars even when left untreated. The staphylococcal toxin is the reason for bullous lesions and the diagnosis is confirmed clinically, by gram staining or culture [2–4]. Herpes infections also lead to development of vesicles and erosions following the symptoms of burning, stinging, and pruritus, which lasts for about 1–2 days. If not treated, herpes lesions take about 1–3 weeks to heal completely [5–7]. On the other hand, epidermolysis bullosa or EB is an autosomal dominant or recessive inherited monogenic disorder composed of several disorders characterized by recurrent mechanical bullae formation due to an increase in skin fragility. The characteristic finding in almost all types of EB is emergence of repetitive blisters or erosions with minor trauma. A majority of patients with mild forms of the disease may not show signs until childhood or early adulthood, while in others, findings may appear at birth or shortly after birth [8].

Juvenile bullous pemphigoid is more common in girls, often before the age of 10, and a significant proportion of patients present in the first year of life [9, 10]. Onset of symptoms is sometimes triggered by vaccination [11–13]. Juvenile bullous pemphigoid is characterized by tense blisters that develop on urticarial or normal-appearing skin, while facial and acral involvement is more common in childhood. In infants, the lesions are specifically distributed in palms, soles and face [9, 10, 14]. Mucosal involvement is frequently observed in juvenile bullous pemphigoid but not during infancy [9, 10, 15].

Q2. What is the next best step to confirm the diagnosis?

A. Histopathology
B. Cytology
C. ELISA BP180 test
D. Direct immunofluorescence test

Answer: *The correct answer is* ***D.***

Specimens for light microscopy studies should be taken from early bullae arising on erythematous skin and placed in formalin solution. Typical findings consist of subepidermal bullae containing eosinophils and/or neutrophils, associated with a dermal infiltrate of eosinophils and/or neutrophils or a marginalization of eosinophils along the dermoepidermal junction. Nevertheless, in the absence of blistering and in non-bullous forms, histopathological findings may be nonspecific, such as the presence of eosinophilic spongiosis [16].

Direct immunofluorescence (DIF) study is critical to make the diagnosis of bullous pemphigoid [17, 18]. Biopsy specimen for DIF should be obtained from perilesional skin and the blistered skin should be avoided. DIF typically demonstrates linear deposits of IgG and/or C3 along the dermoepidermal junction. Occasionally IgA and IgE are also found with a similar pattern [17, 18] (Fig. 63.2). IgG anti-basement membrane antibodies binding to the epidermal side show a n-serration pattern in the DIF analysis. This finding can be helpful and specific in combination with IIF studies [19]. IgG anti-basement membrane antibodies binding to the epidermal, and sometimes dermal, side of the split in IIF microscopy on normal human salt-split skin allows differentiation of bullous pemphigoid from epidermolysis bullosa acquisita, anti-laminin-332 mucous membrane pemphigoid and anti-p200 pemphigoid [17, 19–22].

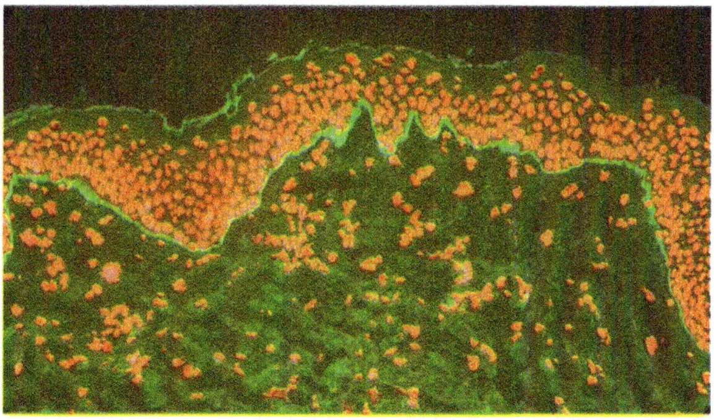

Fig. 63.2 Positive DIF for bullous pemphigoid. Linear deposition of IgG on dermoepidermal junction in a 26-month-old boy

Q3. All of the following are among first-line treatment options in this patient, except:

A. Cyclosporine
B. Systemic corticosteroids
C. Dapsone
D. Topical corticosteroids

Answer: *The correct answer is* ***A.***

Juvenile bullous pemphigoid differs from adult bullous pemphigoid in terms of treatment response and prognosis. Contrary to the chronic course in elderly individuals, pemphigoid cases in childhood can be healed within 1 year after completion of the disease [9, 10, 14]. There is also no accompanying disease that contributes to morbidity. Topical steroids are usually well-tolerated and efficient.

Practical Points

- Juvenile bullous pemphigoid is characterized by tense blisters that develop on urticarial or normal-appearing skin, while facial and acral involvement is more common in childhood
- In infants, the lesions are specifically distributed in palms, soles and face
- Mucosal involvement is frequently observed in juvenile bullous pemphigoid but not during infancy
- Juvenile bullous pemphigoid is more common in girls, often before the age of 10
- Specimens for light microscopy studies should be taken from early bullae arising on erythematous skin and placed in formalin solution

References

1. Rico M. Differential diagnosis of vesiculobullous lesions. In: Textbook of pediatric dermatology. Slovenya: Blackwell Science; 2000.
2. Yaylı S. Common bacterial skin infections in children. Turkderm. 2011;45(2):104–8.
3. Cole C, Gazewood J. Diagnosis and treatment of impetigo. Am Fam Physician. 2007;75:859–64.
4. Sladden M, Johnston G. Common skin infections in children. BMJ Case Rep. 2004;329(7457):95–9.
5. Sarıcaoğlu H. Diseases of viral origin. Türkderm. 2011;45(2):81–6.
6. Madkon V, Sra K, Brantley J, Carrasco D. Human herpes viruses. In: Dermatology. 2nd ed. Philadelphia: Mosby-Elsevier; 2008.
7. James W, Elston D, Berger T. Viral diseases. Andrews' diseases of the skin. 11th ed. Philadelphia: Elsevier Saunders; 2011.
8. Karaduman A. Inherited bullous diseases. Türkderm. 2011;45(2):81–6.
9. Sansaricq F, Stein S, Petronic-Rosic V. Autoimmune bullous diseases in childhood. Clin Dermatol. 2012;30(1):114–27.

10. Marathe K, Lu J, Morel K. Bullous diseases: kids are not just little people. Clin Dermatol. 2015;33(6):644–56.
11. Baroero L, Coppo P, Bertolino L, Maccario S, Savino F. Three case reports of post immunization and post viral bullous Pemphigoid: looking for the right trigger. BMC Pediatr. 2017;17(1):60.
12. Baykal C, Okan G, Sarica R. Childhood bullous pemphigoid developed after the first vaccination. J Am Acad Dermatol. 2001;44:348–50.
13. de la Fuente S, Hernandez-Martin A, de Lucas R, Gonzalez-Ensenat MA, Vicente A, Colmenero I, Gonzalez-Beato M, Sunol M, Torrelo A. Postvaccination bullous pemphigoid in infancy: report of three new cases and literature review. Pediatr Dermatol. 2013;30(6):741–4.
14. Gajic-Veljic M, Nikolic M, Medenica L. Juvenile bullous pemphigoid: the presentation and follow-up of six cases. J Eur Acad Dermatol Venereol. 2010;24(1):69–72.
15. Oranje AP vJT. Pemphigoid in children. Pediatr Dermatol. 1989;6(4):267–74.
16. Machado-Pinto J MT, Golitz LE. Eosinophilic and neutrophilic spongiosis: clues to the diagnosis of immunobullous diseases and other inflammatory disorders. Semin Cutan Med Surg. 1996;15:308–16.
17. Pohla-Gubo G, Hintner H. Direct and indirect immunofluorescence for the diagnosis of bullous autoimmune diseases. Dermatol Clin. 2011;29:365–72.
18. Joly P, Courville P, Lok C, Bernard P, Saiag P, Dreno B, Delaporte E, Bedane C, Picard C, Sassolas B, Plantin P, D'Incan M, Chosidow O, Pauwels C, Lambert D, Loche F, Prost C, Tancrede-Bohin E, Guillaume JC, Roujeau JC, Gilbert D, Tron F, Vaillant L. Clinical criteria for the diagnosis of bullous pemphigoid: a reevaluation according to immunoblot analysis of patient sera. Dermatology. 2004;208(1):16–20.
19. Terra JB, Meijer JM, Jonkman MF, Diercks GF. The n- vs. u-serration is a learnable criterion to differentiate pemphigoid from epidermolysis bullosa acquisita in direct immunofluorescence serration pattern analysis. Br J Dermatol. 2013;169(1):100–5.
20. Gammon W, Kowalewski C, Chorzelski T, Kumar V, Briggaman R, Beutner E. Direct immunofluorescence studies of sodium chloride-separated skin in the differential diagnosis of bullous pemphigoid and epidermolysis bullosa acquisita. J Am Acad Dermatol. 1990;22:664–70.
21. Schmidt E, Zillikens D. Pemphigoid diseases. Lancet (London, England). 2013;381(9863):320–32.
22. Feliciani C, Joly P, Jonkman M, Zambruno G, Zillikens D, Ioannides D, Kowalewski C, Jedlickova H, Kárpáti S, Marinovic B, Mimouni D, Uzun S, Yayli S, Hertl M, Borradori L. Management of bullous pemphigoid: the European dermatology forum consensus in collaboration with the European academy of dermatology and venereology. Br J Dermatol. 2015;172(4):867–77.

Chapter 64
Itchy Skin Rashes

Marzieh Tavakol

A 10-year-old girl was referred to our clinic with itchy skin rashes. The rash had developed about 14 months ago and was extremely pruritic with burning sensation. Occasionally lesions evolved into bulla with bloody oozing after being scratched. She had taken various alleviative topical remedies, none of which were successful. The rash had extended throughout her body and is now impeding her night sleep and daily activities.

She was the second child of unrelated parents and had no family history of skin rashes or other similar disorders. Her first allergic manifestation was an eczematoid rash starting since the age of 4, for which she had received several treatments including emollients, topical steroids and calcineurin inhibitors. She developed asthma with frequent exacerbations, leading to several emergency department admissions, and allergic rhinitis managed by nasal and inhaled corticosteroid and oral leukotriene receptor antagonist.

Physical examination showed widespread maculopapular and blistering skin lesions with excoriation on the abdomen, elbows, thighs, shoulders, axillary area, and buttocks (Fig. 64.1). Laboratory data are shown in Table 64.1.

Given her skin prick test that was positive for weeds (Russian thistle, Ragweed, Mugwort and Chenopodium), grasses (Timothy, Bermuda and Vernal grass) and molds (*Cladosporium*, *Aspergillus*, *Alternaria*, *Mucor* and *Penicillium*), she had adopted comprehensive avoidance measures and was a candidate for subcutaneous immunotherapy.

M. Tavakol (✉)
Non-communicable Diseases Research Center, Alborz University of Medical Sciences, Karaj, Iran

Department of Allergy and Clinical Immunology, Shahid Bahonar Hospital, Alborz University of Medical Sciences, Karaj, Iran

© Springer Nature Switzerland AG 2020
F. Rahmani, N. Rezaei (eds.), *Pediatric Autoimmunity and Transplantation*, https://doi.org/10.1007/978-3-030-26280-8_64

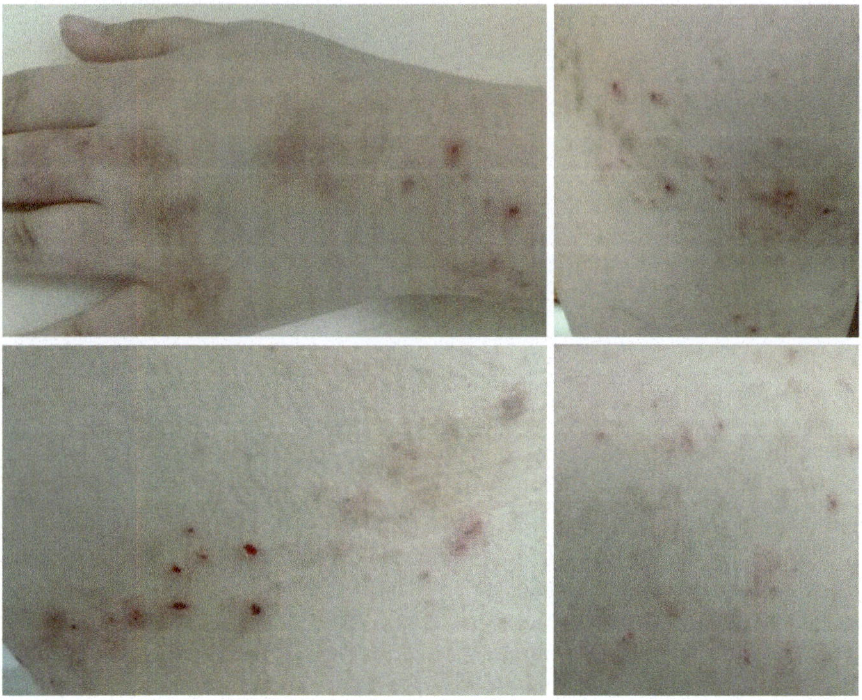

Fig. 64.1 Maculopapular and blistering skin lesions with excoriation on the abdomen, elbows, thighs, shoulders, axillary area, and buttocks in a 10 year-old girl with itchy skin rashes

Table 64.1 Laboratory test results in a 10 year-old girl with itchy skin rashes

White blood cells	8100 /μL (5000–13,000)
Neutrophils	%66
Eosinophils	%2
Lymphocytes	%2
Monocytes	%30
Hemoglobin	13.7 g/dL (reference: 11.5–15.5)
MCV	81.2 fL (reference: 77–95)
Platelet	373,000/μL (170,000-450,000)
ESR	3 (up to 35) mm/h
CRP	4 mg/dL (up to 10)
Cr	0.73 mg/dL (reference: 0.4–1.3)
AST	28 IU/L (up to 37)
ALT	53 IU/L (up to 41)
IgG	988.9 mg/dL (reference: 500–1300)
IgA	<10 mg/dL (reference: 41–297)
IgM	48.7 mg/dL (reference: 55–210)
IgE	85.30 mg/dL (reference: up to 90)

Q1. What is the most likely diagnosis?

A. Contact dermatitis
B. Atopic dermatitis
C. Scabies
D. None of the above

Answer: *The correct answer is* ***D.***

According to the distribution of the lesions and unresponsiveness to topical steroids and calcineurin inhibitors, the diagnosis of atopic and contact dermatitis would be under question [1].There was no index case of scabies in her family history. Also, absence of typical distribution of the scabies attributable skin lesions and lack of barrow along with long duration of the disease are against scabies [2].

Q2. What is the best initial step in the diagnosis of this patient?

A. Radioallergosorbent test for food allergens
B. Skin biopsy
C. Skin scrape test
D. Measurement of serum IgG, IgA, IgM, IgE

Answer: *The correct answer is* ***B.***

Given the high negative predictive value of the skin prick test and considering the negative result of our patient's skin prick test for food allergens, a radioallergosorbent test (RAST) test does not provide more beneficial information in this case [3]. Skin scrape test is used to confirm the diagnosis of scabies and given incompatible findings in this patient, would probably be of low diagnostic value [2].

Skin biopsy was performed revealing superficial perivascular dermatitis with psoriasiform minimal spongiotic epidermal reaction in favor of chronic eczematous dermatitis. Direct immunofluorescence (DIF) examination showed granular deposition of IgA antibody in dermal papilla in support of dermatitis herpetiformis (DH).

Q3. All of the following tests would help to the diagnosis in this patient, except:

A. IgA anti-tissue transglutaminase antibodies
B. IgG antiendomysial antibodies
C. Serum total IgA level
D. Serum total IgG level

Answer: *The correct answer is* ***D.***

Dermatitis herpetiformis is a papulovesicular skin disorder [4]. The pathologic basis of DH is cell-mediated hypersensitivity to gluten, manifested by symmetric distribution of intensely itchy papules and vesicles, predominantly involving the skin and extensor surfaces [5]. Given that the lesions are severely pruritic, intact vesicles are hardly ever seen and excoriated papulovesicles are the most common physical findings [4, 6]. Females outnumber males and the forth decade of life is the usual age of first manifestation [4]. Papular eczema, contact dermatitis, insect bite, papular urticaria, scabies, other cutaneous vesiculobullous disorders such as bullous pemphigoid and linear immunoglobulin A dermatosis are considered in differential diagnoses of DH [4, 6]. IgA anti-tissue transglutaminase antibody (anti-tTG) has been shown to be the most sensitive and specific method of serologic study in patients with DH and is recommended as the initial diagnostic test in these patients. Serum IgA level should be determined simultaneously to rule out IgA deficiency, to identify possible false-negative results of tTG-IgA. IgG and IgA anti-endomysial antibodies (anti-EMA) are valuable to approve the diagnosis. These antibodies are used to evaluate patients' adherence to the gluten-free regimen as well [7].

Q4. What is the first best step in the management of this patient?

A. Systemic corticosteroid
B. Topical steroid
C. Gluten-free diet
D. Dapson

Answer: *The correct answer is* ***C.***

Life-long gluten-free regimen (contained less than 20 ppm gluten) is considered the primary, as well as the most effective therapeutic measure for management of the DH [4, 7]. It is worth mentioning the fact that the DH patients who are under therapeutic regimen, are vulnerable to deficiency of some essential nutrients. Constant monitoring, at least once a year, is a necessary step of their follow-up [8].

Q5. What is the best way to evaluate patient's adherence to treatment?

A. Repeated kin and duodenal biopsy
B. Anti-endomysial antibodies
C. Anti-epidermal transglutaminase antibodies
D. Anti-deamidated synthetic gliadin-derived peptides

Answer: *The correct answer is* ***B.***

Anti-deamidated synthetic gliadin-derived peptides (DGP) have variable sensitivity and specificity but not significantly more than anti-endomysial antibodies (anti-EMA) and anti-tissue transglutaminase antibodies (anti-tTG). This test accessibility is limited to research laboratories and it is not a good test for the patient diagnosis or follow-up. Anti-epidermal transglutaminase (anti-eTG) antibodies are approximately as sensitive and specific as anti-EMA and anti-tTG and given their higher cost, are only used in suspicious cases under 2 years old. Anti-EMA and anti-tTG are more useful as confirmatory tests for the diagnosis of celiac disease. Considering the fact that anti-EMA and anti-tTG antibodies are negative in patients under gluten-free diet, these antibodies are commonly considered as objective sign of patient adherence to diet [7].

Practical Points

- In dermatitis herpetiformis direct immunofluorescent examination shows granular deposition of IgA antibody in dermal papilla
- IgA anti-tissue transglutaminase antibody has been shown to be the most sensitive and specific method of serologic study in patients with dermatitis herpetiformis
- Life-long gluten-free regimen is the primary and the most effective therapeutic measure for management of the dermatitis herpetiformis

References

1. Boguniewicz M, Alexis AF, Beck LA, Block J, Eichenfield LF, Fonacier L, Guttman-Yassky E, Paller AS, Pariser D, Silverberg JI. Expert perspectives on management of moderate-to-severe atopic dermatitis: a multidisciplinary consensus addressing current and emerging therapies. J Allergy Clin Immunol Pract. 2017;5:1519–31.
2. Arlian LG, Morgan MS. A review of Sarcoptes scabiei: past, present and future. Parasit Vectors. 2017;10(1):297.
3. Verstege A, Mehl A, Rolinck-Werninghaus C, Staden U, Nocon M, Beyer K, Niggemann B. The predictive value of the skin prick test weal size for the outcome of oral food challenges. Clin Exp Allergy. 2005;35(9):1220–6.
4. Marathe K, Lu J, Morel KD. Bullous diseases: kids are not just little people. Clin Dermatol. 2015;33(6):644–56.
5. Anna Nowak-Węgrzyn AWB, Sampson HA. Reactions to foods. In: Adkinson NF, Bochner B, Burks AW, Busse WW, Holgate ST, Lemanske Jr RF, O'Hehir RE, editors. Middleton's allergy: principles and practice, vol. 2. 8th ed. Philadelphia, PA: Elsevier Saunders; 2014. p. 1310–39.
6. Joyce JC. Vesiculobullous disorders. In: Robert Kliegman BS, St. Geme J, Schor NF, Behrman RE, editors. Nelson textbook of pediatrics, vol. 2. 20th ed. Phialdelphia, PA: Elsevier; 2015. p. 3140–9.
7. Antiga E, Caproni M. The diagnosis and treatment of dermatitis herpetiformis. Clin Cosmet Investig Dermatol. 2015;8:257.
8. Vici G, Belli L, Biondi M, Polzonetti V. Gluten free diet and nutrient deficiencies: a review. Clin Nutr. 2016;35(6):1236–41.

Chapter 65
Blisters on Back and Upper Extremities

Gulsen Akoglu

A 9-year-old boy presented with multiple blisters filled with clear fluid over his upper chest, back and upper arms. The eruption had begun about 1 month ago, after he was treated with a mucolytic drug containing erdosteine, ibuprofen, and clarithromycin for 2 weeks. His dermatological examination revealed widespread multiple groups of herpetiform vesicles and bulla over an erythematous background on his back and upper extremities. Excoriations and some crusts were observed on his trunk and lower extremities (Fig. 65.1). He also complained of excessive tire and intense pruritus since the onset of symptoms.

On examination, nails, scalp, and mucosal regions were normal, and no organomegaly, lymphadenopathy, or fever was detected. Laboratory examinations including total blood count with differential, renal, liver, and thyroid function tests, fasting glucose, lipids, ESR, CRP, and urinalysis were all within normal limits.

Q1. What is the best initial step in the diagnosis of this patient?

A. Anti-herpes simplex antibodies
B. Skin biopsy for light microscopy and direct immunofluorescence
C. Placebo-controlled drug challenge tests
D. Systemic work up for malignancy

Answer: *The correct answer is* ***B.***

A skin biopsy from a newly blistered skin is mandatory to establish a correct diagnosis and to differentiate mainly autoimmune vesiculobullous diseases, bullous drug reactions, erythema multiforme, or viral eruptions. DIF microscopy of the skin is the gold-standard for diagnosing autoimmune blistering diseases. The level of detachment and possible deposits of immunoglobulins within skin are best observed

G. Akoglu (✉)
Gulhane Training and Research Hospital, Dermatology and Venereology Clinic, University of Health Sciences, Ankara, Turkey

© Springer Nature Switzerland AG 2020

F. Rahmani, N. Rezaei (eds.), *Pediatric Autoimmunity and Transplantation*,
https://doi.org/10.1007/978-3-030-26280-8_65

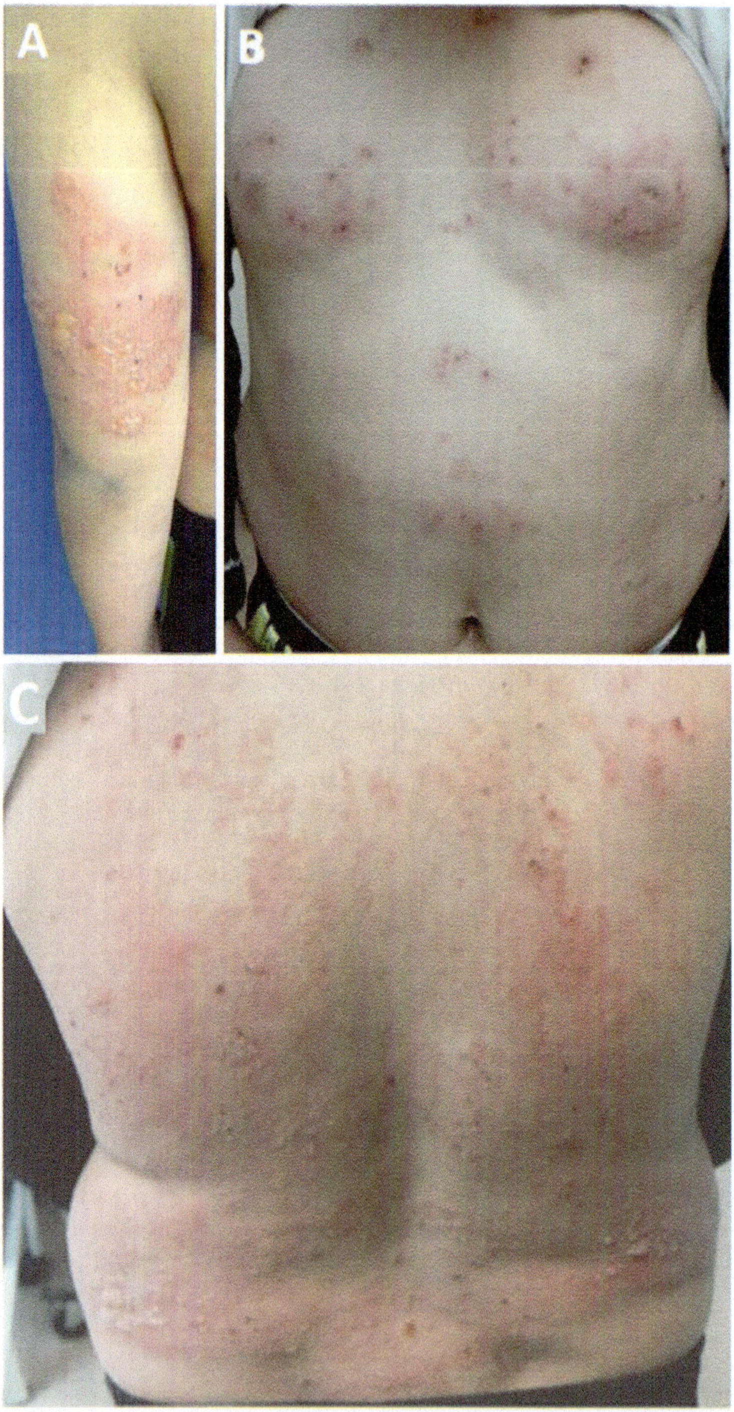

Fig. 65.1 Multiple grouping and herpetiform vesicles and bulla over erythema on the left arm (**a**) and trunk (**b**, **c**)

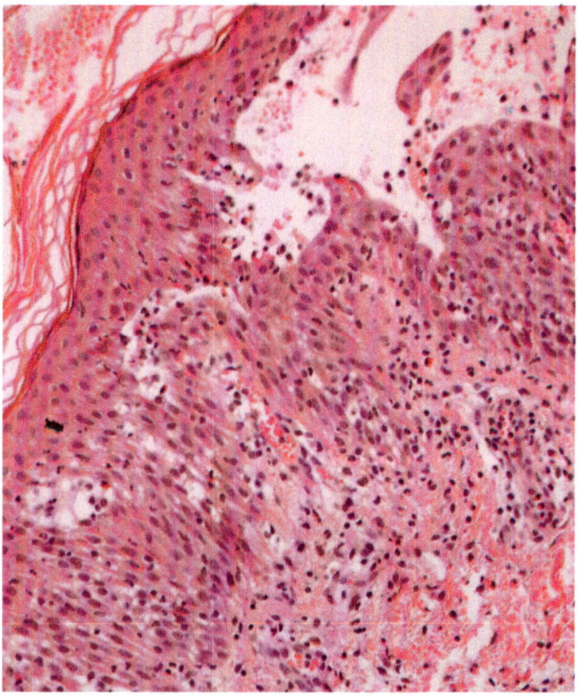

Fig. 65.2 Intraepidermal cleft containing acantholytic cells, epidermal spongiosis, and mixed inflammatory infiltrate with eosinophils in the papillary dermis (H&E, ×200)

when DIF of the periblistered skin specimen is performed [1]. In the present case, histopathological examination of a bulla showed an intraepidermal cleft containing acantholytic cells, epidermal spongiosis, and mixed inflammatory infiltrate with eosinophils in the papillary dermis (Fig. 65.2). Intercellular C3 and IgG deposition within the entire epidermis was observed in DIF of the perilesional skin.

Q2. What is the most likely diagnosis?

A. Bullous pemphigoid
B. Pemphigus
C. Linear IgA bullous disease
D. Dermatitis herpetiformis

Answer: *The correct answer is* ***B.***

Presence of intraepidermal cleft, acantholytic cells, and IgG and C3 deposition helps us establish that this bullous eruption belongs to pemphigus family of autoimmune bullous skin disorders. The major autoantigens in pemphigus are desmogleins that extend from desmosomal plaque to the intercellular space to maintain the integrity of epidermis, forming tight attachments with adjacent cells. Desmoglein 1 antigen is mainly expressed in the upper parts of both epidermis and mucosa while desmoglein 3 antigens are located in the basal parts of the epidermis and throughout the mucosa. Direct immunofluorescence of the perilesional skin typically reveals intercellular deposits of IgG ± C3. The pemphigus group consists of several subtypes: pemphigus vulgaris (PV, the most common with mucocutaneous and mucosal variants), pemphigus foliaceous (PF, with superficial flaccid blisters and scales with anti desmoglein 1 antibody), pemphigus vegetans (with vegetative and papillomatous lesions), pemphigus herpetiformis (with grouped and herpetiform small blisters, mainly with antidesmoglein 1 antibody, without papillary dermal deposits), paraneoplastic (associated with underlying malignancy and more severe painful oral lesions), and drug-induced types [2].

Bullous pemphigoid, linear IgA bullous disease (LABD), and dermatitis herpetiformis or DH are other types of autoimmune bullous skin disorders with different clinical and histopathological features when compared with PV. Bulla are flaccid in PV and tense in bullous pemphigoid. Discrete or herpetiform vesicules and bullae in a chain-like pattern at the edge of inflammatory erythema characterises LABD, and intensely pruritic small papulovesicular are seen in DH. Level of detachment in skin is intraepidermal in PV and subepidermal in bullous pemphigoid, LABD, and DH. PV presents with intraepidermal IgG deposits, while deposition of IgG along basal membrane is seen in bullous pemphigoid and of IgA type in LABD. A granular deposition of IgA in the upper papillary dermis is seen in DH [3]. Depending on the clinicopathological features, our case has a pemphigus eruption.

Q3. What is the next best step in evaluation of this patient?

A. Specific and total IgE levels
B. C3, C4 levels
C. Serum titre of autoantibodies against desmoglein 1 and 3 antigens
D. Ig A, Ig M, Ig G levels

Answer: *The correct answer is* ***C.***

The circulating autoantibodies can be detected by different immunoassays such as indirect immunofluorescence/IIF (when patient's serum is applied on the monkey's esophagus substrate, and the circulating IgG autoantibodies bind to epidermal surfaces), immunoblotting, immunoprecipitation and enzyme-linked immunosorbent assay. If serum is positive for desmoglein 1 but negative for desmoglein 3, a diagnosis of pemphigus foliaceus is suggested. Detection of anti-desmoglein 3 but no anti-desmoglein 1 antibody in turn suggests a diagnosis of the mucosal-dominant type of pemphigus vulgaris. When both anti-desmoglein 1 and anti-desmoglein 3 antibodies are present, a diagnosis of the mucocutaneous type of pemphigus vulgaris is supported. The titre of the autoantibodies often correlates with the clinical activity of pemphigus and beneficial for follow-ups [3]. The majority of the drug induced pemphigus cases show pemphigus foliaceus-type phenotype with anti-desmoglein 1 autoantibodies [4]. Pemphigus herpetiformis is a variant of pemphigus, with intraepidermal herpetiform blisters, different from very superficial blisters and scales of pemphigus foliaceus, associated with IgA and IgG antibodies to desmoglein 1 [5]. In the present case, serum anti-desmoglein 1 antibody was positive at 1:100 dilution. Clinicopathological features with positive anti-desmoglein 1 antibodies support the diagnosis of pemphigus herpetiformis variant in our case.

Q4. What is the most likely triggering cause of this pemphigus eruption?

A. Upper respiratory infection
B. Drug intake
C. Idiopathic
D. Hormonal factors

Answer: *The correct answer is* ***B****.*

Pemphigus may be triggered by exposure to thiol drugs (D-penicillamine, captopril), phenol drugs, or non-thiol non-phenol drugs (peniciline, cephalosporine). When a patient is diagnosed as having pemphigus, taking a detailed and careful history of his medications is mandatory. In the present case, the patient had been administered a mucolytic agent, erdosteine, whose active metabolite has a free thiol group. The mechanism of acantholysis due to thiol groups of the suspected medications is unclear; however, immunological and biochemical mechanisms are suggested to be involved. Thiol containing drugs may directly interfere with enzyme involving cell adhesion or may cause formation of neoantigens that lead to production of pathological autoantibodies against desmosomal antigens [6]. Drug induced pemphigus mostly presents as pemphigus foliaceus-like clinical and histopathological features [4]. In the present case, it is most likely that erdosteine caused drug induced pemphigus by induction of antidesmoglein 1 autoantibody production, intraepidermal cleft formation, and herpetiform blisters. Therefore, the correct diagnosis of our case is pemphigus herpetiformis type drug-induced pemphigus.

Q5. What is the best initial management in this patient?

A. Warning about avoiding thiol drugs
B. Elimination of thiol containing foods in diet
C. Immunosuppressive treatments
D. All of the above

Answer: *The correct answer is* ***D.***

The causative drug or similar medications should not be administered to this patient. The family should be warned that exposure to thiol drugs or thiol containing food, such as onions, garlic, etc., may deteriorate his condition and lead to flares [4, 7]. Treatment aims to suppress the autoimmunity towards to epidermal cells mainly with systemic corticosteroids [4]. In the present case, the child was treated with oral 1 mg/Kg/d methylprednisolone for 2 months and regression of blisters were observed. However, during tapering of steroid dosage, a flare up of new blisters emerged. Since increasing of steroid dosage did not control the flare up, oral weekly 10 mg methotrexate and 5 mg folic acid once a week were added to the therapy. Three months of this combination treatment provided clinical remission and lowered antidesmoglein 1 antibody titre (1:10). Gradual tapering of the agents did not lead to new flare ups. The treatments did not cause any side effects.

Practical Points

- Pemphigus vulgaris is the most common type of pemphigus with mucocutaneous and mucosal variants
- Pemphigus foliaceus presents with superficial flaccid blisters and scales with anti desmoglein 1 antibody
- Pemphigus vegetans presents with vegetative and papillomatous lesions and pemphigus herpetiformis with grouped and herpetiform small blisters and is mainly with antidesmoglein 1 antibody, without papillary dermal deposits
- Paraneoplastic pemphigus is associated with underlying malignancy and more severe painful oral lesions
- Drug-induced types of pemphigus may be triggered by exposure to thiol drugs, such a D-penicillamine and captopril, phenol drugs, or non-thiol non-phenol drugs such as peniciline and cephalosporines

References

1. Jukic IL, Marinovic B. Significance of immunofluorescence in the diagnosis of autoimmune bullous dermatoses. Clin Dermatol. 2011;29(4):389–97.
2. Mihalyi L, Kiss M, Dobozy A, Kemeny L, Husz S. Clinical relevance of autoantibodies in patients with autoimmune bullous dermatosis. Clin Dev Immunol. 2012;2012:369546.
3. Ishii K. Importance of serological tests in diagnosis of autoimmune blistering diseases. J Dermatol. 2015;42(1):3–10.
4. Yoshimura K, Ishii N, Hamada T, Abe T, Ono F, Hashikawa K, Fukuda S, Ohyama B, Koga H, Sogame R, Teye K, Ochiai T, Nakajima H, Nakajima K, Iijima S, Kanzaki M, Kojima K, Nagatani T, Fujimoto W, Karashima T, Nakama T, Ohata C, Furumura M, Tsuruta D, Hashimoto T. Clinical and immunological profiles in 17 Japanese patients with drug-induced pemphigus studied at Kurume University. Br J Dermatol. 2014;171(3):544–53.
5. Kozlowska A, Hashimoto T, Jarzabek-Chorzelska M, Amagai A, Nagata Y, Strasz Z, Jablonska S. Pemphigus herpetiformis with IgA and IgG antibodies to desmoglein 1 and IgG antibodies to desmocollin 3. J Am Acad Dermatol. 2003;48(1):117–22.
6. Ruocco V, De Angelis E, Lombardi ML. Drug-induced pemphigus. II. Pathomechanisms and experimental investigations. Clin Dermatol. 1993;11(4):507–13.
7. Ruocco E, Wolf R, Ruocco V, Brunetti G, Romano F, Lo Schiavo A. Pemphigus: associations and management guidelines: facts and controversies. Clin Dermatol. 2013;31(4):382–90.

Chapter 66
Itchy Blisters

Yan Ling Kong and Emily Yiping Gan

An 8-year-old boy presented with a 2-week history of blisters that started on his lower limbs and feet, but gradually progressed to involve his hands, trunk and scalp. The rashes were intensely itchy. He had experienced an upper respiratory tract infection 2 weeks prior to the onset of the blisters. On examination, there were extensive annular urticated plaques rimmed with vesicles on his trunk, limbs and groin, with larger bullae present on his acral surfaces (Figs. 66.1 and 66.2). There was no mucosal involvement.

Histological examination revealed multilocular subepidermal blisters, containing mainly neutrophils and few eosinophils. Laboratory data revealed leukocyte count of 9900/μL (neutrophils: 44%, lymphocytes: 34%, monocytes: 9.5%, eosinophils 12%, basophils 0.5%), Hb: 13.2 g/dL and platelet count 295,000/μL. Liver function tests including total serum protein (7.1 g/dL), albumin (4.2 g/dL), total bilirubin (0.15 mg/dL), and alkaline phosphatase (135 IU/L) were all within normal range. A skin biopsy was also taken for direct immunofluorescence and this returned positive.

Q1. What is the most likely diagnosis and what are the expected findings in direct immunofluorescence?

A. Bullous pemphigoid: linear IgG and C3 along the basement membrane zone
B. Dermatitis herpetiformis: granular IgA at the dermal papillae
C. Linear IgA bullous dermatosis: linear IgA at the basement membrane zone
D. Epidermolysis bullosa: direct immunofluorescence is negative

Answer: *The correct answer is* ***C.***

Y. L. Kong
National Skin Centre, Singapore, Singapore

E. Y. Gan (✉)
Dermatology Service, KK Women's and Children's Hospital, Singapore, Singapore

© Springer Nature Switzerland AG 2020

F. Rahmani, N. Rezaei (eds.), *Pediatric Autoimmunity and Transplantation*,
https://doi.org/10.1007/978-3-030-26280-8_66

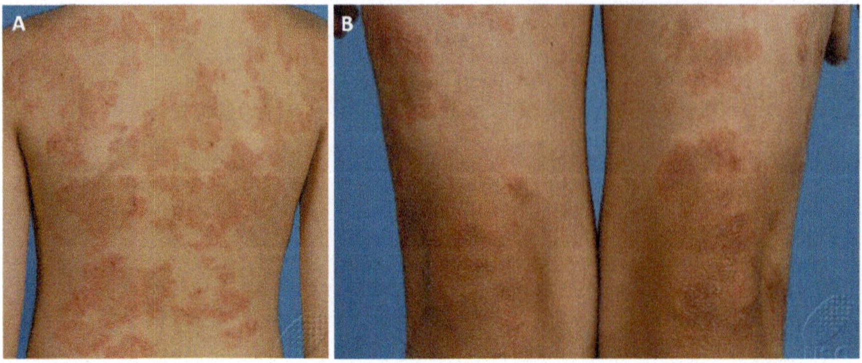

Fig. 66.1 Polycyclic and annular erythematous plaques rimmed with vesicles on the (**a**) back and (**b**) thighs and knees

Fig. 66.2 Close-up of the lesions on the back resembling a "string of beads": Annular erythematous plaques with tense vesicles at the edges

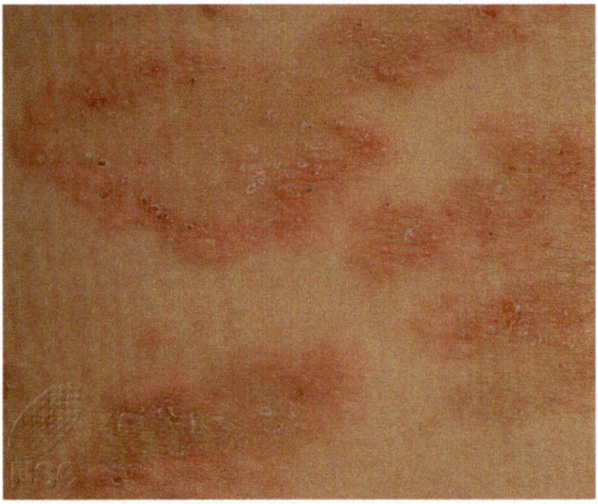

Linear IgA bullous dermatosis (LABD) is a rare, autoimmune subepidermal blistering disease that may affect both adults and children. Historically, the childhood form of LABD was known as chronic bullous disease of childhood [1]. Children typically present with widespread annular or polycyclic erythematous or urticated plaques, with tense vesicles or bullae at the edges. The presentation has been described as a "string of beads" or "cluster of jewels". The lesions are pruritic, and symmetrically distributed, with a predilection for the trunk, thighs, and groin [2]. Histologically, LABD is characterized by the presence of small subepidermal blisters with neutrophil-predominant infiltrates. Direct immunofluorescence demonstrates linear deposits of IgA at the basal membrane zone (BMZ) (Fig. 66.3) [1]. Dermatitis herpetiformis (DH) resembles LABD clinically and histologically, but may be differentiated by its direct immunofluorescence findings of granular IgA deposits at the dermal papillae. Unlike DH, gluten-sensitivity is not a feature of LABD [1].

The patient condition improved with a combination of azathioprine, dapsone and prednisolone.

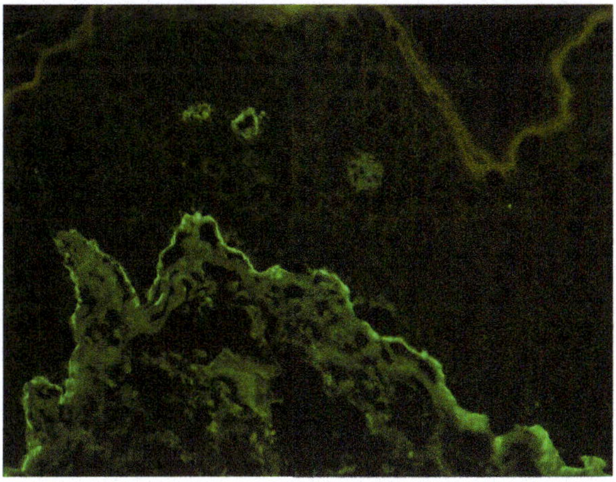

Fig. 66.3 Linear deposits of IgA at the basement membrane zone

Q2. This condition may be induced by the certain drugs. Which antibiotic has been most frequently reported as the inciting agent for the disease?

A. Bactrim
B. Ciprofloxacin
C. Meropenem
D. Vancomycin

Answer: *The correct answer is* ***D.***

Drug exposure has commonly been reported as a precipitant for LABD. Vancomycin is the most common implicated pharmacological agent, but other drugs that have been reported to induce LABD include antibiotics like penicillins, cephalosporins, sulfamethoxazole, non-steroidal anti-inflammatory drugs like naproxen, diclofenac and piroxicam, amiodarone, phenytoin and angiotensin converting enzyme inhibitors like captopril [1, 3, 4].

Drug-induced LABD is usually more severe than the idiopathic variant, and can present atypically. Patients may develop a polymorphic eruption consisting of erythematous papules, erosions and scaly erythematous patches, in addition to the characteristic vesiculobullous lesions [4]. A pseudo-toxic epidermal necrolysis variant has also been described, in which patients present with large erosions and a positive Nikolsky sign [4, 5].

Q3. The patient now presents with a 3-week history of bloody diarrhea associated with abdominal cramps, weight loss and loss of appetite. Which of the following conditions is associated with this disease?

A. Ulcerative colitis
B. Infectious colitis
C. Irritable bowel syndrome
D. Ischemic colitis

Answer: *The correct answer is* ***A.***

Linear IgA bullous dermatosis has been reported in association with inflammatory bowel disease, in particular ulcerative colitis (UC). In most patients, the diagnosis of UC precedes the onset of LABD. It is postulated that the abnormal production of IgA1 by the inflamed bowel cross-reacts with antigens of the lamina lucida and sub-lamina densa in the skin, resulting in the development of LABD [6, 7]. It is unclear why the association between LABD and UC is stronger than with Crohn disease. Reports have demonstrated clinical remission of LABD following surgical intervention for UC [6, 7].

Q4. What is the first-line oral pharmacological agent used in treatment of this condition?

A. Oral glucocorticoids
B. Dapsone
C. Azathioprine
D. Mycophenolate mofetil

Answer: *The correct answer is* ***B.***

Dapsone is a synthetic sulfone that has both antimicrobial and anti-inflammatory features. It is a well-recognized treatment for LABD and remains the mainstay of its management today. The drug inhibits neutrophil toxicity and chemotaxis by blocking myeloperoxidase activity [8]. Dapsone is started at about 0.5–2 mg/Kg/day in children, and the dose is gradually titrated upwards over several weeks to months in accordance to the patient's treatment response [9]. In LABD, the response to treatment can be dramatic, with signs of improvement noted within days of treatment initiation [8]. Alternative immunosuppressants to be used for patients with G6PD deficiency or for patients with dapsone-resistant disease include colchicine, mycophenolate mofetil, cyclosporine and oral glucocorticoids like prednisolone [9–11].

The patient was treated with a combination of oral prednisolone and the drug mentioned above (please refer to question 4). One week later, he complained of shortness of breath, light-headedness and headache. He was found to be tachycardic and cyanotic.

Q5. What do is the most likely cause of his shortness of breath and cyanosis?

A. Methemoglobinemia
B. Pulmonary embolism
C. Heart failure
D. Tracheoesophageal fistula

Answer: *The correct answer is* ***A.***

The patient has developed dapsone-induced methemoglobinemia. Dapsone is metabolized in the liver via the cytochrome P450 pathway to byproducts such as dapsone hydroxylamine, which is a strong oxidant responsible for inducing methemoglobinemia [12]. Methemoglobin is an abnormal form of hemoglobin, which arises from oxidation of iron in the heme molecule from the normal ferrous (Fe^{2+})

to the ferric (Fe^{3+}) state. Ferric heme molecules causes a structural change in the hemoglobin molecule, resulting in an inability to unload oxygen to tissues [13, 14]. Due to the impaired delivery of oxygen to vital organs, patients present with clinical features including dizziness, headache, fatigue, cyanosis and tachycardia. At higher methemoglobin levels, respiratory depression, seizures and death may result [13]. Intravenous injection of methylene blue is effective for emergency therapy. Milder cases can be treated with oral methylene blue, ascorbic acid or cimetidine [14, 15]. Importantly, dapsone-induced methemoglobinemia is not related to the patient's G6PD activity.

Practical Points

- Linear IgA bullous dermatosis (LABD) is an autoimmune subepidermal blistering disorder that presents with annular or polycyclic erythematous plaques associated with tense vesicles or bullae
- A detailed drug history is mandatory, as LABD may be precipitated by drug intake, of which the strongest association is seen with vancomycin
- LABD may also be associated with inflammatory bowel disease, in particular ulcerative colitis
- Patients with LABD respond dramatically to dapsone with improvement often noted within a few days of its initiation

References

1. Fortuna G, Marinkovich M. Linear immunoglobulin A bullous dermatosis. Clin Dermatol. 2012;30(1):38–50.
2. Haneef N, Ramachandra S, Metta A, Srujana L. Chronic bullous disease of childhood with IgG predominance: what is the locus standi? Indian J Dermatol. 2012;57(4):285–7.
3. Kang M, Kim H, Park Y. Vancomycin-induced linear IgA bullous dermatosis: a case report and review of the literature. Ann Dermatol. 2008;20(2):102–6.
4. Chanal J, Ingen-Housz-Oro S, Ortonne N, Duong TA, Thomas M, Valeyrie-Allanore L, Lebrun-Vignes B, Andre C, Roujeau JC, Chosidow O, Wolkenstein P. Linear IgA bullous dermatosis: comparison between the drug-induced and spontaneous forms. Br J Dermatol. 2013;169(5):1041–8.
5. Kakar R, Paugh H, Jaworsky C. Linear IgA bullous disease presenting as toxic epidermal necrolysis: a case report and review of the literature. Dermatology. 2013;227(3):209–13.
6. Watchorn RE, Gulmann C, Keogan M, Okane M. Linear IgA disease associated with ulcerative colitis: the role of surgery. Clin Exp Dermatol. 2014;39(3):327–9.
7. Vargas TJ, Fialho M, Santos LT, Rodrigues PA, Vargas AL, Sousa MA. Linear IgA dermatosis associated with ulcerative colitis: complete and sustained remission after total colectomy. An Bras Dermatol. 2013;88(4):600–3.
8. Han A. A practical approach to treating autoimmune bullous disorders with systemic medications. J Clin Aesthet Dermatol. 2009;5:19–28.
9. Mintz E, Morel K. Treatment of chronic bullous disease of childhood. Dermatol Clin. 2011;29(4):699–700.
10. Marzano A, Ramoni S, Spinelli D, Alessi E, Berti E. Refractory linear IgA bullous dermatosis successfully treated with mycophenolate sodium. J Dermatol Treat. 2008;19(6):364–7.

11. Young H, Coulson I. Linear IgA disease: successful treatment with cyclosporin. Br J Dermatol. 2000;143(1):204–5.
12. Reilly T, Woster P, Svensson C. Methemoglobin formation by hydroxylamine metabolites of sulfamethoxazole and dapsone: implications for differences in adverse drug reactions. J Pharmacol Exp Ther. 1999;288(3):951–9.
13. Burke P, Jahangir K, Kolber M. Dapsone-induced methemoglobinemia: case of the blue lady. Can Fam Physician. 2013;59(9):958–61.
14. Das J, Katyal A, Naunwaar D. Dapsone-induced methemoglobinemia in a patient of leprosy. Indian J Dermatol. 2015;60(1):108.
15. Coleman MD, Rhodes LE, Scott AK, Verbov JL, Friedmann PS, Breckenridge AM, Park BK. The use of cimetidine to reduce dapsone-dependent methaemoglobinaemia in dermatitis herpetiformis patients. Br J Clin Pharmacol. 1992;34(3):244–9.

Chapter 67
Sudden Onset Grouped Blisters

Soner Uzun and Aslı Bilgic-Temel

A 7-year-old boy presented with grouped blisters, starting suddenly on the knees and elbows and spreading to the face, scalp, lower limbs, hands and feet, starting a few days ago (Fig. 67.1). These lesions, usually rising from the urticarial area, were accompanied by severe itching.

Q1. What is the most probable diagnosis?

A. Pemphigus vulgaris
B. Psoriasis
C. Epidermolysis bullosa
D. Childhood linear IgA disease

Answer: *The correct answer is* ***D.***

Childhood linear IgA disease (CLAD) also known as childhood chronic bullous dermatosis is typically an autoimmune bullous disease observed in children and characterized by the accumulation of linear IgA along the basal membrane and subepidermal bullae [1].

The rash resembles juvenile pemphigoid and often occurs in the first decade of life and most often in pre-school children [2–4]. Tense, occasionally hemorrhagic vesicles and bullae which are arranged in annular pattern are characteristic findings of CLAD (Fig. 67.2). Genital area and facial involvement are frequent as well [2].

S. Uzun (✉)
Department of Dermatology and Venereology, School of Medicine, Akdeniz University, Antalya, Turkey
e-mail: sonuzun@akdeniz.edu.tr

A. Bilgic-Temel
Seydisehir State Hospital, Dermatology Clinic, Konya, Turkey

© Springer Nature Switzerland AG 2020

F. Rahmani, N. Rezaei (eds.), *Pediatric Autoimmunity and Transplantation*,
https://doi.org/10.1007/978-3-030-26280-8_67

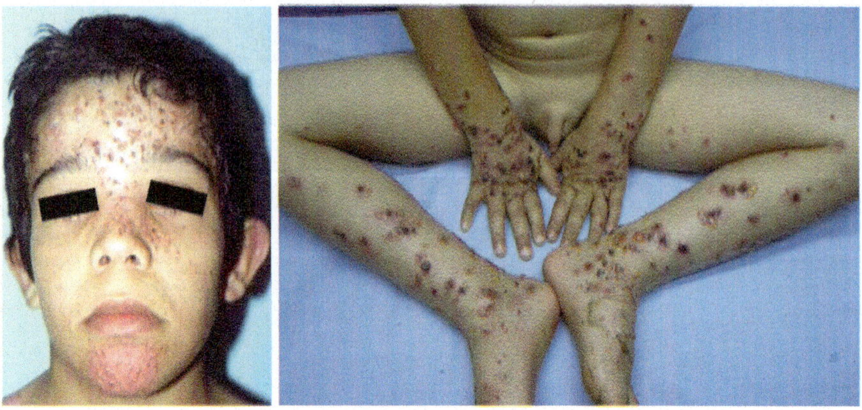

Fig. 67.1 Grouped blisters in a 7-year-old boy

Fig. 67.2 Tense, occasionally haemorrhagic blisters in Childhood linear IgA disease

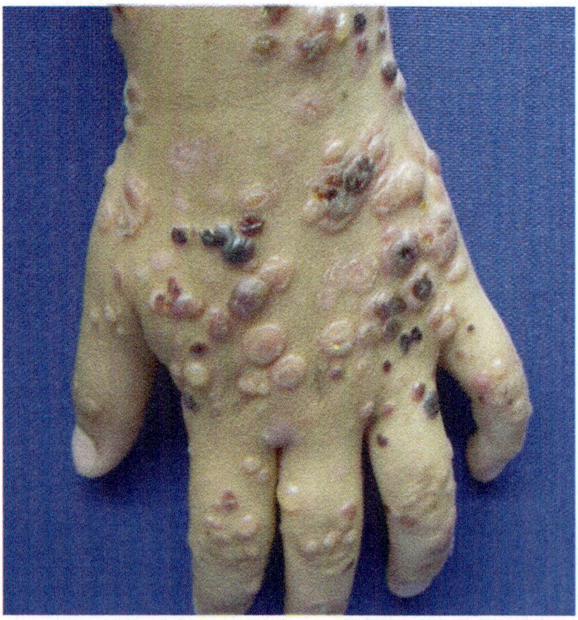

The appearance of a series of vesicles lined up around a central crest is likened to a pearl or jewel cluster is considered typical for the disease (jewel sign). The new vesicles and bulla appear at the periphery of old ones. The onset of disease is immediate and the lesions may be spread or limited in a certain area of the body. The most commonly involved areas are the lower half of the body and the anogenital region, followed by hands, feet and face (Figs. 67.1 and 67.2) [5–7].

Mucosal involvement can be observed and sometimes can be severe [8, 9]. Intact vesicles may show signs of erosion areas with gingivitis and cheilitis as well as eye involvement with photosensitivity, blurred vision, and a spectrum extending from visual perception to visual loss due to cicatrisation [10, 11]. Unlike adult patients, there is no association with hematopoietic system diseases, solid organ malignancy or autoimmune diseases in paediatric cases [11].

Q2. All of the following histopathologic findings are observed in this patient, except: (BMZ: basement membrane zone)

A. Acantholysis
B. Subepidermal blister
C. Dermal neutrophilic infiltration
D. Linear IgA deposition along BMZ

Answer: *The correct answer is* ***A.***

Acantholysis is the main pathologic finding of pemphigus. There are three important diagnostic criteria for CLAD diagnosis; a) biopsy with subepidermal vesicles, b) predominant neutrophil infiltration in subepidermal vesicles, and c) presence of linear IgA deposition along the BMZ in direct immunofluorescence [11, 12]. Pathognomonic for CLAD are the linear IgA deposits along BMZ [11, 12].

Q3. What is the best initial treatment in this patient?

A. Cyclosporine
B. Methotrexate
C. Dapsone
D. Plasmapheresis

Answer: *The correct answer is* ***C.***

CLAD has a better prognosis than adult linear IgA disease. However, it is suggested that treatment should not be delayed for a long time in cases of widespread lesions and mucosal involvement, especially for those at risk of developing scars. The most frequently preferred agents are dapsone and systemic steroids [10, 13]. Dapsone alone or in combination with corticosteroids is the predominant choice starting with a dose of 1 mg/kg/day [10]. Measuring the level of G6PD enzyme to predict possible hemolysis before starting treatment with dapsone provides generally a safe side effect profile. Patients should be followed for development of methemoglobinemia, neuropathy and hepatitis. Laboratory checks are recommended especially in the first 3 months of the use of dapsone, starting at first month then once a week and finally once a month [9, 14]. Response to dapsone is observed in weeks, and following the control of the disease, gradual dose reduction should be done within months. Unilateral vesicles within 1–2 weeks of follow-up are reported to require no new treatment [11]. In some cases, improvement with local corticosteroids may be achieved without systemic treatment [15]. In the case of inadequate control of the disease with dapsone alternative treatment is systemic corticosteroid therapy. There have been reported cases, treated successfully also with azathioprine, mycophenolate mofetil, cyclosporine, erythromycin, dicloxacillin, sulfapyridine, colchicine and intravenous immunoglobulin (IVIG) [3, 14, 16]. Although the disease often recurs, it usually disappears within 2–4 years. However, in some cases the disease can last until puberty [11, 16].

Practical Points

- Childhood linear IgA disease (CLAD) also known as childhood chronic bullous dermatosis is characterized by the accumulation of linear IgA along the basal membrane and subepidermal bullae
- The rash resembles juvenile pemphigoid and often occurs in the first decade of life and most often in pre-school children
- The appearance of a series of vesicles lined up around a central crest is likened to a pearl or jewel cluster is considered typical for the disease (jewel sign)
- Pathognomonic for CLAD are the linear IgA deposits along basement membrane zone
- Dapsone alone or in combination with corticosteroids is the predominant choice with CLAD

References

1. Egan Conleth A, Zone John J. Linear IgA bullous dermatosis. Int J Dermatol. 2001;38(11):818–27.
2. Lara-Corrales I, Pope E. Autoimmune blistering diseases in children. Semin Cutan Med Surg. 2010;29:85–91.
3. Morelli J, Hastalıklar V, Mülayim MK. Nelson Pediatri Türkçe. İstanbul: Nobel Tıp Kitap Evleri; 2015.
4. Cauza K, Hinterhuber G, Sterniczky B, Brugger K, Pieczkowski F, Karlhofer F, Wolff K, Foedinger D. Unusual clinical manifestation of linear IgA dermatosis: a report of two cases. J Am Acad Dermatol. 2004;51(2 Suppl):S112–7.
5. Bickle K, Roark T, Hsu S. Autoimmune bullous dermatoses: a review. Am Fam Physician. 2002;65:1861–70.
6. Küçükoğlu R, Babuna G. Otoimmun büllöz hastalıkların klinik tanısı. Türkderm. 2011;45:16–25.
7. Patricio PFC, Gomes MM, Filipe P. Autoimmune bullous dermatoses: a review. Ann N Y Acad Sci. 2009;1173:203–10.
8. Valle AE, Urizar JA, Sahuquillo AM. Oral manifestations caused by the linear IgA disease. Med Oral. 2004;9:39–44.
9. Fernandes MD, Chiminazzo MD, Tebcherani AJ, Aoki V, Sanchez AP. Inflammatory epidermolysis bullosa acquisita: case report. An Bras Dermatol. 2009;84(2):181–4.
10. Sansaricq F, Stein SL, Petronic-Rosic V. Autoimmune bullous diseases in childhood. Clin Dermatol. 2012;30(1):114–27.
11. Collier P, Wojnarowska F. Chronic bullous disease of childhood textbook of pediatric dermatology. Slovenya: Blackwell Science; 2000.

12. Akman A. Lineer IgA Dermatozu ve Çocukluk Çağının Kronik Büllü Hastalığı. In: Dermatoloji, vol. 3. Baskı. İstanbul: Nobel Tıp Kitapevleri; 2008.
13. Fortuna G, Marinkovich MP. Linear immunoglobulin A bullous dermatosis. Clin Dermatol. 2012;30(1):38–50.
14. Zone J. Clinical spectrum, pathogenesis and treatment of linear IgA bullous dermatosis. J Dermatol. 2001;28:651–3.
15. Sáenz FG, Urdániz GD, Galar MF, Ballester J, Varasa AH, Bordege EG. Topical corticosteroids as a therapeutic alternative in linear immunoglobulin A bullous dermatosis in childhood: case report. Arch Argent Pediatr. 2016;114(6):440–3.
16. Karakaş A. Linear IgA Büllöz Dermatozu. In: Dermatolojide Tedavi. İstanbul: Nobel Tıp Kitapevleri; 2010.

Chapter 68
Pruritic Blisters

Anupam Das and Piyush Kumar

A 5-year-old boy, born from non-consanguineous parents, presented with pruritic blisters all over his body for the preceding month (Fig. 68.1). The lesions used to heal spontaneously, followed by the appearance of a ring of blisters, surrounding the healed lesions. Past history and family history were unremarkable. Cutaneous examination showed tense vesicles and bullae on an erythematous base, along with erosions and crusting. The lesions were distributed all over the body including perioral area, neck, upper limbs, groin, perianal and perigenital regions. They were arranged in an annular configuration around a central crust giving the appearance of a "string of pearls".

Routine investigations were normal. Tzanck smear examination did not reveal any acantholytic cell. Histopathological examination revealed a subepidermal bulla with plenty of neutrophils. Upper dermis was notable for a collection of neutrophils. Direct immunofluorescence study of the perilesional skin showed linear deposits of IgA and C3 at the dermoepidermal junction.

Q1. What is the best initial diagnosis?

A. Childhood bullous pemphigoid
B. Linear IgA disease
C. Chronic bullous disease of childhood
D. Epidermolysis bullosa

Answer: *The correct answer is* ***C.***

Vesiculobullous lesions in children can be attributed to a large number of causes. However, the clinical appearance and the histopathological findings by

A. Das
Department of Dermatology, KPC Medical College, Kolkata, India

P. Kumar (✉)
Department of Dermatology, Katihar Medical College, Katihar, Bihar, India

© Springer Nature Switzerland AG 2020

F. Rahmani, N. Rezaei (eds.), *Pediatric Autoimmunity and Transplantation*,
https://doi.org/10.1007/978-3-030-26280-8_68

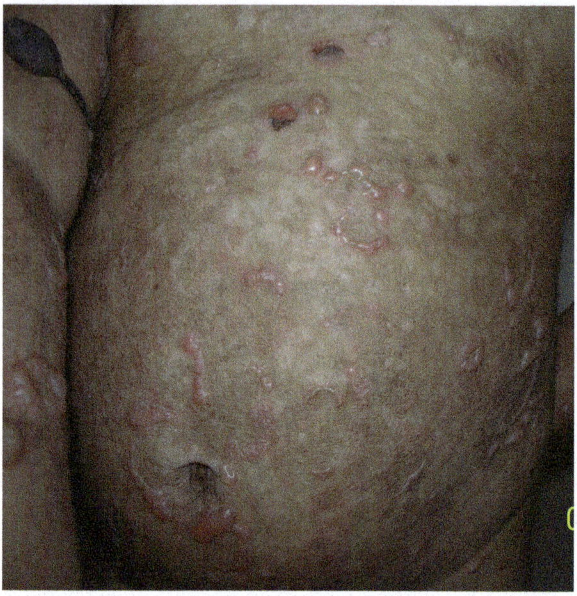

Fig. 68.1 Tense blisters of chronic bullous disease of childhood on trunk

immunofluorescence studies provide the pin-point diagnosis. In this case, the presence of tense blisters on an erythematous base, distribution around the mouth, groin, perianal and perigenital areas, string of pearls appearance are subtle diagnostic clues. Histology showing subepidermal bulla with neutrophilic collection and direct immunofluorescence (DIF) revealing linear deposits of IgA and C3 along the dermoepidermal junction, clinch the diagnosis of chronic bullous disease of childhood (CBDC) [1].

Q2. What is the major target antigen in CBDC?

A. BPAG1
B. BPAG2
C. Keratin 5/14
D. All of the above

Answer: *The correct answer is* ***B.***

The best-characterized antigen is a 97-kilodalton (kD) protein extracted from human epidermis that binds to IgA antibodies from sera of patients with chronic bullous disease of childhood. Initially, this protein was thought to be a unique component of lamina lucida. However, recent studies have shown that the 97-kD protein is actually a portion of the extracellular domain of the 180-kD bullous pemphigoid antigen (BPAg2) [1].

Few other antigenic targets have been reported, including a 285-kD target antigen in the lamina lucida and sublamina densa, a 250-kD antigen corresponding to collagen VII of anchoring fibrils, laminin 332 and etc. [1].

Q3. Which statement is true regarding linear IgA disease?

A. Remission rate in adults is less than that in children
B. Cutaneous lesions usually heal with scarring
C. Drug-induced disease is less severe than spontaneous cases
D. Pathophysiology of disease is different in children from that in adults

Answer: *The correct answer is* ***A.***

Immunologically, linear IgA disease and CBDC are similar to one another. In fact, linear IgA disease can be clinically categorized into two disorders with two distinct presentations: CBDC, which begins in childhood and is also called the childhood linear IgA disease (CLAD), and adult linear IgA disease, which starts later during adulthood. Cutaneous lesions usually heal without scarring. CBCD may show spontaneous remission and mean duration of disease in childhood is about 3.9 years. Remission occurs in 64% of patients, and in most cases within 2 years. However, in adults the disease runs a more protracted course with mean disease duration being 5.6 years and remission rates in adults being lower than in children (48%). Drug-induced cases typically resolve quickly once the causative agent is identified and withdrawn. Drug-induced cases are more severe and erosions are larger [2].

As in this case, the disease usually started below the age of 5 years. The lesions are typically manifested as herpetiform clustering of tense blisters and a "cluster of jewels" like annular arrangement of new, small, tense blisters around a central crusted healing erythematous plaque ("string of pearls" sign). Adult lesions may have flexural and truncal involvement, with a few lesions being linear, sausage-shaped and hemorrhagic. Perineal and perioral involvement are less common in adults. More than 80% of patients have mucosal involvement, most commonly as painful erosions or ulcers. Occasionally, nasal, ocular and laryngeal involvement may occur [3, 4].

Q4. What is the most important differential diagnosis of linear IgA disease in a young child?

A. Dermatitis herpetiformis
B. Bullous pemphigoid
C. Bullous impetigo
D. Epidermolysis bullosa

Answer: *The correct answer is* ***C.***

In a young child, linear IgA disease is most commonly confused with bullous impetigo, while dramatic improvement with oral antibiotics in bullous impetigo, as a differentiating feature.

Dermatitis herpetiformis is characterized by grouped papulovesicles and excoriations over the extensors of limbs, mostly elbows and buttocks. The hallmark finding is presence of granular IgA deposits in the dermal papillae. Bullous pemphigoid, on the other hand is characterized by the presence of a dense infiltrate of eosinophils along with a subepidermal blister, while neutrophilic infiltrates, can distinguish linear IgA disease from bullous pemphigoid. In epidermolysis bullosa, the blisters occur over the areas of friction like elasticted regions of a diaper. When the child starts crawling, lesions tend to appear over the elbows and knees, followed by palms and soles [3].

Q5. Which of the following are among initial treatments for CBDC?

A. Topical steroids
B. Dapsone
C. Oral Corticosteroids
D. All of the above

Answer: *The correct answer is* ***D.***

Linear IgA disease is an immunobullous disease, and the therapy is aimed towards the control of the disease. Mild cases and oral lesions respond well to topical corticosteroids. Severe cases respond to dapsone and sulfapyridine. A response is classically seen with 48–72 hours. Other medications reported to be useful include; prednisolone, tetracycline and niacinamide combination, sulfamethoxypyridazine, colchicine, dicloxacillin, mycophenolate mofetil, IVIG and rituximab [5].

Practical Points

- Chronic bullous disease of childhood (CBDC) and linear IgA disease are similar to one another in histology
- CBDC begins in childhood and is also called the childhood linear IgA disease
- Cutaneous lesions in CBDC usually heal without scarring
- CBCD may show spontaneous remission and mean duration of disease in childhood is about 3.9 years
- Mild cases and oral lesions respond well to topical corticosteroids while severe cases respond to dapsone or sulfapyridine

References

1. Zone JJ, Taylor TB, Meyer LJ, Petersen MJ. The 97 kDa linear IgA bullous disease antigen is identical to a portion of the extracellular domain of the 180 kDa bullous pemphigoid antigen, BPAg2. J Invest Dermatol. 1998;110(3):207–10.
2. Chanal J, Ingen-Housz-Oro S, Ortonne N, Duong TA, Thomas M, Valeyrie-Allanore L, Lebrun-Vignes B, Andre C, Roujeau JC, Chosidow O, Wolkenstein P. Linear IgA bullous dermatosis: comparison between the drug-induced and spontaneous forms. Br J Dermatol. 2013;169(5):1041–8.
3. Jablonska S, Chorzelski TP, Rosinska D, Maciejowska E. Linear IgA bullous dermatosis of childhood (chronic bullous dermatosis of childhood). Clin Dermatol. 1991;9(3):393–401.
4. Verma R, Vasudevan B, Pragasam V, Dabbas D. Linear IgA disease in an adult with unusual clinical features. Indian Dermatol Online J. 2013;4(2):115–8.
5. Norris IN, Haeberle MT, Callen JP, Malone JC. Generalized linear IgA dermatosis with palmar involvement. Dermatol Online J. 2015;21:9.

Chapter 69
Widespread Depigmented and Hypopigmented Patches

Piyush Kumar and Sunil K. Kothiwala

A 5-year-old boy presented with multiple, asymptomatic, depigmented and hypopigmented patches all over body appearing 5 months ago. These lesions developed spontaneously, without a prior history of trauma, contact with chemicals, drugs or any dermatosis. Soon, these lesions progressed in size and number to the present status (Fig. 69.1). Parents noticed development of similar lesions subsequent to superficial trauma on the same site.

There was no remarkable personal or family history of other diseases. Medical and surgical history of the boy were unremarkable. On examination, multiple depigmented patches of various sizes were found to be distributed randomly all over body. Many of these depigmented patches were surrounded by hypopigmented areas. Kobnerization in the form of linear depigmented lesions on the back was recorded. Routine blood investigations, thyroid profile and biochemical profile were within normal range.

Q1. What is the best initial diagnosis?

A. Vitiligo
B. Nevus depigmentosus
C. Oculocutaneous albinism
D. Leukoderma

Answer: *The correct answer is* ***A.***

Vitiligo is an autoimmune condition characterized by selective loss of melanocytes and clinically presents with depigmentation of skin and mucosa [1].

P. Kumar (✉)
Department of Dermatology, Katihar Medical College, Katihar, Bihar, India

S. K. Kothiwala
Consultant Dermatologist, SkinEva Clinic, Jaipur, Rajsthan, India

© Springer Nature Switzerland AG 2020

F. Rahmani, N. Rezaei (eds.), *Pediatric Autoimmunity and Transplantation*,
https://doi.org/10.1007/978-3-030-26280-8_69

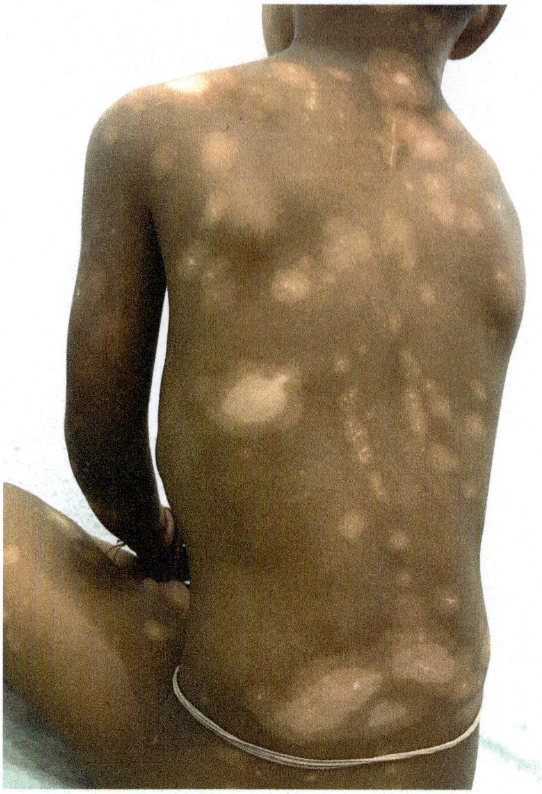

Fig. 69.1 Hypo-depigmented patches on the back

Around one-third to one-half of vitiligo incidence is in pediatric population. Similar to adults, childhood vitiligo may present as segmental form, non-segmental form or mixed form. In non-segmental form, various subphenotypes including acrofacial, mucosal, generalized, and universal forms, have been recognized.

Childhood vitiligo needs to be differentiated from leukoderma and post-inflammatory hypopigmentation, Hansen's disease (associated with sensory loss and nerve trunk thickening), and nevus depigmentosus (nevoid condition with serrated margin) for segmental vitiligo [2] . Other important conditions considered in differentials of childhood vitiligo include oculocutaneous albinism (OCA) and piebaldism. OCA results from a defect in one of the several genes that produce or distribute melanin, resulting in the absence of melanin production, or a reduced amount of melanin production. Piebaldism is an autosomal dominant condition resulting from mutation of c-kit proto-oncogene, which causes impaired embryonic migration and survival of melanocytes in skin [3].

Q2. Which of the following conditions is known to be associated with vitiligo?

A. Thyroid disease
B. Diabetes mellitus

C. Alopecia areata
D. All of the above

Answer: *The correct answer is* ***D.***

Being an autoimmune condition, vitiligo has been found to be associated with many other autoimmune conditions, most commonly with thyroiditis. Female patients with longer duration of disease and patients with extensive involvement are more likely to develop autoimmune thyroid disease, and hence monitoring for thyroid function and anti-thyroid peroxidase (anti-TPO) antibodies is recommended for this group. Other known associations include alopecia areata, diabetes mellitus, Addison disease, and autoimmune polyglandular syndrome type I [2]. Isolated positive anti-nuclear antibody (ANA), is seen in up to 8.6% of vitiligo patients with extensive lesions. ANA positivity is seen more frequently in female patients and in early-onset disease [4].

Q3. Which of the following diseases should be considered as a differential diagnosis if the patient was having concurrent symptomatic ocular disease?

A. Vogt-Koyanagi-Harada syndrome
B. Oculocutaneous albinism
C. Waardenburg syndrome
D. Griscelli syndrome

Answer: *The correct answer is* ***A.***

Other tissues hosting melanocyte are sometimes affected in similar autoimmune process targeting melanocytes. Vogt-Koyanagi-Harada syndrome is one such syndrome with involvement of both anterior and posterior segments of the eye as a hallmark. Diffuse choroiditis, exudative retinal detachment, optic disc edema, bilateral acute iridocyclitis, iris nodules and shallow anterior chamber, and subsequent acute angle closure glaucoma, are prominent ocular findings. Meningeal involvement results in neck stiffness, confusion, headache and cerebrospinal fluid pleocytosis. In severe cases, serious meningeal-encephalic manifestations and focal neurological signs may appear. Inner ear involvement results in dysacusis, hearing loss, tinnitus and vertigo. Skin and hair affection results in vitiligo and poliosis, with patchy grey or white hair, respectively [5].

OCA, Waardenburg syndrome and Griscelli syndrome are hereditary disorders of pigmentary dilution and present with loss of pigmentation since birth, the later being the reason why they are considered as differential diagnoses of childhood vitiligo. The ocular findings in OCA are nystagmus, photophobia and iris translucency [5]. Waardenburg syndrome present with heterochromia iridis, dystopia canthorum, congenital deafness in addition to white forelock and piebaldism like achromic patches [5].

Griscelli syndome, Chediak-Higashi syndrome and Elejalde disease, are rare autosomal recessive conditions, collectively known as “silvery hair syndromes”. These conditions are characterized by pigmentary dilution of skin and hair, and bleeding tendency, neurological defects and features of immune dysregulation [6].

Q4. Which statement is true about the pathogenesis of vitiligo?

A. There is a genetic dysregulation of immunesurveillance against the melanocytic enzyme, tyrosinase
B. Melanocytes in vitiligo patients have intrinsic susceptibility to oxidative stress mediated damage
C. Keratinocytes have low level of catalase, an anti-oxidant responsible for neutralizing hydrogen peroxide (H2O2)
D. All of the above

Answer: *The correct answer is **D.***

The most favored hypothesis about vitiligo pathogenesis is autoimmune theory, supported by association of many other autoimmune conditions with incidence of vitiligo. Several susceptibility loci for generalized vitiligo have been identified and tyrosinase is believed to be major autoantigen. Both innate and adaptive immune system play a role in development and progression of vitiligo [7].

Another favored hypothesis highlights the role of reactive oxygen species (ROS) in destruction of inherently susceptible melanocytes. Some authors have documented low level of catalase in epidermal cells. Catalase, a potent anti-oxidant, is primary agent responsible for neutralization of hydrogen peroxide. With low levels of catalase, H2O2 is not adequately neutralized and causes damage to melanocytes [7].

Q5. Which of the following is the marker of disease activity in vitiligo?

A. Trichrome vitiligo
B. Kobnerization
C. Confetti-like depigmented macules
D. All of the above

Answer: *The correct answer is **D.***

Determining disease activity in vitiligo is important for assessing prognosis, deciding plan of treatment and deciding suitability of patients for surgical management. Clinically, Kobner phenomenon, trichrome vitiligo and appearance of confetti-like lesions are associated with active disease process [8].

Various scoring tools have been developed to assess disease active and prognosis in vitiligo including; Vitiligo Area Scoring Index (VASI), Vitiligo Disease Activity Score (VIDA), and Potential Repigmentation Index (PRI) and Vitiligo European Task Force (VETF) [9].

Q6. What is the best first-line treatment option in localized vitiligo?

A. Topical corticosteroid
B. Oral steroid minipulse
C. Suction blister epidermal grafts
D. Psoralens and ultraviolet A

Answer: *The correct answer is **A.***

The choice of treatment in vitiligo depends on a lot of factors including; localized or generalized disease, stability or instability of the disease, site affected, and age and preference of patient (and parents). Psychological issues, school activities and tendency to develop striae in teenagers, are other specific concerns in childhood vitiligo. Vitiligo affecting less than 20% body surface area is treated with topical medicines. Extensive disease is treated with phototherapy or systemic drugs [10]. Long term cumulative adverse effects and consideration of treatment resistant sites, i.e. areas without hair follicles such as the lips, palms, and soles, should be kept in mind, while deciding treatment plan [11]. Combination therapies, particularly those involving phototherapy are associated with better repigmentation, yet more adverse outcomes, compared to monotherapies. Available treatment options include [9]:

- Cosmetic camouflage
- Topical treatment
  - Topical corticosteroids (mid-potency to high-potency)
  - Calcineurin inhibitors such as tacrolimus and pimecrolimus
  - Topical vitamin D analogue- Calcipotriene (in combination with topical corticosteroids or phototherapy)
- Phototherapy
  - Narrow-band ultraviolet B (NB-UVB)
  - Excimer laser (308 nm)
  - Psoralens and ultraviolet A (PUVA)- rarely used now
- Systemic treatment
  - Oral steroid minipulse- in unstable vitiligo for 3–6 months
- Surgical modalities- for treatment resistant lesions in a case of stable vitiligo. Not preferred as initial step in active disease. Even the stable vitiligo lesions increase in size proportionately with increase in size with body growth.
  - Minipunch grafts
  - Suction blister epidermal grafts (SBEG)
  - Thin Thiersch grafts
  - Transplantation of epidermal cell suspension
  - Cultured and non-cultured melanocyte suspension
- Depigmentation therapy with 20% monobenzyl ether of hydroquinone (MBEH)
- Psychological support

Practical Points

- One-third to one-half of vitiligo incidence is in pediatric population
- Vitiligo is associated with thyroid disease, diabetes mellitus, and alopecia areata
- Female patients with longer duration of disease and patients with extensive involvement are more likely to develop autoimmune thyroid disease
- Anti-nuclear antibody positivity is seen more frequently in female patients and in early-onset disease

References

1. Ezzedine K, Silverberg N. A practical approach to the diagnosis and treatment of Vitiligo in children. Pediatrics. 2016;38(1):e20154126.
2. Taïeb A, Seneschal J, Mazereeuw-Hautier J. Special considerations in children with Vitiligo. Dermatol Clin. 2017;35(2):229–33.
3. Geel NV, Speeckaert M, Chevolet I, Schepper SD, Lapeere H, Boone B, Speeckaert R. Hypomelanoses in children. J Cutan Aesthet Surg. 2013;6(2):65–72.
4. Lim H, Bae M, Jeong K, Shin M, Lee M. Positivity rates of antithyroid antibody, antinuclear antibody and thyroid peroxidase antibody in different types of Vitiligo. Clin Exp Dermatol. 2016;41(3):242–7.
5. Lavezzo M, Sakata V, Morita C, Rodriguez E, Abdallah S, Silva FD, Hirata C, Yamamoto J. Vogt-Koyanagi-Harada disease: review of a rare autoimmune disease targeting antigens of melanocytes. Orphanet J Rare Dis. 2016;11:29.
6. Khemka P, Kundu R, Niyogi P, Tudu J. A case of silvery hair syndrome: Griscelli syndrome. Indian J Paediatr Dermatol. 2015;16:72–4.
7. Ezzedine K, Eleftheriadou V, Whitton M, Geel NV. Vitiligo. Lancet (London, England). 2015;386(9988):74–84.
8. Goh B, Pandya A. Presentations, signs of activity, and differential diagnosis of Vitiligo. Dermatol Clin. 2017;35(2):135–44.
9. Alghamdi K, Kumar A, Taïeb A, Ezzedine K. Assessment methods for the evaluation of Vitiligo. J Eur Acad Dermatol Venereol. 2012;26(12):1463–71.
10. Driessche FV, Silverberg N. Current management of pediatric Vitiligo. Paediatr Drugs. 2015;17(4):303–13.
11. Tamesis M, Morelli J. Vitiligo treatment in childhood: a state of the art review. Pediatr Dermatol. 2010;27(5):437–45.

Chapter 70
Whitish Patches

Gulsen Akoglu

A 6-year-old boy presented with whitish patches on his skin which first appeared at 4 years old. The patches began to emerge first over his buttocks and genital areas, and then over his neck and face. He was an otherwise healthy child without any significant family history of similar eruptions. Dermatological examination revealed multiple whitish patches on his left upper lid, genital skin, and lumbar region. The off-white patches on his neck were surrounded with sharp red-brown borders (Fig. 70.1a, b). On examination, nails, scalp, and mucosal regions were normal, and no organomegaly, lymphadenopathy, or fever were detected.

Q1. What is the best initial step in the diagnosis of this patient?

A. Skin biopsy
B. Wood light examination
C. Skin ultrasonography
D. Searching for viral markers

Answer: *The correct answer is* ***B.***

Wood light examination is a practical, non-invasive, simple initial step to differentiate many aspects of skin disorders including pigmentary disorders, bacterial and fungal cutaneous infections, as well as porphyria. Wood light examination is performed in a dark room by a Wood lamp which is a mercury arc covered by a Wood filter that allows a radiation between 320 to 400 nm. The filtered light from Wood's lamp is absorbed by the tissue and radiation of longer wavelengths, usually visible light, is emitted [1]. Since Wood's light is strongly absorbed by melanin, this tool is very helpful for detection of a dyschromic lesion whether it is hypopigmented, depigmented, or hyperpigmented. Vitiligo patches with a complete loss of epider-

G. Akoglu (✉)
Gulhane Training and Research Hospital, Dermatology and Venereology Clinic, University of Health Sciences, Ankara, Turkey

© Springer Nature Switzerland AG 2020

F. Rahmani, N. Rezaei (eds.), *Pediatric Autoimmunity and Transplantation*,
https://doi.org/10.1007/978-3-030-26280-8_70

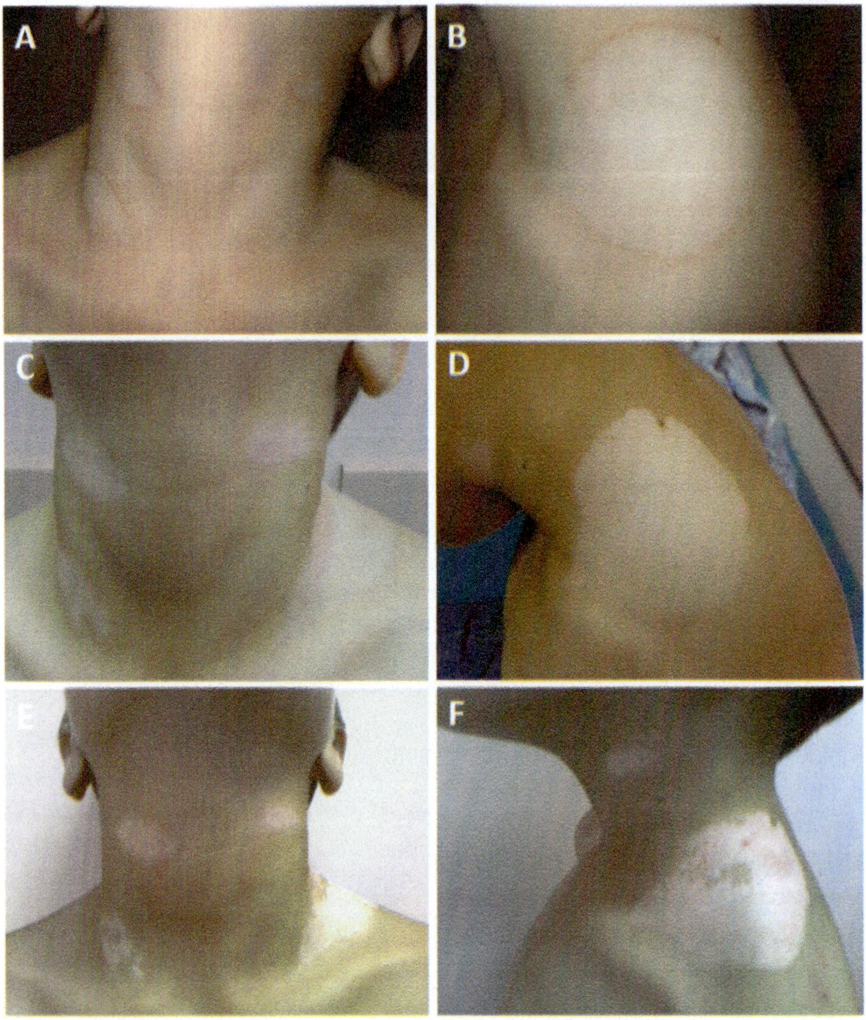

Fig. 70.1 Tan-brown macules and patches on the child's (**a**) chest, abdomen and (**b**) back. (**c** and **d**), enlargement of the patches and disappearance of active borders and halo nevi after 3 months of tacrolimus therapy, and (**e** and **f**) gradual repigmentation of the patches after 5 months of therapy

mal melanin are depigmented, whereas pityriasis alba, nevus anemicus, hypomelanosis of Ito, hypopigmented mycosis fungoides, in which melanocyte activity is little impaired or not affected, are hypopigmented under Wood's light as well. Wood's light makes the subtle ash leaf-shaped white macules more visible in infants and young children and supports the early diagnosis of tuberosclerosis [1–3]. In the present case, Wood light examination showed that these patches were mostly hypopigmented and some of them were quite depigmented.

Q2. What is the next best laboratory examination?

A. Skin biopsy
B. Bacterial culture
C. Magnetic resonance imaging of the brain
D. Systemic work-up for malignancy

Answer: *The correct answer is* ***A.***

The histopathological examination of inflammatory margin adjacent to hypo- or depigmented lesion was needed to differentiate marginal inflammatory vitiligo, hypopigmented mycosis fungoides, discoid lupus erythematosus, annular lichenoid dermatitis of youth (ALDY), and morphea. In the present case, a skin biopsy was obtained from the active border of a patch on the neck. Histopathological examination revealed irregular epidermal acanthosis, exocytosis, dense lymphocytic infiltration in the perivascular and dermal papillary areas, and melanin incontinence in dermoepidermal junction. Fibrosis or atypia were not observed.

Q3. What is the most probable diagnosis?

A. Hypopigmented mycosis fungoides
B. Morphea
C. Marginal inflammatory vitiligo with generalized non-inflammatory type
D. Discoid lupus erythematosus

Answer: *The correct answer is* ***C.***

Vitiligo is an autoimmune skin disorder with loss of melanocytes in the depigmented macules or patches. Marginal inflammatory vitiligo (MIV) is a rare subset of vitiligo characterized by depigmented patches surrounded by a raised, erythematous border, usually associated with pruritus. The border may be present at the onset of disease, or may emerge during the course of disease. Spontaneous regression may be observed, while lesion clearance by topical corticosteroids is commonly achieved. Atopic individuals may present with slightly scaling inflammatory borders of depigmented patches [4]. Histopathological features of MIV reveal dermal and perivascular inflammation with lymphocytes and histiocytes infiltration, exocytosis of lymphocytes, spongiosis, interface dermatitis, and degradation of melanocytes [4, 5]. Psoriasiform hyperplasia, parakeratosis, hyperkeratosis, or lichenoid infiltration are also reported [4]. The clinical aspects of lesions with inflammatory border associated with typical histopathological features helped us diagnose the neck lesions as MIV. Since the patient had other depigmented patches over his body regions, the case was MIV with generalized noninflammatory type vitiligo.

The diagnosis of MIV may be challenging when it is not associated with clearly depigmented vitiligo patches. MIV may be a diagnostic dilemma to physicians who are not aware of this rare entity. There are some important skin disorders to be in the differential diagnosis.

Hypopigmented mycosis fungoides (MF) is a rare variant of cutaneous T cell lymphoma, characterized by hypo- or depigmented patches or plaques accompanied with atrophy, telangiectasia, or hyperpigmentation. Although it is rarely reported in children, differentiation between hypopigmented MF and vitiligo may be difficult. The biopsy from periphery of vitiligo patches may show similarities to hypopigmented MF [2]. Detection of band like lymphocytic infiltration in papillary dermis, fibrosis, Pautrier microabses, and epidermotrophism of atypical lymphocytes within epidermis support hypopigmented MF [2, 6]. In some suspected cases, a T cell gene rearrangement study may be useful although sensitivity and specificity are low [2, 5]. In our case, we did not detect any atypical lymphocytes, epidermotrophism, or fibrosis.

The late lesions of discoid lupus erythematosus (DLE) presents as atrophic depigmented central scarring surrounded by hyperpigmented rim. Hyperkeratosis, thick basal membrane, vacuolar degeneration, dermal lymphocytic infiltration, and deposits of immunoglobulins along with dermoepidermal junction are characteristic histopathological features of DLE [7].

Morphea is a sclerosing disorder of skin and subcutaneous tissue, characterized by erythematous, hypopigmented or hyperpigmented patches and plagues. The spectrum of lesions may lead to misdiagnosis of vitiligo. The hypopigmented lesions may have an erythematous rim as seen in MIV. However, clinically sclerotic texture of patches, presence of thickened and sclerotic collagen bundles in the reticular dermis is not a feature of vitiligo [8].

The lesions of annular lichenoid dermatitis of youth usually observed as persistent annular hypopigmented patches surrounded by red-brown border or erythematous macules on the groins and flanks. The histopathology typically shows a lichenoid dermatitis and keratinocyte necrosis on the tip of rete ridges [9].

Q4. Which of the following laboratory screening tests are indicated in this patient?

A. Total blood count with differential
B. Thyroid stimulating hormone and anti-thyroid autoantibodies
C. Fasting serum glucose levels
D. All of the above

Answer: *The correct answer is* ***D.***

Vitiligo may be associated with other autoimmune disorders including thyroid disease, diabetes mellitus, pernicious anemia, psoriasis, and alopecia areata. Screening of vitiligo patients for associated autoimmune systemic disorders are recommended for an early diagnosis and treatment [10]. In the present case, laboratory examinations including total blood count with differential, renal, liver, and thyroid function tests, fasting glucose and lipids, ESR were all within normal limits. We did not detect any associated systemic or dermatological autoimmune disorder.

Q5. What is the most appropriate first-line management in this patient?

A. Topical immunomodulators and topical corticosteroids
B. Systemic steroids
C. Phototherapy
D. Excimer laser therapy

Answer: *The correct answer is* **A.**

The most commonly used drugs administered for children and adolescents with vitiligo are topical tacrolimus alone or combined with moderate to high potent topical corticosteroids, pimecrolimus, corticosteroids, and calcipotriol [11]. Topical tacrolimus ointment is especially preferred for neck and head region and folds of the body and topical corticosteroids for extrafacial regions [11, 12]. Long-term use of topical steroids should be avoided especially in children since irreversible skin atrophy, striae, acne, and systemic absorption of steroids may occur. Therefore, topical corticosteroids are usually prescribed with a discontinuous regimen, not with a continuous application for a long time. Oral minipulse treatment with methylprednisolone, 308-nm excimer laser therapy, and phototherapy with narrow band ultraviolet B or ultraviolet A are the other treatment strategies for children in special conditions. When vitiligo is widespread and topical treatment is not suitable, and the child has compliance to stand in the cabin, phototherapy option may be decided to apply [12].

In the present case, topical tacrolimus ointment for eyelid and genitalia patches and topical steroid ointment for other patches were administered. The parents of the patient had applied these medications for 1 month and stopped the therapy. After 3 months, on the second visit, enlargement of the patches and disappearance of active borders and some halo nevi were observed (Fig. 70.1c, d). The same treatment was continued for 2 months and gradual repigmentation of the patches was seen in the third visit (Fig. 70.1e, f).

Practical Points

- Wood light examination is a simple initial step to differentiate many aspects of skin disorders including pigmentary disorders, bacterial and fungal cutaneous infections, as well as porphyria
- Marginal inflammatory vitiligo (MIV) is a rare subset of vitiligo characterized by depigmented patches surrounded by a raised, erythematous border, usually associated with pruritus
- The most commonly used drugs administered for children and adolescents with vitiligo are topical tacrolimus alone or combined with moderate to high potent topical corticosteroids, pimecrolimus, corticosteroids, and calcipotriol

References

1. Asawanonda P, Taylor C. Wood's light in dermatology. Review. Int J Dermatol. 1999;38(11):801–7.
2. Gomez-Moyano E, Vera-Casaño A, Gamero A, Sanz-Trelles A, Crespo-Erchiga V. Inflammatory vitiligo or hypopigmented mycosis fungoides? J Pediatr Hematol Oncol. 2010;32(4):338–9.
3. Ruocco E, Baroni A, Donnarumma G, Ruocco V. Diagnostic procedures in dermatology. Clin Dermatol. 2011;29(5):548–56.
4. Verma S. Inflammatory vitiligo with raised borders and psoriasiform histopathology. Dermatol Online J. 2005;11(3):13.
5. Trikha R, McCowan N, Brodell R. Marginal vitiligo: an unusual depigmenting disorder. Dermatol Online J. 2014;21:3.
6. Gameiro A, Gouveia M, Tellechea Ó, Moreno A. Childhood hypopigmented mycosis fungoides: a commonly delayed diagnosis. BMJ Case Rep. 2014;2014:bcr2014208306.
7. Turan E, Bagci IS, Erdemir AT, Gurel MS. Successful treatment of generalized discoid lupus erythematosus with imiquimod cream 5%: a case report and review of the literature. Acta Dermatovenerol Croat. 2014;22(2):150–9.
8. Chu H, Lee J, Lee Y, Kim D. Delayed treatment of generalized morphea due to misdiagnosis as vitiligo at an oriental medical clinic. Ann Dermatol. 2017;29(5):649–50.
9. Annessi G, Paradisi M, Angelo C, Perez M, Puddu P, Girolomoni G. Annular lichenoid dermatitis of youth. J Am Acad Dermatol. 2003;49(6):1029–36.
10. Phiske M. Vitiligo in children: a birds eye view. Curr Pediatr Rev. 2016;12(1):55–66.
11. Menezes AD, Carvalho FO, Barreto R, Silva BS, Shanmugam S, Gurgel R, Araújo AS. Pharmacologic treatment of vitiligo in children and adolescents: a systematic review. Pediatr Dermatol. 2017;34(1):13–24.
12. Taïeb A, Seneschal J, Mazereeuw-Hautier J. Special considerations in children with vitiligo. Dermatol Clin. 2017;35(2):229–33.

Chapter 71
Hyperpigmented Patches

Yan Ling Kong and Emily Yiping Gan

A 5-month-old Chinese girl presented with a 4-month history of hyperpigmented patches that started on her scalp and face. The rash subsequently progressed to involve her trunk and upper limbs. There was relative sparing of her lower limbs. She did not appear to be bothered by its presence. There were no systemic symptoms, and she had normal developmental milestones. On examination, there were tan-brown patches and papules scattered on her scalp, face, trunk and upper limbs (Fig. 71.1a, b). Laboratory data revealed WBC: 10,400/μL (neutrophils: 35%, lymphocytes 60%, monocytes: 4%), Hb: 13.4 g/dL, platelet: 206,000/μL. A punch biopsy was performed from one of the skin lesions.

Q1. What is the most likely diagnosis?

A. Urticaria pigmentosa
B. Langerhans cell histiocytosis
C. Cutaneous plasmacytosis
D. Multiple insect bite marks

Answer: *The correct answer is* ***A.***

Mastocytosis refers to a heterogeneous group of disorders characterized by pathologic infiltration of mast cells in one or multiple organs including the skin, bone marrow, liver, spleen and lymph nodes. It is a clonal disease associated with *KIT* mutations, causing abnormal mast cell accumulation and activation [1]. Mastocytosis is subdivided into two groups: cutaneous mastocytosis (CM) describes the skin-limited forms, and systemic mastocytosis (SM) describes the forms of mastocytosis in which abnormal accumulation of mast cells occur in one or more

Y. L. Kong
National Skin Centre, Singapore, Singapore

E. Y. Gan (✉)
Dermatology Service, KK Women's and Children's Hospital, Singapore, Singapore

© Springer Nature Switzerland AG 2020

F. Rahmani, N. Rezaei (eds.), *Pediatric Autoimmunity and Transplantation*,
https://doi.org/10.1007/978-3-030-26280-8_71

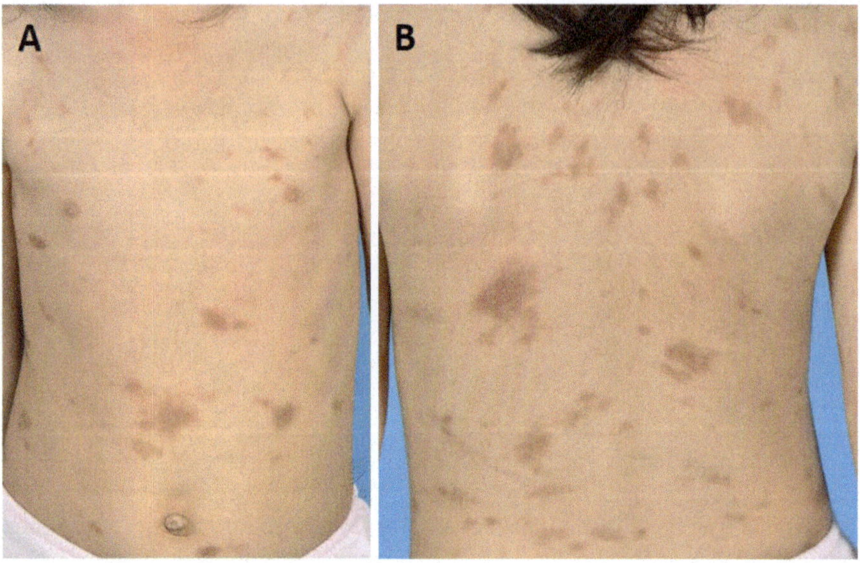

Fig. 71.1 Tan-brown macules and patches on the child's (**a**) chest, abdomen and (**b**) back

extra-cutaneous organs, with or without cutaneous involvement. The main subtypes of CM in children are maculopapular cutaneous mastocytosis, which includes urticaria pigmentosa (UP), mastocytoma and diffuse cutaneous mastocytosis (DCM) [1, 2]. Up to 90% of pediatric mastocytosis occur before the age of 2 years. Prognosis in pediatric mastocytosis is generally good with up to two-thirds of patients demonstrating partial or complete resolution [1]. Having fewer affected areas, smaller lesions and an earlier disease onset are good prognostic factors associated with disease regression [3].

Our patient was diagnosed with UP, which is the most common variant of mastocytosis in the pediatric population [2]. This condition presents with tan-brown macules or papules affecting the distal extremities and trunk. Bullous eruptions with hemorrhage can occur, and there may be associated lymphadenopathy and hepatosplenomegaly [1]. The face and scalp are usually involved in children, unlike adults. Darier's sign, which describes the development of urticaria locally following rubbing or stroking of the lesional skin, is usually present. Cutaneous symptoms include flushing, dermographism and pruritus. Systemic symptoms include nausea, vomiting, abdominal pain, diarrhea, dyspnea, headache, fatigue, lethargy and neuropsychiatric symptoms [1, 4, 5]. These symptoms may occur even in the absence of systemic infiltration.

Q2. Presence of elevated serum concentrations of which of the following biomarkers may be indicative of systemic involvement in UP?

A. Platelets
B. Tryptase
C. Alkaline phosphatase
D. Eosinophils

Answer: *The correct answer is* ***B.***

Systemic mastocytosis/SM is rare in children. No additional evaluation is necessary if systemic symptoms are mild with no evidence of hepatosplenomegaly or lymphadenopathy on physical examination, and baseline CBC and LFT are normal.

If SM is suspected, serum tryptase, which is a protease produced predominantly in mast cells, may be measured. Unlike adults, serum tryptase levels higher than 20 ng/mL in children does not immediately translate to a diagnosis of SM. However, the presence of an elevated serum baseline total tryptase level reflects extensive skin disease and higher risk of severe mast cell activation symptoms [6]. In children with tryptase levels <20 ng/mL, the diagnosis of CM may be decided upon without bone marrow examination (BME), unless other signs of SM are present. If the serum tryptase level is 20–100 ng/mL in children without other signs of SM, the provisional diagnosis "mastocytosis in the skin (MIS)" can be established and monitored until puberty. If MIS remains present after puberty, referral to a pediatric hematologist for further assessment and a BME is recommended. If the baseline tryptase level exceeds 100 ng/mL, a BME should be considered immediately [7].

Q3. What histological stains might help highlight the predominant cell type seen in the skin biopsy of this patient?

A. Toluidine blue, CD-1a
B. Melan-A, Tryptase
C. Crystal violet, CD-117
D. Leder, Giemsa

Answer: *The correct answer is* ***D.***

Histologically, CM is characterized by the presence of perivascular or diffuse dermal mast cells, often with few eosinophils. Dermal edema is usually present, with occasional formation of subepidermal blisters. Mast cells are highlighted on Leder, Giemsa, toluidine blue, CD-117 (c-kit) or tryptase stains [8]. Crystal violet stains acid mucopolysaccharides and amyloid, Melan-A stains for melanocytes and CD-1a highlights Langerhans cells.

Q4. Some medications may trigger or aggravate the child's symptoms. Which of the following options contains drugs from this category?

A. Non-steroidal inflammatory drugs (NSAIDs), vancomycin, narcotics
B. Penicillin, paracetamol, antihistamines
C. Colchicine, prednisone, fluoroquinolones
D. Paracetamol, montelukast, dapsone

Answer: *The correct answer is* ***A.***

A variety of stimuli and agents are known to activate mast cells, as illustrated in Table 71.1 [2]. In children, the main trigger is changes in temperature, followed by irritability, fever and teething [9].

Q5. Assuming that the child has skin-limited disease, what is the best initial oral medication for her?

A. Prednisolone
B. Ketoconazole
C. Cetirizine
D. Acitretin

Answer: *The correct answer is* ***C.***

The treatment of pediatric CM is aimed at suppressing skin and systemic mast cell mediated symptoms, with the anticipation that skin lesions will fade as the child grows. Therapy should be tailored according to the symptom severity in each patient.

A four-grade scale for mastocytosis severity from mast cell degranulation, applicable to children, has been established by consensus guidelines [7].

Table 71.1 Clinically relevant etiologies for mast cell degranulation

Physical stimuli	Heat, cold, sudden changes of temperature, mechanical friction or pressure, sunlight
Emotional factors	Stress, anxiety, sleep deprivation
Infectious diseases with fever	Viral (most commonly upper respiratory tract infections), bacterial (bronchitis, pneumonia)
Drugs	NSAIDs, alcohol, narcotics (morphine, codeine and derivatives), cough medication (dextromethorphan, dimemorfan), acetylsalicylic acid, procaine, polymyxin B, amphotericin B, vancomycin, atropine, thiamine, D-tubocurarine, Quinine, radiographic contrast media containing iodine, scopolamine, gallamine, decamethonium, rederpine
Foods	Aged cheese, alcohol, chocolate, strawberries
Miscellaneous	Dentition (teething and dental procedures), vaccinations, surgery, endoscopic procedures

Grade 0: no symptoms.
Grade 1: mild symptoms, no therapy required.
Grade 2: moderate symptoms, kept under control with antimediator-type drugs.
Grade 3: severe symptoms, not sufficiently controlled with therapy.
Grade 4: severe adverse events that require emergency therapy and hospitalization.

Both H1 and H2 antihistamines are useful in the treatment of CM. H1 antihistamines, like cetirizine and hydroxyzine, have been shown to be useful in decreasing pruritus, flushing, urticaria and tachycardia [2]. H_2 antihistamines such as ranitidine or famotidine can be used to manage gastric hypersecretion and peptic ulcer disease associated with mastocytosis [10, 11]. Oral cromolyn sodium has proven to be effective in some children to control diarrhea, abdominal pain, nausea and vomiting, and useful in some patients for the treatment of cutaneous symptoms including pruritus [12]. Leukotriene antagonist has been used in case reports for both refractory symptoms and standard therapy [13]. Children with extensive cutaneous involvement or elevated baseline serum tryptase may develop anaphylaxis and should carry an epinephrine autoinjector at all times [6].

Practical Points

- Mastocytosis is divided into the systemic and skin-limited forms. The main subtypes of pediatric cutaneous mastocytosis include maculopapular cutaneous mastocytosis which includes urticaria pigmentosa, mastocytoma and diffuse cutaneous mastocytosis.
- The presence of an elevated serum total tryptase level (≥20 ng/mL) reflects more extensive skin disease, higher risk of severe mast cell activation, and may be indicative of systemic involvement
- Physical stimuli, emotional factors, infection, drugs and food may activate mast cells
- In children, common triggers include temperature changes, irritability, fever and teething
- Medications that may be effective in the treatment of cutaneous mastocytosis include H1 and H2 antihistamines, mast cell stabilizers like cromolyn sodium and leukotriene antagonists

References

1. Meni C, Bruneau J, Georgin-Lavialle S, Le Sache de Peufeilhoux L, Damaj G, Hadj-Rabia S, Fraitag S, Dubreuil P, Hermine O, Bodemer C. Paediatric mastocytosis: a systematic review of 1747 cases. Br J Dermatol. 2015;172(3):642–51.
2. Castells M, Metcalfe DD, Escribano L. Diagnosis and treatment of cutaneous mastocytosis in children: practical recommendations. Am J Clin Dermatol. 2011;12(4):259–70.
3. Heinze A, Kuemmet TJ, Chiu YE, Galbraith SS. Longitudinal study of pediatric urticaria pigmentosa. Pediatr Dermatol. 2017;34(2):144–9.

4. Horan RF, Austen KF. Systemic mastocytosis: retrospective review of a decade's clinical experience at the Brigham and Women's Hospital. J Invest Dermatol. 1991;96(3 Suppl):5S–13S; discussion S-4S, 60S–65S
5. Moura DS, Georgin-Lavialle S, Gaillard R, Hermine O. Neuropsychological features of adult mastocytosis. Immunol Allergy Clin N Am. 2014;34(2):407–22.
6. Alvarez-Twose I, Vano-Galvan S, Sanchez-Munoz L, Morgado JM, Matito A, Torrelo A, Jaen P, Schwartz LB, Orfao A, Escribano L. Increased serum baseline tryptase levels and extensive skin involvement are predictors for the severity of mast cell activation episodes in children with mastocytosis. Allergy. 2012;67(6):813–21.
7. Valent P, Akin C, Escribano L, Fodinger M, Hartmann K, Brockow K, Castells M, Sperr WR, Kluin-Nelemans HC, Hamdy NA, Lortholary O, Robyn J, van Doormaal J, Sotlar K, Hauswirth AW, Arock M, Hermine O, Hellmann A, Triggiani M, Niedoszytko M, Schwartz LB, Orfao A, Horny HP, Metcalfe DD. Standards and standardization in mastocytosis: consensus statements on diagnostics, treatment recommendations and response criteria. Eur J Clin Investig. 2007;37(6):435–53.
8. Kirsch R, Geboes K, Shepherd NA, de Hertogh G, Di Nicola N, Lebel S, Mickys U, Riddell RH. Systemic mastocytosis involving the gastrointestinal tract: clinicopathologic and molecular study of five cases. Mod Pathol. 2008;21(12):1508–16.
9. Kettelhut BV, Berkebile C, Bradley D, Metcalfe DD. A double-blind, placebo-controlled, crossover trial of ketotifen versus hydroxyzine in the treatment of pediatric mastocytosis. J Allergy Clin Immunol. 1989;83(5):866–70.
10. Johnson GJ, Silvis SE, Roitman B, Blumenthal M, Gilbert HS. Long-term treatment of systemic mastocytosis with histamine H2 receptor antagonists. Am J Gastroenterol. 1980;74(6):485–9.
11. Berg MJ, Bernhard H, Schentag JJ. Cimetidine in systemic mastocytosis. Drug Intell Clin Pharm. 1981;15(3):180–3.
12. Horan RF, Sheffer AL, Austen KF. Cromolyn sodium in the management of systemic mastocytosis. J Allergy Clin Immunol. 1990;85(5):852–5.
13. Tolar J, Tope WD, Neglia JP. Leukotriene-receptor inhibition for the treatment of systemic mastocytosis. N Engl J Med. 2004;350(7):735–6.

Chapter 72
Outbreaks of Erythematous and Necrotic Papules with Hemorrhagic Crusts

Selcen Kundak and Malik Ergin

A 9-year-old girl presented with erythematous macules, papules and necrotic papules with hemorrhagic crusts located predominantly in trunk and extremities (Fig. 72.1). It was learnt that the patient had three recurrences during a period 5 months. The eruption was associated with mild fever (37–38 °C) and malaise. Her personal and family histories were unremarkable. There was no history of drug intake or episodes of infection before the onset skin eruptions.

Skin examination revealed widely distributed, crusted and scaly papules. Head, soles, palms and oral mucosa were spared. Physical examination was otherwise normal. Complete blood count, hepatic and renal function tests, ESR, complement levels (C3, C4), and serum immunoglobulin levels were normal. Skin biopsy demonstrated focal parakeratosis, orthokeratosis and spongiosis of the epidermis. Degenerated keratinocytes in the upper layers of the epidermis were observed. Moreover, dense and mixed chronic infiltrations of inflammatory cells involved the superficial perivascular, interstitial plexus and papillary dermis (Fig. 72.2). Direct immunofluorescence was negative.

Q1. What is the most likely diagnosis?

A. Lymphomatoid papulosis
B. Pityriasis lichenoides chronica
C. Pityriasis lichenoides et varioliformis acuta
D. Vasculitis

Answer: *The correct answer is* ***C.***

S. Kundak (✉)
Department of Dermatology, Dr. Behçet Uz Children's Hospital, Izmir, Turkey

M. Ergin
Department of Pathology, Dr. Behçet Uz Children's Hospital, İzmir, Turkey

© Springer Nature Switzerland AG 2020

F. Rahmani, N. Rezaei (eds.), *Pediatric Autoimmunity and Transplantation*,
https://doi.org/10.1007/978-3-030-26280-8_72

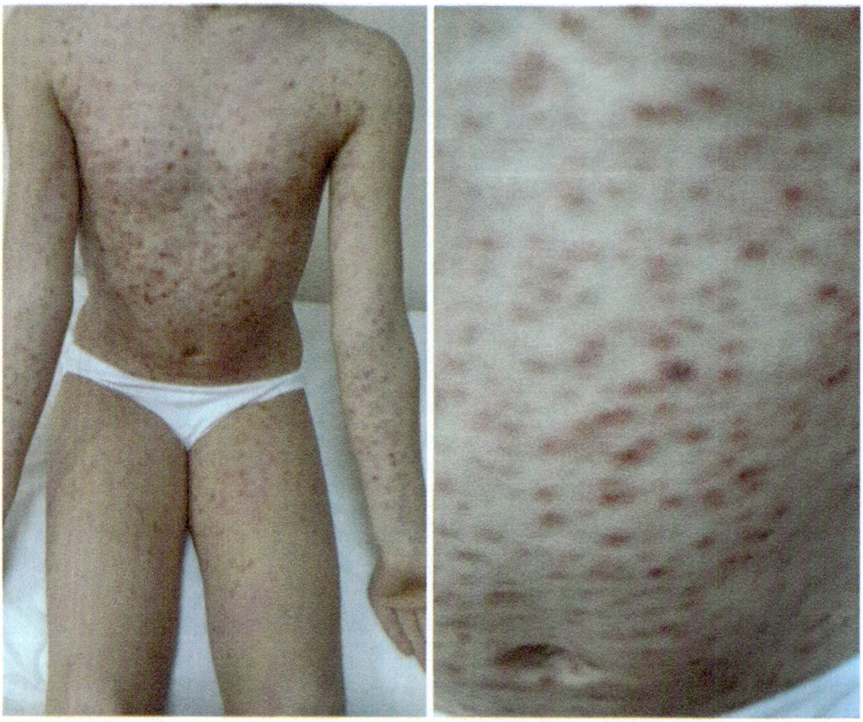

Fig. 72.1 Erythematous macules, papules and necrotic papules with hemorrhagic crusts in trunk and extremities of a 9-year-old girl

Pityriasis lichenoides (PL) which is also called Mucha-Habermann disease is an uncommon type of self-limited lymphocytic inflammatory dermatosis. Currently it has three subtypes: Pityriasis lichenoides chronica (PLC), pityriasis lichenoides et varioliformis acuta (PLEVA) and febrile ulceronecrotic Mucha-Habermann disease (FUMHD). PLEVA presents with erythematous macules and polymorphic lesions of papules which rapidly evolve into vesicopustular lesions with hemorrhagic and adherent crusts. Varioliform scars do not commonly occur. Post-inflammatory hypopigmentation and hyperpigmentation may occur and these alterations are rarely accompanied by malaise, fever, lymphadenopathies and arthritis (Table 72.1) [1–3]. PLEVA should be differentiated from varicella, other necrotic skin infections, vasculitis, pyoderma gangrenosum and lymphomatoid papulosis [4–7].

FUMHD is a rare and severe variant of PLEVA. It is clinically characterized by aggressive ulceronecrotic skin lesions and high fever and histologically described by features which are typical of PLEVA. In PLEVA, the infiltrate may be deep, dense and wedge-shaped, and the epidermis is edematous, with an interface dermatitis comprised of mainly lymphocytes. In addition, necrotic keratinocytes are generally present [5].

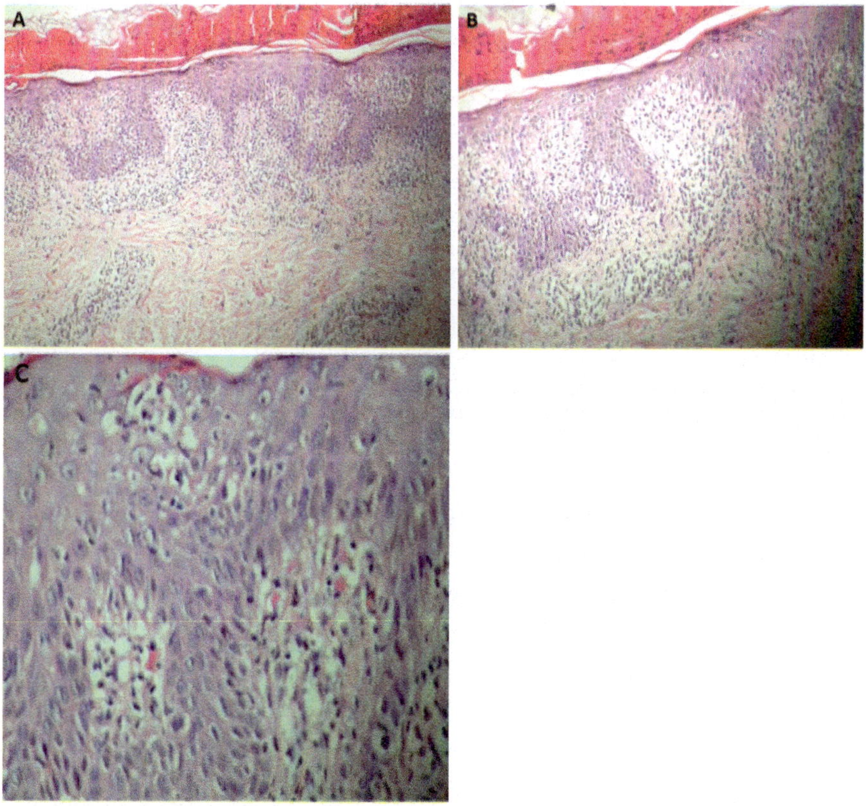

Fig. 72.2 (**a**) Parakeratosis and irregular acanthosis of the epidermis, as well as mix chronic inflammatory cell infiltrations which are mostly composed of lymphocytes in superficial perivascular and interstitial plexus and papillary dermis (H&E, ×100), (**b**) vacuolar degeneration of basal layer with a marked lymphocytic exocytosis (H&E, ×200) and (**c**) necrotic keratinocytes within epidermis (H&E, ×400)

Q2. Which of the following does not exclude the diagnosis of FUMHD in our patient?

A. Fever and constitutional symptoms
B. An acute onset of ulcers and necrotic lesions
C. Histological findings
D. All of the above

Answer: *The correct answer is* ***D.***

FUMHD is a rarely encountered, severe and potentially fatal variant of PLEVA. It is clinically characterized by aggressive ulceronecrotic skin lesions with high fever. It differs by rapid and painful clinical course and its association with systemic signs [7, 8].

Table 72.1 Comparison of pityriasis lichenoides chronica, pityriasis lichenoides et varioliformis acuta and febrile ulceronecrotic Mucha Habermann disease [5]

	Pityriasis lichenoides chronica (PLC)	Pityriasis lichenoides et varioliformis acuta (PLEVA)	Febrile ulceronecrotic Mucha Habermann disease (FUMHD)
Age or sex predominance	More prevalent in the pediatric population/ male predominance	More prevalent in the pediatric population/male predominance	More prevalent in the pediatric population/ male predominance
Clinical features	The papules are erythematous or red–brown and scaly	Individual lesions develop crusts, ulcers, vesicles or pustules which may heal with varioliform scars	Same as PLEVA The development of large coalescent skin necroses which may lead to death
Clinical course	Recurrent crops of spontaneously regressing erythematous to purpuric papules More indolent course	Individual lesions develop crusts, ulcers, vesicles or pustules Malaise, fever and generalized lymphadenopathy	Associated with high fever, systemic symptoms and fatal outcomes
Histopathology	T-cell infiltrates, with a general predominance of CD4+ cells Lymphocytic vasculitis In the infiltrate is less dense and more superficial	T-cell infiltrates, with a general predominance of CD8+ cells Lymphocytic vasculitis in the infiltrate is moderately dense	Same as PLEVA Lymphocytic vasculitis

FUMHD and PLEVA present with similar histological signs and reveal moderate acanthosis with necrotic keratinocytes over epidermis. The basal layer is vacuolated with a marked lymphocytic exocytosis. The superficial dermis is edematous and contains diffuse infiltrations of neutrophils and eosinophils. These infiltrations also spread around the skin appendages and vessels of the middle dermis [1, 2, 4, 5].

In this patient, the eruption was associated with mild fever (37–38 °C) and malaise. During follow-up, these findings did not progress and only skin eruption was observed. It was also notified that the patient had three recurrent outbreaks of erythematous and necrotic papules within 5 months.

Q3. What is the most appropriate next step in evaluation of this patient?

A. Screening for infections
B. Investigate T cell clonality and screen for T cell lymphoproliferative disease
C. Take history of drug intake
D. All of the above

Answer: *The correct answer is* ***D.***

Seasonal peaks of onset and rare familial outbreaks suggest an infectious trigger. Numerous potential infectious triggers including hepatitis B virus, hepatitis C virus,

Toxoplasma gondii, cytomegalovirus, parvovirus B19, adenovirus, Epstein–Barr virus, herpes simplex virus, varicella zoster virus, human immunodeficiency virus, Streptococci, Staphylococci and Mycoplasma [7].

Evidence of T-cell clonality has been detected in most cases of PLEVA and in FUMHD. PLEVA has also been reported in lymphoma. Additionally, PLC-like lesions have been described in patients with typical features of mycosis fungoides [1, 6]. Chemotherapeutic agents, oral contraceptives, astemizole and herbs have been reported to be associated with PLEVA and FUMHD [1, 6].

Q4. Which of the following is an appropriate and effective treatment for this 9-year-old girl?

A. Oral corticosteroids
B. Oral erythromycin
C. Oral tetracycline
D. Methotrexate

Answer: *The correct answer is* ***B.***

Erythromycin and tetracyclines are used for their anti-inflammatory effects rather than antibiotic effects. Erythromycin is preferred in children because tetracyclines have a side effect of dental pigmentation. Other antibiotics may be added if there is a secondary infection. In severe PLEVA or FUMHD, immunosuppressive agents including methotrexate, cyclosporine, dapsone and intravenous immunoglobulin may prove to be successful. Oral erythromycin treatment was administered in this patient as the disease had a mild course and the patient had a relatively younger age [8–11].

Practical Points

- Pityriasis lichenoides (PL) which is also called Mucha-Habermann disease is an uncommon type of self-limited lymphocytic inflammatory dermatosis
- Pityriasis lichenoides et varioliformis acuta (PLEVA) is one form of PL, which presents with erythematous macules and polymorphic lesions of papules which rapidly evolve into vesicopustular lesions with hemorrhagic and adherent crusts
- Febrile ulceronecrotic Mucha-Habermann disease (FUMHD) is a rare and severe variant of PLEVA, characterized by aggressive ulceronecrotic skin lesions and high fever and histologically described by features which are typical of PLEVA
- Erythromycin and tetracyclines are used for their anti-inflammatory effects rather than antibiotic effects in PLEVA
- In severe PLEVA or FUMHD, immunosuppressive agents may prove to be successful

References

1. de Castro BAC, Pereira JMM, Meyer RLB, Trindade FM, Pedrosa MS, Piancastelli ACC. Pityriasis lichenoides et varioliformis acuta after influenza vaccine. An Bras Dermatol. 2015;90(3 Suppl 1):181–4.
2. Markus JR, Carvalho VO, Lima MN, Abagge KT, Nascimento A, Werner B. The relevance of recognizing clinical and morphologic features of pityriasis lichenoides: clinicopathological study of 29 cases. Dermatol Pract Concept. 2013;3(4):7–10.
3. Virdi S, Kanwar A, Saikia U. Pityriasis lichenoides with ulceronecrosis and hyperthermia: a rare variant of pityriasis lichenoides et varioliformis acuta. Indian J Dermatol Venereol Leprol. 2010;76(2):172–5.
4. Child Fiona WSJ. Lymphocytic infiltrates. In: Christopher G, Barker J, editors. Rook's textbook of dermatology. 9th ed. Oxford: Wiley Blackwell; 2016. p. 3685–8.
5. Wood Gary S, Reizner G. Other papulosquamous disorders. In: Bolognia Jean L, Jorizzo JL, Rapini Ronald P, editors. Dermatology. 2nd ed. Edinburgh: Elsevier; 2008. p. 156–61.
6. Pereira N, Brinca A, Manuel Brites M, José Julião M, Tellechea O, Gonçalo M. Pityriasis Lichenoides et Varioliformis Acuta: case report and review of the literature. Case Rep Dermatol. 2012;4(1):61–5.
7. Lejuste FX, Michaux C, Lehners C, Calteux N. Febrile ulceronecrotic Mucha-Habermann disease. BMJ Case Rep. 2013;2013:bcr2013009739.
8. Meziane L, Caudron A, Dhaille F, Jourdan M, Dadban A, Lok C, Chaby G. Febrile Ulceronecrotic Mucha-Habermann disease: treatment with infliximab and intravenous immunoglobulins and review of the literature. Dermatology. 2012;225(4):344–8.
9. Bulur I, Kaya Erdoğan H, Nurhan Saracoglu Z, Arık D. Methotrexate treatment in children with febrile ulceronecrotic Mucha-Habermann disease: case report and literature review. Case Rep Dermatol Med. 2015;2015:357973.
10. Sotiriou E, Patsatsi A, Tsorova C, Lazaridou E, Sotiriadis D. Febrile ulceronecrotic Mucha-Habermann disease: a case report and review of the literature. Acta Derm Venereol. 2008;88(4):350–5.
11. Alzolibani AA, Zedan K. Macrolides in chronic inflammatory skin disorders. Mediat Inflamm. 2012;2012:159354.

Chapter 73
Persistent, Annular Urticarial Plaque

Selcen Kundak and Malik Ergin

A 12-year-old girl patient presented with erythematous, violaceous, annular and serpiginous urticarial plaques, located on the shoulders, thighs, buttocks and trunk (Fig. 73.1). Her lesions were accompanied by burning sensation and itching. It was learnt that she had recurrent episodes of these wheals for the last 6 months and each episode lasted for 4–5 weeks. Use of antihistamines and NSAIDs had resulted in very limited improvement. Her medical and family histories as well as her physical examination was unremarkable.

Complete blood cell count, hepatic and renal function tests, thyroid function tests, ESR, complement levels (C3, C4), IgA, IgG, IgM, IGE and other immunological tests (anti-nuclear antibody (ANA), anti-neutrophil cytoplasmic antibodies (p-ANCA and c-ANCA), anti-double stranded DNA antibody (anti-dsDNA), rheumatoid factor (RF)) were normal. Skin biopsy demonstrated prominent edema of the upper dermis as well as perivascular infiltration of inflammatory cells and eosinophils (Fig. 73.2). Direct immunofluorescence (DIF) showed fibrinogen deposition along the basement membrane.

Q1. What is the most likely diagnosis?

A. Erythema gyratum repens
B. Erythema annulare centrfigum
C. Urticarial vasculitis
D. Cutaneous lupus erythematosus

Answer: *The correct answer is* ***C.***

S. Kundak (✉)
Department of Dermatology, Dr. Behçet Uz Children's Hospital, İzmir, Turkey

M. Ergin
Department of Pathology, Dr. Behçet Uz Children's Hospital, İzmir, Turkey

© Springer Nature Switzerland AG 2020

F. Rahmani, N. Rezaei (eds.), *Pediatric Autoimmunity and Transplantation*,
https://doi.org/10.1007/978-3-030-26280-8_73

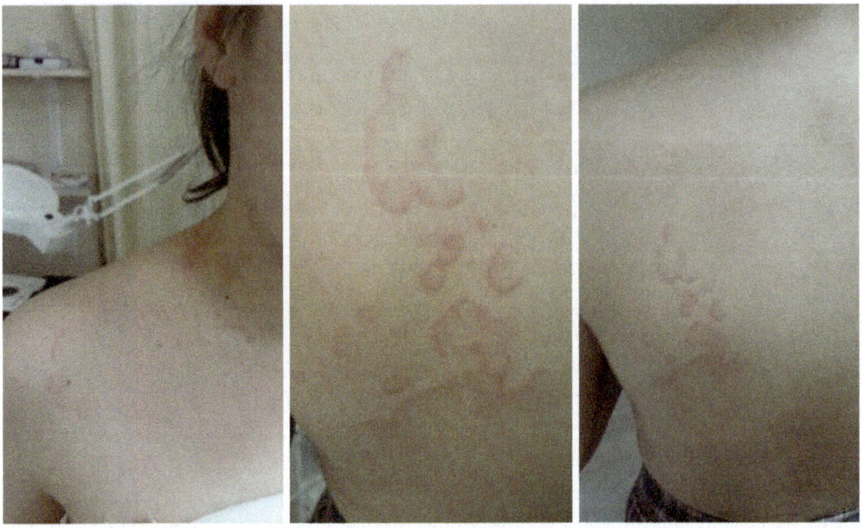

Fig. 73.1 Erythematous, violaceous and annular urticarial plaques in a 12-year-old girl

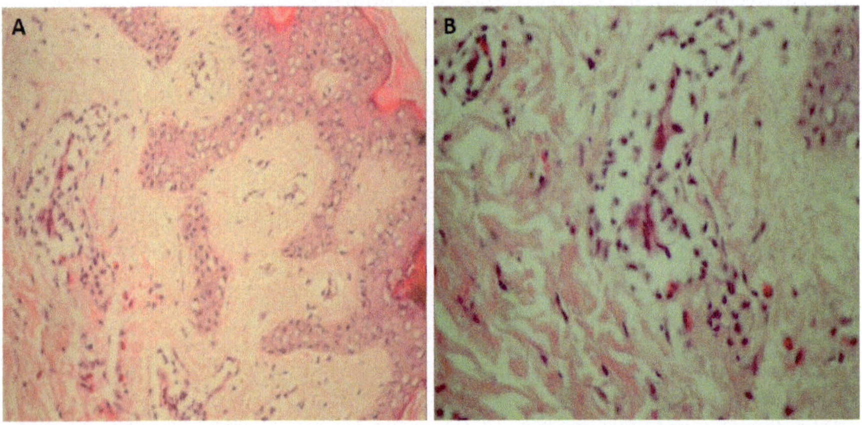

Fig. 73.2 (**a**) Prominent edema of the upper dermis and perivascular infiltration of mix inflammatory cells (H&E, ×200) and (**b**) perivascular infiltration of inflammatory cells with eosinophils in the superficial plexus (H&E, ×400)

Urticarial vasculitis is an uncommonly encountered type of chronic urticaria which is associated with vasculitic features. Urticarial vasculitis typically presents as erythematous wheals that resemble urticarial lesions and last more than 24 h. The most important clue for the diagnosis of urticarial vasculitis is the existence of urticarial lesions that last longer than 24 h. The diagnosis of urticarial vasculitis can be challenging due to uncommon presentations which resemble erythema gyratum repens-like eruptions [1–3]. Erythema gyratum repens-like skin lesions are characterized with centrifugal and annular eruption that expand in a zebra-like pattern. Such eruptions might appear in some autoimmune conditions [3].

As for this case, there were annular, erythematous and violoceous urticarial plaques as erythema gyratum repens–like eruption. Histological features of the case disclosed leukocytoclastic vasculitis with perivascular infiltration with eosinophils (Fig. 73.2). Based on the clinical and histological findings, this patient was diagnosed with urticarial vasculitis. Annular or gyrate urticarial lesions should be differentiated from erythema multiforme, urticaria multiforme, common urticaria, erythema marginatum, erythema annulare centrifugum and annular erythema in childhood [3, 4]. A skin biopsy should help differentiate these conditions. Prominent edema of the upper dermis is usually observed in skin biopsies. Some authors believe that lymphocytic infiltrate in association with endothelial swelling, erythrocyte extravasation and fibrin deposition are sufficient for the diagnosis [5, 6]. DIF may reveal deposits of immunoglobulins or fibrin around blood vessels.

It should be remembered that urticarial vasculitis, systemic lupus erythematosus (SLE), Sjogren syndrome, dermatomyositis, mixed connective tissue disease, juvenile rheumatoid arthritis, Churg-Strauss disease, Wegener granulomatosis, polyarteritis nodosa, or neutrophilic urticarial dermatosis might manifest with urticarial skin lesions. The clinicians should distinguish between urticaria and systemic urticarial syndromes (Table 73.1) [6, 7].

Q2. Which is the most appropriate long-term follow-up test for this patient?

A. Repetitive biopsies
B. Complement levels (C3,C4)
C. ANA, p-ANCA, c-ANCA, anti-dsDNA, and RF
D. DIF examination

Answer: *The correct answer is* ***B.***

Table 73.1 Differentiation between urticaria and systemic urticarial syndromes [7]

Common urticaria	Urticarial lesions (one or more of the following)
• Urticarial lesions (one or more of the following) • Only typical wheals: Erythematous edematous lesions • Transient (24–36 h) • Asymmetric distribution resolution without signs • No associated different elementary lesions (papules, vesicles, purpura, or crustae, etc.) • Pruritic (rarely stinging/burning) • Possibly associated with angioedema • No associated systemic symptoms	• Atypical "wheals": Infiltrated plaques • Persistent (24–36 h) • Symmetric distribution • Resolution with signs (hypo/hyperpigmentation, bruising, or scarring) • Associated different elementary lesions (papules, vesicles, purpura, scaling, or crustae, etc.) • Not pruritic; rather painful or burning • Usually no associated angioedema • Often associated with systemic symptoms (fever, malaise, arthralgia, abdominal pain, weight loss, acral circulatory abnormalities, or neurologic signs)

Three forms of urticarial vasculitis have been described. The first form is normocomplementemic urticarial vasculitis (NUV), the second form is hypocomplementemic urticarial vasculitis (HUV) and the third form is hypocomplementemic urticarial vasculitis syndrome (HUVS). In accordance, the patients with hypocomplementemia tend to have more frequent systemic involvement, more severe clinical course and longer disease duration compared to patients with normocomplementemia. Hypocomplementemia of C3 and C4 is usually observed and the HUV subtype can be associated with autoimmune connective tissue diseases including Sjögren's syndrome and SLE [5, 6, 8–10]. There may be transition between these forms of urticarial vasculitis within a period of time. HUVS is a distinct and severe clinical syndrome which is associated with systemic symptoms and identified in about 5% of patients with urticarial vasculitis. Since more than 50% of patients with HUVS develop SLE over time, patients with urticarial vasculitis need a full screening for vasculitis, including serum complement assays and exclusion of SLE [5].

Q3. What is the most appropriate next step in evaluation and management of this patient?

A. Investigate infections including hepatitis B and C viruses, Lyme disease and infectious mononucleosis
B. Ask about drug history
C. Investigate both benign and malignant hematological disorders
D. All of the above

Answer: *The correct answer is* ***D.***

In a majority of patients with urticarial vasculitis, the etiology is unknown. However, some antigens may trigger the circulating immune complexes and can activate the classical pathway of complement. Hepatitis B, hepatitis C, *Mycoplasma pneumonia*, Coxsackie infections, lyme disease and infectious mononucleosis are among accompanying conditions that are reported [5–7, 11]. Rarely, urticarial vasculitis may be linked with a drug such as cimetidine, diltiazem, sulfamethoxazole-trimethoprim, procainamide, infliximab, BCG vaccine, fluoxetine, paroxetine, sodium valproate, atenolol, thiazides, procarbazine, sulfonamides, ciprofloxacin, penicillin and potassium iodide [4, 7]. Hypergammaglobulinemia, hematological disorders, IgM or IgG monoclonal gammopathies, and IgA multiple myeloma have been described in association with urticarial vasculitis as well [4, 5, 7].

Q4. What is the most effective treatment for this 12-year-old girl?

A. Oral corticosteroids
B. Oral colchicine or dapson
C. Intravenous rituximab
D. Oral hydroxychloroquine

Answer: *The correct answer is* ***B.***

Table 73.2 Therapeutic algorithm in urticarial vasculitis [5]

First line treatment	Second line treatment	Third line treatment
• Non-sedating H1 antihistaminics • Non-steroidal anti-infl ammatory drugs	• Dapsone • Colchicine • Hydroxychloroquine • Short trials of corticosteroids	• Azathioprine • Cyclosporines • Mycophenolate mofetil • Methotrexate • Intravenous immunoglobulins • Cyclophosphamide interleukin antagonists (malizumab)

There are no universally effective treatment modalities for urticarial vasculitis. The variations in individual responses might affect the treatment success. Anti-histamines and NSAIDs may reduce the swelling and pain but these drugs are only sufficient in mild cases [4, 5]. As expected, anti-histamines and NSAIDs provided very limited improvement in this case. Oral corticosteroids are effective but the duration of use should be kept to a minimum in an attempt to prevent long-term side effects in children. Corticosteroid-sparing agents might provide benefits including; oral dapsone, colchicine, hydroxychloroquine and mycophenolate mofetil [4]. Rituximab may be a useful therapy for hypocomplementemic urticarial vasculitis [4]. When histopathological examination predominantly points out to neutrophilic and eosinophilic infiltrates, neutrophil inhibiting agents such as colchicine may be beneficial. The skin biopsy of this patient showed perivascular infiltration of inflammatory cells with eosinophils. Considering the age of the patient and the duration of the treatment, the most appropriate and effective treatment was specified as colchicine or dapson (Table 73.2) [5]. Colchicine treatment was preferred for this patient because the duration of corticosteroid treatment should be kept to a minimum in children. On the other hand, the relatively shorter duration of corticosteroid treatment may be insufficient for patients who experience long lasting and recurring episodes.

Practical Points

- Urticarial vasculitis is one type of chronic urticaria associated with vasculitic features
- Urticarial vasculitis typically presents as erythematous wheals that resemble urticarial lesions and last more than 24 h
- Patients with urticarial vasculitis and hypocomplementemia tend to have more frequent systemic involvement
- Hypocomplementemia of C3 and C4 is usually observed and the hypocomplementemic urticarial vasculitis (HUV) subtype can be associated with autoimmune connective tissue diseases including Sjögren's syndrome and systemic lupus erythematosus (SLE)
- HUV is identified in about 5% of patients with urticarial vasculitis and more than 50% of these patients develop SLE over time

References

1. Emer JJ, Bernardo SG, Kovalerchik O, Ahmad M. Urticaria multiforme. J Clin Aesthet Dermatol. 2013;6(3):34–9.
2. Pique E, Palacios S, Santana Z. Leukocytoclastic vasculitis presenting as an erythema gyratum repens-like eruption on a patient with systemic lupus erythematosus. J Am Acad Dermatol. 2002;47(5 Suppl):S254–6.
3. Fukunaga M, Harada K, Mae K, Wakamatsu K, Kiriyama N, Tsuboi R, Okubo Y. Erythema gyratum repens-like purpura in a patient with Sjögren syndrome. Case Rep Dermatol. 2017;9(2):40–3.
4. Imbernón-Moya A, Vargas-Laguna E, Burgos F, Fernández-Cogolludo E, Aguilar-Martínez A, Gallego-Valdés MÁ. Urticaria vasculitis in a child: a case report and literature review. Clin Case Rep. 2017;5(8):1255–7.
5. Borzova E, Grattan CEH. Urticarial vasculitis. In: Griffiths Christopher EM, Barker J, editors. Rook's textbook of dermatology. 9th ed. Oxford: Wiley Blackwell; 2016. p. 1321–7.
6. Lorinda Chung BK, Fiorentino DF. Cutaneous vasculitis. In: Bolognia Jean L, Jorizzo JL, Rapini Ronald P, editors. Dermatology. 2nd ed. Spain: Elsevier; 2008. p. 374–5.
7. Peroni A, Colato C, Zanoni G, Girolomoni G. Urticarial lesions: if not urticaria, what else? The differential diagnosis of urticaria. J Am Acad Dermatol. 2010;62(4):557–70.
8. Al Mosawi ZSA, Al Hermi BEA. Hypocomplementemic urticarial vasculitis syndrome in an 8-year-old boy: a case report and review of literature. Oman Med J. 2013;28(4):275–7.
9. Loricera J, Calvo-Río V, Mata C, Ortiz-Sanjuán F, González-López MA, Alvarez L, González-Vela MC, Armesto S, Fernández-Llaca H, Rueda-Gotor J, González-Gay MA, Blanco R. Urticarial Vasculitis in northern Spain: clinical study of 21 cases. Medicine. 2014;93(1):53–60.
10. Ghazanfar MN, Thomsen SF. Omalizumab for urticarial vasculitis: case report and review of the literature. Case Rep Dermatol Med. 2015;2015:576893.
11. Kulthanan K, Cheepsomsong M, Jiamton S. Urticarial vasculitis: etiologies and clinical course. Asian Pac J Allergy Immunol. 2009;27(2–3):95–102.

Chapter 74
Yellow, Reddish Brown Skin Lesions

Alireza Shafiei

A 9-month-old boy was referred to our clinic due to yellow to reddish brown papules and nodules and similar plaque-like lesions since 1 month old. Rubbing of the lesions by the tip of a pen lead to urtication and erythema around the lesions.

Q1. What is the most probable diagnosis?

A. Delayed pressure urticaria
B. Urticarial pigmentosa
C. Urticarial vasculitis
D. Muckle-Wells syndrome

Answer: *The correct answer is* ***B.***

Urticaria pigmentosa lesions are cutaneous manifestations of mastocytosis and appear as small yellowish-tan to reddish-brown macules or slightly raised papules and plaque.

Q2. What is the name of the above maneuver "urtication by rubbing of the lesions"?

A. Dermatographism
B. Darier's sign
C. Nikolsky sign
D. Pathergy test

Answer: *The correct answer is* ***B.***

Rubbing of the skin lesions in urticaria pigmentosa usually leads to urtication and erythema over and around the macules, known as Darier's sign [1].

A. Shafiei (✉)
Bahrami Children's Hospital, Tehran, Iran

© Springer Nature Switzerland AG 2020

F. Rahmani, N. Rezaei (eds.), *Pediatric Autoimmunity and Transplantation*,
https://doi.org/10.1007/978-3-030-26280-8_74

Q3. Which of the following tests would help confirm the diagnosis?

A. Skin biopsy
B. Serum tryptase level
C. Bone marrow aspiration
D. Serum histamine level

Answer: *The correct answer is* ***A.***

Diagnosis should be confirmed by skin biopsy. In infants bone marrow biopsy is indicated if there are specific findings to suggest extra-cutaneous organ involvement.

Practical Points

- Urticaria pigmentosa lesions are cutaneous manifestations of mastocytosis and appear as small yellowish-tan to reddish-brown macules or slightly raised papules and plaque
- Rubbing of the skin lesions in urticaria pigmentosa usually leads to urtication and erythema over and around the macules, known as Darier's sign
- Diagnosis should be confirmed by skin biopsy

Reference

1. Galen BT, Rose MG. Darier's sign in mastocytosis. Blood. 2014;123(8):1127.

Chapter 75
Erythroderma

Wojciech Baran and Jacek Szepietowski

A 4-year-old boy presented with erythroderma. He was healthy and doing well until 3 weeks before consultation, when he had symptoms of a viral infection of the upper respiratory tract. Seven days later, erythematous skin lesions appeared around the mouth and on the face and within the next 2 weeks the lesions spread to the trunk and proximal extremities. His past medical history revealed asthma since 1 year old which was well controlled. His family history was relevant for atopic dermatitis and asthma in mother. On examination erythrodermic appearance was present (Fig. 75.1a), and in some areas of healthy skin small perifollicular papules were noted (Fig. 75.1b). Keratoderma was present on both palms and soles (Fig. 75.2a, b). Itching was mild (numeric rating scale = 3). Laboratory data revealed only elevated IgE: 1040 IU/mL.

Q1. Which of the following tests will most probably give you the underlying diagnosis?

A. Antinuclear antibody testing
B. Specific IgE levels
C. Search for mutation in SPINK5 gene coding serine peptidase inhibitor LEKTI
D. Skin biopsy with histopathological evaluation

Answer:** The correct answer is **D.

Pityriasis rubra pilaris (PRP) is an idiopathic, papulosquamous disease. The age distribution of PRP has two peaks in the first and fifth decade of life. Most cases are acquired and familial variants are very rare with recently described heterozygous gene mutations in *CARD14* which encodes the caspase recruitment domain family,

W. Baran (✉) · J. Szepietowski
Department of Dermatology, Venereology and Allergology, Wroclaw Medical University, Wrocław, Poland
e-mail: wojciech.baran@umed.wroc.pl

© Springer Nature Switzerland AG 2020

F. Rahmani, N. Rezaei (eds.), *Pediatric Autoimmunity and Transplantation*,
https://doi.org/10.1007/978-3-030-26280-8_75

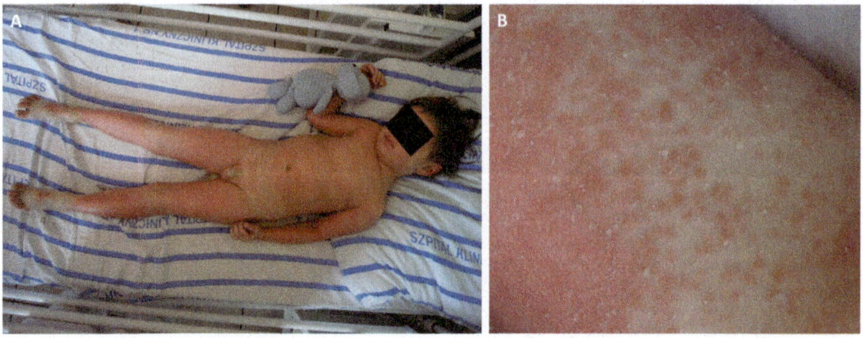

Fig. 75.1 (**a**) erythroderma covering almost the whole body and (**b**) perifollicular papules with fine scale on the islands of sparing

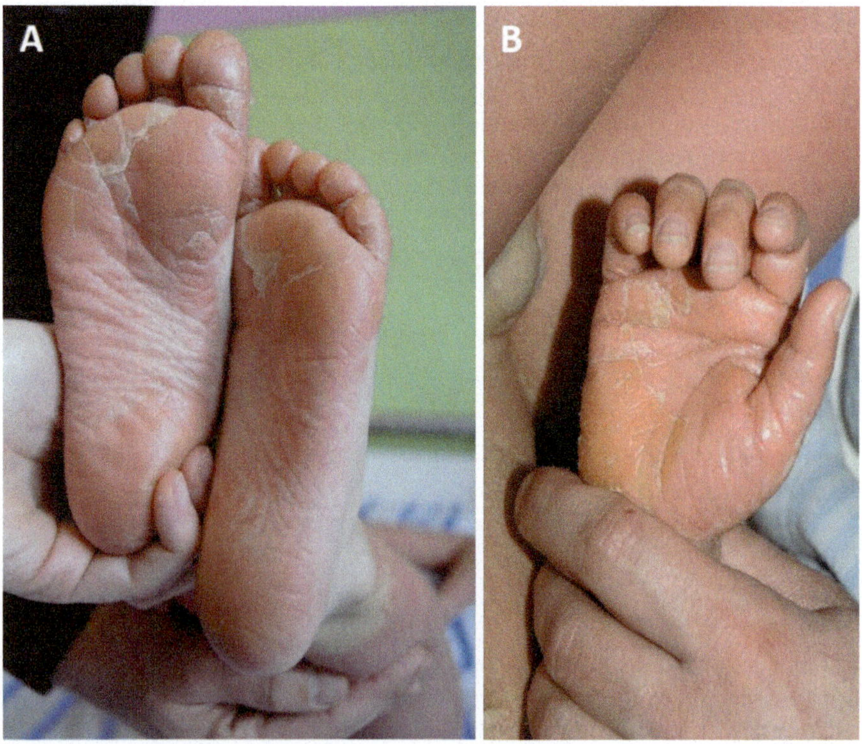

Fig. 75.2 (**a**, **b**) Orange-yellow palmoplantar keratoderma

member 14 [1]. PRP is classified into six types with three types presenting in childhood. Type III, called "juvenile classical", can result in erythroderma with islands of sparing called "nappes claires". Diagnosis is made based on clinical features and is supported by histology. Histopathological examination reveals follicular plugging, acanthosis with exaggerated follicular shoulders, spotty parakeratosis and mild upper dermal inflammatory infiltrate [2]. The boy's parents are worried about future outcome of the disease and his prognosis.

Q2. Which statement is true regarding the disease course and prognosis?

A. Lifelong disease with slow progression over the years
B. Lifelong disease with slow regression over the years
C. Disease occurs once in a lifetime and may clear spontaneously
D. Disease occurs once in a lifetime but always requires aggressive systemic treatment

Answer: *The correct answer is* ***C.***

Disease course and prognosis depends on the type of PRP. Classical juvenile PRP, as diagnosed in our patient typically resolves in an average of 1 year. In severe cases, patients might require few months of systemic treatment, however the prognosis is good. Circumscribed juvenile PRP is a localized variant of PRP affecting pediatric population which has uncertain prognosis and in some cases may last several years [2].

Q3. What is the best initial treatment?

A. Systemic corticosteroids
B. Systemic acitretin
C. Systemic antibiotics
D. Systemic azathioprine

Answer: *The correct answer is* ***B.***

Several therapeutic approaches for treating PRP have been suggested, however considering the self-limited nature of the disease, risk benefit ratio must be balanced. In pediatric population with localized lesions topical corticosteroids and emollients should be considered as a first line. In more severe cases of erythrodermic PRP patients may need supportive care to prevent hypothermia, electrolyte imbalance and protein loss. The use of acitretin as first-line treatment of severe adult-onset PRP is well established and this drug should be considered also in childhood cases of severe PRP. Other therapeutic options include methotrexate and cyclosporine [3].

Practical Points

- Pityriasis rubra pilaris (PRP) is an idiopathic, papulosquamous disease with two age peaks in the first and fifth decade of life
- Type III PRP, called "juvenile classical", can result in erythroderma with islands of sparing called "nappes claires"

- Classical juvenile PRP, as diagnosed in our patient typically resolves in an average of 1 year
- In severe cases, patients might require few months of systemic treatment
- In more severe cases of erythrodermic PRP patients may need supportive care to prevent hypothermia, electrolyte imbalance and protein loss

References

1. Fuchs-Telem D. Familial pityriasis rubra pilaris is caused by mutations in CARD14. Am J Hum Genet. 2012;91(1):163–70.
2. Allison D. Pityriasis rubra pilaris in children. J Am Acad Dermatol. 2002;47(3):386–9.
3. Eastham A. Treatment options for pityriasis rubra pilaris including biologic agents: a retrospective analysis from an academic medical center. JAMA Dermatol. 2014;150(1):92–4.

Chapter 76
Erythematous Scaly Plaques

Sunil K. Kothiwala and Piyush Kumar

An 11-year-old girl presented with multiple itchy erythematous scaly plaques over trunk, scalp, palms and soles since 4 years ago (Fig. 76.1a–c). She was apparently well 4 years back, when lesions gradually appeared, and later increased in size and number and associated with fissure formation over sole. Patient had applied topical medications on and off to which lesions used to partially respond, yet slight thickening and scaling were still present. When she presented to our clinic, she had well-defined multiple erythematous scaly indurated plaques all over her body, whitish, thick, adherent scaly plaques over scalp and hyperkeratotic scaly plaques and fissures over palm and sole. Scales were centrally adherent, white and coarse. There was also a history of winter exacerbation of the symptoms. There was no history of preceding upper respiratory tract infection, no history of nail involvement, pustular lesions, erytheroderma or joint pain. Patient had not received systemic treatment in past. Skin biopsy showed acanthosis, parakeratosis and mononuclear infiltrate. Her anti-streptolysin O titer was normal.

Q1. What is the most likely diagnosis?

A. Pitryiasis rubra pilaris
B. Plaque psoriasis
C. Progressive symmetric erythrokeratoderma
D. Atopic Dermatitis

Answer: *The correct answer is* ***B.***

Type of scale, which is coarse, white and centrally adherent, and the distribution of plaques over scalp, trunk with palmoplantar hyperkeratotic lesions and fissure are

S. K. Kothiwala
Consultant Dermatologist, SkinEva Clinic, Jaipur, Rajsthan, India

P. Kumar (✉)
Department of Dermatology, Katihar Medical College, Katihar, Bihar, India

© Springer Nature Switzerland AG 2020

F. Rahmani, N. Rezaei (eds.), *Pediatric Autoimmunity and Transplantation*,
https://doi.org/10.1007/978-3-030-26280-8_76

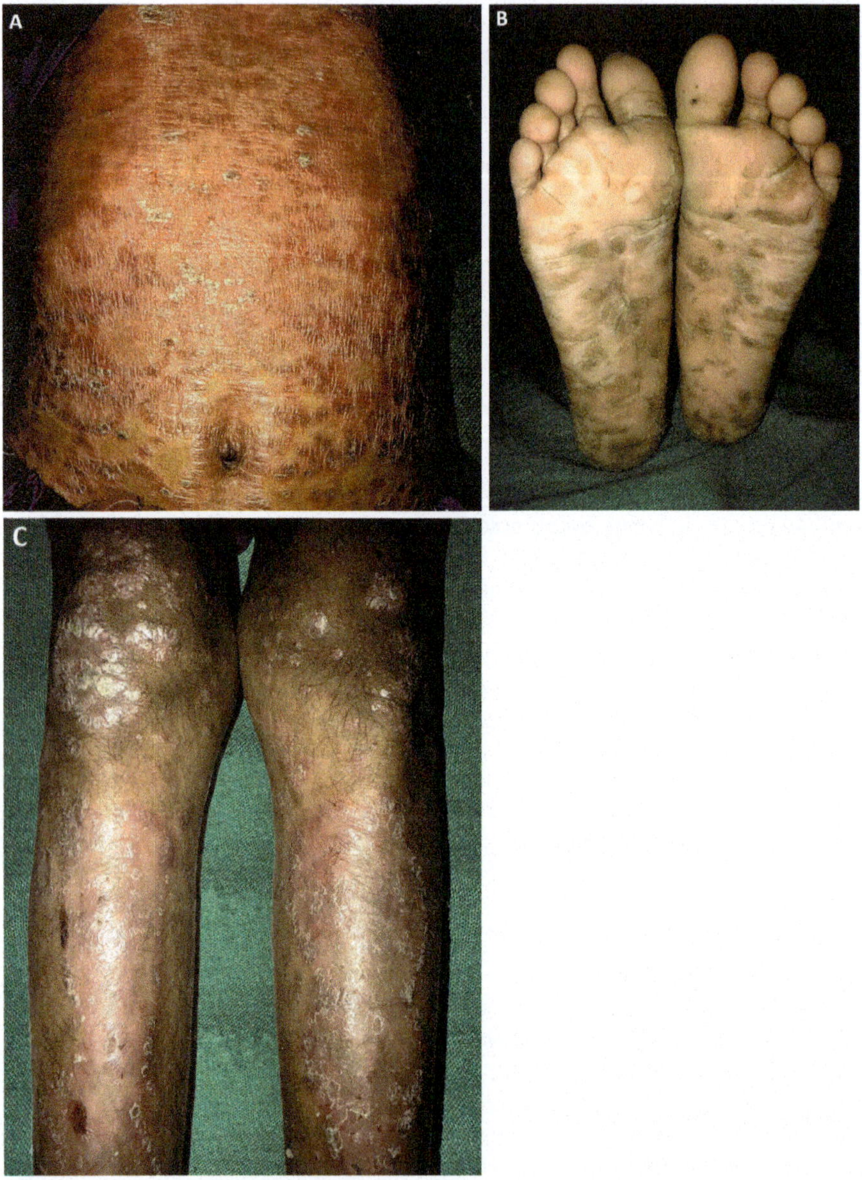

Fig. 76.1 Itchy erythematous scaly plaques over trunk (**a**), sole (**b**) and leg (**c**) of an 11-year-old girl

all suggestive of plaque psoriasis as the most likely diagnosis. Psoriasis is a relatively common immune-mediated disorder that accounts for 4% of all dermatoses seen in children under 16 years of age. Classical lesions of plaque psoriasis are well defined, round, intensely erythematous covered with silver white scale. Lesions are usually bilaterally symmetrical with predominant extensor involvement. Other presentations are inverse psoriasis, facial psoriasis, guttate psoriasis, diaper area psoriasis and nail psoriasis. Other common forms of the disease are pustular psoriasis, either generalized or palmoplantar, and erythrodermic psoriasis. Histopathology show regular acanthosis, acanthosis with elongation of rete ridges, parakeratosis, hypogranulosis, dilated capillaries and perivascular infiltrate composed of lymphocytes, neutrophils and macrophages. Accumulation of neutrophils within a pustule is referred to as a "spongiform pustule of Kogoj" and the accumulation of neutrophils remnants in stratum corneum surrounded by parakeratosis is called "micro abscess of Munro". These findings are both pathognomonic for psoriasis [1].

Pitryiasis rubra pilaris (PRP) is an important condition to differentiate from psoriasis. The follicular accentuation, islands of skipping areas, and salmon color of lesions over palm and sole favor the diagnosis of PRP over psoriasis. Biopsy of PRP lesions may show perifollicular inflammation as well. Progressive symmetric erythrokeratoderma is a dominantly inherited ichthyosis usually noted during infancy and yellow to brown scaly lesions, limited to the extremities, buttocks and face. Atopic dermatitis is an immunologically mediated, chronic relapsing skin disorder, clinically characterized by eczematous eruptions involving extensor surfaces of extremities, trunk, face, and neck in infants and flexors areas of wrists, ankles, antecubital fossae, popliteal fossae, and neck in older children and adolescents.

Q2. Which of the following signs support the diagnosis above?

A. Positive Auspitz sign
B. Positive Woronoff ring
C. Koebner phenomenon
D. All of the above

Answer: *The correct answer is* ***D.***

Auspitz sign is the appearance of pin-point bleeding spots when scale is removed from plaque, caused by rupture of dilated capillaries beneath the thinned suprapapillary epidermis. This is a characteristic feature of psoriasis [2]. Woronoff ring is blanched halo (white ring) of approximately uniform width, surrounding erythematous lesions. This sign can develop after phototherapy or topical treatments for psoriasis [3]. Koebner phenomenon is characterised by formation of new psoriatic lesions in otherwise healthy skin. Lesions developed by Koebner phenomenon are often linear in shape, as they follow the route of cutaneous injury. Koebner is also known as an isomorphic response as lesions show similar clinical and histopathological features to the original psoriatic lesions. Koebner is noted to be more common in unstable psoriasis, patients with younger age of onset, patients who have received multiple treatments for psoriasis and emotionally disturbed patients [4], and might even happen in patients without pre-existing skin lesions.

Q3. All statements are correct regarding childhood psoriasis, except:

A. Childhood psoriasis is more likely to be associated with positive family history than late-onset psoriasis
B. Human leukocyte antigen Cw6 is associated with severe early-onset disease

C. Psoriasis in children is frequently precipitated by infections and manifests as acute guttate psoriasis
D. Elevated anti-streptolysin O titters are more common in patients with guttate psoriasis and are associated with subsequent progression to plaque psoriasis and long-term disease

Answer: *The correct answer is* ***D.***

Childhood or early onset psoriasis, as compared to late onset disease, has more inclination to a positive family history. Based on a large survey, having one parent with psoriasis can increase risk of developing disease by 14% and if both parents are affected, risk of developing psoriasis is as high as 41% [5]. Researchers have identified at least nine chromosomal loci with statistically significant linkage to psoriasis. These loci care called psoriasis susceptibility 1 through 9 (PSORS1 through PSORS9), PSORS1 (located on chromosome 6) being the major genetic determinant (35–50% of patients) [6]. Early-onset psoriasis has been linked to HLA-Cw6 antigen and 73.7% of patients with guttate psoriasis show positive HLA-Cw6 antigen. Many environmental factors have been implicated in initiation as well as exacerbation of pre-existing disease. These include trauma, infection, drugs, psychogenic factors, smoking, alcohol consumption, and obesity. In children, preceding or concurrent pharyngeal streptococcal infection is a common trigger of guttate psoriasis. Patients with guttate psoriasis who have early onset, as well as those with recurrent upper respiratory tract infection and/or raised anti-streptolysin O titers, are found to have a rapid involution and are surprisingly less prone to recurrence [7].

Q4. The patient is showing poor response to treatment with topical steroids and moisturizers. All of the following options are included in your second-line treatments, except:

A. Educating the parents about chronicity of disease and time consuming therapy
B. Initiation of phototherapy with continuation of topical medicines
C. Reserve systemic agents for recalcitrant disease
D. Use of oral steroids

Answer: *The correct answer is* ***D.***

Patient education about chronic nature of disease and slow response to treatment, is a key element in successful treatment of psoriasis. Selection of treatment modality depends on disease severity in terms of area of involvement, erythema, induration and response to early treatments. Therapeutic modalities for psoriasis are topical therapy, photochemotherapy and systemic therapy. Topical therapy includes corticosteroids, vitamin D_3 analogues, anthralin, tazarotene, salicylic acid, coal tar and calcineurin inhibitors. Although patients with limited disease respond well to topical therapy, patients with moderate to severe psoriasis should be considered for additional phototherapy for further management. Photochemotherapy is first line treatment as monotherapy or in combination for moderate to severe psoriasis. Narrow-band ultraviolet B (NBUVB, 311 nm) has a higher ratio of therapeutic-to-toxic wavelength than broadband UVB light (290–320 nm). Application of oils or ointment prior to exposure of phototherapy increase the efficacy of phototherapy. As photochemotherapy and phototherapy require frequent visits to clinic, children may be asked to expose themselves to natural sunlight, i.e. PUVA solarization, however, PUVA solarization appears to be less effective than PUVA.

Systemic intervention with methotrexate, cyclosporine, acitretin, and biologic agent should be reserved for children with erythrodermic and pustular forms of psoriasis or for those with moderate to severe plaque psoriasis recalcitrant to other modalities. In general, systemic corticosteroid should be avoided as withdraw of steroid therapy may result in flares of psoriasis or trigger of pustular psoriasis [8].

Q5. All statements are correct regarding comorbidities of pediatric psoriasis, except:

A. The risk of developing ulcerative colitis is higher in pediatric psoriasis
B. The most common comorbidity of pediatric psoriasis is obesity
C. Recent evidences suggest an association between metabolic syndrome and psoriasis
D. Asymmetric anterior uveitis is seen in patients with juvenile psoriatic arthritis

Answer: *The correct answer is* ***A.***

Pediatric psoriasis patients have higher risk of developing Crohn disease, but not ulcerative colitis [9]. Obesity appears to be a frequent co-morbidity both in children as well as adults [10]. Comorbidities like impaired quality of life, decreased tendency to participate in physical activities because of pruritus and visible lesions increase the risk of developing obesity. Increasing evidence support an association between pediatric psoriasis and metabolic syndrome. Approximately two to four times the rate of comorbidity from hyperlipidemia, hypertension, and diabetes have been reported in children with psoriasis compared to unaffected children [11], and evidence suggests screening for such comorbidities in pediatric patients with psoriasis. Joint pain has been described in 10% of children with moderate to severe psoriasis. The diagnosis of juvenile psoriatic arthritis (JPsA) when typical psoriatic skin lesions and inflammatory articular disease are both present is pretty straightforward. In absence of typical psoriatic skin lesions, the definitive diagnosis of juvenile psoriatic arthritis requires presence of any three of the following added to inflammatory arthritis: dactylitis, nail pitting or onycholysis, psoriasis-like rash, and history of psoriasis in a first-degree relative (Vancouver criteria) [12]. Children with JPsA have a high risk of developing uveitis and up to 14–17% of children with JPsA may develop asymmetric anterior uveitis [13].

Practical Points

- Psoriasis accounts for 4% of all dermatoses seen in children under 16 years of age
- Classical lesions of plaque psoriasis are well defined, round, intensely erythematous covered with silver white scale

- In histology, accumulation of neutrophils within a pustule is referred to as a "spongiform pustule of Kogoj" and the accumulation of neutrophils remnants in stratum corneum surrounded by parakeratosis is called "micro abscess of Munro"
- Auspitz sign is appearance of pin-point bleeding spots when scale is removed from plaque caused by rupture of dilated capillaries beneath the thinned suprapapillary epidermis
- Koebner phenomenon is characterised by formation of new psoriatic lesions in otherwise healthy skin
- Therapeutic modalities for psoriasis are topical therapy, photochemotherapy and systemic therapy
- Topical therapy includes corticosteroids, vitamin D_3 analogues, anthralin, tazarotene, salicylic acid, coal tar and calcineurin inhibitors
- Obesity, metabolic syndrome and higher risk for developing Crohn's disease are future complications of childhood psoriasis

References

1. Silverberg N. Update on pediatric psoriasis, part 1: clinical features and demographics. Cutis. 2010;86:118–24.
2. Bernhard J. Clinical pearl: Auspitz sign in psoriasis scale. J Am Acad Dermatol. 1997;36(4):621.
3. Penneys N, Ziboh V, Simon P, Lord J. Pathogenesis of Woronoff ring in psoriasis. Arch Dermatol. 1976;112:955–7.
4. Thappa D. The isomorphic phenomenon of Koebner. Indian J Dermatol Venereol Leprol. 2004;70(3):187–9.
5. Andressen C, Henseler T. Inheritance of psoriasis. Analysis of 2035 family histories. Hautarzt. 1982;33(4):214–7.
6. Bowcock A, Krueger J. Getting under the skin: the immunogenetics of psoriasis. Nat Rev Immunol. 2005;5(9):699–711.
7. Ko H, Jwa S, Song M, Kim M, Kwon K. Clinical course of guttate psoriasis: long-term follow-up study. J Dermatol. 2010;37(10):894–9.
8. Silverberg N. Update on pediatric psoriasis, part 2: therapeutic management. Cutis. 2010;86(4):172–6.
9. Augustin M, Glaeske G, Radtke M, Christophers E, Reich K, Schafer I. Epidemiology and comorbidity of psoriasis in children. Br J Dermatol. 2010;162(3):633–6.
10. Paller A, Mercy K, Kwasny M, Choon S, Cordoro K, Girolomoni G. Association of pediatric psoriasis severity with excess and central adiposity: an international cross-sectional study. JAMA Dermatol. 2013;149(2):166–76.
11. Mahe E, Maccari F, Beauchet A, Lahfa M, Barthelemy H, Reguiai Z, Beneton N, Estève E, Chaby G, Ruer-Mulard M, Steiner H, Pauwels C, Avenel-Audran M, Goujon-Henry C, Descamps V, Begon E, Sigal ML, Resopso GEM. Childhood-onset psoriasis: association with future cardiovascular and metabolic comorbidities. Br J Dermatol. 2013;169(4):889–95.
12. Southwood T, Petty R, Malleson P, Delgado E, Hunt D, Wood B, Schroeder M. Psoriatic arthritis in children. Arthritis Rheum. 1989;32(8):1007–13.
13. Twilt M, Swart van den Berg M, van Meurs JC, ten Cate R, van Suijlekom-Smit LW. Persisting uveitis antedating psoriasis in two boys. Eur J Pediatr. 2003;162(9):607–9.

Chapter 77
Multiple Circinate, Sterile, Flaccid, Relapsing Pustules

Selcen Kundak and Malik Ergin

An 8-year-old girl presented with recurring pustular lesions with serpiginous and grouped appearance intensely located on the neck and body folds. She reports recurrent episodes of same lesions in the last 2 years, each lasting for 4–5 weeks. Her past and family history and the rest of her physical examination are unremarkable. Dermatological examination revealed 2 to 10-mm flaccid pustules on normal or erythematous bases (Fig. 77.1a, b) These pustules had coalesced in the axillary and groin folds and some had eroded. Palms, soles and mucous membranes were spared. Healed pustules had resulted in hyperpigmentation.

Laboratory analysis revealed hemoglobin: 9.6 g/dL, leukocyte count: 14,090/μL, ESR: 70 mm/h, CRP: 7 mg/dL. Liver and renal function tests, thyroid function tests, and complement levels (C3, C4) were normal. Repetitive cultures obtained from pustular lesions were negative. Skin biopsy revealed spongiosis in epidermis, sucorneal pustules filled with abundant polymorphonuclear leukocytes, acantholytic cells and a few eosinophils (Fig. 77.2). Direct immunofluorescence analysis were negative.

Q1. What is the most likely diagnosis?

A. Deficiency of IL-1 receptor antagonist
B. Subcorneal pustular dermatosis/Sneddon-Wilkinson disease
C. IgA pemphigus
D. Pustular psoriasis

Answer: *The correct answer is* ***B.***

Subcorneal pustular dermatosis (SPD), also known as Sneddon-Wilkinson disease, is a rare chronic and recurring flaccid sterile pustular eruption, characterized

S. Kundak (✉)
Department of Dermatology, Dr. Behçet Uz Children's Hospital, İzmir, Turkey

M. Ergin
Department of Pathology, Dr. Behçet Uz Children's Hospital, İzmir, Turkey

© Springer Nature Switzerland AG 2020

F. Rahmani, N. Rezaei (eds.), *Pediatric Autoimmunity and Transplantation*,
https://doi.org/10.1007/978-3-030-26280-8_77

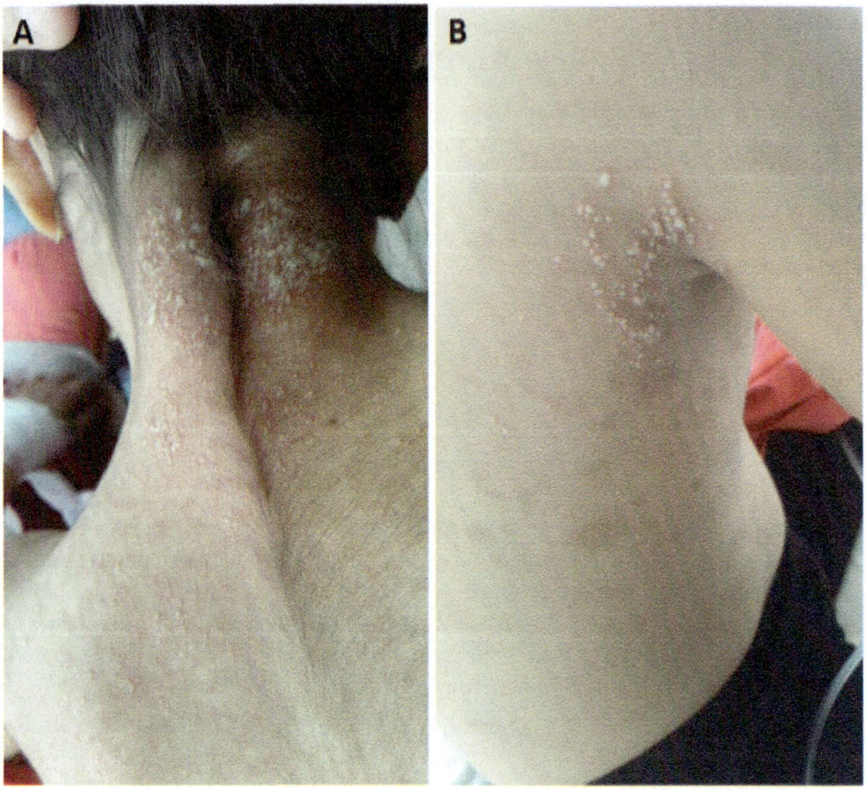

Fig. 77.1 (**a**) flaccid pustules serpiginous and grouped apperance intensely located on the neck, and body folds, and (**b**) pustules varying in size from 2 to 7 mm serpiginous and grouped appearance intensely located on the neck, and body folds

by annular or serpiginous structures involving the trunk and body fold [1, 2]. SPD is classified within the "neutrophilic dermatoses" [2]. SPD is histopathologically characterized by a neutrophil predominant infiltrate in the blister with pustules situated immediately below stratum corneum [2, 3]. It develops mainly in middle-aged women, although the disease has been reported in children as well [4].

Deficiency of interleukin 1 receptor antagonist (DIRA) is characterized by pustular lesions resembling pustular psoriasis. It is accompanied with aseptic osteomyelitis, periostitis, leukocytosis and elevated acute phase reactants. DIRA is characterized by perinatal onset. It appears between birth and 2.5 weeks of age [2].

In IgA pemphigus, circulating IgA autoantibodies can be identified and DIF analysis reveals intercellular, intrapustular or subcorneal IgA deposition. IgA pemphigus gives rise to intraepidermal bulla in either of the two forms identified: SPD-type or intraepidermal neutrophilic type. Immunological evaluation is necessary for distinguishing between IgA pemphigus and SPD as these two entities are clinically and histopathologically inrecognizable [1–5]. In this case DIF examination were negative.

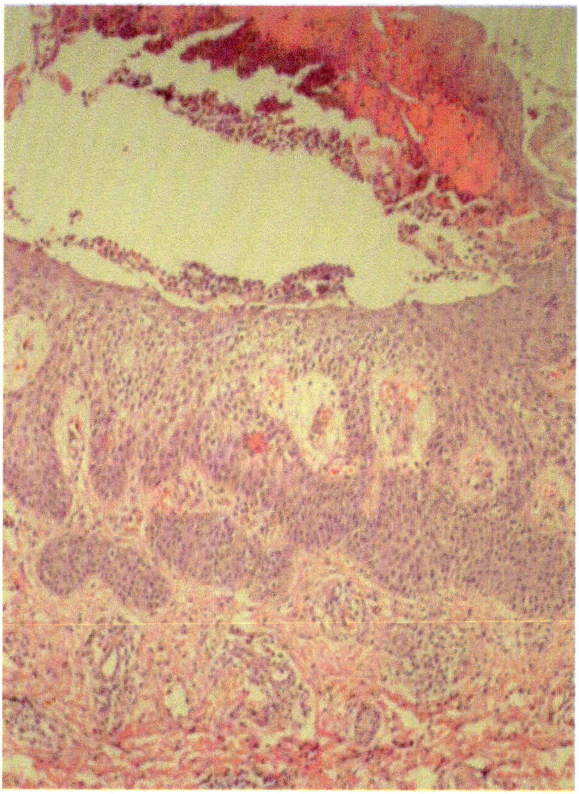

Fig. 77.2 The subcorneal pustule formation filled with neutrophils and mixed superficial perivascular inflammatory cell infiltrate in the underlying dermis (H&E, ×100)

Pustular psoriasis composes a spectrum of pustular dermatoses [1], ranging from palmoplantar pustulosis to generalized disorders including von Zumbusch pustular psoriasis and impetigo herpetiformis. SPD is clinically and histologically similar to both SPD-type IgA pemphigus and annular pustular psoriasis [1, 2, 6, 7]. Immunologic studies are needed for differential diagnose of SPD from pustular psoriasis and SPD-type IgA pemphigus [1, 2, 6, 8]. DIF examination is negative in SPD. In pustular psoriasis Kogoj's spongiform pustules are histopathologically confirmed [2].

Based on the clinical features, histopathological characteristics and direct immunofluorescence analysis results the patient was diagnosed with SPD.

Q2. What is the most appropriate next step in evaluation of this patient?

A. Investigation for autoimmune disorders
B. Investigation for IgA gammopathy and IgA myeloma
C. Investigation for underlying infections
D. All of the above

Answer: *The correct answer is* ***D.***

The etiology of the SPD is still obscure. Infectious and autoimmune factors have been implicated [7]. Immunological disturbance resulting from abnormal cytokine profile has been generally accepted as the underlying cause for this dermatosis. There are well-documented cases of SPD associated with benign IgA gammopathy or IgA elevation without gammopathy. There are also reports in association with IgA myeloma and marginal zone lymphoma [1, 5, 9]. This relationship between gammopathy and SPD might indicate a possible predisposition for immune dysregulation. SPD can be associated with disorders such as pyoderma gangrenosum, rheumatoid arthritis, systemic lupus erythematosus, inflammatory bowel diseases, hyperthyroidism, and apudoma [1, 5]. These conditions can develop many years after the SPD diagnosis, hence long-term follow-up is suggested. Due to the distinct relationship between SPD and autoimmune disorders, many authors have recommended to screen SPD patients for monoclonal gammopathy, systemic lupus erythematosus and rheumatoid arthritis [1, 5, 7–9].

Q3. What is the most appropriate and effective treatment for this 8-year-old girl with SPD?

A. Oral corticosteroids
B. Dapsone
C. Rituximab
D. Intravenous immunoglobulin

Answer: *The correct answer is* ***B.***

Dapsone is the first line treatment for SPD. In pediatric patients, it should be used carefully because of its hematologic adverse effects. Systemic or topical steroids are used as monotherapy or in combination with dapsone. In addition to dapsone, anti-neutrophilic drugs such as colchicine, sulfapyridine and sulfamethoxypyrazine have also been used successfully [1, 4, 9]. Topical steroids are only sufficient in mild cases. In this patient, we preferred dapson in combination with topical steroids and sufficient response to this management was observed. In recalcitrant cases, variable results have been reported with infliximab, acitretin, adalimumab, etanercept, IVIG.

Q4. Which one of the following conditions is among the differential diagnoses of SPD?

A. Pustular psoriasis
B. Dermatophyte infection
C. Immunobullous diseases
D. All of the above

Answer: *The correct answer is* ***D.***

The differential diagnoses include dermatitis herpetiformis, IgA pemphigus, acute generalized exanthematous pustulosis (AGEP), impetigo, pemphigus foliaceus, pustular psoriasis and dermatophyte infection. In pustular psoriasis, the presence of spongiform pustules, formation of microabscess and elongation of rete ridges are characteristic in the histology and are not found in SPD [1, 2]. A dermatophyte infection can be easily excluded with a direct microscopic examination.

Table 77.1 Differentiation between IgA pemphigus and subcorneal pustular dermatosis [1, 3, 5, 8]

	SPD type IgA pemphigus	Intraepidermal neutrophilic type IgA pemphigus	(SPD) Subcorneal pustular dermatosis
Age/sex	Mostly affects adults, there are reports of pediatric cases	Chiefly affects adults childhood cases have been reported	Affects adults mainly elderly woman, childhood cases have been reported
Clinical features	Characterized by loose pustular lesions that appear in the body folds and scalp	Characterized by loose pustular lesions that appear in the body folds and scalp	Characterized by loose pustular lesions that appear in the body folds
Histopathology	Pustules primarily in the upper epidermis	Pustule formation throughout the entire epidermis	Accumulation of subcorneal neutrophils
Direct immunofluorescence analysis	Intrapustular or subcorneal IgA accumulation	IgA accumulation throughout the epidermis	Negative

DIF examination is crucial in differantial diagnosis between SPD and IgA pemphigus. Table 77.1 summarizes immunoflurescence and clinical findings of these entities [1, 2, 5, 8].

Practical Points

- Subcorneal pustular dermatosis (SPD), also known as Sneddon-Wilkinson disease, is a rare chronic and recurring flaccid sterile pustular eruption
- SPD is classified within the "neutrophilic dermatoses" and develops mainly in middle-aged women, although the disease has been reported in children as well
- SPD has been associated with benign IgA gammopathy or IgA elevation without gammopathy, monoclonal gammopathy, pyoderma gangrenosum, rheumatoid arthritis, systemic lupus erythematosus, inflammatory bowel diseases, hyperthyroidism, and apudoma
- Systemic or topical steroids are used as monotherapy or in combination with dapsone, are first choice treatments for SPD

References

1. Scalvenzi M, Palmisano F, Annunziata MC, Mezza E, Cozzolino I, Costa C. Subcorneal pustular dermatosis in childhood: a case report and review of the literature. Case Rep Dermatol Med. 2013;2013:424797.
2. Naik HB, Cowen EW. Autoinflammatory pustular neutrophilic diseases. Dermatol Clin. 2013;31(3):405–25.

3. Khachemoune A, Blyumin ML. Sneddon-Wilkinson disease resistant to dapsone and colchicine successfully controlled with PUVA. Dermatol Online J. 2003;9(5):24.
4. Afsar FS, Ortac R, Diniz G. Asitretin tedavisi sonrasinda hafif alevlenmeler ile seyreden bir juvenil subkomeal dermatoz olgusu/A juvenile subcorneal pustular dermatosis case with a course of mild exacerbations after acitretin treatment. Turkish J Dermatol. 2010;4(3):84–8.
5. Ratnarathorn M, Newman J. Subcorneal pustular dermatosis (Sneddon-Wilkinson disease) occurring in association with nodal marginal zone lymphoma: a case report. Dermatol Online J. 2008;14(8):6.
6. Abreu-Velez AM, Smith JG, Howard MS. Subcorneal pustular dermatosis an immnohistopathological perspective. Int J Clin Exp Pathol. 2011;4(5):526–9.
7. Lombart F, Dhaille F, Lok C, Dadban A. Subcorneal pustular dermatosis associated with *Mycoplasma pneumoniae* infection. J Am Acad Dermatol. 2014;71(3):e85–e6.
8. Kasha EE, Epinette WW. Subcorneal pustular dermatosis (Sneddon-Wilkinson disease) in association with a monoclonal IgA gammopathy: a report and review of the literature. J Am Acad Dermatol. 1988;19(5):854–8.
9. Kretschmer L, Maul JT, Hofer T, Navarini AA. Interruption of Sneddon-Wilkinson subcorneal pustulation with infliximab. Case Rep Dermatol. 2017;9(1):140–4.

Chapter 78
Purpuric Macules and Oral Erosions

Dipak Kr. Agarwalla and Piyush Kumar

A 14-year-old girl presented with dusky erythematous macules with purpuric centers all over the body for 5 days (Fig. 78.1a). She also had painful oral erosions and hemorrhagic crusts on lips (Fig. 78.1b), along with conjunctival congestion. The lesions first started over the face followed by trunk and upper limb and progressed to involve the lower limb within 4 days. The lesions gradually increased in size and

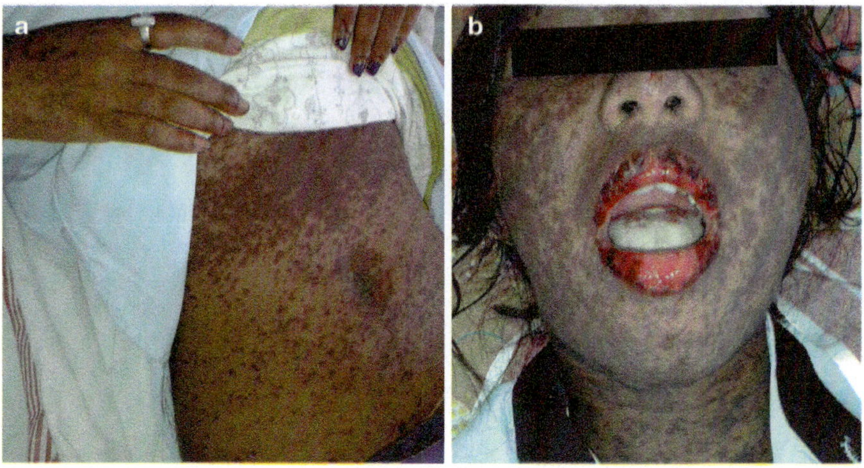

Fig. 78.1 (**a**) Dusky erythematous macules with purpuric centers all over the body and (**b**) painful oral erosions and hemorrhagic crusts on lips

D. K. Agarwalla
Department of Dermatology, Gauhati Medical College and Hospital, Guwahati, Assam, India

P. Kumar (✉)
Department of Dermatology, Katihar Medical College, Katihar, Bihar, India

© Springer Nature Switzerland AG 2020

F. Rahmani, N. Rezaei (eds.), *Pediatric Autoimmunity and Transplantation*,
https://doi.org/10.1007/978-3-030-26280-8_78

coalesced. Soon, vesicles and bullae developed within the lesions, few of which ruptured to leave behind erosions. Nikolsky sign was positive. Her palms and soles were involved with atypical target lesions. There was a history of fever, sore throat and malaise 1–2 days prior to the onset of skin lesions, but no history of similar lesions in the past. The patient was on tablet escitalopram and tablet sodium valproate for the last 6 months, with tablet carbamazepine added since 20 days ago on her recent admission to psychiatry department.

Laboratory data revealed: serum urea: 12 mmol/L, aspartate aminotransferase: 183 IU/L, alanine transaminase: 158 IU/L, alkaline phosphatase: 155 IU/L, CRP: 8.6 mg/dL, ESR: 90 mm/h, serum sodium: 131 mmol/L, and serum potassium: 3.2 mmol/L. HIV ELISA was negative.

Q1. What is the most likely diagnosis?

A. Erythema multiforme major
B. Stevens-Johnson syndrome/toxic epidermal necrolysis
C. Pemphigus vulgaris
D. Staphylococcal scalded skin syndrome

Answer: *The correct answer is* ***B****.*

Stevens-Johnson syndrome (SJS) and toxic epidermal necrolysis (TEN) are rare, potentially life-threatening mucocutaneous adverse reactions, usually appearing in response to drugs. SJS/TEN are characterized by blistering and epithelial sloughing. The terms SJS, TEN and overlap SJS/TEN may be variants of the same spectrum of disease, in which SJS is the less extensive form and TEN is more extensive [1]. Presence of widespread purpuric macules and patches, and atypical target lesions along with erosive and hemorrhagic mucositis of the mouth, eyes, nose and genitalia suggest the clinical diagnosis of SJS/TEN [1].

Erythema multiforme major (EMM) is a close clinical differential. In EMM, the lesions consist of typical targets, predominantly localized on the limbs and extremities while in SJS, the lesions are in atypical target form with a predilection for the torso. EMM occurs commonly following herpes simplex virus reactivation and rarely as a reaction to drugs, in contrast to SJS/TEN [1].

Pemphigus vulgaris is characterized by intraepidermal/suprabasal autoimmune vesicobullous disease with mucocutaneous erosions and positive direct immunofluorescence (DIF) [2].

Staphylococcal scalded skin syndrome (SSSS) is primarily a disease of infants and young children and has a good prognosis. SSSS is characterized by generalized erythema, skin tenderness, superficial blistering, shedding of large areas of epidermis leaving a moist erythematous base, and typical sparing of mucous membrane. Patients are usually not toxic. Performing a frozen section to evaluate the level of split, which is subcorneal in SSSS but subepidermal in TEN, is a quick tool for differentiating between these diseases [3].

Q2. All of the following molecules are key mediators in the pathogenesis of this condition, except:

A. Granulysin
B. Fas ligand
C. Granzyme B
D. Cathepsin G

Answer: *The correct answer is* ***D****.*

SJS/TEN mostly results from complex interactions between the structure of a drug and patient's genetic predisposition including human leukocyte antigen alleles, drug metabolism characteristics, and T cell clonotypes (Fig. 78.2). Widespread keratinocyte necrosis of both skin and mucous membranes is induced by cytotoxic T-lymphocytes (CTLs) [4]. Drug antigens can activate the

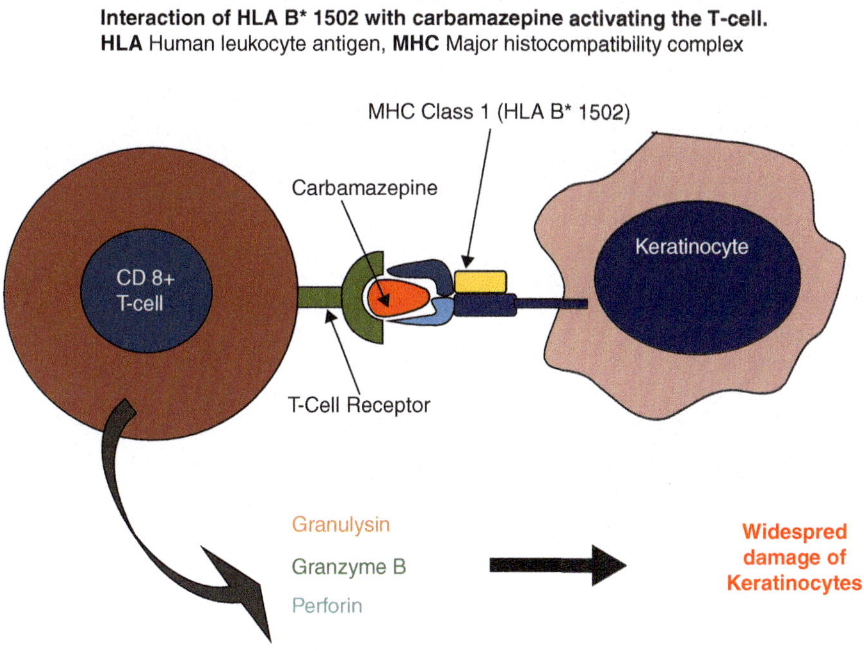

Fig. 78.2 Schematic diagram: Pathogenesis of toxic epidermal necrolysis

immune system by binding to the MHC 1 complex and T cell receptors [5]. Activated lymphocytes may induce keratinocytes apoptosis via an interaction between the fas ligand (FasL), expressed on the surface of lymphocytes and fas antigen on keratinocytes. Pro-apoptotic molecules, including tumor necrosis factor-α, interferon-γ and inducible nitric oxide synthase, may link drug induced immune responses to keratinocyte damage [4, 6]. Soluble fas ligand, perforin and granzyme B have all been implicated in induction of keratinocytes apoptosis [7, 8], however, granulysin is suggested as the key mediator of apoptosis in SJS/TEN [9].

Cathepsin G, a polymorphonuclear leukocyte proteinase plays an important role in eliminating intracellular pathogens as well as in connective tissue remodeling at sites of inflammation and is not involved in the pathogenesis of SJS/TEN [10].

Q3. What is the most probable culprit for SJS/TEN in this patient?

A. Tab escitalopram
B. Tab valproate
C. Tab carbamazepine
D. A viral infection a few days ago

Answer: *The correct answer is* ***C.***

SJS/TEN is primarily a drug-induced phenomenon (in >95% cases), with the culprit drug being demonstrated in approximately 85% of cases [11]. SJS/TEM may rarely be caused by infections as well and Mycoplasma-induced SJS has been reported [12]. A latent period of 7–10 days, ranging from 5 to 28 days, occurs between initiation of the culprit drug and onset of SJS/TEN [11].

Some of the commonest drugs causing SJS/TEN are [13]:

- Allopurinol
- Carbamazepine
- Phenytoin
- Lamotrigine
- Nevirapine
- Oxicam and NSAIDS
- Phenobarbitol
- Sulfamethoxazole and other sulfa antibiotics
- Sulfasalazine
- Aminopenicillins
- Cephalosporins, fluoroquinolones

Q4. Which of the following parameters is associated with poor prognosis in this patient?

A. Age of 14 years
B. Serum urea: 12 mmol/L
C. AST: 183 IU/L
D. CRP: 8.6 mg/dL

Answer: *The correct answer is* ***B.***

SCORTEN is a disease specific severity of illness score developed by Bastuji-Garin et al. to determine the severity of disease and predict mortality. SCORTEN is calculated on the first day of hospitalization and on third day and includes seven independent parameters associated with increased mortality. Presence of each parameter receives a score of one and SCORTEN is calculated by summing up the number of abnormal parameters [14]. The seven parameters included in SCORTEN are [14]:

- Age greater than 40 years
- Presence of malignancy
- Heart rate >120 beats/min
- Epidermal attachment >10% of BSA at admission
- Serum urea >10 mmol/L
- Serum glucose >14 mmol/L
- Bicarbonate level <20 mmol/L

SCORTEN score is a reliable and validated tool to assess severity of disease and predict mortality. For example. SCORTEN score of 1 is associated with 3.9% mortality, while cases with SCORTEN score of 5 or more have around 90% mortality.

The overall SJS/TEN mortality is 22%. Mortality in SJS is less than 10% and in TEN the mortality is estimated to be about 30% [14].

Q5. All of the following could be used in management of this patient, except?

A. Institute supportive care
B. Systemic steroids
C. Intravenous immunoglobulin
D. Tapering the dose of culprit drug

Answer: *The correct answer is* ***D.***

As soon as the diagnosis of SJS/TEN has been made, discontinuation of the culprit drug is an essential and immediate management.

Management of SJS/TEN [15]**:**
General and supportive measures:

- Immediate withdrawal of offending drug.
- Patients with skin loss involving more than 10% BSA need to be admitted in ICU/ burn unit
  - Supportive care including Temperature maintenance at 30–32 °C
  - Frequent monitoring of vital signs
  - Fluid and electrolytes replacement*
  - Nutritional care
  - Antacids, analgesics, anxiolytics and antipyretics
  - Preventing/treating secondary infection
  - Psychological support
- Skin and orifices care with a goal to prevent sepsis and ensure healing

Specific treatment is needed to halt the immunological processes leading to keratinocyte apoptosis. These agents can improve the outcome if given in the early stages of the acute phase. Such disease modifying agents include:

- Systemic steroids (e.g. prednisolone 0.5–1 mg/kg/day for few days, and tapered). They should not be used late in the course of disease or for longer periods as they might increase the risk of sepsis and hence, mortality.
- Cyclosporine (3–5 mg/kg body weight in divided doses for 7–10 days and tapered). Recent evidences favor cyclosporine as preferred agent as results have shown superiority of cyclosporine over other therapies including intravenous immunoglobulin, corticosteroids, cyclophosphamide and supportive care alone.
- Intravenous immunoglobulin (0.5–1 g/kg/day for 3–4 consecutive days)

Oral care: Use of frequent normal saline or antiseptic swishes or mouth washes should be advocated. Saline compresses followed by lubrication helps soften hemorrhagic lip crusts and promotes faster epithelization.

Ophthalmic care: Ophthalmological consultation should be sought. Lubrication and antibiotic eye drops/ointments with or without corticosteroids are needed frequently (every 2 h). Eyelid adhesions should be cautiously removed daily.

Prevention of Recurrences

- Written information about drug(s) and related compounds to be avoided is provided.

∗Fluid replacement: The approximate fluid required during the initial 24 h is calculated using the Parkland's formula: fluid requirement = 4 mL/kg body weight × percentage of body surface area involved determined by the rule of nine. Three-fourths of this amount is required for a patient with TEN. Half the calculated fluid is administered in the first 8 h and the other half in the next 16 h. Ringer lactate is frequently used. For maintenance, the total replacement (i.e., oral and intravenous fluids) should be the urine output + 500 mL, with the urine output being maintained at more than 1000–1500 mL/day.

Practical Points

- Presence of widespread purpuric macules and patches, and atypical target lesions along with erosive and hemorrhagic mucositis of the mouth, eyes, nose and genitalia suggest the clinical diagnosis of Stevens-Johnson syndrome and toxic epidermal necrolysis (SJS/TEN)
- SJS/TEN is primarily a drug-induced phenomenon with the culprit drug being demonstrated in approximately 85% of cases
- A latent period of 7–10 days, ranging from 5 to 28 days, occurs between initiation of the culprit drug and onset of SJS/TEN
- SCORTEN score is a reliable and validated tool to assess severity of disease and predict mortality of SJS/TEN

References

1. Dodiuk-Gad RP, Chung WH, Valeyrie-Allanore L, Shear NH. Stevens-Johnson syndrome and toxic epidermal necrolysis: an update. Am J Clin Dermatol. 2015;16(6):475–93.
2. Kasperkiewicz M, Ellebrecht CT, Takahashi H, Yamagami J, Zillikens D, Payne AS, Amagai M. Pemphigus. Nat Rev Dis Primers. 2017;3:17026.
3. Handler MZ, Schwartz RA. Staphylococcal scalded skin syndrome: diagnosis and management in children and adults. J Eur Acad Dermatol Venereol. 2014;28(11):1418–23.
4. Roujeau JC. Immune mechanisms in drug allergy. Allergol Int. 2006;55(1):27–33.
5. Schwartz RA, McDonough PH, Lee BW. Toxic epidermal necrolysis: Part I. Introduction, history, classification, clinical features, systemic manifestations, etiology, and immunopathogenesis. J Am Acad Dermatol. 2013;69(2):173.e1–13; quiz 85–6
6. Viard-Leveugle I, Gaide O, Jankovic D, Feldmeyer L, Kerl K, Pickard C, Roques S, Friedmann PS, Contassot E, French LE. TNF-alpha and IFN-gamma are potential inducers of Fas-mediated keratinocyte apoptosis through activation of inducible nitric oxide synthase in toxic epidermal necrolysis. J Invest Dermatol. 2013;133(2):489–98.
7. Viard I, Wehrli P, Bullani R, Schneider P, Holler N, Salomon D, Hunziker T, Saurat JH, Tschopp J, French LE. Inhibition of toxic epidermal necrolysis by blockade of CD95 with human intravenous immunoglobulin. Science (New York, NY). 1998;282(5388):490–3.
8. Khalili B, Bahna SL. Pathogenesis and recent therapeutic trends in Stevens-Johnson syndrome and toxic epidermal necrolysis. Ann Allergy Asthma Immunol. 2006;97(3):272–80; quiz 81–3, 320
9. Chung WH, Hung SI, Yang JY, Su SC, Huang SP, Wei CY, Chin SW, Chiou CC, Chu SC, Ho HC, Yang CH, Lu CF, Wu JY, Liao YD, Chen YT. Granulysin is a key mediator for disseminated keratinocyte death in Stevens-Johnson syndrome and toxic epidermal necrolysis. Nat Med. 2008;14(12):1343–50.
10. Burster T, Macmillan H, Hou T, Boehm BO, Mellins ED. Cathepsin G: roles in antigen presentation and beyond. Mol Immunol. 2010;47(4):658–65.
11. Sassolas B, Haddad C, Mockenhaupt M, Dunant A, Liss Y, Bork K, Haustein UF, Vieluf D, Roujeau JC, Le Louet H. ALDEN, an algorithm for assessment of drug causality in Stevens-Johnson syndrome and toxic epidermal necrolysis: comparison with case-control analysis. Clin Pharmacol Ther. 2010;88(1):60–8.
12. Vujic I, Shroff A, Grzelka M, Posch C, Monshi B, Sanlorenzo M, Ortiz-Urda S, Rappersberger K. Mycoplasma pneumoniae-associated mucositis--case report and systematic review of literature. J Eur Acad Dermatol Venereol. 2015;29(3):595–8.
13. Harr T, French LE. Toxic epidermal necrolysis and Stevens-Johnson syndrome. Orphanet J Rare Dis. 2010;5:39.
14. Bastuji-Garin S, Fouchard N, Bertocchi M, Roujeau JC, Revuz J, Wolkenstein P. SCORTEN: a severity-of-illness score for toxic epidermal necrolysis. J Invest Dermatol. 2000;115(2):149–53.
15. Gupta LK, Martin AM, Agarwal N, D'Souza P, Das S, Kumar R, Pande S, Das NK, Kumaresan M, Kumar P, Garg A, Singh S. Guidelines for the management of Stevens-Johnson syndrome/toxic epidermal necrolysis: an Indian perspective. Indian J Dermatol Venereol Leprol. 2016;82(6):603–25.

Chapter 79
Diffuse Skin Rash and Mucosal Lesions

Marzieh Tavakol

A 12-year-old boy was admitted to our hospital with a diffuse erythema and pruritic rash which had started about 5 days before his admission. He had received three doses of outpatient cefazolin due to upper respiratory tract infection in his primary care physician outpatient clinic with fever, rhinorrhea and cough, where he was advised to take bed rest and was prescribed with three doses of intramuscular injection of cefazolin. He developed erythema and itchy skin eruptions 48 h after administration of the last dose of cefazolin and was therefore admitted to another hospital where he received cefotaxim plus metronidazole. His rash expanded rapidly and he started to develop mucosal ulcers, progressive skin exfoliation, gradually leading to abrasions and laceration. He also had nasal congestion, conjunctival injection, as well as meatal ulcer.

He was lethargic and anorexic and was apparently ill a day after mucosal ulcers appeared. Nikolsky sign was positive and his skin was easily removed by rubbing. His lips were covered by thick and bloody crust and ophthalmic mucosal membranes were ulcerated as well (Fig. 79.1). His sclera was icteric but there was no hepatomegaly or liver tenderness on physical examination. None of his lymph nodes were significantly enlarged. There was no abnormal findings in his lung or heart auscultation.

His laboratory findings were as follows: WBC: 5400/μL (PMN: %68, lymph: %28, monocyte: %2, and eosinophil: %2), Hb: 13.1 g/dL, MCV: 78.4 fL, platelet count: 159,000/μL, ESR: 3 mm/h (reference <15), CRP: 3 mg/L (reference: 0–10), BUN: 7 mg/dL, Cr: 0.7 mg/dL, AST: 856 IU/L, ALT: 1025 IU/L, total bilirubin: 4.1 mg/dL with direct portion: 2.6 mg/dL, γ-GT: 386 IU/L (reference <49).

M. Tavakol (✉)
Non-communicable Diseases Research Center, Alborz University of Medical Sciences, Karaj, Iran

Department of Allergy and Clinical Immunology, Shahid Bahonar Hospital, Alborz University of Medical Sciences, Karaj, Iran

© Springer Nature Switzerland AG 2020

F. Rahmani, N. Rezaei (eds.), *Pediatric Autoimmunity and Transplantation*, https://doi.org/10.1007/978-3-030-26280-8_79

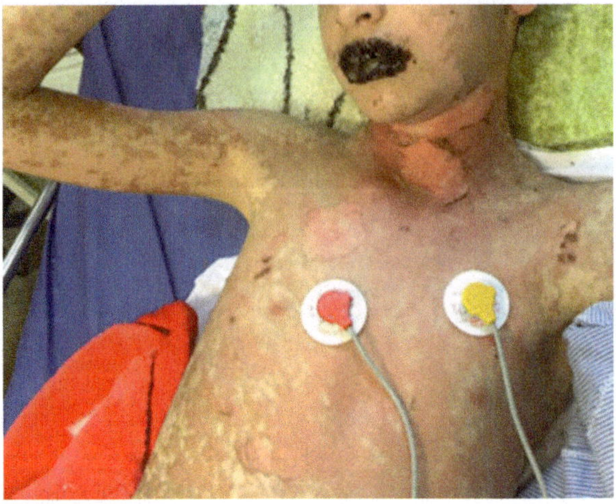

Fig. 79.1 Generalized cutaneous rash and skin detachment in a 12-year-old boy

Q1. What is the most probable diagnosis?

A. Infectious mononucleosis
B. Stevens-Johnson syndrome
C. Drug reaction with eosinophilia and systemic symptoms
D. Serum sickness

Answer: *The correct answer is* ***B.***

Infectious mononucleosis is not an appropriate diagnosis with no spleen enlargement or lymphadenopathy on physical examination and absence of lymphocytosis or atypical lymphocytes in peripheral blood smear [1]. Drug reaction with eosinophilia and systemic symptoms (DRESS) syndrome is diagnosed by different scoring systems which are based on the clinical and paraclinics of the patient. Involvement of internal organs other than skin, high grade fever (≥38 °C), enlargement of the lymph nodes (at least in one zone and as a minimum of 2 cm), characteristic skin rash that starts at least 3 weeks after the drug exposure, lymphocytosis (>11,000/μL and raised atypical lymphocytes above 5%), eosinophilia greater than 10% or absolute blood eosinophil count more than 700/μL, as well as prolonged skin rash more than 2 weeks after the last dose of the culprit drug, are diagnostic for DRESS [2, 3]. The short duration of latent phase between usage of the suspect drug and onset of cutaneous eruptions, as well as rapid progression of the lesions and considerable mucosal involvement makes the diagnosis of DRESS less likely [2]. The presence of fever, rash and malaise in addition to the history of receiving drugs are in agreement with pseudo-serum sickness reaction, nevertheless, absence of arthralgia and mucosal involvement are against this diagnosis [4]. Given the relatively short duration between drug consumption and severe cutaneous reactions with positive Nikolsky sign, added to involvement of more than two mucosal membranes, Stevens-Johnson syndrome is probably the most likely diagnosis [5].

The patient was admitted to the intensive care unit and received supporting treatment including intravenous fluids and topical emollients in addition to IVIG.

Q2. Which of the following cutaneous drug reactions is related to reactivation of human herpesvirus 6 (HHV6)?

A. Stevens-Johnson syndrome/SJS
B. Toxic epidermal necrolysis/TEN
C. Drug reaction with eosinophilia and systemic symptoms/DRESS
D. Acute generalized exanthematous pustulosis/AGEP

Answer: *The correct answer is* ***C.***

Recrudescence of the members of herpesvirus family)HHV6, HHV7, EBV, CMV) and parvovirus B19 is seen commonly in DRESS, while SJS has been reported to be accompanied by *Mycoplasma pneumonia* [6].

Q3. Which statement is correct?

A. SJS/TEN is an immune complex -mediated and partly antibody-mediated hypersensitivity reaction
B. Graded challenge test is the most objective method to confirm the diagnosis of SJS/TEN
C. After confirmation of the culprit drug, rapid desensitization to the drug is the selective therapeutic method
D. HLA haplotype of the patient as well as drug structure are both predisposing factors for SJS/TEN

Answer: *The correct answer is* ***D.***

SJS/TEN belongs to the delayed type hypersensitivity reactions, mediated by cytotoxic T cells and NK cells through the perforin-granzyme pathway. Fas-fasL interaction induces apoptosis of the keratinocytes which is a core finding in SJS pathology. Granulysin derived from cytotoxic $CD8^+$ T and NK cell has been shown to be the most important cytotoxic mediator in SJS/TEN [7].

Q4. Which option is <u>least</u> effective in treatment of SJS/TEN?

A. Intravenous immunoglobulin infusion
B. Discontinuing the culprit drug as soon as possible
C. Starting systemic corticosteroid therapy
D. Supportive care and monitoring of the patient

Answer: *The correct answer is* ***C.***

A crucial, primary step in management of a patient with SJS/TEN is discontinuation of the responsible drug. The patient should be treated as a patient with burn-wound and aggressive fluid and electrolytes balance should be exerted. Special wound care would help re-epithelialization and prevent secondary infection. There is controversy about debridement of the detached skin, while petrolatum saturated gauze is generally recommended to help the skin repair. Application of local antibiotics is not recommended. Special attention should also be given to ophthalmic mucosal ulcers to avoid long-lasting ophthalmic complications. Adjuvant therapy with IVIG, TNF-α antagonists, cyclosporine and plasmapheresis have been recently proposed. As the most frequently used therapy, IVIG is recommended by most guidelines. Nevertheless, the efficacy of IVIG has not been precisely approved by credible evidences especially in adults, and use of IVIG should be balanced by its possible complications. TNF inhibitors such as infliximab have been shown to be beneficial in reducing mortality of patients with SJS/TEN. Cyclosporine has been recently applied in treatment of patients with SJS/TEN with controversial outcomes. Plasmapheresis has been used in isolated cases and has not shown a significant efficacy in improvement of patients with SJS/TEN [7].

Q5. Which statement is correct?

A. Carbamazepine induced SJS/TEN occurs at least 6 month after regular drug consumption
B. HLA typing is recommended in patients who have been using carbamazepine for at least 3 months
C. Carbamazepine prescription is considered completely safe in patients with negative genetic study
D. Carbamazepine induced SJS/TEN is unlikely after the first 3 months of the treatment

Answer: *The correct answer is* ***D.***

Patients taking carbamazepine for the first time are at increased risk to develop SJS/TEN, by an incidence of 1–6 per 10,000 that could increase to up to 1–6 per 1000 in some Asian communities. According to the Food and Drug Administration (FDA), genetic evaluation is generally recommended for all first-time prescribed patients. Considering the fact that SJS/TEN development is most frequent during the first 3 months, patients are unlikely to develop SJS/TEN in response to carbamazepine beyond this period. Similarly, genetic assessment is not recommended in patients who have used the drug for at least 3 months without any sever complications [8].

Practical Points

- Recrudescence of the members of herpesvirus family (HHV6, HHV7, EBV, CMV) and parvovirus B19 is commonly associated with drug reaction with eosinophilia and systemic symptoms (DRESS)
- While Stevens-Johnson syndrome (SJS) has been reported to be accompanied by *Mycoplasma pneumonia*
- A crucial, primary step in management of a patient with SJS is discontinuation of the responsible drug
- Patient with SJS should be treated as a patient with burn-wound and aggressive fluid and electrolytes balance should be exerted
- Special wound care and ophthalmologic care is recommended, but not application of local antibiotics

References

1. Welch JL, Holland D. What elements suggest infectious mononucleosis? Ann Emerg Med. 2018;71(4):521–2.
2. Cho Y-T, Yang C-W, Chu C-Y. Drug reaction with eosinophilia and systemic symptoms (DRESS): an interplay among drugs, viruses, and immune system. Int J Mol Sci. 2017;18(6):1243.
3. Choudhary S, McLeod M, Torchia D, Romanelli P. Drug reaction with eosinophilia and systemic symptoms (DRESS) syndrome. J Clin Aesthet Dermatol. 2013;6(6):31–7.
4. Karmacharya P, Poudel DR, Pathak R, Donato AA, Ghimire S, Giri S, Aryal MR, Bingham CO. Rituximab-induced serum sickness: a systematic review. In: Seminars in arthritis and rheumatism, vol. 3. Philadelphia: Elsevier; 2015. p. 334–40.
5. Verma R, Vasudevan B, Pragasam V. Severe cutaneous adverse drug reactions. Med J Armed Forces India. 2013;69(4):375–83.
6. Duong TA, Valeyrie-Allanore L, Wolkenstein P, Chosidow O. Severe cutaneous adverse reactions to drugs. Lancet. 2017;390(10106):1996–2011.
7. Schneider JA, Cohen PR. Stevens-Johnson syndrome and toxic epidermal necrolysis: a concise review with a comprehensive summary of therapeutic interventions emphasizing supportive measures. Adv Ther. 2017;34(6):1235–44.
8. Dean L. Carbamazepine therapy and HLA genotypes. In: Medical genetics summaries. Bethesda: National Center for Biotechnology Information; 2015.

Chapter 80
Painful Facial Ulceration

Dario Didona and Biagio Didona

A 6-year-old girl presented to our department with a 10-month history of painful ulceration on the right cheek (Fig. 80.1). A well-circumscribed ulcer with a necrotic floor and undermined, dusky purple edge was observed. There was no evidence of other mucosal lesions. The lesion started as an erythematous pustule at the site of minor trauma and rapidly progressed to become a large ulcer with a deep erythematous border over 3 weeks. The girl was also irritable and febrile and her parents complained about reduced oral intake. Her past medical history was positive for

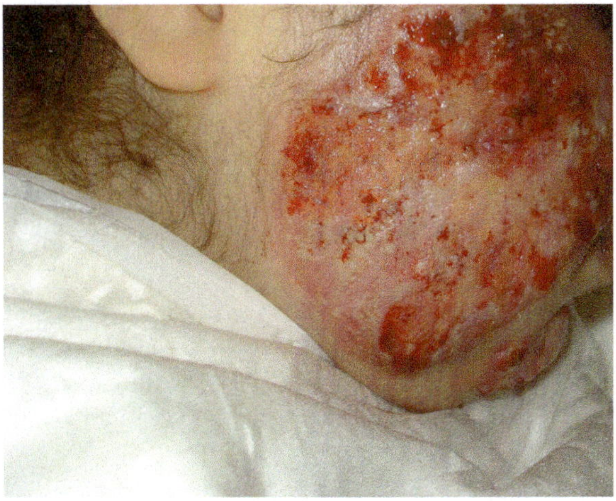

Fig. 80.1 Painful ulceration on the cheek with undermined, dusky purple edge in a 6-years-old girl

D. Didona (✉)
Department of Dermatology and Allergology, Philipps University, Marburg, Germany

B. Didona
First Division of Dermatology, Istituto Dermopatico dell'Immacolata-IRCCS, Rome, Italy

© Springer Nature Switzerland AG 2020

F. Rahmani, N. Rezaei (eds.), *Pediatric Autoimmunity and Transplantation*,
https://doi.org/10.1007/978-3-030-26280-8_80

bacterial pneumonia, but negative for autoimmune skin diseases and skin infections. Parents denied any new exposures to drugs. Her family history was negative for autoimmune or inherited diseases.

Q1. What is the most likely diagnosis?

A. Drug reaction
B. Vasculitis
C. Pyoderma gangrenosum
D. Cutaneous *Leishmaniosis*

Answer: *The correct answer is* ***C.***

According to the clinical features, the most likely diagnosis is pyoderma gangrenosum (PG). PG is member of primarily sterile inflammatory neutrophilic dermatosis, a group of rare diseases that include also Sweet's syndrome, neutrophilic eccrine hidradenitis, erythema elevatum diutinum, Behcet's disease, and bowel bypass syndrome [1]. At the beginning, PG is clinically characterized by painful, erythematous pustules, bullae, or nodules that enlarge concentrically. The lesions usually develop at sites of incidental or surgical superficial trauma, due to a phenomenon called pathergy, which may occur in up to 20% of cases [1]. Pathergy phenomenon is more frequent in pediatric than in adults. PG could occur in association with hematologic, rheumatologic, or gastrointestinal diseases, yet most PG cases are spontaneous. Indeed, it has been speculated that PG may be a systemic disorder [1, 2]. Lesions in PG may evolve into necrotic plaques with raised edges or into violaceous deep ulcers with undermined dusky purple borders, healing with atrophic or cribriform scars [1]. Several clinical subtypes have been described, including ulcerative, pustular, bullous, and vegetating lesions [1, 2]. Visceral involvement is also possible. Pediatric patients account for only 4% of all PG cases and involve more often the head and perineal area [1]. Several differential diagnoses should be taken into the account, including vascular occlusive disease, thrombophilic conditions, vasculitis, malignancies, infections, exogenous tissue injury, insect bites, and pustular drug reactions [1].

Q2. What is the best initial step in the diagnosis of this patient? (ANA: antinuclear antibody; ENA: extractable nuclear antigen)

A. Punch biopsy
B. Serum ANA and ENA
C. MRI or CT scan
D. Antibody screening

Answer: *The correct answer is* ***A.***

Although some clinicians have concerns about performing biopsies in children with PG because of the risk of inducing new lesions, skin punch biopsy is recommended to rule out other differential diagnoses [1, 2]. More specifically, a punch biopsy from the edge of the ulcer could help rule out vasculitis, whereas a punch biopsy from the ulcer itself could be useful to rule out an infection by submitting the specimen for culture. Pathologically, pustular PG is characterized by a dense neutrophilic infiltrate extending to the base of the lesion without vasculitis. PG ulceration on the other hand shows necrosis of epidermis and dermis down to subcutaneous fat, a mixed inflammatory cell infiltrate composed of neutrophils, lymphocytes, and prominent reactive histiocytes extending from the papillary and reticular dermis down to the subcutis [1, 2].

Q3. What is the chief underlying mechanisms of PG?

A. Neutrophil dysfunction
B. Humoral autoimmunity
C. Cellular autoimmunity
D. Monogenic disorders with infectious trigger

Answer: *The correct answer is* ***A.***

Although PG pathogenesis is not fully understood, neutrophil dysfunction has been suggested as main cause of PG. Abnormal neutrophil trafficking and metabolic oscillations have been described to be responsible in the pathogenesis of PG [3]. Furthermore, IL-8, a potent chemotactic agent, has been shown to be overexpressed in PG [3]. Additionally, in the "pyogenic sterile arthritis, PG and acne" (PAPA) syndrome an overproduction of IL-16, which is chemotactic to neutrophils, has been reported [3]. PG is probably multifactorial, including genetic predisposition, and inflammatory phenomena.

Q4. What is the best therapeutic approach?

A. Systemic glucocorticoids as monotherapy
B. Cyclosporine as monotherapy
C. Systemic glucocorticoids and topical corticosteroids
D. Treat the underlying condition and use topical corticosteroids

Answer: *The correct answer is* ***C.***

Treatment of PG in pediatric population is challenging. Local treatment of skin lesions is based on wound care and avoidance of trauma [1, 2]. Swabs for bacterial and fungal cultures should be taken from active lesions to prevent infections [1, 2]. Regular cleansing of ulcers with saline solution, application of nonirritant antibacterial cream, and covering with a non-adhesive dressing are indicated. Topical or intralesional glucocorticoids, and tacrolimus have been reported as effective in the literature [1, 2].

Systemic therapy is usually required to control the disease in this age group. Oral glucocorticoids are the first choice, although intravenous glucocorticoids are also used [1, 2]. Several other medications have been trialed in the literature, including dapsone, colchicine, cyclosporine, and azathioprine [4].

Q5. Which of the following conditions is most likely associated with PG?

A. Hematopoietic malignancies
B. Inflammatory bowel disease

C. Ankylosing spondylitis
D. Type 1 diabetes mellitus

Answer: *The correct answer is* ***B.***

Once the diagnosis of PG is confirmed, the search for an underlying disease should be undertaken. Pediatric PG could be the first presentation of a systemic disease, most frequently underlying inflammatory bowel disease (IBD), which is usually associated with ulcerative PG [4]. In order to perform adequate evaluation of gastrointestinal symptoms endoscopic evaluation should be performed if justified, by the clinician. The second most common group of underlying disorders are hematological diseases such as myelodysplastic syndrome, leukemia, and lymphoma [4]. In these cases, hepatosplenomegaly and palpable lymph nodes on physical exam can give the first clues for a through hematological workup.

Practical Points

- Pediatric pyoderma gangrenosum accounts for 4% of all cases
- A punch biopsy should be performed to rule out other skin diseases
- Systemic steroids and local wound care represent the first line approach

References

1. Kechichian E, Haber R, Mourad N, Khoury RE, Jabbour S, Tomb R. Pediatric pyoderma gangrenosum: a systematic review and update. Int J Dermatol. 2017;56:486–95.
2. McAlee M, Powell F, Devaney D, O'Donnell B. Infantile pyoderma gangrenosum. J Am Acad Dermatol. 2008;58(2 Suppl):S23–8.
3. Ruocco E, Sangiuliano S, Gravina A, Miranda A, Nicoletti G. Pyoderma gangrenosum: an updated review. J Eur Acad Dermatol Venereol. 2009;23:1008–17.
4. Schoch J, Tolkachjov S, Cappel J, Gibson L, Davis D. Pediatric pyoderma gangrenosum: a retrospective review of clinical features, etiologic associations, and treatment. Pediatr Dermatol. 2017;34:39–45.

Chapter 81
Patchy Hair Loss

Anupam Das and Piyush Kumar

A 10-year-old boy, presented with hair loss of 1 year duration. It started as a small patch of hair loss appearing all of a sudden 1 year back and progressed to the present status (Fig. 81.1). There was no prior history of drugs intake, trauma or pustules/nodules. Cutaneous examination showed a diffuse non-scarring alopecia affecting the frontal area and vertex, progressing along the hairline in parietal and occipital regions (Fig. 81.1). The overlying skin was smooth and shiny and there were no

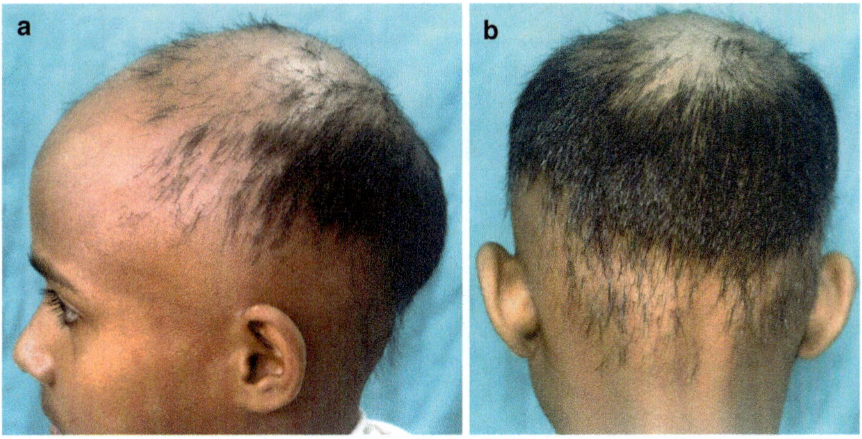

Fig. 81.1 Hair loss on vertex and along hairline, in parietal (**a**) and occipital area (**b**)

A. Das
Department of Dermatology, KPC Medical College, Kolkata, India

P. Kumar (✉)
Department of Dermatology, Katihar Medical College, Katihar, Bihar, India

© Springer Nature Switzerland AG 2020

F. Rahmani, N. Rezaei (eds.), *Pediatric Autoimmunity and Transplantation*,
https://doi.org/10.1007/978-3-030-26280-8_81

similar looking lesions elsewhere in the body. Nails showed geometric pitting. KOH examination did not reveal any fungal hyphae.

Routine investigations and thyroid profile were within normal limits. Histopathological examination of a biopsy specimen taken from the bald patch revealed a peribulbar lymphocytic infiltrate, similar to a swarm of bees.

Q1. What is the best initial diagnosis?

A. Tinea capitis
B. Trichotillomania
C. Alopecia areata
D. Pseudopelade of Brocq

Answer: *The correct answer is* ***C.***

Alopecia areata (AA) manifests as well-demarcated patches of non-scarring alopecia. AA is usually noticed suddenly and may present as single or multiple patches. Scalp is the most common site, while nail changes can be more varied including; geometric pitting, i.e. multiple, small, superficial pits regularly distributed along transverse and longitudinal lines, geometric punctate leukonychia, i.e. multiple white spots in a grill pattern, and trachyonychia, i.e. sandpaper nails. AA may be associated with atopy, autoimmune thyroiditis, vitiligo, psoriasis, diabetes mellitus, Down's syndrome, Addison's disease, autosomal recessive autoimmune polyglandular syndrome, systemic lupus erythematosus, celiac disease, ulcerative colitis, and multiple sclerosis, etc. [1].

Alopecia areata is considered an autoimmune disease, and hair follicle-specific antibodies have been found in peripheral blood of AA patients [2]. Clinical presentation of AA is a myriad which has been classified:

- Based on extent of involvement [1]:
  - Patchy alopecia: one or multiple patches of AA
  - Alopecia totalis: involvement of complete scalp
  - Alopecia universalis: loss of complete body hairs, including scalp, eyebrows, eyelashes, axillary and pubic hair
- Based on pattern of involvement [2]:
  - Reticular: hair loss resembling a net
  - Ophiasis: hair loss along the posterior occipital and temporal margins
  - Sisaipho/Ophiasis inversus: hair loss involving the frontal, temporal, and parietal scalp but spares hair along the scalp periphery and hairline.
  - Diffuse: newly described form characterized by generalized thinning of hair. It can be diagnosed by dermoscopy and histopathology.
  - Linear

Common clinical differentials for patchy AA include tinea capitis, trichotillomania and pseudopelade of Brocq. Tinea capitis is characterized by erythema, scaling, crusting and easy pluckability of hair. Trichotillomania is characterized by loss of hair from accessible areas of scalp, and the hallmark finding is the presence of multiple broken hairs at different lengths. Pseudopelade on the other hand, is manifested as hyperpigmented atrophic patches of hair loss [1, 2].

Q2. Which of the following options is a possible dermoscopic finding in alopecia areata?

A. Yellow and black dots
B. Broken and tapering hairs
C. Short villus hairs
D. All of the above

Answer: *The correct answer is* ***D.***

Dermoscopy is an easy and handy technique of diagnosis of alopecia (including alopecia areata) and obviates the need for biopsy in many cases. Characteristic features of AA in dermoscopy include yellow dots, black dots, broken hairs, tapering hair (i.e. exclamation marks) and short vellus hairs. Presence of black dots, broken hair, and tapering hair suggest an underlying activity. The number of black dots and yellow dots are directly proportional to the severity of disease. A single feature may not be pathognomonic, but a constellation of findings leads to the corroborative diagnosis. Presence of exclamatory mark hairs at periphery, positive hair pull test (>6 hairs), daily hair loss count (>100 hairs), predominance of telogen hairs in pluck test and black dots, broken hair, and tapering hair in dermoscopy, suggest active disease [3, 4].

Q3. Which of the following is <u>not</u> a poor prognostic marker of alopecia areata?

A. Younger age of onset in the patient
B. Alopecia involving the temporal and occipital areas and vertex and leaving the ophiasis regions intact
C. Presence of atopy
D. Presence of nail changes

Answer: *The correct answer is* ***B.***

Poor prognostic factors of alopecia areata has been identified and includes [5, 6]:

- Younger age of onset
- Family history of disease
- Presence of atopy
- Alopecia totalis and alopecia universalis
- Ophiasis pattern
- Duration more than 1 year
- Presence of nail changes
- Associated autoimmune diseases

Q4. All of the following statements are correct regarding the histopathology of alopecia areata, except:

A. Horizontally-sectioned scalp biopsy is helpful in confirming the diagnosis
B. Best place to take a biopsy is at the advancing border of hair loss
C. Mean count of less than one follicle in mm^2 indicates a lower chance of regrowth
D. Terminal to vellus hair ratio is reduced to 7:1

Answer: *The correct answer is* ***C.***

Diagnosis is always made on clinical grounds. Biopsy is seldom required but is helpful when clinical diagnosis is uncertain.

Horizontal sections are usually preferred to vertical sections because they allow examination of multiple hair follicles in a single frame. Best place to take a biopsy is at the advancing border of hair loss. This helps to quantify the hair follicle density, follicle diameter, and assess the proportion of hair follicles in various stages. A mean count of less than one follicle/mm^2 usually indicates lower chances of regrowth. Characteristic feature of an acute case is peribulbar lymphocytic infiltrate akin to a swarm of bees. In chronic cases, follicular miniaturization with variable inflammatory infiltrate are observed in the upper dermis. The terminal to vellus hair ratio is decreased to 1:1 in contrast to 7:1 in normal population [7, 8].

Q5. Which of the following options is used in the management of alopecia areata?

A. Topical steroids
B. Immunotherapy
C. Phototherapy
D. All of the above

Answer: *The correct answer is* ***D.***

Therapeutic options available are topical agents including; corticosteroids, anthralin, minoxidil, immunotherapy, phototherapy, prostaglandin analogues; systemic therapy including; steroids, sulfasalazine, PUVA and others like cyclosporine, methotrexate, capsaicin, topical bexarotene, calcineurin inhibitors, and narrow band UVB etc. [5, 9, 10].

The treatment of choice depends on the extent of disease, co-morbidities and lifestyle of patient, previous treatment history etc. The treatment plan include:

- For patchy alopecia areata:
  - Topical corticosteroids (Class I-III) and intralesional triamcinolone (2.5–5 mg/ml)
  - Topical retinoids
  - Topical anthralins—short contact therapy
  - Phototherapy and photochemotherapy (PUVA)
  - Immunotherapy with diphenylcyclopropenone (DPCP)

  - Topical minoxidil
  - 308-nm Excimer laser

- For alopecia totalis or universalis, or extensive disease recalcitrant to topical therapy;
  - Oral corticosteroids (pulse therapy)
  - Other immunosuppressive agents such as methotrexate, azathioprine, and cyclosporine
  - Wigs and other hair camouflage

Recently, Topical Janus kinase inhibitor, tofacitinib and ruxolitinib, have been used successively to treat pediatric alopecia areata [11].

Practical Points

- Alopecia areata (AA) manifests as well-demarcated patches of non-scarring alopecia. AA is usually noticed suddenly
- Nail changes are common and include geometric pitting, punctate leukonychia, and trachyonychia, i.e. sandpaper nails
- AA may be associated with atopy, autoimmune thyroiditis, vitiligo, psoriasis, diabetes mellitus, autosomal recessive autoimmune polyglandular syndrome, among other autoimmune conditions
- Dermoscopy is an easy and handy technique of diagnosis of alopecia
- Characteristic features of AA in dermoscopy include yellow dots, black dots, broken hairs, tapering hair and short vellus hairs
- Presence of exclamatory mark hairs at periphery, positive hair pull test (>6 hairs), daily hair loss count (>100 hairs), predominance of telogen hairs in pluck test and black dots, broken hair, and tapering hair in dermoscopy, suggest active disease

References

1. Seetharam K. Alopecia areata: an update. Indian J Dermatol Venereol Leprol. 2013;79:563–75.
2. Strazzulla L, Wang E, Avila L, Sicco KL, Brinster N, Christiano A, Shapiro J. Alopecia areata: disease characteristics, clinical evaluation, and new perspectives on pathogenesis. J Am Acad Dermatol. 2018;78(1):1–12.
3. Tosti A, Whiting D, Iorizzo M, Pazzaglia M, Misciali C, Vincenzi C, Micali G. The role of scalp dermoscopy in the diagnosis of alopecia areata incognita. J Am Acad Dermatol. 2008;59(1):64–7.
4. Inui S, Nakajima T, Nakagawa K, Itami S. Clinical significance of dermoscopy in alopecia areata: analysis of 300 cases. Int J Dermatol. 2008;47(7):688–93.
5. Alkhalifah A, Alsantali A, Wang E, McElwee KJ, Shapiro J. Alopecia areata update: part I. Clinical picture, histopathology, and pathogenesis. J Am Acad Dermatol. 2010;62(2):177–88. quiz 89–90
6. McDonald KA, Shelley AJ, Colantonio S, Beecker J. Hair pull test: evidence-based update and revision of guidelines. J Am Acad Dermatol. 2017;76(3):472–7.

7. Chaitra V, Rajalakshmi T, Kavdia R. Histopathologic profile of alopecia areata in Indian patients. Int J Trichol. 2010;2(1):14–7.
8. Dy LC, Whiting DA. Histopathology of alopecia areata, acute and chronic: why is it important to the clinician? Dermatol Ther. 2011;24(3):369–74.
9. Hordinsky MK. Treatment of alopecia areata: "what is new on the horizon?". Dermatol Ther. 2011;24(3):364–8.
10. Peloquin L, Castelo-Soccio L. Alopecia areata: an update on treatment options for children. Paediatr Drugs. 2017;19(5):411–22.
11. Bayart C, DeNiro K, Brichta L, Craiglow B, Sidbury R. Topical Janus kinase inhibitors for the treatment of pediatric alopecia areata. J Am Acad Dermatol. 2017;77(1):167–70.

Chapter 82
Concerning Weight Loss Over Three Weeks

Farzaneh Rahmani and Nima Rezaei

A 3.5-year-old boy was brought to the clinic due to her mother's concern of his abrupt weight loss over a course of 3 weeks. They boy was apparently healthy and normally thriving, and had no history of recent infections or chronic illnesses. His mother said that his mouth was dry all the time and that she had to put on him a diaper as he became incontinent with his urine twice in the past week. She explained that he was fully toilet trained almost 2 months ago.

Q1. What is the best initial workup is this patient?

A. Order CBC, fasting blood glucose and urine analysis
B. Order CBC, peripheral blood smear and ESR
C. Order CBC and refer to a dietician
D. Order urine analysis and sport urine glucose

Answer: *The correct answer is* ***A***.

Recent onset of enuresis in a previously toilet-trained child and abrupt weight loss over 2–6 weeks, should prompt investigation for clinical and laboratory signs of

F. Rahmani
Student's Scientific Research Center (SSRC), Tehran University of Medical Sciences, Tehran, Iran

NeuroImaging Network (NIN), Universal Scientific Education and Research Network (USERN), Tehran, Iran

N. Rezaei (✉)
Department of Immunology, School of Medicine, Research Center for Immunodeficiencies (RCID), Children's Medical Center, Tehran University of Medical Sciences (TUMS), Tehran, Iran

Network of Immunity in Infection, Malignancy and Autoimmunity (NIIMA), Universal Scientific Education and Research Network (USERN), Tehran, Iran
e-mail: rezaei_nima@tums.ac.ir

© Springer Nature Switzerland AG 2020

F. Rahmani, N. Rezaei (eds.), *Pediatric Autoimmunity and Transplantation*,
https://doi.org/10.1007/978-3-030-26280-8_82

diabetes. This patient presented with both non-emergent and emergent presentations of diabetes. Up to 80% of children with diabetes have type 1 diabetes mellitus (T1DM) and more than half of children and adolescents with type 1 diabetes are diagnosed during their first diabetic ketoacidosis (DKA) attack. It is therefore of utmost importance to identify evidence of DKA in patients with high degree of suspicion. These evidence could range from moderate dehydration and repeated vomiting to acetone-smelling breath and tachypnea, altered mentation, hypotension and shock in severe cases. Older children might be able to express abdominal pain or thirst, while younger children might only appear dehydrated, agitated or confused. Among other clinical clue to underlying diabetes is vaginal candidiasis is a prepubertal girl, abrupt weight loss or failure of weight gain over a short period of time and recurrent skin infections [1].

The initial work up should be directed towards early diagnosis of T1DM, while investigating other differential diagnoses including urinary tract infections, gastroenteritis, meningitis, etc. Even the slightest suspicion for DKA should prompt measurement of spot blood glucose and urine ketones with a test tape and immediate treatment. Initial work-up returns with no evidence of urinary tract infection, low positive urine ketone levels, and high fasting blood glucose (>140 g/dL) in this patient.

Q2. Complementary work-up was ordered, including glucose tolerance test, as well as serum C-peptide and insulin levels. All of the following statements are correct, except:

A. Obesity is a good indicator of insulin resistance and type 2 DM in children with a probable diagnosis of DM
B. Persistent low levels of C-peptide in a patient with T2DM features should draw attention to T1DM associated with insulin resistance or obesity
C. Patients with maturity onset diabetes of the young are often misdiagnosed as T1DM or T2DM
D. Screening for DM-associated complications should commence right after the diagnosis of T2DM in children
E. Autoantibody screening against glutamic-acid-decarboxylase, IA2, and zinc transporter 8 has the highest diagnostic accuracy for T1DM in pediatric population

***Answer**: The correct answer is **A**.*

Although nearly all children with type 2 DM are obese, something up to 25% of children with T1DM are also overweight or obese. There is also a reported increase in the number of patients with signs of insulin resistance (T2DM) and positive T1DM autoantibodies. These patients are variable in BMI and clinical manifestations and mandate a full autoantibody workup to complete the diagnosis. Low C-peptide levels in a drug naïve patient with insulin resistance might indicate β-cell glucose toxicity. C-peptide levels tend to resolve with insulin therapy in this group of patients with T1DM [1]. Maturity onset diabetes of the young (MODY) is an important differential diagnosis of type 1 and type 2 DM in pediatric population. Multigenerational onset of DM under 25 years of age should prompt genetic investigation for MODY. Patients with MODY are optimally managed with oral sulfonylureas [1]. Importantly, early onset and rapid progression of microvascular and macrovascular complications of T2DM mandates surveillance for these complications at the time of diagnosis. In contrast, children with T1DM can delay these screening for 3–5 years into the onset of the disease or through adolescence.

Q3. All of the following statements regarding T1DM are correct, except:

A. Celiac disease screening is mandatory in all patients with T1DM at diagnosis, to be repeated at 2–5 years after the diagnosis
B. Unpredictable and brittle blood glucose control with recurrent episodes of hypoglycaemia and growth failure necessitate screening for celiac disease in patients with T1DM
C. Prevalence of celiac disease in T1DM ranges between 20–40% worldwide
D. A higher prevalence of T1DM is seen in patients with Graves' disease orbitopathy

Answer: *The correct answer is* ***C***.

Current guidelines suggest screening for celiac disease at the time T1DM is diagnosed in children, when there is clinical evidence for co-existing celiac disease or poor glycemic control [2]. The screening should typically repeat after 2–5 years, as most cases are diagnosed within this time period. Prevalence of celiac varies from 1.6% to 16.4% in T1DM patients worldwide [2]. Recurrent hypoglycemic episodes in a patient with T1DM might also point to the presence of hypothyroidism [3]. No clinical guideline is yet established to screen for autoimmune thyroid diseases in patients with DM.

Practical Points

- Recent onset of enuresis in a previously toilet-trained child should prompt investigation for diabetes mellitus
- Screening for celiac disease is indicated at the time of the type 1 diabetes mellitus diagnosis in children
- Screening for autoantibodies like against glutamic-acid-decarboxylase, IA2, and zinc transporter 8, does not help differentiate type 1 from type 2 diabetes mellitus in pediatric population

References

1. Amed S, Pozzilli P. Diagnosis of diabetes type in children and young people: challenges and recommendations. Lancet Diabetes Endocrinol. 2016;4(5):385–6.
2. Pham-Short A, Donaghue KC, Ambler G, Phelan H, Twigg S, Craig ME. Screening for celiac disease in Type 1 diabetes: a systematic review. Pediatrics. 2015;136(1):e170–6.
3. Hage M, Zantout MS, Azar ST. Thyroid disorders and diabetes mellitus. J Thyroid Res. 2011;2011:439463.

Chapter 83
Toddler with Bruising on Knees

Farzaneh Rahmani and Nima Rezaei

Mother of a 9-month-old infant brought her daughter to the pediatric general clinic as she noticed appearance of irregularly distributed areas of pin-point bruises on her both knee caps. The girl was a result of an uneventful pregnancy and had reached her developmental milestones on time, with no significant past medical history. The mother remembered an episode of cold 2 weeks prior to the appearance of bruising. Physical examination disclosed nothing, but a healthy baby, with no fever, palor, signs of infection, bleeding or bruises at other sites, or organomegaly. The girl was not taking any medications and the family history was negative for coagulation defects. A complete blood count was ordered, which returned with WBC: 9600/μL, Hb: 11.5, and platelets: 18,000/μL.

Q1. What test(s) would you initially order to confirm the most probable diagnosis?

A. Bone marrow aspiration, HIV, HCV serology, thyroid function tests
B. Direct coombs test, PT, PTT, INR

F. Rahmani (✉)
Student's Scientific Research Center (SSRC), Tehran University of Medical Sciences, Tehran, Iran

NeuroImaging Network (NIN), Universal Scientific Education and Research Network (USERN), Tehran, Iran
e-mail: f-rahmani@alumnus.tums.ac.ir

N. Rezaei
Department of Immunology, School of Medicine, Research Center for Immunodeficiencies (RCID), Children's Medical Center, Tehran University of Medical Sciences (TUMS), Tehran, Iran

Network of Immunity in Infection, Malignancy and Autoimmunity (NIIMA), Universal Scientific Education and Research Network (USERN), Tehran, Iran

© Springer Nature Switzerland AG 2020
F. Rahmani, N. Rezaei (eds.), *Pediatric Autoimmunity and Transplantation*,
https://doi.org/10.1007/978-3-030-26280-8_83

C. Peripheral blood smear
D. Bone marrow biopsy and PT/INR

Answer: *The correct answer is* ***C.***

The case described here is a typical presentation of the idiopathic/immune thrombocytopenic purpura (ITP). The term purpura can be misleading as patients might present with low platelet counts on routine laboratory investigation, typically below 100,000/μL, and not always as a result of appearance of petechiae or purpura. Meanwhile, purpura is almost always the presenting syndrome in cases not spontaneously discovered. Immune-mediated antibody production is by far the most commonly accepted mechanism underlying ITP. ITP is most common in children between 1 and 7 years of age and is usually preceded by a common cold or recent immunization with mumps, measles and rubella (MMR) vaccine, by up to several weeks and in up to two thirds of children [1].

The diagnosis of ITP is one of exclusion. CBC should reveal no evidence of anemia or leukopenia, no lymphadenopathy or organomegaly should be found in physical examination, and peripheral blood smear (PBS) should indicate no abnormal cells. Basic coagulation profile with prorthrombin time (PT), international normalized ratio (INR), and partial thromboplastin time (PTT) should also be ordered only if there is a possibility of inherited bleeding disorders or if the child is ill and febrile and there is a possibility of acute meningococcal infection [2].

The PBS of this girl returned normal except for low platelet count, with no platelet aggregation or abnormal cells.

Q2. Which type of hypersensitivity is a culprit in the pathogenesis of this disorder?

A. Type I
B. Type II
C. Type III
D. Type IV

Answer: *The correct answer is* ***B.***

Immune thrombocytopenic purpura (ITP) is a good example of type II hypersensitivity reaction.

Q3. Imagine there was something wrong in the results of the initial workup. What option does <u>not</u> correctly link the symptoms/finding with the proper diagnostic strategy?

A. Bone pain → perform bone marrow aspiration
B. Recent MMR vaccination → check anti-platelet antibody level
C. Anemia → perform bone marrow aspiration
D. Chronic, recalcitrant ITP → check antinuclear antibodies (ANA)
E. Microthrombocytopenia → check immunoglobulin levels and lymphocyte subset enumeration

Answer: *The correct answer is* ***B.***

One important differential diagnosis of ITP is acute leukemia. Presence of bone pain, anemia, hepatosplenomegaly or hyperleukocytosis should prompt through investigation of the patient with bone marrow aspiration and/or biopsy. ITP can also be associated with HIV infection, systemic lupus erythematosus or anti-phospholipid syndrome, specially in older children. Moreover, chronic ITP, i.e. one that persists over 6 months despite adequate initial therapy, is an important clinical clue to investigate for systemic lupus or anti-phospholipid syndrome. Microthrombocytopenia, along with immunodeficiency and eczema, point to the diagnosis of Wiskott-Aldrich syndrome, while skeletal abnormalities and anemia should raise suspicion for inherited bone marrow failure syndromes such as Fanconi.

Enough evidence is collected to diagnose the girl with ITP. You are now thinking about therapeutic options on table.

Q4. Which statement is correct?

A. Children with severe gastrointestinal bleeds, mucous membrane bleeding, or severe epistaxis comprise about 10% of all children with ITP and should receive therapy
B. Intracranial haemorrhage is uncommon in ITP but prompts immediate high dose corticosteroids and intrvenous immunoglobulin (IVIG) therapy
C. A clinical response to IVIG is usually seen by 7 days in 85% of children
D. Standard initial corticosteroid dose is given as prednisolone 1–2 mg/kg/day for up to 2 weeks, followed by 1 week of tapering
E. IVIG is a desired choice when there is need to rise platelet counts rapidly with a dose of 0.8–1 gm/kg/day

Answer: *The correct answer is* **A.**

A key question to be answered is to whether treat ITP in patients who present only with mild petechiae or bruising, or not. Severe bleeding from the GI tract or other mucosal surfaces, a platelet count below 10,000, intracranial haemorrhage, or a fall in hemoglobin more than 2 g/dL which indicate sever ITP, are seen in less than 5% of patients at initial presentation. Presence of these symptoms/signs is an absolute indication to start treatment. ITP typically resolves within 6 months of the onset of symptoms even without any treatment. This is the exact time course that takes to be able to mark a patient receiving proper treatment as having chronic ITP. IVIG and prednisolone collectively resolve symptoms and improve platelet counts within a week in about 75%–80% of patients. The remaining 20–25% are considered to receive higher doses of IVIG, which is also associated with higher rate of side effects such as headache, vomiting and aseptic meningitis.

The girl was discharged after receiving 20 g of IVIG over 2 days and a short, 5-day course of prednisolone, with platelet count of 120,000/μL and no ecchymosis or bleeding. A control CBC, 2 weeks after discharge revealed relapse of thrombocytopenia (platelet count: 41,000/μL). You admit the girl to start a more prolonged course of IVIG and the mother is worried whether she would ever be able to live a normal life without needing methylprednisolone or IVIG.

Q5. Which statement is correct?

A. Bone marrow aspiration is indicated in all patients with persistent ITP
B. Rituximab is a generally safe alternative for high dose corticosteroids in refractory ITP
C. The next dose of MMR vaccine should not be given to the patient due to risk of recurrence
D. She would be eligible for splenectomy if she remains unresponsive within the next 12 months

Answer*: The correct answer is* ***C****.*

Bone marrow aspiration is indicated only in case of persistent ITP, with no prior remission. Persistent ITP is defined as patients not reaching complete remission after 3–12 months of the diagnosis, which is further defined as platelet counts higher than 100,000/μL over two consecutive measures 1 day apart and off drugs. Chronic ITP is as mentioned, defined as reaching no response with platelet counts less than 30,000 or reaching less than two fold increase from base line measured twice 1 day apart. Patients are not considered as having chronic ITP under 6–12 months of the diagnosis, even if several relapses occur or no complete remission is achieved. Our patients is by none of these definitions, a case of persistent or no-response ITP [3]. She would not be eligible for splenectomy until the age 5-years-old and even then, other second line therapy options, including rituximab, high dose dexamethasone, or thrombopoietin receptor agonists should be tested. Booster MMR vaccination is not generally banned, unless there is evidence that ITP has followed within 3 weeks of first dose MMR and the patient is proved to be immune via serology.

The girl was given high dose IVIG and upon discharge, her parents were advised to protect her from trauma, avoid further infections and return within a week after discharge.

Practical Points

- Immune thrombocytopenic purpura (ITP) is commonly preceded by a viral infection, usually a common cold and has a presumed autoimmune origin
- Presence of bone pain, anemia, hepatosplenomegaly or hyperleukocytosis should prompt further investigation with bone marrow aspiration and/or biopsy.
- Up to 80% of the pediatric patients with ITP respond to the immunomodulatory therapy with intravenous immunoglobulin after the first therapy course

References

1. O'Leary ST, Glanz JM, McClure DL, Akhtar A, Daley MF, Nakasato C, Baxter R, Davis RL, Izurieta HS, Lieu TA, Ball R. The risk of immune thrombocytopenic purpura after vaccination in children and adolescents. Pediatrics. 2012;129(2):248–55.
2. Kime C, Klima J, Rose MJ, O'Brien SH. Patterns of inpatient care for newly diagnosed immune thrombocytopenia in US children's hospitals. Pediatrics. 2013;131(5):880–5.
3. Cuker A, Neunert CE. How I treat refractory immune thrombocytopenia. Blood. 2016;128(12):1547–54.

Index

A

Abdominal distension, 133
Abdominal pain, 139
Acantholysis, 395
Acantholytic cells, 359
Acute cutaneous lupus erythematosus (ACLE), 330–331
Acute GVHD (aGVHD), 242
Acute lung injury, 260, 262
Acute myeloid leukemia (AML)
  HLA typing, 217, 218
  linkage disequilibrium, 218
  patient history, 203–206, 217
Acute respiratory distress
  dextran, 257
  DMSO toxicity, 256
  IgA deficiency, 257
  patient history, 255
  physical examination, 255
  treatment, 257
Acute rheumatic fever (ARF), 43
Acute tubular necrosis (ATN), 321
AIDS-related KS, 162
Allogenic transplant, 140
Alopecia areata (AA), 470–472
American College of Rheumatology (ACR), 99
Amyopathic dermatomyositis, 92, 93
Anaphylaxis, 252, 253
Anemia, 57, 59
Angiotensin converting enzyme inhibitors, 354
Annular blisters and erosions
  acatholytic cells, 359
  clinical findings, 358
  dermatological examination, 357
Annular erythematous plaques, 71–73, 75
Annular rash
  diagnosis, 73
  laboratory findings, 71
  neonatal lupus erythematosus
    anti-La/SSB antibody, 73
    anti-Ro/SSA antibody, 73
    CHB, 73, 74
    deranged liver function tests, 74
    electocardiogram, 74
    hydroxychloroquine, 75
Anterior uveitis, 105
Antibody-mediated rejection (AMR), 320, 321, 323
Anti-CD3 monoclonal antibody, 314, 317
Anti-chimeric antibodies, 296
Anti-citrullinated protein antibody (ACPA), 33
Anti-double stranded DNA antibody (anti-dsDNA), 54
Anti-endomysial antibodies (anti-EMA), 378
Antigen presenting cells (APC), 6
Anti-La/SSB antibody, 75
Anti-MDA-5 antibodies, 94
Anti-melanoma differentiation-associated gene 5 (MDA5) antibodies, 80
Anti-Mi-2 antibodies, 80–81
Anti-nuclear antibody (ANA), 31, 54, 97, 100
Anti-retroviral therapy (ART), 122
Anti-RNP antibodies, 66
Anti-Ro/La antibodies, 66
Anti-Ro/SSA antibody, 73, 75
Antisynthetase antibodies, 80
Anti-topoisomerase I, 99, 100
Aplastic anemia, 128
Aplastic crisis, 150
Aspergillus fumigatus, 135, 136

© Springer Nature Switzerland AG 2020

F. Rahmani, N. Rezaei (eds.), *Pediatric Autoimmunity and Transplantation*,
https://doi.org/10.1007/978-3-030-26280-8

Asthenia, fatigue
anti-tTG, 175
clinical and laboratory findings, 175
CMV testing, 174
cystic fibrosis, 175
diagnosis, 174
differential diagnosis, 176
Gilbert's syndrome, 174
IgE, 173, 176
incidental benzodiazepine, 175
laboratory investigations, 175
liver transaminases, 174, 175
long-term management, 176
management, 174
marsh, 175
micro-array testing, 174
past medical history, 173
pediatric celiac disease, 176
prevalence of, 176
routine laboratory examination, 173
ultrasound sonography, 175
Asymptomatic atrophic plaque
diagnosis, 103
ECDS, 104 (*see* En coup de sabre (ECDS))
examination, 103
Audiovestibular dysfunction, 116, 117, 119
Autoimmunity, 2
Autologous blood donation, 253, 254
Autosomal recessive disease, 181

B
Bacillus Calmette–Guérin (BCG) stimulation, 192
Basal vacuolar degeneration, 91, 93
Basement membrane zone, 395
Basement membrane zone (BMZ), 340
Basiliximab, 296, 297
β-agonists, 67
Biologics, 56
Blaschko lines, 92
Blisters, 339
dermatological examination, 381
histological examination, 387
LABD (*see* Linear IgA bullous dermatosis (LABD))
laboratory examination, 381, 387
patient history, 387
physical examination, 387
See also Bullous systemic lupus erythematosus (BSLE)
Bone marrow hemophagocytosis, 275
Bone marrow transplantation (BMT), 247–249
Bradycardia
dexamethasone to mother, 67, 68
initial diagnosis, 65
laboratory findings, 65
physical examination, 65
Brain-derived natriuretic peptide (BNP), 22
Breathlessness
chest X-ray, 122
physical examination, 121
treatment, 121
Bruising
diagnosis, 479
hypersensitivity type, 480
ITP, 480–482
IVIG, 481, 482
patient history, 479
PBS, 480
Bull's eye maculopathy, 333
Bullous impetigo, 370, 401
Bullous pemphigoid, 401
clinical findings, 370
DIF, 371
treatment, 372
Bullous systemic lupus erythematosus (BSLE)
diagnostic criteria, 340
epidermolysis bullosa acquisita, 340

C
C1q analyses, 317
C1q assay, 323
Calcineurin, 134, 296, 297
Calcinosis cutis, 87, 88
Cartilage matrix protein (CMP), 340
Castleman's disease, 199
CCR5 chemokine receptors, 123
CD195 receptors, 123
CD45RO phenotype, 290–292
$CD8^+$ T lymphocytes, 276
Chediak-Higashi syndrome, 405
Childhood chronic bullous dermatosis, *see* Childhood linear IgA disease (CLAD)
Childhood Health Assessment Questionnaire (CHAQ), 88
Childhood linear IgA disease (CLAD), 401
dapsone, 395
diagnostic criteria, 395
haemorrhagic blisters, 393, 394
mucosal involvement, 394
pearl/jewel cluster appearance, 394
systemic corticosteroid therapy, 395
therapy, 402

Childhood Myositis Assessment Scale (CMAS), 88
Chondrodysplasia, 66
Chronic band-like lichenoid lymphohistiocytic inflammation, 93
Chronic bullous disease of childhood (CBDC), 346
  BPAg2, 400
  herpetiform clustering, 401
  linear IgA disease, 401
    bullous impetigo, 401, 402
    in childhood, 401
    remission in adults, 401
    therapy, 402
Chronic cutaneous lupus erythematosus (CCLE), 331
Clinically amyopathic juvenile dermatomyositis (CAJDM), 92, 93
  assessments, 94
  follow-up test, 93
Cogan's syndrome (CS)
  autoimmunologic mechanism, 116
  cochlea and vestibular labyrinths, 116
  differential diagnosis, 117
  endolymphatic hydrops, 117
  incidence, 116
  MRI and CT scan, 117
  prognosis, 118
  systemic corticosteroid treatment, 118
Cold-ischemic time, 295
Complement deficiencies, 58
Congenital deficiency, 58
Congenital heart block (CHB), 66, 68
Congenital hypothyroidism, 67
Congenital long QT syndrome (LQTS), 67
Congenital rubella, 116
Creatine kinase, 88
Crusted lesions, 337–339
Cryptosporidiosis, 124
Cutaneous lupus erythematosus, 330
Cutaneous telangiectasia, 66
Cuticular dystrophy, 91, 94
CXCR4 chemokine receptors, 123
Cyclophosphamide, 342
Cytomegalovirus (CMV), 198
Cytotoxic T-lymphocytes (CTLs), 453

D

Dedicator of cytokinesis (DOCK8) deficiency
  anti-GVHD medication, 238
  $CD34^+$ hematopoietic stem cells, 238
  laboratory parameters, 237
  management option, 237, 238
  mismatched unrelated donor transplant, 238
  T lymphocyte depletion, 239
Deficiency of interleukin 1 receptor antagonist (DIRA), 446
Depigmentation
  combination therapies, 407
  Griscelli syndrome, 405
  Hansen's disease, 404
  initial diagnosis, 403
  innate and adaptive immune system, 406
  OCA, 404
  patient history, 403, 404
  piebaldism, 404
  poliosis, 405
  ROS, 406
  silvery hair syndromes, 405
  symptomatic ocular disease, 405
  vitiligo, 403–407
  Vogt-Koyanagi-Harada syndrome, 405
  Waardenburg syndrome, 405
Deranged liver function tests, 74
Dermatitis herpetiformis (DH), 388, 401
  anti-endomysial antibodies, 378
  anti-tissue transglutaminase antibodies, 378
  anti-tTG, 378
  differential diagnoses, 378
  direct immunofluorescence examination, 377
  gluten-free diet, 378
Desmogleins, 352
Dextran, 257
Diabetic ketoacidosis (DKA) attack, 476
Dilapidated brick wall appearance, 350
Direct antiglobulin test (DAT), 259
Direct immunofluorescence (DIF), 80, 331
Discoid lupus erythematosus (DLE), 331, 333, 412
  annual screening, 333
  bull's eye maculopathy, 333
  DIF, 331
  hydroxychloroquine, 332
  risk factors, 333
  skin biopsy, 331, 332
  SLE progression, 333
Disease Activity Scale, 88
DMSO toxicity, 256
DNase 1 protein, 62
Donor-specific antibodies (DSA), 295
D-penicillamine, 385, 386

Drug reaction with eosinophilia and systemic symptoms (DRESS)/drug induced hypersensitivity syndrome (DIHS), 460
  anti-herpesvirus medications, 112
  aromatic anticonvulsants, 110, 111
  hepatic necrosis and liver failure, 112
  HHV-6, 111
  RegiSCAR, 110

E

Edema and hypopigmented lesions, 143
  diagnosis, 99
  laboratory evaluation, 97
  nail fold capillaroscopy, 99, 100
  patient history, 97
  physical examination, 97
  Raynaud's phenomenon and proximal skin induration, 99
  treatment, 98
Elejalde disease, 405
En coup de sabre (ECDS), 104–106
  anterior uveitis, 105
  epilepsy, 104
  interface dermatitis, 105
  treatment, 106
  UVA-1 phototherapy, 106
Endocardial fibroelastosis (EFE), 66–68
Enthesitis-related arthritis (ERA), 37
Enzyme-linked immunosorbent assay (ELISA), 136
Epidermal atrophy, 92–94
Epidermolysis bullosa, 340, 347, 402
Epilepsy, 104
Epstein-Barr virus (EBV), 150, 198, 276
Erythema and pruritic rash, 459
Erythema multiforme major (EMM), 452
Erythematous macules
  EMM, 452
  keratinocyte apoptosis, 456
  ophthalmological consultation, 456
  oral care, 456
  pathogenesis, 453
  patient history, 451, 452
  pemphigus vulgaris, 452
  polymorphonuclear leukocyte proteinase, 454
  prevention, 456
  SCORTEN, 455
  SJS/TEN, 452–456
  SSSS, 452, 453
Erythematous papules, 77
Erythematous scaly plaques
  Auspitz sign, 441
  Koebner phenomenon, 441
  patient history, 439, 440
  plaque psoriasis, 440–443
  PRP, 441
Erythrocyte sedimentation rate (ESR), 88
Erythroderma
  diagnosis, 435
  patient history, 435, 436
  PRP, 435–437
Ethambutol, 154
European League Against Rheumatism (EULAR) 2013 Classification Criteria, 99
Extra-corporal membrane oxygenation (ECMO), 311, 313, 315, 316
Extracorporeal photopheresis (ECP), 244
Extractable nuclear antigens (anti-ENAs), 54

F

Familial benign chronic pemphigus, 350
Fever, 128
  anti-IFN-γ autoantibodies, 192, 193
  clinical and pathological features, 189
  clinical history, 191
  and cutaneous nodules
    abdominal examination, 149
    blood transfusion, 149
    encapsulated organisms, 151
    hemoglobin electrophoresis, 149
    parvoviruses, 150
    pathogens, 150
    penicillin prophylaxis, 151
    sickle cell anemia, 150, 151
    vaccination, 151
  excision biopsy, 190
  genetic mutations, 192
  immunodeficiency, 192
  laboratory findings, 189, 281, 282
  malaise, laryngitis and
    allogeneic hematopoietic cell transplantation, 200
    AML inv(16), 200
    bone marrow aspirate, 199
    chemotherapy, 198, 200
    clinical manifestations, 198
    CMV, 198
    CNS involvement, 201
    diagnosis, 199
    diagnostic workup, 197

DNMT3A, BRAF, and SRSF2 mutations, 199
EBV, 198
FACS, 198
massive leukocytosis, 198
patient history, 197
peripheral blood smear, 198
radiographic imaging, 199
reinduction chemotherapy, 201
serological testing, 198
MAS/HLH (*see* Macrophage activation syndrome (MAS)/hemophagocytic lymphohistiocytosis (HAH))
MSMD, 192
Mycobacterium abscessus infections, 191
neck stiffness and
diagnosis, 153
lumbar puncture results, 154
physical examination, 153
TBM, 154
treatment option, 154
NTM infections, 191, 194
oral ulcers, 189
outpatient reviews, 190
physical examination, 189, 190, 281
secondary immunodeficiencies, 192
serology, 190
skin lesions, 189
tissue culture, 190, 191
Fluorescence-activated cell sorting (FACS), 198
Fluorescence cytometric crossmatch (FCXM), 295, 306, 313, 314, 320, 323–324
Fluorescence in-situ hybridization (FISH) analysis, 291
Focal segmental glomerulosclerosis (FSGS), 325, 327, 328
Focal segmental membranoproliferative glomerulonephritis (FS-MPGN), 59
Fogo selvagem, 347
Febrile ulceronecrotic Mucha-Habermann disease (FUMHD), 422–425

G
GATA2 deficiency, 128, 129
Generalized body pains
diagnosis, 157
herpes zoster, 158
HIV test, 158
treatment, 158
vesicular rash, 157
Giant cell arteritis, 117–118
Giardia lamblia, 248
Gottron's papules, 86, 87, 92, 94
Graft versus host disease (GVHD), 10, 298, 301
Granulocyte, monocyte colony stimulating factor (GM-CSF), 136, 137
Griscelli syndome, 405
Griscelli type 2, 275
Grouped blisters, 394

H
Haemophilus influenza, 248, 266
Hailey-Hailey disease, 350
Hair loss
alopecia areata, 470–472
dermoscopy, 471
diagnosis, 470, 472
examination of, 472
patient history, 469, 470
treatment plan, 472, 473
vellus hair ratio, 472
Heart transplantation
ABO incompatible organs, 314
anti-HLA antibody studies, 312
C1q analyses, 317
C4d detection, 316
DSA MFI values, 316
endomyocardial biopsy, 316
IgG anti-HLA, 315–316
patient and donor HLA typing, 312
positive anti-class I DSA, 316, 317
positive crossmatch, 315
pre-transplantation anti-HLA antibody studies, 312, 313
Heliotrope eruption, 78
Heliotrope rash, 87, 94
Hematopoietic stem cell transplantation (HSCT), 129
aggressive management, 231
APC, 6
complications, 234
donor chimerism, 233, 234
donor-patient selection, 8
donor search, 231, 232
donor selection
issues, 10, 11
NMDP search results, 12
process of, 11, 12
serologic level typing, 13
solid organ transplantation, 12, 13
donor typing results, 7
fluid overloaded, 234
gene sequencing, 7, 8
granulocyte-monocyte colony, 232

Hematopoietic stem cell transplantation (HSCT) (*cont.*)
guidelines, 233
GVHD prophylaxis options, 232
HLA, 3–6, 207–209, 219–221
human papillomavirus vaccination, 266
inactivated vaccination, 266, 267
live-attenuated immunizations, 267, 269
long-term toxicity, 235
maternal engraftment, 233
mature blood cells and progenitors, 231
measles exposure, 269
medication plan, 234
Mendelian genetics, 7
Msc, 7
myeloablation and immunosuppression, 233
neutrophils, 234
nomenclature, 8–10
patient history, 203–206, 265
polymorphisms, 7
post-transplant schedule of immunizations, 267, 268
prophylactic medications, 234
serologic determination, 7, 8
special care, 231
survival rate, 231, 232
T cell generation, 232
TCR alpha-beta T cell depletion, 232
treatment, 231
Hematuria, 139
Hemolytic uremic syndrome (HUS), 49
Hemophagocytic lymphohistiocytosis (HLH)
CD163, 284
corticosteroids + cyclosporin A + IL-1 inhibition, 277
Epstein-Barr virus, 276
etoposide-based regimens, 277
familial HLH, 276
ferritin level, 283
gene testing, 275
hereditary causes, 285
HSCT, 286
molecular diagnosis, 275
NK cells and $CD8^+$ T lymphocytes, 276
primary immune test for, 284
sIL-2Rα levels, 283
triglyceride level, 283
See also Macrophage activation syndrome (MAS)
Hemophagocytosis, 284
Hemorrhagic crusts, erythematous and necrotic papules
diagnosis, 421
erythromycin and tetracyclines, 425
FUMHD, 422–425
patient history, 421–423
PL, 422
Hepatosplenomegaly, 290, 291
Herpes zoster
cardinal symptoms, 158
classic findings, 158
clinical manifestations, 158
diagnosis, 158
low $CD4^+$ count, 158
risk factors, 158
shingles, 158
treatment options, 158
HHV8, 163
Highly active ART (HAART) therapy, 124
HIV infection, 3
ART, 125
CD195 receptors, 123
cryptosporidium infection, 124
Hofbauer cells, 123
nucleic acid testing, 125
stage 4 infection, 122
treatment, 122
vitamin A supplementation, 124
zinc supplementation, 124
HLA-matched mesenchymal stem cells (MSCs), 244
Hofbauer cells, 123
Human herpesvirus 6 (HHV6), 111, 461
Human leukocyte antigen (HLA) DQA1∗0501, 79
Humanized monoclonal antibody, 39
Humoral rejection, 321
Hyaline fibromatosis syndrome (HFS), 181
Hyalinoses, 182
Hydroxychloroquine, 56, 75, 332, 342
Hydroxyl radical (OH), 140
Hyperpigmented patches
bullous eruptions, 416
H1 antihistamines, 419
H_2 antihistamines, 419
histological stains, 417
leukotriene antagonist, 419
mast cell degranulation, 418
mastocytosis, 415, 416
medications, 418
oral cromolyn sodium, 419
patient history, 415
serum concentrations, 417
SM, 417
systemic symptoms, 416

Hypertrophied gingiva, 182
Hypocomplementemia, 59
Hypocomplementemic urticarial vasculitis syndrome (HUVS), 430
Hypofractionated radiation treatment, 140, 141
Hypofunctioning T cells, 290
Hypomyopathic dermatomyositis, 93

I
Idiopathic/immune thrombocytopenic purpura (ITP), 480
IFN-γ inhibition, 194
IgA anti-tissue transglutaminase antibody (anti-tTG), 175, 378
IgA deficiency, 252, 253
Immune defects, 3
Immune thrombocytopenic purpura (ITP), 480–482
Immunohistochemistry (IHC) panel, 181
Immunosenescence, 248
Immunosuppression
  edema, 134, 135
  nephrotic syndrome, 134
  tacrolimus and cyclosporine, 134
  vaccines, 134
Indapamide, 354
Indirect immunofluorescence (IIF), 340
Infantile systemic hyalinosis, 181
Infectious mononucleosis, 460, 461
Inflammatory bowel disease (IBD), 468
Interface dermatitis, 80, 331
Intermittent fever, 53
International League of Associations for Rheumatology (ILAR) classification criteria, 282
International Prognostic Scoring System (IPSS), 129
Interstitial keratitis, 115, 116, 119
Intestinal perforation, 81
Intraepidermal blister, 346–348
Intra-lesional steroid injection, 182
Intravenous immunoglobulin (IVIG), 179
Isoniazid, 154
Itchy facial rash
  juvenile dermatomyositis
    direct immunofluorescence, 80
    etiology, 78, 79
    HLA DQA1∗0501, 79
    interface dermatitis, 80
    intestinal perforation, 81
    MDA5 antibody, 80
    methotrexate, 81
  laboratory findings, 77
  physical examination, 77
Itchy skin rashes
  laboratory findings, 375, 376
  patient history, 375
  physical examination, 375
  radioallergosorbent test, 377
  skin biopsy, 377
  skin prick test, 377
Itchy violaceous plaques
  laboratory findings, 329
  physical examination, 329
Intravenous immunoglobulin (IVIG), 17, 19–22, 28, 29, 44, 112, 179, 181, 234, 241, 248, 266, 267, 269, 270, 289, 396, 402, 448, 461, 481, 482

J
Juvenile bullous pemphigoid, 370–372
Juvenile dermatomyositis (JDM)
  cutaneous features, 79
  direct immunofluorescence, 80
  etiology, 78
  HLA DQA1∗0501, 79
  interface dermatitis, 80
  intestinal perforation, 81
  MDA5 antibody, 80
  methotrexate, 81
  muscle weakness and fever
    calcinosis cutis, 88
    CMAS, 88
    corticosteroids, 88
    creatine kinase, 88
    criteria for, 86
    erythematous violaceous rash, 87
    erythrocyte sedimentation rate, 88
    gottron papules, 87
    intravenous immunoglobulin, 89
    MRI, 88
    mycophenolate mofetil, 89
    physiotherapy, 89
    symptomatic lung disease, 87
  pruritic erythematous rashes
    cuticular dystrophy, 94
    lilac erythema, 94
    nail fold telangiectasia, 94
    poikiloderma, 94
    SCLE, 92
    treatment, 95

Juvenile hyaline fibromatosis, 181
Juvenile idiopathic arthritis (JIA), 2, 31, 32
  ILAR classification, 32
  polyarthritis, 32
  positive ANA test, 33
  symptoms, 32
  systemic-onset, 32, 33
Juvenile pemphigus, 357
Juvenile psoriatic arthritis (JPsA), 33, 443

K

Kaposi sarcoma (KS)
  definitive diagnosis, 162
  popular/nodular lesions/blotches, 162
  treatment modality, 163
Kawasaki disease (KD), 26–28
  aggressive initial treatment, 20
  American Heart Association consensus guidelines, 21
  BCG scar erythema, 17, 18
  BNP, 22
  cervical lymphadenopathy, 19
  clinical criteria, 19
  clinical findings, 19
  coronary artery lesions, 19
  diagnosis, 17
  hepatosplenomegaly, 21
  intravenous immunoglobulin administration, 19
  IVIG resistance, 20
  laboratory tests, 17
  MAS, 21, 22
  principal clinical features, 22
  refractory disease, 20
  renal impairment, 20
  TNF-α inhibitors, 21
Kidney transplantation
  AMR response, 323
  anti-HLA antibody, 307–309, 322
  C1q assay, 323
  donor-specific antibodies, 307, 308, 322
  DSA, 323
  ESRD
    ABO matching, 326
    anti-HLA antibody testing, 325
    FCXM, 320
    FSGS recurrence rate, 327
    HLA haplotype, 326
    HLA-typing, 320, 325
    humoral rejection, 321
    membranoproliferative glomerulonephritis, 326
    physician and patient communication, 328
    potential donor HLA, 320
    remission, 327
    SLE, 326
  HLA matching criteria, 307
  IgA anti-HLA antibodies, 309
  typing and anti-HLA antibody studies, 305, 306
  virtual cross-matching, 306
Knee and ankle pain
  evaluation and management, 35, 36
  JIA, 37, 38
  patient's presentations, 36
  treatment option, 38, 39
Knee swelling and rash
  abdominal pain, 50
  arthralgia/arthritis, 50
  clinical syndrome, 48
  CNS vasculitis, 50
  diagnosis, 47
  Henoch-Schönlein Purpura, 48
  history, 47
  HUS, 49
  hypersensitivity vasculitis, 48
  initial treatment, 50
  long-term morbidity, 49
  long-term therapy, 50
  mutations in the familial Mediterranean fever, 48
  PAN, 49
  physical examination, 47
  prognosis, 49
  serum sickness, 48
  severity of disease, 50
  triggering events, 48
Kwashiorkor disease, 144

L

Lamina lucida, 400
Lamotrigine, 111
Lesions
  laboratory findings, 337
  physical examination, 337
  SLE (*see* Systemic lupus erythematosus (SLE))
Leukapheresis, 265
Lilac erythema, 91, 94
Linear IgA bullous dermatosis (LABD), 384
  childhood, 388
  dapsone, 390
  dermatitis herpetiformis, 388

drug-induced, 389
methemoglobinemia, 390, 391
oral prednisolone, 390
ulcerative colitis, 390
vancomycin, 389
Linear morphea, 103
Live vaccines, 134
Localized scleroderma (LSc), 103
histological features, 105
methotrexate, 106
ocular abnormalities, 105
UVA-1 phototherapy, 106
Lower limbs, edema
patient care, 170
physical examination, 169
respiratory distress, 169
severe acute malnutrition, 170
weight for height index, 169, 170
Luminex® technology, 298
Lupus band test, 331
Lymphocyte transformation test (LTT) response, 179
Lymphopenia, 290

M

Macrophage activation syndrome (MAS)/ hemophagocytic lymphohistiocytosis (HAH), 21, 22, 63
CD163, 284
corticosteroids + cyclosporin A + IL-1 inhibition, 277
cytokine targeted biologic therapies, 277
definition, 283
diagnosis, 283
ferritin level, 283
HSCT, 286
laboratory findings, 274
in SJIA, 275, 286
sIL-2Rα levels, 283
triglyceride level, 283
Malaise, 53
Marginal inflammatory vitiligo (MIV), 411, 412
Maternal engraftment syndrome, 290, 292
Maternal T lymphocyte engraftment, 291
Mean fluorescence intensity (MFI), 320
Mean upper arm circumference (MUAC), 170
cell-mediated immunity, 167
child's nutritional status, 165
lymphopenia, 167
moderate acute malnutrition, 166
subcutaneous fat, 166
tuberculin skin test, 166, 167
weight-for-height index, 166
Megaloblastic anemia, 127, 128
Membrane attack complex (MAC), 58
Membranoproliferative glomerulonephritis, 326
Mendelian susceptibility to mycobacterial disease (MSMD), 192
Mesenchymal stem cells (Msc), 7
Methemoglobinemia, 390, 391
Methotrexate, 81, 95
Microhematuria, 57
Microscopic polyangiitis, 59
Mid upper arm circumference (MUAC), 143
Molecular genetic testing, 182
Mononuclear cell infiltrates, 331
Morphea, *see* Localized scleroderma (LSc)
Mucha-Habermann disease, 422
Multi-organ dysfunction syndrome (MODS), 274, 277
Muscle weakness and fever
JDM
calcinosis cutis, 88
CMAS, 88
corticosteroids, 88
creatine kinase, 88
criteria for, 86
erythematous violaceous rash, 87
erythrocyte sedimentation rate, 88
gottron papules, 87
heliotrope rash, 87
intravenous immunoglobulin, 89
MRI, 88
mycophenolate mofetil, 89
physiotherapy, 89
symptomatic lung disease, 87
laboratory findings, 85
physical examination, 85
Mycobacterium avium disease, 247
Mycophenolate mofetil, 89
Mycosis fungoides (MF), 412
Myelodysplastic syndrome (MDS)
HSCT, 129
laboratory/genetic findings, 128
morphologic features, 128
peripheral blood dysgranulopoiesis, 128
survival/progression, 129, 130
Myocarditis, 66
Myositis, 100
Myositis-specific autoantibodies (MSAs), 80

N

Nail fold capillaroscopy, 99
Nail fold telangiectasia, 91, 94
Neck swelling, 127
Neonatal lupus erythematosus (NLE)
annular rash
anti-La/SSB antibody, 73
anti-nuclear antibody, 71–73
anti-Ro/SSA antibody, 73
CHB, 73
deranged liver function tests, 74
electocardiogram, 74
hydroxychloroquine, 75
CHB, 66, 68
clinical manifestations, 66
intrauterine viral infections, 67
intrauterine/perinatal death, 68
LQTS, 67
multiple neurological manifestations, 66
rash, 66
symptoms, 67
Nikolsky sign, 459, 460
Non-alcoholic steatohepatitis (NASH)
anti-IgA measurements, 253
IgA deficiency, 252
immunofixation electrophoresis, 253
patient history, 251
pre-transplant screening, 251
severe allergic reactions, 252
washed RBC and platelets, 253
Non-exposed epitopes, 307–309
Non-SCID primary immunodeficiencies (PIDs), 231
Non-steroidal anti-inflammatory drugs (NSAIDs), 38–40, 50, 56, 418, 427, 431
Non-tuberculous mycobacterial (NTM) infections, 191, 194
Normocomplementemic urticarial vasculitis (NUV), 430
Nucleic acid testing (NAT), 125

O

Oculocutaneous albinism (OCA), 404
Odynophagia, 61
Omenn's syndrome (OS), 290
Organ procurement organization (OPO), 313
Orthotopic liver transplantation (OLT)
basiliximab, 296, 297
cold-ischemic time, 295
cyclosporine, 297
donor chimerism, 300
GVHD, 298, 299
HLA Class I, 301, 302
patient and donor HLA typing, 299
patient history, 295
tacrolimus, 296, 297
transportation, 296

P

P450 system, 111
Pancytopenia, 298
Paraneoplastic pemphigus, 384
Parry-Romberg syndrome (PRS), 104
Pemphigus
anti-desmoglein 1 and 3 antibodies, 384
desmoglein 1 antigen, 383
DIF, 383
LABD, 384
skin biopsy, 381
thiol drugs, 385
treatment, 385
Pemphigus foliaceus (PF), 346, 384, 385
anti-dsg 1 IgG autoantibodies, 366
corticosteroids, 347
dapsone, 347, 361
desmoglein, 358
desmogleins 1 and 3, 348
DIF, 360, 361
differentiating features, 346
direct and indirect immunofluorescence, 366
enzyme-Linked Immunosorbent Assay, 360
fogo selvagem, 347
hydroxychloroquine, 347
intact bullous lesions, 359
pathophysiology, 357
vs. pemphigus vulgaris, 364
serum anti-dsg 1 and 3 autoantibodies, 364
Simulium (black fly) bites, 347
sporadic PF, 359
subcorneal acantholytic blister, 365
sunlight and drugs, 347
symptoms, 364
systemic corticosteroid therapy, 360
topical corticosteroids, 361
Tzanck smear, 359
Pemphigus herpetiformis, 384–386
Pemphigus vegetans, 384
Pemphigus vulgaris (PV), 346, 365, 384, 386
active phase, 352
angiotensin converting enzyme inhibitors, 354

anti-Dsg antibodies, 352, 353
childhood PV, 354
corticosteroids, 353
dapsone, 366
diagnosis, 365
glucocorticoids, 366
H&E staining, 365
pediatric PF, 364
vs. pemphigus foliaceus, 364
prognostic factors, 354
Penicillamine, 347, 348
Perforin pathway genes, 276
Peripheral blood smear (PBS), 480
Peripheral blood stem cell transplantation (PBSCT), 265–266
Peripheral lymphocyte subsets, 290
Photosensitivity, 337
Pityriasis lichenoides (PL), 422
Pityriasis rubra pilaris (PRP), 435–437, 441
Platelet transfusion, 259, 261
Pneumococcal polysaccharide vaccine (PPSV), 151
Pneumocystis jirovecii pneumonia (PCP), 122, 229, 290
Pneumocystis pneumonia, 122
Poikiloderma, 94
Post hematopoietic stem cell transplantation (HSCT)
aGVHD, 242
diarrhea, 242–244
patient history, 241, 242
Premature ovarian failure, 342
Primary/familiar HLH (FHLH), 284
Primary immunodeficiency disorders (PID), 180
Protein kinase C-delta (PKCδ), 62
Protein losing enteropathy (PLE), 181
Proteinuria, 57
Pruriginous morbiliform eruption
laboratory findings, 109
physical examination, 109
Pruritic blisters, 399
Pruritic erythematous rashes, face and eyelids
CAJDM
follow-up test, 93
interstitial lung disease, 94
methotrexate with hydroxychloroquine, 95
oral corticosteroid, 95
topical corticosteroid, 95
JDM
clinical findings, 92
cuticular dystrophy, 94
lilac erythema, 94
nail fold telangiectasia, 94
poikiloderma, 94
SCLE, 92
laboratory findings, 91
physical examination, 91
Pulmonary edema, 260
Pustular lesions
diagnosis, 445
DIRA, 446
IgA pemphigus, 446
patient history, 445–447
pustular psoriasis, 447
SPD, 445–449
Pyoderma gangrenosum (PG)
diagnosis, 466
differential diagnoses, 466
hematological diseases, 468
incidental/surgical superficial trauma, 466
mechanisms, 467
papillary and reticular dermis, 467
pathergy phenomenon, 466
pathogenesis, 467
patient history, 465, 466
pediatric PG, 468
therapeutic approach, 467
visceral involvement, 466
Pyrazinamide, 154

R

Radioimmunotherapy
in children, 140
growth disturbances, 141
mammalian cells, 139, 140
total body irradiation, 140
Raynaud's phenomenon (RP), 97, 99, 100
Reactive oxygen species (ROS), 406
Recurrent pneumonia
chronic granulomatous disease, 186
clinical presentation and history, 186
combined immunodeficiencies, 186
cutaneous and systemic infections, 186
hypogammaglobulinemia, 186, 187
IgG levels, 187
IgG replacement, 187
patient history, 185
primary tests, 186
respiratory tract infections, 186
rituximab, 187
serum immunoglobulin concentrations, 186
treatment option, 187

Refractory high fever
bone marrow aspiration, 27
characteristics, 27
coronary artery aneurysms, 26
diagnosis, 25
differential diagnoses, 27
drug reactions, 27
echocardiography, 27
evaluations, 27
initial laboratory investigations, 25
Kawasaki disease, 26–28
laboratory tests, 26
physical examination, 25
recommendations, 29
treatment, 28, 29
vasculitis, 26
RegiSCAR, 110
Renal biopsy, 58
Renal disease, 55
biopsy, 55
initial therapy, 55
International Society of Nephrology/Renal Pathology Society, 55
Rheumatologic disorders, 2, 63, 64
Rifampicin, 154
Rituximab, 353
Rowell syndrome, 340
rSSO technique, 298

S
Sarcoidosis, 118
Scleroderma, 103, 107
SCORTEN, 455
Secondary immunodeficiency disorders, 2, 3
Serum ferritin, 275
Serum sickness-like reaction (SSLR), 43
Severe acute malnutrition (SAM)
acute gastroenteritis, 145
in children, 146
congestive cardiac failure, 144
definition, 144
diagnosis, 143
edema, 144
hepatic failure, 144
hypoglycemia and amino acid imbalances, 146
medical complications, 144
micronutrients, 146, 147
nephrotic syndrome, 144
physiologic and metabolic changes, 145
shock, 145
treatment of, 144
WHO recommendations, 144
Severe combined immunodeficiency (SCID)
BMT
antibiotic prophylaxis, 248
common variable immunodeficiency, 248
diagnosis, 248
follow up, 248
genetic test, 248
IVIG, 248
laboratory findings, 248
patient history, 247
clinical presentation, 230
FISH analysis, 291
HLA class I and II typing, 211–214, 291
HLA-DQ6, 214
laboratory test, 230
maternal T-cells, 213
maternal T lymphocyte engraftment, 291
Omenn's syndrome, 290
patient history, 211
PCR based STR analysis, 291
rotavirus vaccine strain, 230
T cell engraftment, 290
T cell immunodeficiencies, 290
treatment, 230, 292
Short tandem repeat (STR) analysis, 291
Simulium (black fly) bites, 347
Sjögren syndrome, 66, 73
Skin disease, 56
Skin papules
IVIG, 179
skin manifestations, 180
whitish papules, 180
Staphylococcal scalded skin syndrome (SSSS), 452, 453
Staphylococcus aureus, 363, 364
Stevens-Johnson syndrome (SJS)/toxic epidermal necrolysis (TEN), 452–456, 461, 462
Streptococcus pneumoniae, 248
Subacute cutaneous lupus erythematosus (SCLE), 92, 330, 331
Subcorneal acantholytic blister, 365
Subcorneal pustular dermatosis (SPD), 445–449
Subcutaneous nodules
evaluation and management, 180
excisional biopsy, 180
features, 181
gingival hypertrophy, 179, 180
HFS, 181
IHC panel, 181
infantile systemic hyalinosis, 181
rectal prolapse, 179

Subepidermal blister, 387, 388
Subepidermal bullae, 371
Suprabasilar acantholysis, 349
Systemic inflammatory response syndrome (SIRS), 277
Systemic juvenile idiopathic arthritis (SJIA), 274–275, 282, 283
Systemic lupus erythematosus (SLE), 53, 54, 73, 326, 330, 331, 333, 334, 429
  BSLE (*see* Bullous systemic lupus erythematosus (BSLE))
  chest X-ray, 338
  cyclophosphamide, 342
  diagnosis, 62
  juvenile SLE, 62
  LE associated autoimmune bullous disorders, 340
  LE-specific skin lesions, 340
  molecular defect, 62
  non-specific LE cutaneous lesion, 340
  partial C4 deficiency, 58
  pediatric SLE, 341, 342
  steroid treatment, 342
  24-hours urinary protein, 339
  ultrasonography of whole abdomen, 339
Systemic lupus international collaborating clinics (SLICC) criteria, 337–338
Systemic mastocytosis (SM), 417
Systemic sclerosis (SSc)
  antibodies, 99
  autoantibodies, 100
  nail fold capillaroscopy, 99
  overlap syndromes, 100
  treatment, 101
Systemic tacrolimus therapy, 136

T

Tacrolimus, 296–298
Takayasu arteritis, 118
TB meningitis (TBM), 154
T cell epitopes (TCE), 10, 220
T cell lymphoblastic leukemia/lymphoma
  autologous HCT, 224
  diagnosis and treatment, 224
  donor selection process, 225
  hematologic malignancy, 223
  HLA-A, -B, -C, and -DRB1 matching, 225
  HLA-DPB1 TCE group, 225, 226
  HLA-DRB3, -DRB4, and -DRB5, 225, 226
  HLA typing results, 224
  patient history, 223
  surveillance, 224
T cell receptor excision circles (Trec) level, 290
Thiopurine methyltransferase (TPMT) enzyme, 135
Tombstone pattern, 349–350
Toxic epidermal necrolysis (TEN), 340, 452–456
Transfusion-associated lung injury (TRALI)
  anti-HLA class 1 antibodies, 261
  anti-HLA class II antibodies, 261
  definition, 260
  granulocyte crossmatch, 262
  HLA type of the patient, 262
  oxygen supplementation, 262
  PAF receptor, 261
  septic reaction, 261
Transient hypogammaglobulinemia of infancy (THI), 181, 182
Tzanck smear, 359

U

Ulcerative colitis (UC), 390
Umbilical cord stem cells, 255–257
United Network for Organ Sharing (UNOS), 313
Urticaria pigmentosa lesions, 433, 434
Urticarial rash
  clinical findings, 44
  diagnosis, 43–45
  paraclinic evaluation, 44
Urticarial vasculitis, 430
  centrifugal and annular eruption, 429
  diagnosis, 428
  edema, 429
  evaluation and management, 430
  features, 428
  histological features, 429
  HUVS, 430
  hypersensitivity reaction, 430
  long-term follow-up test, 429
  patient history, 427, 428
  treatment, 430, 431
  urticaria and systemic urticarial syndromes, 429
UVA-1 phototherapy, 106

V

Vancomycin, 389
Vascular rejection, 321
Veno-occlusive disease (VOD), 233
Vesicular pruriginous lesions, 363
Vesiculobullous rash, 369

Violet macular rash, HIV-positive
  diagnosis, 161
  Kaposi sarcoma, 161–163
  microorganism, 161
  treatment, 162
Virtual cross-matching, 306

W

Wegener's granulomatosis, 117
Weight loss, 53
  glucose tolerance test, 476
  initial workup, 475, 476
  patient history, 475
  patient presentation, 476
  T1DM, 477
  type 2 DM, 476, 477
Whitish patches
annular lichenoid dermatitis, 412
diagnosis, 409, 411
DLE, 412
histopathological examination, 411
MIV, 411, 412
morphea, 412
patient history, 409, 410
vitiligo, 412, 413
wood light examination, 409–411

The manufacturer's authorised representative in the EU is Springer Nature Customer Service Centre GmbH, Europaplatz 3, 69115 Heidelberg, Germany. If you have any concerns regarding our products, please contact ProductSafety@springernature.com

Printed and bound by CPI Group (UK) Ltd, Croydon, CR0 4YY
30/07/2026
02181689-0001